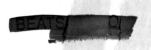

Cancer

Principles & Practice of Oncology

Primer of the Molecular Biology of Cancer

Cancer

Principles & Practice of Oncology

Primer of the Molecular Biology of Cancer

EDITORS

Vincent T. DeVita, Jr., MD

Amy & Joseph Perella Professor of Medicine, Yale Comprehensive Cancer Center and Smilow Cancer Hospital at Yale-New Haven, Yale University School of Medicine, Professor of Epidemiology and Public Health, Yale University School of Public Health, New Haven, Connecticut

Theodore S. Lawrence, MD, PhD

Isadore Lampe Professor and Chair, Department of Radiation Oncology, University of Michigan, Ann Arbor, Michigan

Steven A. Rosenberg, MD, PhD

Chief of Surgery, National Cancer Institute, National Institutes of Health, Professor of Surgery, Uniformed Services University of the Health Sciences School of Medicine, Bethesda, Maryland, Professor of Surgery, George Washington University School of Medicine, Washington, DC

ASSOCIATE SCIENTIFIC ADVISORS

Robert A. Weinberg, PhD

Member, Whitehead Institute for Biomedical Research, Daniel K. Ludwig Professor of Biology, Massachusetts Institute of Technology, Cambridge, Massachusetts

Ronald A. DePinho, MD

Director, Center for Applied Cancer Science, Belfer Institute for Innovative Cancer Science, Dana-Farber Cancer Institute, American Cancer Society Research Professor, Professor of Medicine and Genetics, Harvard Medical School, Boston, Massachusetts

With 70 Contributing Authors

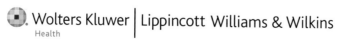

Wolters Kluwer | Lippincott Williams & Wilkins
Health
Philadelphia · Baltimore · New York · London
Buenos Aires · Hong Kong · Sydney · Tokyo

Executive Editor: Jonathan W. Pine, Jr.
Senior Product Manager: Emilie Moyer
Vendor Manager: Alicia Jackson
Senior Manufacturing Manager: Benjamin Rivera
Senior Marketing Manager: Angela Panetta
Senior Designer: Stephen Druding
Cover Designer: Stephen Druding
Production Service: Aptara, Inc.

Printed in China

Library of Congress Cataloging-in-Publication Data
[978-1-4511-1897-1]
[1-4511-1897-X]
CIP data available upon request

Care has been taken to confirm the accuracy of the information presented and to describe generally accepted practices. However, the authors, editors, and publisher are not responsible for errors or omissions or for any consequences from application of the information in this book and make no warranty, expressed or implied, with respect to the currency, completeness, or accuracy of the contents of the publication. Application of the information in a particular situation remains the professional responsibility of the practitioner.

The authors, editors, and publisher have exerted every effort to ensure that drug selection and dosage set forth in this text are in accordance with current recommendations and practice at the time of publication. However, in view of ongoing research, changes in government regulations, and the constant flow of information relating to drug therapy and drug reactions, the reader is urged to check the package insert for each drug for any change in indications and dosage and for added warnings and precautions. This is particularly important when the recommended agent is a new or infrequently employed drug.

Some drugs and medical devices presented in the publication have Food and Drug Administration (FDA) clearance for limited use in restricted research settings. It is the responsibility of the health care provider to ascertain the FDA status of each drug or device planned for use in their clinical practice.

To purchase additional copies of this book, call our customer service department at (800) 638-3030 or fax orders to (301) 223-2320. International customers should call (301) 223-2300.

Visit Lippincott Williams & Wilkins on the Internet: at LWW.com. Lippincott Williams & Wilkins customer service representatives are available from 8:30 am to 6 pm, EST.

10 9 8 7 6 5 4 3 2

CONTRIBUTORS

Anupriya Agarwal, PhD
Postdoctoral Fellow
Department of Hematology/Oncology
Center for Hematologic Malignancies
Oregon Health & Science University
Portland, Oregon

Nishant Agrawal, MD
Department of Otolaryngology-Head and
　Neck Surgery
Johns Hopkins Medical Institutions
Baltimore, Maryland

Matthew L. Anderson, MD, PhD
Assistant Professor
Division of Gynecologic Oncology
Baylor College of Medicine
Attending Surgeon
Texas Cancer Institute
Saint Luke's Episcopal Hospital
Houston, Texas

Cristina R. Antonescu, MD
Department of Pathology
Memorial Sloan-Kettering Cancer Center
New York, New York

Vivek K. Arora, MD, PhD
Fellow
Human Oncology & Pathogenesis Program
Memorial Sloan-Kettering Cancer Center
New York, New York

David A. Barbie, MD
Massachusetts General Hospital
Boston, Massachusetts

Alberto Bardelli, PhD
Laboratory of Molecular Genetics
Institute for Cancer Research and Treatment
University of Torino Medical School
Candiolo, Italy

John C. Byrd, MD
Division of Hematology and Comprehensive
　Cancer Center
The Ohio State University
Columbus, Ohio

Joseph Califano, MD
Department of Otolaryngology-Head and
　Neck Surgery
Johns Hopkins Medical Institutions
Milton J. Dance Head and Neck Center
Greater Baltimore Medical Center
Baltimore, Maryland

Lewis C. Cantley, PhD
Clinical Oncology
Merck Research Laboratories
Upper Gwynned, Pennsylvania

David P. Carbone, MD, PhD
Professor of Medicine & Cancer Biology
Department of Medicine/Hematology &
　Oncology
Vanderbilt University
Nashville, Tennessee

Chris L. Carpenter, PhD
Division of Signal Transduction
Department of Medicine
Beth Israel Deaconess Medical Center
Boston, Massachusetts

Webster K. Cavenee, PhD
Director and Distinguished Professor
Ludwig Institute for Cancer Research
University of California, San Diego
La Jolla, California

Jan Cerny, MD, PhD
Assistant Professor of Medicine
Department of Medicine
Division of Hematology and Oncology
University of Massachusetts
University of Massachusetts Memorial
　Medical Center
Worchester, Massachusetts

Yu Chen, MD, PhD
Fellow
Human Oncology & Pathogenesis Program
Fellow
Department of Medicine
Memorial Sloan-Kettering Cancer Center
New York, New York

Lynda Chin, MD
Professor of Dermatology
Department of Medical Oncology
Dana-Farber Cancer Institute
Boston, Massachusetts

Gina G. Chung, MD
Assistant Professor
Department of Internal Medicine
Yale Cancer Center
Yale University School of Medicine
Smilow Cancer Hospital
Yale-New Haven Hospital
New Haven, Connecticut

Riccardo Dalla-Favera, MD
Professor and Director
Institute for Cancer Genetics
Columbia University
New York, New York

Alan D. D'Andrea, MD
Dana Farber Cancer Institute
Boston, Massachusetts

Michael W. Deininger, MD, PhD
Maxwell M. Wintrobe, MD Presidential
    Endowed Chair in Internal Medicine
Chief, Division of Hematology and
    Hematologic Malignancies
Department of Internal Medicine University of
    Utah/Huntsman Cancer Institute
Salt Lake City, Utah

Ronald A. DePinho, MD
Director
Belfer Institute for Applied Cancer Science
Dana-Farber Cancer Institute
Harvard Medical School
Professor
Department of Medicine
Brigham & Women's Hospital
Boston, Massachusetts

John E. Dick, PhD
Professor
Department of Molecular Biology
University of Toronto
Canada Research Chair in Stem Cell Biology,
    Senior Scientist
Department of Cellular and Molecular Biology
University Health Network
Toronto, Ontario, Canada

Lee M. Ellis, MD
Professor of Surgery and Cancer Biology
Department of Surgical Oncology and Cancer
    Biology
University of Texas
M. D. Anderson Cancer Center
Houston, Texas

Levi A. Garraway, MD, PhD
Assistant Professor of Medicine, Harvard
    Medical School
Department of Medical Oncology
Dana-Farber Cancer Institute
Boston, Massachusetts
Senior Associate Member, The Broad Institute
    of Harvard and MIT
Cambridge, Massachusetts

David J. Gordon, MD, PhD
Instructor
Department of Pediatrics
Harvard Medical School
Department of Hematology/Oncology
Dana-Farber Cancer Institute
Boston, Massachusetts

Joe W. Grisham, MD
Senior Scientist
Laboratory of Experimental
    Carcinogenesis
Center for Cancer Research, NCI, National
    Institutes of Health
Bethesda, Maryland

Patrick K. Ha, MD
Department of Otolaryngology-Head and
    Neck Surgery
Johns Hopkins Medical Institutions
Milton J. Dance Head and Neck Center
Greater Baltimore Medical Center
Baltimore, Maryland

William C. Hahn, MD, PhD
Associate Professor
Department of Medicine
Harvard Medical School
Division Chief
Department of Molecular and Cellular
    Oncology
Dana-Farber Cancer Institute
Boston, Massachusetts

Lyndsay N. Harris, MD
Associate Professor
Yale Cancer Center, Section of Medical
    Oncology
Co-Director Breast Disease Unit
Smilow Cancer Hospital
Yale-New Haven Hospital
New Haven, Connecticut

Lee J. Helman, MD
Scientific Director for Clinical Research
Center for Cancer Research
National Cancer Institute
Bethesda, Maryland

Erin W. Hofstatter, MD
Assistant Professor
Yale Cancer Center, Section of Medical
  Oncology
Yale University
Smilow Cancer Hospital
Yale-New Haven Hospital
New Haven, Connecticut

Leora Horn, MD, MS
Assistant Professor
Department of Internal Medicine
Vanderbilt University
Nashville, Tennessee

Ralph H. Hruban, MD
Department of Pathology
Johns Hopkins University
Baltimore, Maryland

C. David James, PhD
Professor
Department of Neurological Surgery
University of California, San Francisco
San Francisco, California

Peter A. Jones, MD
Distinguished Professor
Department of Urology, Biochemistry
  and Molecular Biology
Keck School of Medicine of
  University of Southern California
Director, Cancer Center
University of Southern California/Norris
  Comprehensive Cancer Center
Los Angeles, California

Vassiliki Karantza, MD, PhD
Assistant Professor
Department of Medicine-Medical
  Oncology
Cancer Institute of New Jersey
Attending Physician
Robert Wood Johnson University Hospital
New Brunswick, New Jersey

Jacob Kaufman
Vanderbilt University Medical Center
Nashville, Tennessee

Robert S. Kerbel, PhD
Professor
Department of Biophysics
Senior Scientist
Department of Molecular & Cellular
  Biology Research
Sunnybrook Health Sciences Centre
Toronto, Ontario, Canada

Scott E. Kern, MD
Professor
Department of Oncology
Johns Hopkins University
Baltimore, Maryland

Margaret A. Knowles, PhD
Professor of Experimental Cancer Research
Section of Experimental Oncology
Leeds Institute of Molecular Medicine
St. James's University Hospital
University of Leeds
Leeds, United Kingdom

Raju Kucherlapati, PhD
Paul C. Cabot Professor of Genetics
Department of Genetics
Havard Medical School
Professor of Medicine
Departments of Medicine and Genetics
Brigham and Women's Hospital
Boston, Massachusetts

W. Marston Linehan, MD
Chief
Urologic Oncology Branch
National Cancer Institute
National Institute of Health
Bethesda, Maryland

Carlos López-Otín
Departamento de Bioquímica y Biología
  Molecular
Instituto Universitario de Oncología
  (IUOPA)
Universidad de Oviedo
Oviedo, Spain

David N. Louis, MD
James Homer Wright Pathology Laboratories
Massachusetts General Hospital and
  Harvard Medical School
Pathology
Massachusetts General Hospital
Boston, Massachusetts

David Malkin, MD, FRCPC
Professor
Department of Pediatrics
Universtiy of Toronto
Senior Staff Oncologist
Division of Hematology/Oncology
The Hospital for Sick Children
Toronto, Ontario

Joan Massagué, PhD
Member and Chair
Cancer Biology and Genetics Program
Memorial Sloan-Kettering Cancer Center
New York, New York

Matthew Meyerson, PhD
Department of Medical Oncology and Center for
   Genome Discovery
Dana-Farber Cancer Institute
Boston, Massachusetts
Broad Institute of Cambridge, Massachusetts
Broad Institute of Harvard and M.I.T.
Cambridge, Massachusetts

Karin B. Michels, ScD, PhD
Associate Professor
Harvard Medical School
Co-Director
Obstetrics and Gynecology
Epidemiology Center
Brigham and Women's Hospital
Boston, Massachusetts

Andy J. Minn, MD, PhD
Assistant Professor, Assistant Investigator
Department of Radiation Oncology
Abramson Family Cancer Research Institute
University of Pennsylvania
Philadelphia, Pennsylvania

Torsten O. Nielsen, MD, PhD, FRCPC
Associate Professor
Department of Pathology and
   Laboratory Medicine
University of British Columbia
Pathologist
Provincial Pathology Program
British Columbia Cancer Agency
Vancouver, Canada

Urban Novak, MD
Research Scientist
Institute for Cancer Genetics
Columbia University
New York, New York
Klinik und Poliklinik für Medizinische
   Onkologie
INSELSPITAL, Universitätsspital Bern
Freiburgstrasse
Switzerland

Kunle Odunsi, MD, PhD
Professor and Chairman
Department of Gynecologic Oncology
Roswell Park Cancer Institute
Buffalo, New York

Laura Pasqualucci, MD
Associate Professor
Department of Pathology and
   Cell Biology
Institute for Caner Genetics
Columbia University
New York, New York

Tanja B. Pejovic, MD, PhD, FACOG
Assistant Professor, Division Chief
Gynecological Oncologist
Department of Obstetrics and Gynecology
Kinght Cancer Institute
Oregon Health & Science University
Portland, Oregon

David Pellman, MD
Massachusetts General Hospital
Boston, Massachusetts

Glen D. Raffel, M.D., Ph.D.
Assistant Professor of Medicine
Department of Medicine
Division of Hematology and Oncology
University of Massachusetts Medical School
Worchester, Massachusetts

Steven I. Reed, PhD
Professor
Department of Molecular Biology
The Scripps Research Institute
La Jolla, California

Anil K. Rustgi, MD
T. Grier Miller Professor of Medicine and Genetics
Chief of Gastroenterology
University of Pennsylvania
Philadelphia, Pennsylvania

Yardena Samuels, PhD
Assistant Professor
Cancer Genetics Branch
National Human Genome Research Institute
National Institutes of Health
Bethesda, Maryland

Charles L. Sawyers, MD
Investigator
Howard Hughes Medical Institute
Chairman
Human Oncology & Pathogenesis Program
Memorial Sloan-Kettering Cancer Center
New York, New York

Laura S. Schmidt, PhD
Principal Scientist
SAIC-Frederick, Inc.
NCI-Frederick
National Cancer Institute
National Institutes of Health
Bethesda, Maryland

Norman E. Sharpless, MD
Associate Professor
Department of Medicine and Genetics
The University of North Carolina
Chapel Hill, North Carolina

Ramesh A. Shivdasani, MD, PhD
Associate Professor
Department of Medicine
Harvard Medical School
Associate Professor
Department of Medical Oncology
Dana-Farber Cancer Institute
Boston, Massachusetts

Samuel Singer, MD
Professor of Surgery
Department of Surgery
Weill Cornell Medical College
Member with Tenure-of-Title
Chief, Gastric and Mixed
  Tumor Service
Department of Surgery
Memorial Sloan-Kettering
  Cancer Center
New York, New York

Snorri S. Thorgeirsson, MD, PhD
Chief
Laboratory of Experimental
  Carcinogenesis
Center for Cancer Research
National Cancer Institute
Bethesda, Maryland

Matthew G. Vander Heiden, MD
Koch Institute for Integrative Cancer Research
  at M.I.T.
Dana-Farber Cancer Institute
Boston, Massachusetts

Jean C.Y. Wang, MD, PhD
Assistant Professor
Department of Medicine
University of Toronto
Affiliate Scientist
Division of Stem Cell and Developmental Biology
Ontario Cancer Institute
Toronto, Ontario, Canada

Samuel A. Wells, Jr., MD
Senior Clinician
Medical Oncology Branch
National Cancer Institute
Center for Cancer Research
National Institutes of Health
Bethesda, Maryland

Eileen White, PhD
Professor
Department of Molecular Biology and
  Biochemistry
Rutgers University
Associate Director for Basic Science
Cancer Institute of New Jersey
New Brunswick, New Jersey

Kwok-Kin Wong, MD, PhD
Associate Professor
Department of Medical Oncology
Dana Farber Cancer Institute
Harvard Medical School
Attending Physician
Department of Medicine
Brigham & Women's Hospital
Boston, Massachusetts

The development of information in molecular biology has had a profound influence on understanding the nature of malignant transformation and the unique behavior of cancer cells. Virtually every area of cancer research has been transformed by the increased understanding of biologic processes at a molecular level. The translation of this revolution in molecular biology has infiltrated into every aspect of clinical oncology and spans prevention, screening, precise diagnosis and choice of appropriate therapy. New molecular information is accumulating rapidly and research scientists as well as practicing oncologists often struggle to keep abreast of this developing information.

In this *Primer of the Molecular Biology of Cancer*, we have brought together the basic scientific information of the molecular biology of cancer. The format is designed to be useful both to research scientists interested in the study of cancer and to oncologists who need to understand these new developments that are having a profound impact on the care of patients with cancer.

Leading scientists and clinicians in the field of molecular biology and clinical oncology have lent their expertise to this project. The text has been divided into two parts. Part I includes 13 chapters that deal with the general principles of the molecular biology of cancer that provide the basic framework for an understanding of the behavior of cancer cells. Part II includes an up-to-date description of how this new information has affected the understanding of the biology of 19 of the most common cancers, with an emphasis on how these new findings have been translated to impact the management of cancer patients. The current volume has been distilled from our comprehensive textbook, *Cancer: Principles and Practice of Oncology*, to provide a single concise source of information for scientists and clinicians in this rapidly developing field.

Vincent T. DeVita, Jr., MD
Theodore S. Lawrence, MD, PhD
Steven A. Rosenberg, MD, PhD

CONTENTS

xi

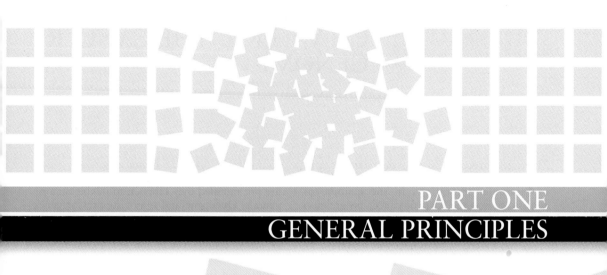

PART ONE
GENERAL PRINCIPLES

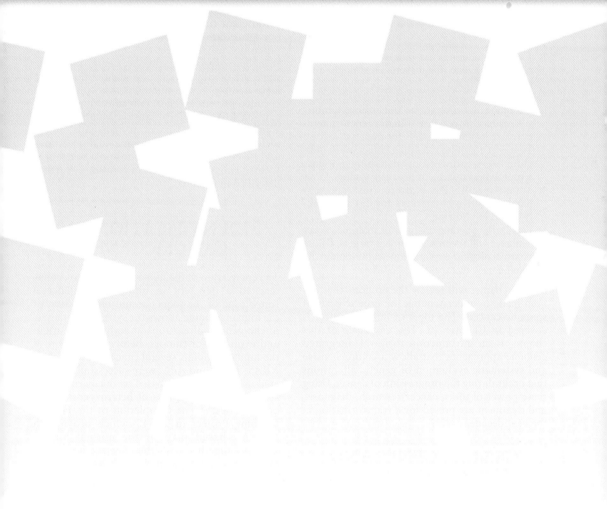

CHAPTER 1 THE CANCER GENOME

YARDENA SAMUELS, ALBERTO BARDELLI, AND CARLOS LÓPEZ-OTÍN

There is a broad consensus that cancer is, in essence, a genetic disease, and that accumulation of molecular alterations in the genome of somatic cells is the basis of cancer progression (Fig. 1.1).[1] In the past 5 years the availability of the human genome sequence and progress in DNA sequencing technologies has dramatically improved knowledge of this disease. These new insights are transforming the field of oncology at multiple levels:

1. The genomic maps are redesigning the tumor taxonomy by moving it from a histologic- to a genetic-based level.
2. The success of cancer drugs designed to target the molecular alterations underlying tumorigenesis has proven that somatic genetic alterations are legitimate targets for therapy.
3. Tumor genotyping is helping clinicians to individualize treatments by matching patients with the best treatment for their tumors.
4. Tumor-specific DNA alterations represent highly sensitive biomarkers for disease detection and monitoring.
5. Finally, the ongoing analyses of multiple cancer genomes will identify additional targets, whose pharmacological exploitation will undoubtedly result in new therapeutic approaches.

This chapter will review the progress that has been made in understanding the genetic basis of sporadic cancers. The topic of familial cancer is covered in Chapter 12. The emphasis of this chapter is an introduction to novel integrated genomic approaches that allow a comprehensive and systematic evaluation of genetic alterations that occur during the progression of cancer. Using these powerful tools, cancer research, diagnosis, and treatment are poised for a transformation in the next decade.

CANCER GENES AND THEIR MUTATIONS

Cancer genes are broadly grouped into oncogenes and tumor suppressor genes. Using a classical analogy, oncogenes can be considered as the car accelerator, so that a mutation in an oncogene would be the equivalent of having the accelerator continuously pressed.[2] Tumor suppressor genes, in contrast, act as "brakes,"[2] so that when they are not mutated they function to inhibit tumorigenesis. Oncogene and tumor suppressor genes may be classified by the nature of their somatic mutations in tumors.[1] Mutations in oncogenes typically occur at specific hotspots, often affecting the same codon or clustered at neighboring codons in different tumors. Furthermore, mutations in oncogenes are almost always missense, and the mutations usually affect only one allele, making them heterozygous. In contrast, tumor suppressor genes are usually mutated throughout the gene; a large number of the mutations may truncate the encoded protein and generally affect both alleles, causing loss of heterozygosity. Major types of somatic mutations present in malignant tumors include nucleotide substitutions, small insertions and deletions (*indels*), chromosomal rearrangements, and copy number alterations (further described in Chapter 2).

IDENTIFICATION OF CANCER GENES

The completion of the human genome project has marked a new era in biomedical sciences.[3] Knowledge of the sequence and organization of the human genome allows the systematic analysis of the genetic alterations underlying the origin and evolution of tumors. Before elucidation of the human genome, several cancer genes, such as *KRAS*, *TP53*, and *APC*, were successfully discovered using approaches based on oncovirus analysis, linkage studies, loss of heterozygosity, and cytogenetics.[4,5] The completion of the Human Genome Project in 2004,[3] which provided a sequence-based map of the normal human genome, together with the construction of HapMap, containing single nucleotide polymorphisms (SNPs), and the underlying genomic structure of natural human genomic variation,[6,7] allowed an extraordinary throughput in cataloging somatic mutations in cancer. These projects now offer an unprecedented opportunity: the identification of all the genetic changes associated with a human cancer. This ambitious goal is for

A metastatic cancer genome requires decades to develop

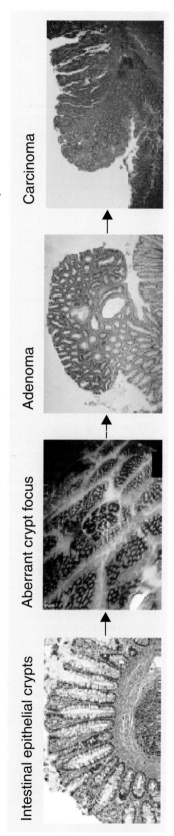

Intestinal epithelial crypts   Aberrant crypt focus   Adenoma   Carcinoma

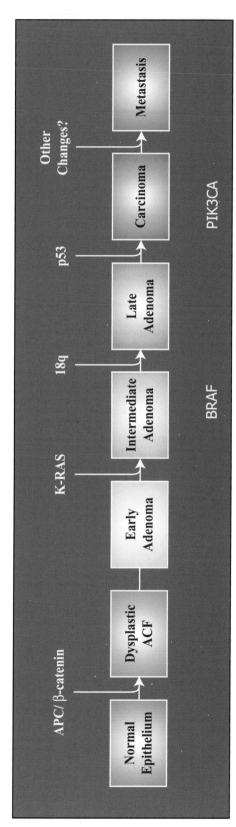

FIGURE 1.1 Schematic representation of the genomic and histopathological steps associated to tumor progression: from the occurrence of the initiating mutation in the founder cell to metastasis formation. It has been convincingly shown that the genomic landscape of solid tumors such as that of pancreatic and colorectal requires the accumulation of many genetic events, a process which requires decades to complete This timeline offers an incredible window of opportunity for the early detection (often associated to excellent prognosis) of this disease.

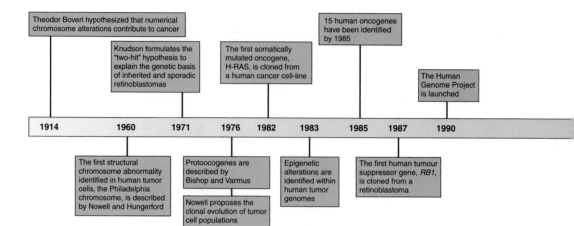

FIGURE 1.2 Timeline of seminal hypotheses, research discoveries, and research initiatives that have led to an improved understanding of the genetic etiology of human tumorigenesis within the past century. The consensus cancer gene data were obtained from the Wellcome Trust Sanger Institute Cancer Genome Project website (http://www.sanger.ac.uk/genetics/CGP). Redrawn from ref. 80.

the first time within reach of the scientific community. Already a number of studies have demonstrated the usefulness of strategies aimed at the systematic identification of somatic mutations associated with cancer progression. Notably, the Human Genome Project, the HapMap project, as well as the candidate and family gene approaches described below, utilized capillary-based DNA sequencing (first-generation sequencing, also known as Sanger sequencing).[8] Figure 1.2 clearly illustrates the developments in the search of cancer genes, its increased pace, as well as the most relevant findings in this field.

CANCER GENOME INVESTIGATION: TOOLS AND QUALITY CONTROLS

In order to perform mutational analysis of cancer genomes it is imperative to acquire high-quality reagents and to perform several quality controls to verify that the derived data are reliable. To detect somatic (i.e., tumor-specific) mutations in cancer both the tumor DNA and the germline DNA from the same individual are required, especially because knowledge of the variations in the normal human genome is as yet incomplete. Normal genomic DNA from the same individual may be derived either from blood or from tumor neighboring tissue in cases where solid tumors are investigated.

A cancer sample (either from bioptic or surgical origin) typically contains both malignant and nonmalignant (stromal) cells. Most genomic analyses require that samples are highly enriched for tumor tissue. These can either be generated by deriving early passage tumor cell lines, mouse xenografts, or through a pathologist-guided selective macro- or microdissection of neoplastic tissue. This allows the isolation of tumor-derived genomic DNA and sensitive detection of somatic mutations that would otherwise be masked by contamination of normal tissue. Importantly, the quality of the derived genomic DNA may be affected by its source. Surgical resection specimens are usually large and therefore appropriate for these studies. However, biopsies from patients usually contain few cells, thus reducing the quantity of genomic DNA available. Although whole-genome amplification may be a possibility when low genomic DNA amounts are available, this method can give rise to artifactual genetic alterations.[9] Another reason that negatively affects the quality of genomic DNA is that cancer samples (for example, liver metastases) often contain significant numbers of necrotic or apoptotic cells. These issues might also be resolved by increased genetic coverage utilizing second-generation sequencing approaches,[10] as detailed below.

Prior to genomic analysis multiple key quality controls should be applied to the tumor and normal tissues. These include verification that the tumor sample contains at least 75% cancer cells, a threshold that allows the identification of homozygous and hemizygous deletions, copy-neutral loss of heterozygosity, duplication, and amplification.[11–13] To unequivocally assess the somatic tumor-specific nature of sequence changes, genotyping of SNPs in the tumor and normal tissue is also required to prove that both are derived from the same individual.

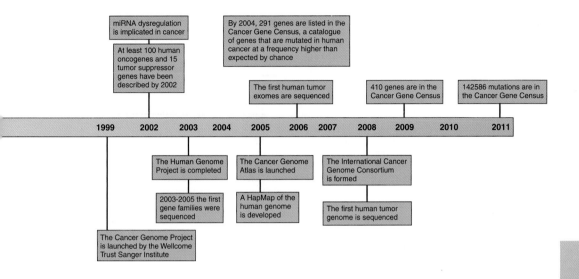

Cancer Gene Discovery by Sequencing Candidate Gene Families

The availability of the human genome sequence provides new opportunities to comprehensively search for somatic mutations in cancer on a larger scale than previously possible. Progress in the field has been closely linked to improvements in the throughput of DNA analysis and the continuous reduction in sequencing costs. Below some of the achievements in this research area are described, as well as how they affected knowledge of the cancer genome.

A seminal work in the field was the systematic mutational profiling of the genes involved in the RAF-RAS pathway in multiple tumors. This candidate gene approach led to the discovery that *BRAF* is frequently mutated in melanomas and is mutated at a lower frequency in other tumor types.[14] Follow-up studies quickly revealed that mutations in *BRAF* are mutually exclusive with alterations in *KRAS*,[14,15] genetically emphasizing that these genes function in the same pathway, a concept that had been previously demonstrated in lower organisms such as *Caenorhabditis elegans* and *Drosophila melanogaster*.[16,17]

In 2003, identification of cancer genes shifted from a candidate gene approach to the mutational analyses of gene families. The first gene families to be completely sequenced were those that involved protein[18,19] and lipid phosphorylation.[20] The rationale for focusing initially on these gene families was threefold:

1. The corresponding proteins were already known at that time to play a pivotal role in signaling and proliferation of normal and cancerous cells.
2. Multiple members of the protein kinases family had already been linked to tumorigenesis.

3. Kinases are clearly amenable to pharmacological inhibition, making them attractive drug targets.

The mutational analysis of all the tyrosine kinase domains in colorectal cancers revealed that 30% of cases had a mutation in at least one tyrosine kinase gene, and overall mutations were identified in eight different kinases, most of which had not previously been linked to cancer.[18] An additional mutational analysis of the coding exons of 518 protein kinase genes in 210 diverse human cancers, including breast, lung, gastric, ovarian, renal, and acute lymphoblastic leukemia, identified approximately 120 mutated genes that probably contribute to oncogenesis.[19] A recent somatic mutations interrogation of the protein tyrosine kinases in cutaneous melanoma identified *ERBB4* to be mutated in 19% of cases, making it the most highly mutated protein tyrosine kinase in melanoma.[21] *ERBB4* is a member of the ERBB/HER family of receptor tyrosine kinases. Other family members, including *ERBB1* (EGFR) and *ERBB2* (HER-2), have been implicated by mutations or amplifications in a number of cancers, including lung, colon, and breast cancers. The high mutation frequency as well as the nonsynonymous (NS) to synonymous (S) ratio, which was 24:3, significantly higher than the NS:S ratio predicted for non-selected mutations ($P < .01$)[22] indicated that *ERBB4* mutations are selected for during tumorigenesis and therefore contribute to melanoma tumorigenesis.

As kinase activity is attenuated by enzymes that remove phosphate groups called phosphatases, the rational next step in these studies was to perform a mutation analysis of the protein tyrosine phosphatases. Mutational investigation of this family in colorectal cancer identified that 25% of cases had mutations in six different phosphatase genes (*PTPRF, PTPRG, PTPRT, PTPN3, PTPN13,* or *PTPN14*).[23] Combined analysis of the protein tyrosine kinases and the protein tyrosine phosphatases showed that 50% of colorectal cancers had mutations in a tyrosine kinase gene, a protein tyrosine phosphatase gene, or both, further emphasizing the pivotal role of protein phosphorylation in neoplastic progression. Many of the identified genes had previously been linked to human cancer, thus validating the unbiased comprehensive mutation profiling. These landmark studies led to additional gene family surveys.

The phosphatidylinositol 3-kinase (*PI3K*) gene family, which also plays a role in proliferation, adhesion, survival, and motility, was also comprehensively investigated.[24] Sequencing of the exons encoding the kinase domain of all 16 members belonging to this family pinpointed *PIK3CA* as the only gene to harbor somatic mutations. When the entire coding region was analyzed, *PIK3CA* was found somatically mutated in 32% of colorectal cancers. At that time, the *PIK3CA* gene was certainly not a newcomer in the cancer arena, as it had previously been shown to be involved in cell transformation and metastasis.[24] Strikingly, its staggering high mutation frequency was discovered only through systematic sequencing of the corresponding gene family.[20] Subsequent analysis of *PIK3CA* in other tumor types identified somatic mutations in this gene in additional cancer types, including 36% of hepatocellular carcinomas, 36% of endometrial carcinomas, 25% of breast carcinomas, 15% of anaplastic oligodendrogliomas, 5% of medulloblastomas and anaplastic astrocytomas, and 27% of glioblastomas.[25-29] It is known that *PIK3CA* is one of the two (the other being *KRAS*) most commonly mutated oncogenes in human cancers. Further investigation of the *PI3K* pathway in colorectal cancer showed that 40% of tumors had genetic alterations in one of the *PI3K* pathway genes, emphasizing the central role of this pathway in colorectal cancer pathogenesis.[30] The relevance and the functional role of the PI3K pathway in tumorigenesis is further described in Chapter 5.

Although most cancer genome studies of large gene families have focused on the kinome, recent analyses have revealed that members of other families highly represented in the human genome are also a target of mutational events in cancer. This is the case of proteases, a complex group of enzymes consisting of at least 569 components that constitute the so-called human degradome.[31] Proteases exhibit an elaborate interplay with kinases and have traditionally been associated with cancer progression because of their ability to degrade extracellular matrices, thus facilitating tumor invasion and metastasis.[32,33] However, recent studies have shown that these enzymes hydrolyze a wide variety of substrates and influence many different steps of cancer, including early stages of tumor evolution.[34] These functional studies have also revealed that beyond their initial recognition as prometastatic enzymes, they play dual roles in cancer, as assessed by the identification of a growing number of tumor-suppressive proteases.[35]

These findings emphasized the possibility that mutational activation or inactivation of protease genes occurs in cancer. The first clear evidence of this is derived from systematic analysis of genetic alterations in breast and colorectal cancers, which revealed that proteases from different catalytic classes were candidate cancer genes that had somatically mutated in cancer.[36] These results have prompted the mutational analysis of entire protease families such as MMPs (matrix metalloproteinases), ADAMs (a disintegrin and metalloproteinase) and ADAMTSs (ADAMs with thrombospondin domains) in different tumors. These studies led to identification of protease genes frequently mutated in cancer, such as *MMP8*, which is mutated and functionally inactivated in 6.3% of human melanomas.[37,38] Other MMP genes, including *MMP2, MMP9, MMP14,* and *MMP27*, are also somatically mutated in melanomas and other malignant tumors, albeit at low frequency.[37,39] Systematic mutational analysis of all members of the ADAM family of membrane-bound metalloproteases has shown that *ADAM7* and *ADAM29* are also often mutated in melanoma, whereas parallel studies of the ADAMTS family have revealed that *ADAMTS15* is mutated in colorectal carcinomas and *ADAMTS18* and *ADAMTS20* in melanomas.[40,41] Functional analyses have indicated that *ADAM7, ADAM29,* and *ADAMTS18* mutations affect adhesion of melanoma cells to specific extracellular matrix proteins and in some cases increase their migrating and invasive properties, suggesting that these mutated genes play a role in melanoma progression.[41,42] In contrast, functional studies of *ADAMTS15* mutations in colorectal cancer cells have revealed that this metalloprotease restrains tumor growth and invasion, further validating the concept that secreted proteases may have tumor-suppressor properties.[40]

The mutational status of caspases has also been extensively analyzed in different tumors as these proteases play a fundamental role in execution of apoptosis, one of the hallmarks of cancer.[43] These studies demonstrated that *CASP8* is deleted in neuroblastomas and inactivated by somatic mutations in a variety of human malignancies, including head and neck, colorectal, lung, and gastric carcinomas.[44-46] Likewise *CASP3, CASP4, CASP5, CASP6, CASP7, CASP10,* and *CASP14* are occasionally inactivated by mutation in different human cancers.[47-54] Other large protease families whose components are often mutated in cancer are the deubiquitylating enzymes (DUBs), which catalyze the removal of ubiquitin and ubiquitinlike modifiers of their target proteins.[55] Some DUBs were initially identified as oncogenic proteins, but recent work has shown that other deubiquitylases such as CYLD, A20, and BAP1 are tumor suppressors inactivated in cancer. *CYLD* is mutated in patients with familial cylindromatosis, a disease characterized by the formation of multiple tumors of skin appendages.[56] A20 is a DUB family member encoded by the *TNFAIP3* gene, which is mutated in a large number of Hodgkin's lymphomas and primary mediastinal B-cell lymphomas.[57–60] Finally, the *BAP1* gene, encoding an ubiquitin C-terminal hydrolase, has been found to be somatically mutated in 86% metastasizing uveal melanomas of the eye.[61]

Mutational Analysis of Exomes Using Sanger Sequencing

Although the gene family approach for the identification of cancer genes has proven extremely valuable, it still is a candidate approach and thus biased in its nature. The next step forward in the mutational profiling of cancer has been the sequencing of exomes, which is the entire coding portion of the human genome (18,000 protein-encoding genes). As of today the exomes of breast, colorectal, pancreatic, and ovarian clear cell carcinomas, glioblastoma multiforme, and medulloblastoma have been analyzed using Sanger sequencing. These large-scale analyses for the first time allowed researchers to describe and understand the genetic complexity of human cancers.[22,36,62–65] The declared goals of these exome studies were to provide for the first time methods for exome-wide mutational analyses in human tumors, to characterize their spectrum and quantity of somatic mutations, and, finally, to discover new genes involved in tumorigenesis as well as novel pathways that have a role in these tumors. In these studies, sequencing data were complemented with gene expression and copy number analyses, thus providing for the first time a comprehensive view of the genetic complexity of human tumors.[62–65] A number of conclusions can be drawn from these analyses:

1. Cancer genomes have an average of 30 to 100 somatic alterations per tumor, which was a higher number than previously thought. Although the alterations included point mutations, small insertions, deletions, or amplifications, the great majority of the mutations observed were single-base substitutions.[62,63]
2. Even within a single cancer type, there is a significant intertumor heterogeneity. This means that multiple mutational patterns (encompassing different mutant genes) are present in tumors that cannot be distinguished based on histological analysis. The concept that individual tumors have a unique genetic milieu is highly relevant for personalized medicine, a concept that will be discussed below.
3. The spectrum and nucleotide contexts of mutations differ between different tumor types. For example, over 50% of mutations in colorectal cancer were C:G to T:A transitions, and 10% were C:G to G:C transversions. In contrast, in breast cancers, only 35% of the mutations were C:G to T:A transitions, and 29% were C:G to G:C transversions. Knowledge of mutation spectra is vital as it allows insight into the mechanisms underlying mutagenesis and repair in the various cancers investigated.
4. A considerably larger number of genes that had not been previously reported to be involved in cancer were found to play a role in the disease.
5. Solid tumors arising in children, such as medulloblastoma, harbor on average five to ten times less gene alterations compared to a typical adult solid tumor. These pediatric tumors also harbor fewer amplifications and homozygous deletions within coding genes compared to adult solid tumors.

Importantly, to deal with the large amount of data generated in these genomic projects, it was necessary to develop new statistical and bioinformatic tools. Furthermore, examination of the overall distribution of the identified mutations allowed the development of a novel view of cancer genome landscapes and a novel definition of cancer genes. These new concepts in the understanding of cancer genetics are further discussed below. The compiled conclusions derived from these analyses have led to a paradigm shift in the understanding of cancer genetics.

A clear indication of the power of the unbiased nature of the whole exome surveys was revealed by the discovery of recurrent mutations in the active site of *IDH1*, a gene with no known link to gliomas, in 12% of tumors analyzed.[63] As malignant gliomas are the most common and lethal tumors of the central nervous system, and glioblastoma multiforme (GBM; World Health Organization grade IV astrocytoma) is the most biologically aggressive subtype, the unveiling of *IDH1* as a novel GBM gene is extremely significant. Importantly, mutations of *IDH1* predominantly occurred in younger patients (median age of 34 versus 56 years for anaplastic astrocytomas and 32 versus 59 years for GBMs) and were associated with a better prognosis, as patients with *IDH* mutations have a median overall survival of 31 months, and patients with wild type *IDH1* and *IDH2* have a median 15-month survival.[66] Follow-up studies showed that mutations of *IDH1* occur early in glioma progression, the R132 somatic mutation is harbored by the majority (greater than 70%) of grades II and III astrocytomas and oligodendrogliomas, as well as in secondary GBMs that develop from these lower grade lesions.[66–72] In contrast, less than 10% of primary GBMs harbor these alterations. Furthermore, analysis of the associated *IDH2* revealed recurrent somatic mutations in the R172 residue, which is the exact analog of the frequently mutated R132 residue of *IDH1*. These mutations occur mostly in a mutually exclusive manner with *IDH1* mutations,[66,68] suggesting that they have equivalent phenotypic effects. Subsequently, *IDH1* mutations have been reported in additional cancer types such as myeloid leukemia samples,[73–75] a single case of colorectal cancer, two prostate carcinomas,[71] one melanoma case,[76] and a few cases of adult supratentorial primitive neuroectodermal tumors.[69] Further description of the function of *IDH1* and *IDH2* mutations in cancer is found in Chapter 8.

Next-Generation Sequencing and Cancer Genome Analysis

The introduction in 1977 of the Sanger method for DNA sequencing with chain-terminating inhibitors has transformed biomedical research.[8] Over the past 30 years, this first-generation technology has been universally used for elucidating the nucleotide sequence of DNA molecules. However, the launching of new large-scale projects, including those implicating whole-genome sequencing of cancer samples, has made necessary the development of new methods that are widely known as next-generation sequencing technologies.[77–79] These approaches have significantly lowered the cost and the time required to determine the sequence of the 3×10^9 nucleotides present in the human genome. Moreover, they have a series of advantages over Sanger sequencing, which are of special interest for the analysis of cancer genomes.[80] First, next-generation sequencing approaches are more sensitive than Sanger methods and can detect somatic mutations even when they are present only in a subset of tumor cells.[81] Moreover, these new sequencing strategies are quantitative and can be used to simultaneously determine both nucleotide sequence and copy number variations.[82] They can also be coupled to other procedures such as those involving paired-end reads, allowing the identification of multiple structural alterations, such as insertions, deletions, and rearrangements, commonly occurring in cancer genomes.[81] Nonetheless, next-generation sequencing still presents some limitations mainly derived from the relatively high error rate in the short reads generated during the sequencing process. In addition, these short reads make the task of *de novo* assembly of the generated sequences and the mapping of the reads to a reference genome extremely complex. To overcome some of these current limitations, deep coverage of each analyzed genome is required and a

careful validation of the identified variants must be performed, typically using Sanger sequencing. As a consequence, there is a substantial increase in both cost of the process and time of analysis. Therefore, it can be concluded that whole-genome sequencing of cancer samples is already a feasible task but not yet a routine process. Further technical improvements will be required before the task of decoding the entire genome of any malignant tumor of any cancer patient can be applied to clinical practice.

The number of next-generation sequencing platforms has substantially grown over the past few years and currently includes technologies from Roche/454, Illumina/Solexa, Life/APG's SOLiD3, Helicos BioSciences/HeliScope, and Pacific Biosciences/PacBio RS.[79] Noteworthy also are the recent introduction of the Polonator G.007 instrument, an open source platform with freely available software and protocols, the Ion Torrent's semiconductor sequencer, as well as those involving self-assembling DNA nanoballs or nanopore technologies.[83–85] These new machines are driving the field toward the era of third-generation sequencing, which brings enormous clinical interest as it can substantially increase speed and accuracy of analysis at reduced costs and facilitate the possibility of single-molecule sequencing of human genomes. A comparison of next-generation sequencing platforms is shown in Table 1.1. These various platforms differ in the method utilized for template preparation and in the nucleotide sequencing and imaging strategy, which finally result in their different performance. Ultimately, the most suitable approach depends on the specific genome sequencing projects.[79]

Current methods of template preparation first involve randomly shearing genomic DNA into smaller fragments from which a library of either fragment templates or mate-pair templates are generated. Then, clonally amplified templates from single DNA molecules are prepared by either emulsion polymerase chain reaction (PCR) or solid-phase amplification.[86,87] Alternatively, it is possible to prepare single-molecule templates through methods that require less starting material and do not involve PCR amplification reactions, which can be the source of artifactual mutations.[88] Once prepared, templates are attached to a solid surface in spatially separated sites, allowing thousands to billions of nucleotide sequencing reactions to be performed simultaneously.

The sequencing methods currently used by the different next-generation sequencing platforms are diverse and have been classified into four groups: cyclic reversible termination, single-nucleotide addition, real-time sequencing, and sequencing by ligation[79,89] (Fig. 1.3). These sequencing strategies are coupled with different imaging methods, including those based on measuring bioluminescent signals or involving

TABLE 1.1

COMPARATIVE ANALYSIS OF NEXT-GENERATION SEQUENCING PLATFORMS

Platform	Library/Template Preparation	Sequencing Method	Average Read-Length (Bases)	Run Time (Days)	Gb Per Run	Instrument Cost (US$)	Comments
Roche 454 GS FLX	Fragment, Mate-pair Emulsion PCR	Pyrosequencing	400	0.35	0.45	500,000	Fast run times High reagent cost
Illumina HiSeq2000	Fragment, Mate-pair Solid-phase	Reversible terminator	100–125	8 (mate-pair run)	150–200	540,000	Most widely used platform Low multiplexing capability
Life/APG's SOLiD 5500xl	Fragment, Mate-pair Emulsion PCR	Cleavable probe, sequencing by ligation	35–75	7 (mate-pair run)	180–300	595,000	Inherent error correction Long run times
Helicos BioSciences HeliScope	Fragment, Mate-pair Single molecule	Reversible terminator	32	8 (fragment run)	37	999,000	Non-bias template representation Expensive, high error rates
Pacific Biosciences PacBio RS	Fragment Single molecule	Real-time sequencing	1,000	1	0.075	NA	Greatest potential for long reads Highest error rates
Polonator G.007	Mate-pair Emulsion PCR	Non-cleavable probe, sequencing by ligation	26	5 (mate-pair run)	12	170,000	Least expensive platform Shortest read lengths

NA, not available.
(Data represent an update of information provided in ref. 78.)

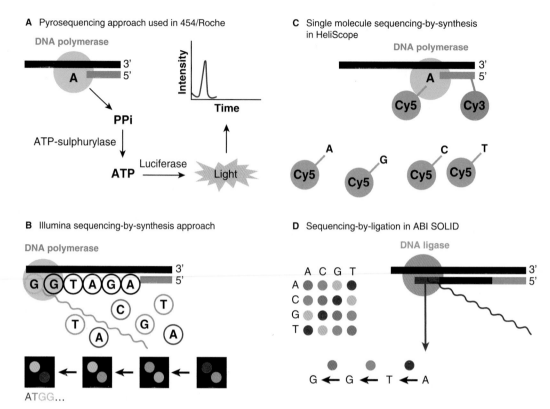

FIGURE 1.3 Advances in sequencing chemistry implemented in next-generation sequencers. **A:** The pyrosequencing approach implemented in 454/Roche sequencing technology detects incorporated nucleotides by chemiluminescence resulting from PPi release. **B:** The Illumina method utilizes sequencing-by-synthesis in the presence of fluorescently labeled nucleotide analogs that serve as reversible reaction terminators. **C:** The single-molecule sequencing-by-synthesis approach detects template extension using Cy3 and Cy5 labels attached to the sequencing primer and the incoming nucleotides, respectively. **D:** The SOLiD method sequences templates by sequential ligation of labeled degenerate probes. Two-base encoding implemented in the SOLiD instrument allows for probing each nucleotide position twice. (From ref. 88.)

four-color imaging of single molecular events. Finally, the extraordinary amount of data released from these nucleotide sequencing platforms is stored, assembled, and analyzed using powerful bioinformatic tools that have been developed in parallel with next-generation sequencing technologies.[90]

Next-generation sequencing approaches represent the newest entry into the cancer genome decoding arena and have already been applied to cancer analysis. The first research group to apply these methodologies to whole cancer genomes was that of Ley et al.,[91] who reported in 2008 the sequencing of the entire genome of a patient with acute myeloid leukemia (AML) and its comparison with the normal tissue from the same patient, using the Illumina/Solexa platform. As further described below, this work has allowed the identification of point mutations and structural alterations of putative oncogenic relevance in AML and represents proof-of-principle of the relevance of next-generation sequencing for cancer research.

Whole-Genome Analysis Utilizing Second-Sequencing

The sequence of the first whole cancer genome was reported in 2008, where an AML and skin from the same patient were described.[91] Numerous additional whole-genomes, together with the corresponding normal genomes of patients with a variety of malignant tumors, have been reported since then.[73,92–95] The first available whole-genome of a cytogenetically normal AML subtype M1 (AML-M1) revealed eight genes with novel mutations along with another 500 to 1,000 additional mutations found in noncoding regions of the genome. Most of the identified genes were not previously associated with cancer. Validation of the novel mutations identified no novel recurring mutations.[91] Concomitantly, with the expansion in the use of next-generation sequencers, other whole-genomes have been evaluated in a similar manner, including malignant melanoma, small cell lung cancer bone metastasis, lung adenocarcinoma, and a second AML.

In contrast to the first AML whole genome, the second did observe a recurrent mutation in *IDH1*, encoding isocitrate dehydrogenase.[73] Follow-up studies extended this finding and reported that mutations in *IDH1* and the related gene *IDH2* occur at a 20% to 30% frequency in AML patients and are associated with a poor prognosis in some subgroups of patients.[96–98] A good example illustrating the high pace at which second-generation technologies and their accompanying analytical tools are found is demonstrated by the following finding derived from reanalysis of the first AML whole genome. Thus, when improvements in sequencing techniques were available, the first AML whole genome described above, which identified no recurring mutations and had a 91.2% diploid coverage, was re-evaluated by deeper sequence coverage, yielding 99.6% diploid coverage of the genome. This improvement together with more advanced mutation naming algorithms allowed the discovery of several nonsynonymous mutations that had not been identified in the initial sequencing. This included a frameshift mutation in the DNA methyltransferase gene *DNMT3A*. Validation of *DNMT3A* in 280 additional *de novo* AML patients to define recurring mutations led to the significant discovery that a total of 22.1% of AML cases had mutations in *DNMT3A* that were predicted to affect translation. The median overall survival among patients with *DNMT3A* mutations was significantly shorter than that among patients without such mutations (12.3 months vs. 41.1 months; $P < .001$).

Shortly after this study, complete sequences of a series of cancer genomes together with matched normal genomes of the same patients have been reported.[73,92,93,99] These works have opened the way to more ambitious initiatives, including those involving large international consortia, aimed at decoding the genome of malignant tumors from thousands of cancer patients. In addition to these direct applications of next-generation sequencing technologies for the mutational analysis of cancer genomes, these methods have an additional range of applications in cancer research. Thus, genome sequencing efforts have begun to elucidate the genomic changes that accompany metastasis evolution through comparative analysis of primary and metastatic lesions from breast and pancreatic cancer patients.[94,100–102] Likewise, massively parallel sequencing has been used to analyze the evolution of a tongue adenocarcinoma in response to selection by targeted kinase inhibitors.[103] Detailed information of several of these whole genome projects is found below.

The first solid cancer to undergo whole-genome sequencing was a malignant melanoma that was compared to a lymphoblastoid cell line from the same person.[92] Impressively, a total of 33,345 somatic base substitutions were identified, with 187 nonsynonymous substitutions in protein-coding sequences, at least one order of magnitude

higher than any other cancer type. Most somatic base substitutions were C:G greater than T:A transitions and of the 510 dinucleotide substitutions, 360 were CC.TT/GG.AA changes, which is consistent with ultraviolet light exposure mutation signatures previously reported in melanoma.[19] Such results from the most comprehensive catalog of somatic mutations not only provide insight into the DNA damage signature in this cancer type but can also be useful in determining the relative order of some acquired mutations. Indeed, this study shows that a significant correlation exists between the presence of a higher proportion of C.A/G.T transitions in early (82%) compared to late mutations (53%). Another important aspect that the comprehensive nature of this melanoma study provided was that cancer mutations are spread out unevenly throughout the genome, with a lower prevalence in regions of transcribed genes, suggesting that DNA repair occurs mainly in these areas.

An interesting example of the power of whole-genome sequencing in deciphering the mutation evolution in carcinogenesis was seen in a study in which a basal-like breast cancer tumor, a brain metastasis, a tumor xenograft derived from the primary tumor, and the peripheral blood from the same patient were compared (Fig. 1.4).[94] This analysis showed a wide range of mutant allele frequencies in the primary tumor, which was narrowed in the metastasis and xenograft samples. This suggested that the primary tumor was significantly more heterogeneous in its cell populations compared to its matched metastasis and xenograft samples as these underwent selection processes whether during metastasis or transplantation. The clear overlap in mutation incidence between the metastatic and xenograft cases suggests that xenografts undergo similar selection as metastatic lesions and are therefore a reliable source for genomic analyses. The main conclusion of this whole-genome study was that although metastatic tumors harbor an increased number of genetic alterations, the majority of the alterations found in the primary tumor are preserved.

Whole-Exome Analysis Utilizing Second-Generation Sequencing

Another application of second-generation sequencing involves utilizing nucleic acid "baits" to capture regions of interest in the total pool of nucleic acids. These could either be DNA, as described above,[104,105] or RNA.[106] Indeed, most areas of interest in the genome can be targeted, including exons and noncoding RNAs. Despite inefficiencies in the exome targeting process, including the uneven capture efficiency across exons, which results in not all exons being sequenced, and the occurrence of some off-target hybridization events,

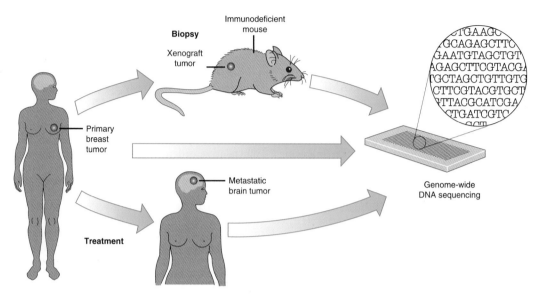

FIGURE 1.4 Covering all the bases in metastatic assessment. Ding et al.[94] performed genome-wide analysis on three tumor samples: a patient's primary breast tumor; her metastatic brain tumor, which formed despite therapy; and a xenograft tumor in a mouse, originating from the patient's breast tumor. They find that the primary tumor differs from the metastatic and xenograft tumors mainly in the prevalence of genomic mutations (permission from Gray et al. Nature 2010).

the higher coverage of the exome makes it highly suitable for mutation discovery in cancer samples.

A recent study using exome capture followed by massively parallel sequencing surveyed somatic mutations in metastasizing uveal melanoma,[61] which is the most common primary cancer of the eye and is at high risk for fatal metastasis.[107] In this impressive study only two class II uveal melanoma tumors and their matching normal DNA were investigated. Although not much is known about the genetic basis of uveal melanoma, class II tumors are strongly associated with monosomy 3.[108] The authors therefore chose to specifically survey tumors that were monosomic for chromosome 3 to see whether loss of one copy of chromosome 3 could unmask a mutant gene on the remaining copy that promotes metastasis. This strategy was extremely fruitful as it allowed the identification of inactivating somatic mutations in *BAP1*, located at chromosome 3p21.1 and encoding a deubiquitylating enzyme. Further functional studies have implicated mutational inactivation of *BAP1* as a key event in uveal melanoma metastasis, thus expanding the relevance of DUBs as potential therapeutic targets in cancer.[61]

Use of Next-Generation Sequencing for Additional Cancer Genome Applications

Next-generation sequencing of RNA extracted from tumor cells can be used for the precise and complete characterization of cancer transcriptomes to sample the expressed part of the genome.[109] This approach, called RNA-seq, has higher sensitivity than methods of RNA profiling based on DNA microarrays and can be also useful to find novel genes mutated in cancer, as illustrated by the identification of a recurrent *FOXL2* mutation in granulose-cell ovarian tumors.[109] An additional example of the power of RNA-seq was a survey in which the whole transcriptome of 18 ovarian clear-cell carcinomas and 1 ovarian clear-cell carcinoma cell line were sequenced, leading to the discovery of somatic mutations in *ARID1A* in 6 of the samples.[110] Validation analyses of *ARID1A* identified it to be somatically mutated in 46% of ovarian clear-cell carcinomas and 30% of endometrioid carcinomas. The spectrum of the identified mutations suggested that *ARID1A*, which encodes BAF250a, part of the SWI–SNF chromatin remodeling complex, is a novel tumor suppressor.

Next-generation sequencing technologies have also been relevant in the identification of noncoding RNAs, including both microRNAs and large noncoding RNAs, which are encoded by a new class of genes of growing importance in cancer.[89,111,112] Likewise, RNA-seq data have also proven to be useful for detecting alternative splicing events or novel fusion transcripts in cancer samples.[113,114] Finally, several large-scale approaches such as ChIP-seq, which involves chromatin immunoprecipitation coupled with massively parallel sequencing, have facilitated the genome-wide identification of epigenetic alterations in cancer cells.[115,116]

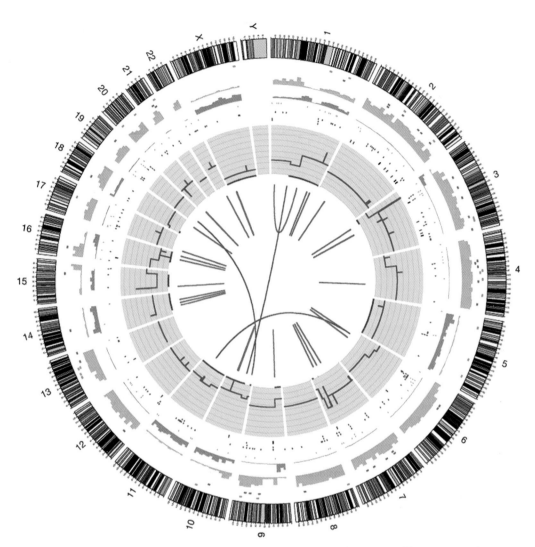

FIGURE 1.5 The catalog of somatic mutations in COLO-829. Chromosome ideograms are shown around the outer ring and are oriented pter–qter in a clockwise direction with centromeres indicated in red. Other tracks contain somatic alterations (*from outside to inside*): validated insertions (*light green rectangles*); validated deletions (*dark green rectangles*); heterozygous (*light orange bars*), and homozygous (*dark orange bars*) substitutions shown by density per 10 megabases; coding substitutions (*colored squares: silent in gray, missense in purple, nonsense in red, and splice site in black*); copy number (*blue lines*); regions of loss of heterozygosity (LOH) (*red lines*); validated intrachromosomal rearrangements (*green lines*); validated interchromosomal rearrangements (*purple lines*). (From ref. 92.)

SOMATIC ALTERATION CLASSES DETECTED BY CANCER GENOME ANALYSIS

Whole-genome sequencing of cancer genomes has an enormous potential to detect all major types of somatic mutations present in malignant tumors. This large repertoire of genomic abnormalities includes single nucleotide changes, small insertions and deletions, large chromosomal reorganizations, and copy number variations (Fig. 1.5).

Nucleotide substitutions are the most frequent somatic mutations detected in malignant tumors, although there is a substantial variability in the mutational frequency among different cancers.[78] On average, human malignancies have one nucleotide change per million bases, but melanomas reach mutational rates tenfold higher and tumors with mutator phenotype caused by DNA mismatch repair deficiencies may accumulate tens of mutations per million nucleotides. By contrast, tumors of hematopoietic origin have less than one base substitution per million. Several bioinformatic tools and pipelines have been developed to efficiently detect somatic nucleotide substitutions through comparison of the genomic information obtained from paired normal and tumor samples from the same patient. Likewise, there are a number of publicly available computational methods to predict the functional relevance of the identified mutations in cancer specimens.[78] Most of these bioinformatic tools exclusively deal with nucleotide changes in protein coding regions and evaluate the putative structural or functional effect of an amino acid substitution in a determined protein, thus obviating changes in other genomic regions, which can also be of crucial interest in cancer. In any case, current computational methods used in this regard are far from being optimal, and experimental validation is finally required to assess the functional relevance of nucleotide substitutions found in cancer genomes.

Small insertions and deletions (*indels*) represent a second category of somatic mutations that can be discovered by whole-genome sequencing of cancer specimens. These mutations are about tenfold less frequent than nucleotide substitutions but may also have an obvious impact in cancer progression. Accordingly, specific bioinformatic tools have been created to detect these *indels* in the context of the large amount of information generated by whole-genome sequencing projects.[117]

The systematic identification of large chromosomal rearrangements in cancer genomes represents one of the most successful applications of next-generation sequencing methodologies. Previous strategies in this regard had mainly been based on the utilization of cytogenetic methods for the identification of recurrent translocations in hematopoietic tumors. More recently, a combination of bioinformatics and functional methods has allowed the finding of recurrent translocations in solid epithelial tumors such as *TMPRSS2–ERG* in prostate cancer and *EML4–ALK* in non-small cell lung cancer.[118,119] Now, by using next-generation sequencing analysis of genomes and transcriptomes, it is possible to systematically search for both intrachromosomal and interchromosomal rearrangements occurring in cancer specimens. These studies have already proven their usefulness for cancer research through the discovery of recurrent translocations involving genes of the *RAF* kinase pathway in prostate cancer, gastric cancer, and melanoma.[120] Likewise, massively parallel paired-end genome and transcriptome sequencing has already been used to detect new gene fusions in cancer and to catalog all major structural rearrangements present in some tumors and cancer cell lines.[81,113,121,122] The ongoing cancer genome projects involving thousands of tumor samples will likely lead to the detection of many other chromosomal rearrangements of relevance in specific subsets of cancers. It is also remarkable that whole-genome sequencing may also facilitate the identification of other types of genomic alterations, including rearrangements of repetitive elements, such as active retrotransposons or insertions of foreign gene sequences, such as viral genomes, which can contribute to cancer development. Indeed, next-generation sequencing analysis of the transcriptome of Merkell cell carcinoma samples has revealed the clonal integration within the tumor genome of a previously unknown polyomavirus likely implicated in the pathogenesis of this rare but aggressive skin cancer.[123]

Finally, next-generation sequencing approaches have also demonstrated their feasibility to analyze the pattern of copy number alterations in cancer, as they allow researchers to count the number of reads in both tumor and normal samples at any given genomic region and then to evaluate the tumor-to-normal copy number ratio at this particular region. These new methods offer some advantages when compared with those based on microarrays, including much better resolution, precise definition of the involved breakpoints, and absence of saturation, which facilitates the accurate estimation of high-copy number levels occurring in some genomic loci of malignant tumors.[78]

PATHWAY-ORIENTED MODELS OF CANCER GENOME ANALYSIS

Genome-wide mutational analyses suggest that the mutational landscape of cancer is made up of a handful of genes that are mutated in a high fraction of tumors, otherwise know as "mountains," and most mutated genes are altered at relatively low frequencies, otherwise known as "hills"[36] (Fig. 1.6). The mountains probably give a high selective advantage to the mutated cell, and the hills might provide a lower advantage, making it hard to distinguish them from passenger mutations. As the hills differ between cancer types, it seems that the cancer genome is more complex and heterogeneous than anticipated. Although highly heterogeneous, bioinformatic studies suggest that the mountains and hills can be grouped into sets of pathways and biologic processes. Some of these pathways are affected by mutations in a few pathway members and others by numerous members. For example, pathway analyses have allowed the stratification of mutated genes in pancreatic adenocarcinomas to 12 core pathways that have at least one member mutated in 67% to 100% of the tumors analyzed[62] (Fig. 1.7). These core pathways deviated to some that harbored one single highly mutated gene, such as in *KRAS* in the G_1/S cell cycle transition pathway and pathways where a few mutated genes were found, such as the transforming growth factor (TGF-β) signaling pathway. Finally, there were pathways in which many different genes were mutated, such as invasion

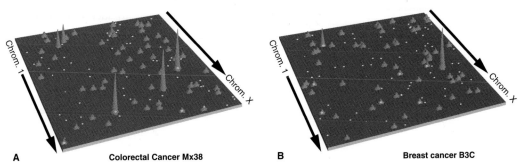

A   Colorectal Cancer Mx38   **B**   Breast cancer B3C

FIGURE 1.6 Cancer genome landscapes. Nonsilent somatic mutations are plotted in two-dimensional space representing chromosomal positions of RefSeq genes. The telomere of the short arm of chromosome 1 is represented in the rear left corner of the green plane and ascending chromosomal positions continue in the direction of the arrow. Chromosomal positions that follow the front edge of the plane are continued at the back edge of the plane of the adjacent row, and chromosomes are appended end to end. Peaks indicate the 60 highest-ranking CAN-genes for each tumor type, with peak heights reflecting CaMP scores (7). The dots represent genes that were somatically mutated in the individual colorectal (Mx38) (**A**) or breast tumor (B3C) (**B**) displayed. The dots corresponding to mutated genes that coincided with hills or mountains are black with white rims; the remaining dots are white with red rims. The mountain on the right of both landscapes represents TP53 (chromosome 17), and the other mountain shared by both breast and colorectal cancers is PIK3CA (upper left, chromosome 3). (Redrawn from ref. 36. Reprinted with permission from AAAS.)

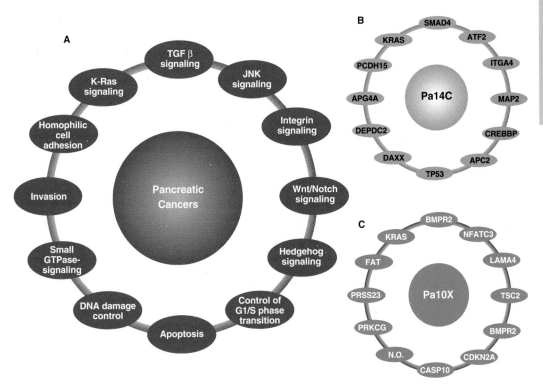

FIGURE 1.7 Signaling pathways and processes. **A:** The 12 pathways and processes whose component genes were genetically altered in most pancreatic cancers. **B, C:** Two pancreatic cancers (Pa14C and Pa10X) and the specific genes that are mutated in them. The positions around the circles in (B) and (C) correspond to the pathways and processes in (A). Several pathway components overlapped, as illustrated by the BMPR2 mutation that presumably disrupted both the SMAD4 and hedgehog signaling pathways in Pa10X. Additionally, not all 12 processes and pathways were altered in every pancreatic cancer, as exemplified by the fact that no mutations known to affect DNA damage control were observed in Pa10X. NO, not observed. (Redrawn from ref. 61. Reprinted with permission from AAAS.)

regulation molecules, cell adhesion molecules, and integrin signaling. Importantly, independent of how many genes in the same pathway are affected, if they are found to occur in a mutually exclusive fashion in a single tumor, they most likely give the same selective pressure for clonal expansion.

The idea of genetically analyzing pathways rather than individual genes has been applied previously, revealing the concept of mutual exclusivity. Mutual exclusivity has been shown elegantly in the case of *KRAS* and *BRAF* where a *KRAS* mutated cancer generally does not also harbor a *BRAF* mutation, as *KRAS* is upstream of *BRAF* in the same pathway.[14] A similar concept was applied for *PIK3CA* and *PTEN*, where both mutations do not usually occur in the same tumor.[30]

"Passenger" and "Driver" Mutations

By the time a cancer is diagnosed, it is comprised of billions of cells carrying DNA abnormalities, some of which have a functional role in malignant proliferation but also many genetic lesions acquired along the way that have no functional role in tumorigenesis.[19] The emerging landscapes of cancer genomes include thousands of genes that were not previously linked to tumorigenesis but are found to be somatically mutated. Many of these changes are likely to be "passengers" or neutral in that they have no functional effects on the growth of the tumor.[19] Only a small fraction of the genetic alterations are expected to drive cancer evolution by giving cells a selective advantage over their neighbors. Passenger mutations occur incidentally in a cell that later or in parallel develops a "driver" mutation, but are not ultimately pathogenic.[124] Although neutral, cataloging passengers mutations is important as they incorporate the signatures of previous exposures the cancer cell underwent as well as DNA repair defects the cancer cell has. As in many cases passenger and driver mutations occur at similar frequencies, and identification of drivers versus the passenger is of utmost relevance and remains a pressing challenge in cancer genetics.[125-127] This goal will eventually be achieved through a combination of genetic and functional approaches, some of which are listed below.

The most reliable indicator that a gene was selected for and therefore is highly likely to be pathogenic is identification of recurrent mutations, whether at the same exact amino acid position or in neighboring amino acid positions in different patients. Further than that, if somatic alterations in the same gene occur very frequently (mountains in the tumor genome landscape), these can be confidently classified as drivers. For example, cancer alleles that are identified in multiple patients and different tumors types such as those found in *KRAS*, *TP53*, *PTEN*, and *PIK3CA* are clearly selected for during tumorigenesis.

However, most genes discovered thus far are mutated in a relatively small fraction of tumors (hills), and it has been clearly shown that genes that are mutated in less than 1% of patients can still act as drivers.[128] The systematic sequencing of newly identified putative cancer genes in the vast number of specimens from cancer patients will help in this regard. However, even if examination of large numbers of samples can provide helpful information to classify drivers versus passengers, this approach alone is limited by the marked variation in mutation frequency among individual tumors and individual genes. The statistical test utilized in this case calculates the probability that the number of mutations in a given gene reflects a mutation frequency that is greater than expected from the nonfunctional background mutation rate,[36,129] which is different between different cancer types. These analyses incorporate the number of somatic alterations observed, the number of tumors studied, and the number of nucleotides that were successfully sequenced and analyzed.

Another approach often used to distinguish driver from passenger mutations exploits statistical analysis of synonymous versus nonsynonymous changes.[130] In contrast to nonsynonymous mutations, synonymous mutations do not alter the protein sequence. Therefore, they do not usually apply a growth advantage and would not be expected to be selected during tumorigenesis. This strategy works by comparing the observed-to-expected ratio of synonymous with that of nonsynonymous mutation. An increased proportion of nonsynonymous mutations from the expected two-to-one ratio implies selection pressure during tumorigenesis.

Other approaches are based on the concept that driver mutations may have characteristics similar to those causing Mendelian disease when inherited in the germ line and may be identifiable by constraints on tolerated amino acid residues at the mutated positions. In contrast, passenger mutations may have characteristics more similar to those of nonsynonymous SNPs with high minor allele frequencies. Based on these premises, supervised machine learning methods have been used to predict which missense mutations are drivers.[131] Additional approaches to decipher drivers from passengers include identification of mutations that affect locations that have previously been shown to be cancer causing in protein members of the same gene family. Enrichment for mutations in evolutionarily conserved residues and algorithms, such as SIFT (sorting intolerant from tolerant),[132] estimate the effects of the different mutations identified.

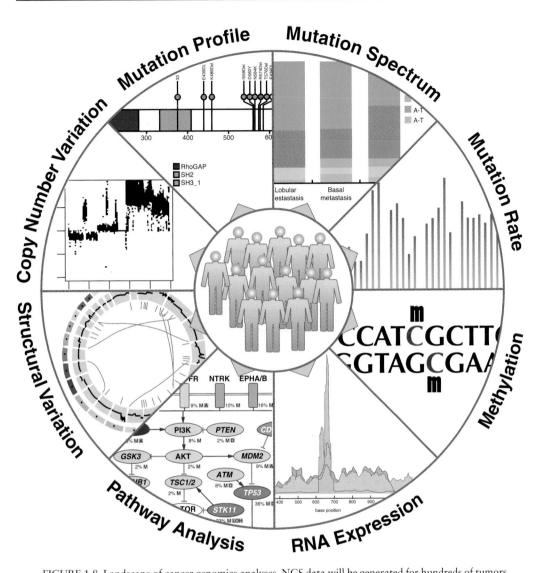

FIGURE 1.8 Landscape of cancer genomics analyses. NGS data will be generated for hundreds of tumors from all major cancer types in the near future. The integrated analysis of DNA, RNA and methylation sequencing data will help elucidate all relevant genetic changes in cancers. (Permission from ref. 94.)

Probably the most conclusive methods to identify driver mutations will be rigorous functional studies using biochemical assays as well as model organisms or cultured cells, using knock-out and knock-in of individual cancer alleles.[133] Unfortunately, these methods are not well suited to the analysis of the hundreds of gene candidates that arise from every large-scale cancer genome project. In conclusion, it is fair to say that sequencing cancer genomes is only the beginning of a journey that will ultimately be completed when the thousands of the newly discovered alleles are annotated as being the drivers of this disease. A summary of the various next-generation applications and approaches for their analysis is summarized in Figure 1.8 and Table 1.2.

NETWORKS OF CANCER GENOME PROJECTS

The first large-scale studies of genes mutated in malignant tumors have allowed the identification of new cancer genes that represent potential targets for therapy in different types of cancer. However, these analyses have also demonstrated that the repertoire of oncogenic mutations is extremely heterogeneous, suggesting that it would be difficult for independent cancer genome initiatives to address the generation of comprehensive catalogs of mutations in the wide spectrum of human malignancies. Accordingly, there have been different efforts to coordinate the cancer genome

GENERAL PRINCIPLES

TABLE 1.2

COMPUTATIONAL TOOLS AND DATABASES USEFUL FOR CANCER GENOME ANALYSIS

Category	Tool/Database	URL	Refs.
Alignment	MAQ	http://maq.sourceforge.net	1
	BWA	http://bio-bwa.sourceforge.net	2
Mutation calling	SNVMix	http://www.bcgsc.ca/platform/bioinfo/software/SNVMix	3
	Samtools	http://samtools.sourceforge.net	4
	VarScan	http://varscan.sourceforge.net	5
Indel calling	Pindel	http://www.ebi.ac.uk/~kye/pindel	6
Copy number analysis	CBS	http://www.bioconductor.org	7
	SegSeq	http://www.broadinstitute.org/cgi-bin/cancer/publications/pub_paper.cgi?mode=view&paper_id=182	8
Functional effect	SIFT	http://blocks.fhcrc.org/sift/SIFT.html	9
	Polyphen-2	http://genetics.bwh.harvard.edu/pph2	10
Visualization	CIRCOS	http://mkweb.bcgsc.ca/circos	11
	IGV	http://www.broadinstitute.org/igv	12
Repository	Cosmic	http://www.sanger.ac.uk/genetics/CGP/cosmic	13
	CGP	http://www.sanger.ac.uk/genetics/CGP	14
	dbSNP	http://www.ncbi.nlm.nih.gov/SNP	15
	Gene Ranker	http://cbio.mskcc.org/tcga-generanker/	16

(Table based on Table 2 from Meyerson M, Stacey G, and Getz G. Advances in understanding cancer genomes through second generation sequencing. *Nature Rev Genet* 2010;11:685–696.)

1. Li H, Durbin R. Fast and accurate short read alignment with Burrows–Wheeler transform. *Bioinformatics* 2009;25:1754–1760.
2. Li H, Durbin R. Fast and accurate long-read alignment with Burrows–Wheeler transform. *Bioinformatics* 2010;26:589–595.
3. Goya R, et al. SNVMix: predicting single nucleotide variants from next-generation sequencing of tumors. *Bioinformatics* 2010;26:730–736.
4. Li H, et al. The Sequence Alignment/Map format and SAMtools. *Bioinformatics* 2009;25:2078–2079.
5. Koboldt DC, Chen K, Wylie T, et al. VarScan: variant detection in massively parallel sequencing of individual and pooled samples. *Bioinformatics* 2009;25(17):2283–2285.
6. Ye K, Schulz MH, Long Q, et al. Pindel: a pattern growth approach to detect break points of large deletions and medium sized insertions from paired-end short reads. *Bioinformatics* 2009;25:2865–2871.
7. Venkatraman ES, Olshen AB. A faster circular binary segmentation algorithm for the analysis of array CGH data. *Bioinformatics* 2007;23:657–663.
8. Chiang DY, et al. High-resolution mapping of copy-number alterations with massively parallel sequencing. *Nature Methods* 2009;6:99–103.
9. Ng PC, Henikoff S. Predicting deleterious amino acid substitutions. *Genome Res.* 2001;11:863–874.
10. Idzhubei IA, et al. A method and server for predicting damaging missense mutations. *Nature Methods* 2010;7:248–249.
11. Krzywinski M, et al. Circos: an information aesthetic for comparative genomics. *Genome Res.* 2009;19:1639–1645.
12. Robinson JT, Thorvaldsdóttir H, Winckler W, et al. Integrative Genomics Viewer. *Nature Biotechnol* 2010 (In Press).
13. Forbes SA, Bhamra S, Dawson E, et al. The catalogue of somatic mutations in cancer (COSMIC). *Curr Protoc Hum Genet.* 2008; Chapter 10:Unit 10.11
14. Futreal PA, Coin L, Marshall M, et al. A census of human cancer genes. *Nat Rev Cancer.* 2004;4;177–183.
15. Sherry ST, Ward MH, Kholodov M, et al. dbSNP: The NCBI Database of genetic variation. *Nucleic Acids Res.* 2001;29(1):308–311.
16. The Cancer Genome Atlas Research Network. Comprehensive genomic characterization defines human glioblastoma genes and core pathways. *Nature* 2008;455:1061–1068.

sequencing projects being carried out around the world. The first initiative in this regard was the Cancer Genome Project (CGP) of the Wellcome Trust Sanger Institute launched in the United Kingdom, which has been followed by two large and ambitious projects called the Cancer Genome Atlas (TCGA) and the International Cancer Genome Consortium (ICGC). Besides these three large cancer genome projects, there are other initiatives that are more focused on specific tumors, such as that lead by scientists at St. Jude Children's Research Hospital in Memphis, and Washington University, which aims at sequencing 600 pediatric-cancer genomes.

The CGP initially focused on the systematic search for somatic alterations in human tumors and cancer cell lines, analyzing large sets of candidate cancer genes as well as whole genomes. This project has already completed the whole-genome sequencing of several cancer patients and tumor-derived cell lines, including lung carcinomas and melanomas,[92,93] and intends to extend these studies to a total of 2,000 to 3,000 cases over the next 5 years.

TCGA began in 2006 at the United States as a comprehensive program in cancer genomics supported by the U.S. National Institutes of Health (NIH). The initial project focused on three tumors: glioblastoma multiforme, serous cystadenocarcinoma of the ovary, and lung squamous carcinoma. These studies have already generated novel and interesting information regarding genes mutated in these malignancies.[134] On the basis of these positive results, the NIH has recently announced an expansion of the TCGA program with the aim to produce genomic data sets for at least 10 additional cancers by the end of 2011 and 20 to 25 cancers over the next 5 years.

The ICGC was formed in 2008 to coordinate the generation of comprehensive catalogs of genomic abnormalities in tumors from 50 different cancer types or subtypes that are of clinical and societal importance across the world.[135] The project aims to perform systematic studies of over 25,000 cancer genomes at the genomic level and integrate this information with epigenomic and transcriptomic studies of the same cases as well as with clinical features of patients. At present, ten countries and two European consortia have already initiated cancer genome projects coordinated by the ICGC. These projects will deal with at least 500 samples per cancer type from cancers affecting a variety of human organs and tissues, including blood, brain, breast, kidney, liver, pancreas, stomach, oral cavity, and ovary.[135] All participating countries and scientists have adhered to a series of predetermined procedures for ethical approval, sample quality, clinical annotation, study design, statistical issues, data storage, and intellectual property. In this regard, the ICGC has made the commitment to make the data available to the entire research community as rapidly as possible to accelerate the understanding of cancer biology and translate these discoveries into clinical practice.

All these coordinated projects have already provided new insights into the catalog of genes mutated in cancer and have unveiled specific signatures of the mutagenic mechanisms, including carcinogen exposures or DNA-repair defects, implicated in the development of different malignant tumors.[92,93,136] Furthermore, these cancer genome studies have also contributed to define clinically relevant subtypes of tumors for prognosis and therapeutic management, and in some cases have identified new targets and strategies for cancer treatment.[66,73,95,137,138] Nevertheless, and similar to the doubts raised at the first stages of the Human Genome Project, the proposal to sequence large numbers of cancer genomes has also generated some controversy because of the high cost of these projects, the lack of novel functional hypotheses driving these projects, or their failure to characterize the mutational heterogeneity within individual tumors.[139,140] However, the rapid technological advances in DNA sequencing will likely drop the costs of sequencing cancer genomes to a small fraction of the current price and will allow researchers to overcome some of the current limitations of these global sequencing efforts. Hopefully, worldwide coordination of cancer genome projects with those involving large-scale functional analysis of genes in both cellular and animal models will likely provide us with the most comprehensive collection of information generated to date into the causes and molecular mechanisms of cancer.

THE GENOMIC LANDSCAPE OF CANCERS

Examination of the overall distribution of the identified mutations redefined the cancer genome landscapes whereby the mountains are the handful of commonly mutated genes and the hills represent the vast majority of genes that are infrequently mutated. One of the most striking features of tumor genomic landscape is that it involves different sets of cancer genes that are mutated in a tissue-specific fashion.[141,142] To continue with the analogy, the scenery is very different if we observe a colorectal, a lung, or a breast tumor. This indicates that mutations in specific genes cause tumors at specific sites, or are associated with specific stages of development, cell differentiation, or tumorigenesis, despite many of those genes being expressed in various fetal and adult tissues. Moreover, different types of tumors follow specific genetic pathways in terms of the combination of genetic alterations that it must acquire. For example, no cancer outside the bowel has been shown to follow the classic genetic pathway of colorectal tumorigenesis. Additionally, *KRAS* mutations are almost always present in pancreatic cancers but are very rare or absent in breast cancers. Similarly, *BRAF* mutations are present in 60% of melanomas but are very infrequent in lung cancers.[1] Another intriguing feature is that alterations in ubiquitous housekeeping genes, such as those involved in DNA repair or energy production, occur only in particular types of tumors.

In addition to tissue specificity, the genomic landscape of tumors can also be associated with the gender and the hormonal status. For example *HER-2* amplification and *PIK3C2A* mutations, two genetic alterations associated with breast cancer development, are correlated with the estrogen-receptor hormonal status.[143] The molecular basis for the occurrence of cancer mutations in tissue- and gender-specific profiles is still largely unknown. Organ-specific expression profiles and cell-specific neoplastic transformation requirements are often mentioned as possible causes for this phenomenon. Identifying tissue and gender cancer mutations patterns is relevant as it may allow the definition of individualized therapeutic avenues.

THE CANCER GENOME AND THE NEW TAXONOMY OF TUMORS

The deciphering of the cancer genome has already impacted clinical practice at multiple levels. On the one hand, it allowed the identification of new cancer genes such as *IDH1*, a gene involved in glioma, which was discovered recently (see above), and on the other hand, it is redesigning the taxonomy of tumors.

Until the genomic revolution, tumors had been classified based on two criteria: their localization (site of occurrence) and their appearance (histology). These criteria are also currently used as primary determinants of prognosis and to establish the best treatments. For many decades it has been known that patients with histologically similar tumors have different clinical outcomes. Furthermore, tumors that cannot be distinguished based on histological analysis can respond very differently to identical therapies.[144]

It is becoming increasingly manifest that the frequency and distribution of mutations affecting cancer genes can be used to redefine the histology-based taxonomy of a given tumor type. Lung and colorectal tumors represent paradigmatic examples. Genomic analysis led to the identification of activating mutations in the receptor tyrosine kinase *EGFR* in lung adenocarcinomas.[145] The occurrence of *EGFR* mutations molecularly defines a subtype of non–small cell lung cancer (NSCLC) that occur mainly in nonsmoker women, tend to have a distinctly enhanced prognosis, and typically respond to EGFR-targeted therapies.[146–148] Similarly, the

recent discovery of the *EML4-ALK* fusion identifies yet another subset of NSCLC that is clearly distinct from those that harbor *EGFR* mutations, have distinct epidemiologic and biological features, and respond to ALK inhibitors.[119,149]

The second example is colorectal cancers (CRC), the tumor type for which the genomic landscape has been refined with the highest accuracy. CRCs can be clearly categorized according to the mutational profile of the genes involved in the *KRAS* pathway (Fig. 1.9). It is now known that *KRAS* mutations occur in approximately 40% of CRCs. Another subtype of CRC (approximately 10%) harbors mutations in *BRAF*, the immediate downstream effectors of *KRAS*.[15]

In CRC and other tumor types, *KRAS* and *BRAF* mutations are known to be mutually exclusive. The mutual exclusivity pattern indicates that these genes operate in the same signaling pathway. Large epidemiologic studies have shown that the prognosis of tumors harboring wild type *KRAS/BRAF* genes is distinct, typically more favorable, than that of the mutated ones.[150,151] Of note, *KRAS* and *BRAF* mutations have been recently shown to impair responsiveness to the anti-EGFR monoclonal antibodies therapies in CRC patients.[152–154] Clearly distinct subgroups can be genetically identified in both NSCLC and CRC with respect to prognosis and response to therapy. It is likely that, as soon as the genomic landscapes of other tumor types are defined, molecular subgroups like those described above will also become defined.

In conclusion, the taxonomy of tumors is being rewritten using the presence of genetic lesions as major criteria. Genome-based information will improve diagnosis and will be used to determine personalized therapeutic regimens based on the genetic landscape of individual tumors.

CANCER GENOMICS AND DRUG RESISTANCE

Cancer genomics has dramatically impacted disease management, as its application is helping researchers determine which patients are likely to benefit from which drug. As discussed in great detail in Chapters 12 and 13, good examples for such treatment include targeted therapy using imatinib for chronic myeloid leukemia (CML) patients and use of gefitinib and erlotinib for NSCLC patients.

Key to the successful development and application of anticancer agents is a better understanding of the effect of the therapeutic regimens and of resistance mechanisms that may develop. In most tumor types, a fraction of patients' tumors are refractory to therapies (intrinsic resistance). Even if an initial response to therapies is obtained, the vast majority of tumors subsequently become refractory (i.e., acquired resistance) and patients

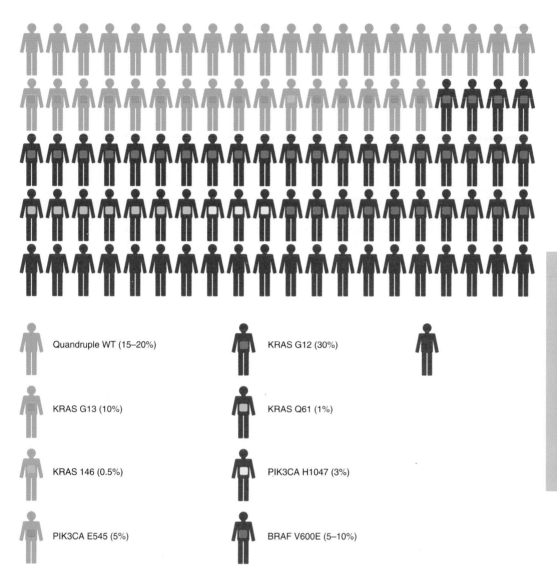

FIGURE 1.9 Graphic representation of a cohort of 100 patients with colorectal cancer treated with cetuximab or panitumumab. The genetic milieu of individual tumors and their impacts on the clinical response are listed. *KRAS, BRAF,* and *PIK3CA* somatic mutations as well as loss of PTEN protein expression are indicated according to different color codes. Molecular alterations mutually exclusive or coexisting in individual tumors are indicated using different color variants. The relative frequencies at which the molecular alterations occur in colorectal cancers are described. (Redrawn from Bardelli A, Siena S. Molecular mechanisms of resistance to cetuximab and panitumumab in colorectal cancer. *J Clin Oncol* 2009;22:6043.)

eventually succumb to disease progression. Secondary resistance should therefore be regarded as a key obstacle to treatment progress. The analysis of the cancer genome represents a powerful tool both for the identification of chemotherapeutic signatures as well as to understand resistance mechanisms to therapeutic agents. Examples for each of these are described below.

An important application of systematic sequencing experiments is identification of the effects of chemotherapy on the cancer genome. For example, gliomas that recur after temozolo-mide treatment have been shown to harbor large numbers of mutations with a signature typical of a DNA alkylating agent.[155,156] Since these alterations were detected using Sanger sequencing, which as described above has limited sensitivity, the data suggested that the detected alterations were clonal. The model that unfolds from this study indicates that although temozolomide has limited efficacy, almost all of the cells in a glioma respond to the drug. However, a single cell that was resistant to the chemotherapy proliferated and formed a cell clone. Later genomic analyses

GENERAL PRINCIPLES

of the cell clone allowed the identification of the underlying mutated resistance genes.[155,156]

Single-molecule targeted therapy is almost always followed by acquired drug resistance.[157–159] Genomic analyses can be successfully exploited to decipher resistance mechanisms to such inhibitors. Below a few paradigmatic examples are presented that will be discussed extensively in other chapters. Despite the effectiveness of gefitinib and erlotinib in EGFR mutant cases of NSCLC,[160] drug resistance develops within 6 to 12 months after initiation of therapy. The underlying reason for this resistance was identified as a secondary mutation in *EGFR* exon 20, T790M, detectable in 50% of patients who relapse.[161–163] Importantly, some studies have shown the mutation to be present before the patient was treated with the drug,[164,165] suggesting that exposure to the drug selected for these cells.[166] As the drug resistant *EGFR* mutation is structurally analogous to the mutated gatekeeper residue T315I in BCR-ABL, T670I in c-KIT, and L1196M in EML4-ALK, which have been shown previously to confer resistance to imatinib and other kinase inhibitors,[158,167,168] this mechanism of resistance represent a general problem that needs to be overcome.

A recent elegant study, which also represents the use of genomics in understanding drug resistance mechanisms, focused on the inhibition of activating *BRAF* (V600E) mutations, which occur in 7% of human malignancies and 60% of melanomas.[14] Clinical trials using PLX4032, a novel class I RAF-selective inhibitor, showed an 80% antitumor response rate in melanoma patients with *BRAF* (V600E) mutations, however, cases of drug resistance were observed.[169] Use of microarray and sequencing technologies showed that in this case the resistance was not due to secondary mutations in *BRAF*, but due rather to either up-regulation of *PDGFRB* or *NRAS* mutations.[170]

It was, however, the introduction of two anti-EGFR monoclonal antibodies, cetuximab and panitumumab, for the treatment of metastatic colorectal cancer that provided the largest body of knowledge on the relationship between tumors' genotypes and response to targeted therapies. The initial clinical analysis pointed out that only a fraction of metastatic colorectal cancer patients benefited from this novel treatment. Different from the NSCLC paradigm, it was found that EGFR mutations do not play a major role in the response. On the contrary, from the initial retrospective analysis it became clear that somatic *KRAS* mutations, thought to be present in 35% to 45% of metastatic colorectal cancers, are important negative predictors of efficacy in patients who are given panitumumab or cetuximab.[152–154] Among tumors carrying wild type *KRAS*, mutations of *BRAF* or *PIK3CA*, or loss of PTEN expression may also predict resistance to EGFR-targeted monoclonal antibodies, although the latter biomarkers require further validation before they can be incorporated into clinical practice. From these few examples, it is clear that future deeper genomic understanding of targeted drug resistance is crucial to the effective development of additional as well as alternative therapies to overcome this resistance.

PERSPECTIVES OF CANCER GENOME ANALYSIS

The completion of the human genome project has marked a new beginning in biomedical sciences. As human cancer is a genetic disease, the field of oncology has been one of the first to be impacted by this historic revolution. Knowledge of the sequence and organization of the human genome allows the systematic analysis of the genetic alterations underlying the origin and evolution of tumors. High throughput mutational profiling of common tumors, including lung, skin, breast, and colorectal cancers, and the application of next-generation sequencing to whole genome, whole exome, and whole transcriptome of cancer samples has allowed substantial advances in the understanding of this disease by facilitating the detection of all main types of somatic cancer genome alterations. These have also led to historical results such as the identification of genetic alterations that are likely to be the major drivers of these diseases.

However, the genetic landscape of cancers is by no means complete, and what has been learned so far has raised new and exciting questions that must be addressed. There are still important technical challenges for the detection of somatic mutations.[78] Clinical tumor samples often contain large amounts of nonmalignant cells, which makes the identification of mutations in cancer genomes more challenging when compared with similar analyses of peripheral blood samples for germline genome studies. Moreover, the genomic instability inherent to cancer development and progression largely increases the complexity and diversity of genomic alterations of malignant tumors, making it necessary to distinguish between driver and passenger mutations. Likewise, the fact that malignant tumors are genetically heterogeneous and contain several clones simultaneously growing within the same tumor mass raises additional questions regarding the quality of the information currently derived from cancer genomes. Hopefully, in the near future, advances in third-generation sequencing technologies will make it feasible to obtain high-quality sequence data of a genome isolated from a single cell, an aspect of crucial relevance for cancer research.

One of the next imperatives is the definition of the oncogenomic profile of all tumor types. Particularly the less common—though not less lethal—ones are still largely mysterious to scientists and untreatable to clinicians. For some of these diseases few new therapeutically amenable molecular targets have been discovered in the past years. For example, identification of druggable genetic lesions associated with pancreatic and ovarian cancers could help define new therapeutic strategies for these aggressive diseases. To achieve this, detailed oncogenomic maps of the corresponding tumors must be drafted. The latter will hopefully be completed in the coming years, thanks to the systematic cancer genome projects that are presently being performed.

Even in the case of common cancers, a lot of genomic profiling efforts still lay ahead. For example, in a significant fraction of breast and lung tumors the mutations that are likely to be drivers have not yet been found. This is not surprising considering that even in these tumor types only a limited number of samples have been systematically analyzed so far. Therefore, low incidence mutations that could represent potentially key therapeutic targets in a subset of tumors might have escaped detection. Consequently, the scaling up of the mutational profiling to large number of specimens for each tumor type is warranted.

Finally, understanding the cellular properties imparted by the hundreds of recently discovered cancer alleles is another area that must be developed. As a matter of fact, compared to the genomic discovery stage, the functional validation of putative novel cancer alleles, despite their potential clinical relevance, is substantially lagging behind. To achieve this, high-throughput functional studies in model systems that accurately recapitulate the genetic alterations found in human cancer must be developed.

To conclude, the eventual goal of profiling the cancer genome is not only to further understand the molecular basis of the disease, but also to discover novel diagnostic and drug targets. One might anticipate that the most immediate application of these new technologies will be noninvasive strategies for early cancer detection. Considering that oncogenic mutations are present only in cancer cells, screening for tumor-derived mutant DNA in patients' blood holds great potential and will progressively substitute current biomarkers, which have poor sensitivity and lack specificity.[171] Further improvements in next-generation sequencing technologies are likely to reduce their cost as well as make these analyses more facile in the future. Once this happens, most cancer patients will undergo in-depth genomic analyses as part of their initial evaluation and throughout their treatment. This will offer more precise diagnostic and prognostic information, which will affect treatment decisions. Although many challenges remain, the information gained from next-generation sequencing platforms is laying a foundation for personalized medicine, in which patients are managed with therapies that are tailored to the specific gene mutations found in their tumors. Ultimately, these should lead to therapeutic successes similar to the ones attained for chronic myelogenous leukemia patients with imatinib,[172,173] melanoma patients with PLX4032,[169] and NSCLC patients with gefitinib and erlotinib.[160] Clearly, this is the absolute goal for all of this work.

GENERAL PRINCIPLES

Selected References

The full list of references for this chapter appears in the online version.

1. Vogelstein B, Kinzler KW. Cancer genes and the pathways they control. *Nat Med* 2004;10(8):789.
2. Kinzler KW, Vogelstein B. Lessons from hereditary colon cancer. *Cell* 1996;87(2):159.
3. International Human Genome Sequencing Consortium. Finishing the euchromatic sequence of the human genome. *Nature* 2004;431(7011): 931.
5. Rous P. Transmission of a malignant new growth by means of a cell-free filtrate. *JAMA* 1911;56:198.
7. International HapMap Consortium. A haplotype map of the human genome. *Nature* 2005;437(7063):1299.
14. Davies H, Bignell GR, Cox C, et al. Mutations of the BRAF gene in human cancer. *Nature* 2002;417(6892):949.
18. Bardelli A, Parsons DW, Silliman N, et al. Mutational analysis of the tyrosine kinome in colorectal cancers. *Science* 2003;300(5621):949.
19. Greenman C, Stephens P, Smith R, et al. Patterns of somatic mutation in human cancer genomes. *Nature* 2007; 446(7132):153.
20. Samuels Y, Wang Z, Bardelli A, et al. High frequency of mutations of the PIK3CA gene in human cancers. *Science* 2004;304(5670):554.
21. Prickett TD, Agrawal NS, Wei X, et al. Analysis of the tyrosine kinome in melanoma reveals recurrent mutations in ERBB4. *Nat Genet* 2009;41(10):1127.
22. Sjoblom T, Jones S, Wood LD, et al. The consensus coding sequences of human breast and colorectal cancers. *Science* 2006;314(5797):268.
23. Wang Z, Shen D, Parsons DW, et al. Mutational analysis of the tyrosine phosphatome in colorectal cancers. *Science* 2004;304(5674):1164.
33. López-Otín C, Hunter T. The regulatory crosstalk between kinases and proteases in cancer. *Nat Rev Cancer* 2010; 10(4):278.
35. López-Otín C, Matrisian LM. Emerging roles of proteases in tumour suppression. *Nat Rev Cancer* 2007;7(10):800.
36. Wood LD, Parsons DW, Jones S, et al. The genomic landscapes of human breast and colorectal cancers. *Science* 2007;318(5853):1108.
37. Palavalli LH, Prickett TD, Wunderlich JR, et al. Analysis of the matrix metalloproteinase family reveals that MMP8 is often mutated in melanoma. *Nat Genet* 2009;41(5):518.
43. Hanahan D, Weinberg RA The hallmarks of cancer. *Cell* 2000;100(1):57.
44. Teitz T, Wei T, Valentine MB, et al. Caspase 8 is deleted or silenced preferentially in childhood neuroblastomas with amplification of MYCN. *Nat Med* 2000;6(5):529.

54. Ghavami S, Hashemi M, Ande SR, et al. Apoptosis and cancer: mutations within caspase genes. *J Med Genet* 2009;46(8):497.

56. Bignell GR, Warren W, Seal S, et al. Identification of the familial cylindromatosis tumour-suppressor gene. *Nat Genet* 2000;25(2):160.

59. Kato M, Sanada M, Kato I, et al. Frequent inactivation of A20 in B-cell lymphomas. *Nature* 2009;459(7247):712.

61. Harbour JW, Onken MD, Roberson ED, et al. Frequent mutation of BAP1 in metastasizing uveal melanomas. *Science* 2010;330(6009):1410.

62. Jones S, Zhang X, Parsons DW, et al. Core signaling pathways in human pancreatic cancers revealed by global genomic analyses. *Science* 2008;321(5897):1801.

63. Parsons DW, Jones S, Zhang X, et al. An integrated genomic analysis of human glioblastoma multiforme. *Science* 2008;321(5897):1807.

64. Jones S, Wang TL, Shih Ie M, et al. Frequent mutations of chromatin remodeling gene ARID1A in ovarian clear cell carcinoma. *Science* 2010;330(6001):228.

65. Parsons DW, Li M, Zhang X, et al. The genetic landscape of the childhood cancer medulloblastoma. *Science* 2010; (in press).

66. Yan H, Parsons DW, Jin G, et al. IDH1 and IDH2 mutations in gliomas. *N Engl J Med* 2009;360(8):765.

73. Mardis ER, Ding L, Dooling DJ, et al. Recurring mutations found by sequencing an acute myeloid leukemia genome. *N Engl J Med* 2009;361(11): 1058.

77. Mardis ER, Wilson RK. Cancer genome sequencing: a review. *Hum Mol Genet* 2009;18(R2):R163.

78. Meyerson M, Gabriel S, Getz G. Advances in understanding cancer genomes through second-generation sequencing. *Nat Rev Genet* 2010;11(10):685.

79. Metzker ML. Sequencing technologies—the next generation. *Nat Rev Genet* 2010;11(1):31.

80. Bell DW. Our changing view of the genomic landscape of cancer. *J Pathol* 2010;220(2):231.

81. Campbell PJ, Pleasance ED, Stephens PJ, et al. Subclonal phylogenetic structures in cancer revealed by ultra-deep sequencing. *Proc Natl Acad Sci U S A* 2008;105(35): 13081.

82. Kidd JM, Cooper GM, Donahue WF, et al. Mapping and sequencing of structural variation from eight human genomes. *Nature* 2008;453(7191):56.

85. Schadt EE, Turner S, Kasarskis A. A window into third-generation sequencing. *Hum Mol Genet* 2010;19(R2): R227.

89. Morozova O, Hirst M, Marra MA. Applications of new sequencing technologies for transcriptome analysis. *Annu Rev Genomics Hum Genet* 2009;10:135.

91. Ley TJ, Mardis ER, Ding L, et al. DNA sequencing of a cytogenetically normal acute myeloid leukaemia genome. *Nature* 2008;456(7218):66.

92. Pleasance ED, Cheetham RK, Stephens PJ, et al. A comprehensive catalogue of somatic mutations from a human cancer genome. *Nature* 2010;463(7278):191.

93. Pleasance ED, Stephens PJ, O'Meara S, et al. A small-cell lung cancer genome with complex signatures of tobacco exposure. *Nature* 2010;463(7278):184.

94. Ding L, Ellis MJ, Li S, et al. Genome remodelling in a basal-like breast cancer metastasis and xenograft. *Nature* 2010;464(7291):999.

95. Ley TJ, Ding L, Walter MJ, et al. DNMT3A mutations in acute myeloid leukemia. *N Engl J Med* 2010;363(25): 2424.

99. Lee W, Jiang Z, Liu J, et al. The mutation spectrum revealed by paired genome sequences from a lung cancer patient. *Nature* 2010;465(7297):473.

100. Yachida S, Jones S, Bozic I, et al. Distant metastasis occurs late during the genetic evolution of pancreatic cancer. *Nature* 2010;467(7319):1114.

101. Shah SP, Morin RD, Khattra J, et al. Mutational evolution in a lobular breast tumour profiled at single nucleotide resolution. *Nature* 2009;461(7265):809.

102. Campbell PJ, Yachida S, Mudie LJ, et al. The patterns and dynamics of genomic instability in metastatic pancreatic cancer. *Nature* 2010;467(7319):1109.

110. Wiegand KC, Shah SP, Al-Agha OM, et al. ARID1A mutations in endometriosis-associated ovarian carcinomas. *N Engl J Med* 2010;363(16):1532.

111. Farazi TA, Spitzer JI, Morozov P, et al. miRNAs in human cancer. *J Pathol* 2011;223(2):102.

112. Huarte M, Rinn JL. Large non-coding RNAs: missing links in cancer? *Hum Mol Genet* 2010;19(R2):R152.

113. Maher CA, Kumar-Sinha C, Cao X, et al. Transcriptome sequencing to detect gene fusions in cancer. *Nature* 2009;458(7234):97.

115. Park PJ. ChIP-seq: advantages and challenges of a maturing technology. *Nat Rev Genet* 2009;10(10):669.

116. Laird PW. Principles and challenges of genome-wide DNA methylation analysis. *Nat Rev Genet* 2010;11(3):191.

118. Tomlins SA, Rhodes DS, Perner S, et al. Recurrent fusion of TMPRSS2 and ETS transcription factor genes in prostate cancer. *Science* 2005;310(5748):644.

119. Soda M, Choi YL, Enomoto M, et al. Identification of the transforming EML4-ALK fusion gene in non-small-cell lung cancer. *Nature* 2007; 448(7153):561.

120. Palanisamy N, Ateeq B, Kalyana-Sundaram S, et al. Rearrangements of the RAF kinase pathway in prostate cancer, gastric cancer and melanoma. *Nat Med* 2010; 16(7):793.

121. Leary RJ, Kinde I, Diehl F, et al. Development of personalized tumor biomarkers using massively parallel sequencing. *Sci Transl Med* 2010;2(20):20ra14.

122. Stephens PJ, McBride DJ, Lin ML, et al. Complex landscapes of somatic rearrangement in human breast cancer genomes. *Nature* 2009;462(7276): 1005.

123. Feng H, Shuda M, Chang Y, et al. Clonal integration of a polyomavirus in human Merkel cell carcinoma. *Science* 2008;319(5866):1096.

127. Kaminker JS, Zhang Y, Waugh A, et al. Distinguishing cancer-associated missense mutations from common polymorphisms. *Cancer Res* 2007;67(2):465.

128. Futreal PA. Backseat drivers take the wheel. *Cancer Cell* 2007;12(6):493.

129. Greenman C, Wooster R, Futreal PA, et al. Statistical analysis of pathogenicity of somatic mutations in cancer. *Genetics* 2006;173(4):2187.

134. The Cancer Genome Atlas Research Network. Comprehensive genomic characterization defines human glioblastoma genes and core pathways. *Nature* 2008; 455(7216):1061.

135. Hudson TJ, Anderson W, Artez A, et al. International network of cancer genome projects. *Nature* 2010; 464 (7291):993.

136. Bignell GR, Greenman CD, Davies H, et al. Signatures of mutation and selection in the cancer genome. *Nature* 2010;463(7283):893.

137. Dalgliesh GL, Furge K, Greenman C, et al. Systematic sequencing of renal carcinoma reveals inactivation of histone modifying genes. *Nature* 2010;463(7279): 360.

142. Benvenuti S, Frattini M, Arena S, et al. PIK3CA cancer mutations display gender and tissue specificity patterns. *Hum Mutat* 2008;29(2):284.

144. Bleeker FE, Bardelli A. Genomic landscapes of cancers: prospects for targeted therapies. *Pharmacogenomics* 2007;8(12):1629.

145. Paez JG, Janne PA, Lee JC, et al. EGFR mutations in lung cancer: correlation with clinical response to gefitinib therapy. *Science* 2004;304(5676):1497.

146. Ciardiello F, Tortora G. EGFR antagonists in cancer treatment. *N Engl J Med* 2008;358(11):1160.

149. Gerber DE, Minna JD. ALK inhibition for non-small cell lung cancer: from discovery to therapy in record time. *Cancer Cell* 2010;18(6):548.

152. Bardelli A, Siena S. Molecular mechanisms of resistance to cetuximab and panitumumab in colorectal cancer. *J Clin Oncol* 2010;28(7):1254.

153. Siena S, Sartore-Bianchi A, Di Nicolantonio F, et al. Biomarkers predicting clinical outcome of epidermal growth factor receptor-targeted therapy in metastatic colorectal cancer. *J Natl Cancer Inst* 2009;101(19):1308.
158. Gorre ME, Mohammed M, Ellwood K, et al. Clinical resistance to STI-571 cancer therapy caused by BCR-ABL gene mutation or amplification. *Science* 2001; 293(5531): 876.
169. Flaherty KT, Puzanov I, Kim KB, et al. Inhibition of mutated, activated BRAF in metastatic melanoma. *N Engl J Med* 2010;363(9):809.
173. Druker BJ, Guilhot F, O'Brien SG, et al. Five-year follow-up of patients receiving imatinib for chronic myeloid leukemia. *N Engl J Med* 2006;355(23):2408.

CHAPTER 2 MECHANISMS OF GENOMIC INSTABILITY

DAVID J. GORDON, DAVID A. BARBIE, ALAN D. D'ANDREA, AND DAVID PELLMAN

Cancer arises from a series of genetic alterations that promote resistance to apoptosis, self-sufficiency in growth, cellular immortalization and escape from cell-cycle exit. The acquisition of these properties ultimately facilitates angiogenesis, invasion, and metastasis.[1] It has been recognized for more than a century that genetic instability might represent an important pathway for the development of these disease characteristics. Von Hansemann[2] identified abnormal mitotic figures in cancers, leading Boveri[3] to propose that genetic instability, manifest in his experiments as whole-chromosome aneuploidy, could have a causal role in tumor development. The recognition that mutation of genes involved in monitoring genomic integrity underlies inherited cancer syndromes such as hereditary nonpolyposis colon cancer (HNPCC) and familial *BRCA*-mutant breast cancer provides clear evidence that genomic instability due to a so-called mutator phenotype can be the starting point for tumor development.[4,5]

However, many important questions remain. Does genomic instability play a central role in oncogenesis in common sporadic tumors? When during tumorigenesis does genetic instability develop, and what are the dominant mechanisms in specific cancer types? Why do inherited mutations in caretaker genes such as *BRCA1* and *BRCA2* lead to breast and ovarian cancer when their repair function is presumed to be ubiquitous? What is the relative contribution of telomere shortening to the development of genomic instability? Finally, what is the specific role of aneuploidy in cancer development, and what are the defects that promote chromosomal instability?

This chapter will outline the basic mechanisms involved in the maintenance of genomic integrity and will address these questions. One theme that has emerged from recent work in this area is that the development of genomic instability during cancer progression involves evolutionary tradeoffs.[6–8] Loss of genetic stability is expected to increase the rate of growth-promoting or survival-promoting mutations that could drive tumor growth. However, genomic instability will also increase the rate of deleterious mutations that could kill cells before they develop into tumors. Understanding how these factors balance out will ultimately be the key to understanding tumor development via genome destabilization. Perhaps most importantly, understanding this balance may also have implications for cancer therapeutics. If deleterious, genome-destabilizing mutations are found in the population of developing cancer cells, these defects may provide an "Achilles heel" for therapeutic attack.

BASIC DEFENSES AGAINST GENOMIC INSTABILITY

The roughly 10^{14} cells in the human body are continually exposed to sources of genomic injury, both spontaneous injury accompanying normal cell division and metabolism and external sources of damage. In addition to the oxidative stresses that are a by-product of cellular metabolism, cell populations that undergo constant turnover are subject to errors that may arise during the processes of DNA replication, mitosis, and telomere maintenance. Cells are also exposed to a variety of exogenous genotoxic insults. Examples include ultraviolet and gamma irradiation and certain chemicals (as detailed in other chapters). As a result, mechanisms have evolved at a number of different levels to guard against genomic instability and prevent the propagation of cancer-promoting and/or deleterious mutations.

At an organismal level, tissues are designed to prevent the accumulation of cells with sustained disruption of genomic integrity.[4] For example, those cell types in constant contact with the outside world, including the skin, gastrointestinal tract, and bronchial epithelium, undergo continuous self-renewal, with shedding of those differentiated cells that are exposed most directly to a potentially deleterious environment. In addition to being shielded from this stress, the stem cell compartment undergoes cell division fairly infrequently, with the bulk of exponential growth occurring in transit-amplifying cells that are ultimately discarded at the surface. Thus, in tissues such as the colon, stem cells are normally protected within the crypts, and those cells that proliferate and migrate toward the lumen are ultimately eliminated. Nevertheless, this process is imperfect and subject to persistence of dysplastic clones if a cell sustains a mutation that affords a proliferative advantage.

Many cells also possess physiologic characteristics that can shield them from genotoxic injury.[4,9] For example, melanin in the skin absorbs ultraviolet radiation, while antioxidants and enzymes such as catalase and superoxide dismutase reduce concentrations of reactive oxygen species generated as a result of cell metabolism. In addition, cytochrome P-450 enzymes detoxify a variety of chemicals, and glutathione-S-transferases (GSTs) conjugate glutathione with electrophilic compounds, neutralizing their mutagenic potential. Defective GST function has been observed in lung, breast, and prostate cancer and has been shown to predispose patients to myelodysplastic syndrome. Conversely, drugs that inhibit GST function are being tested in combination with chemotherapy in an attempt to enhance toxicity to cancer cells.

BARRIERS TO GENOMIC INSTABILITY

Cell Cycle Checkpoints

Coordinated progression through the cell cycle is crucial for the maintenance of genome stability.[4,10,11] This is particularly the case for the main tasks of the cell cycle—DNA replication and mitosis. Either incomplete DNA replication or overreplication of DNA would generate lesions that could lead to chromosome breaks and rearrangements. Mitotic errors produce chromosome mis-segregation and whole-chromosome aneuploidy. These types of errors do not occur in isolation; a defect in one process can lead to a cascade of downstream events. Chromosome breaks can lead to translocations, chromosomes with two centromeres (dicentric chromosomes), anaphase bridges, and chromosome mis-segregation. Likewise, mitotic errors leading to aneuploidy will generate gene expression imbalances that could, in principle, compromise DNA replication, telomere maintenance, or DNA repair. Both DNA replication/repair and mitotic errors can cause cytokinesis to fail, resulting in tetraploid cells that contain extra centrosomes and are themselves genetically unstable. Although an extensive review of the cell cycle is beyond the scope of this chapter, selected features of the normal cell cycle that are crucial for preventing genome instability and cancer are described here. In particular, the following sections will focus on the restriction point, the DNA damage checkpoint, and the spindle assembly checkpoint. More extensive summaries of the eucaryotic cell cycle can be found in other chapters and in recent reviews.

Restriction Point

The decision to commit to cell division is controlled by a complex signaling system, the retinoblastoma protein (RB) pathway, that is the major target of human cancer-causing mutations.[11,12] RB represses the transcription of genes involved in cell cycle progression by binding to the E2F family of transcription factors and altering the expression of E2F target genes, blocking E2F-mediated transactivation and recruiting active repressor complexes to promoters.[13,14] E2F target genes include components of the nucleotide synthesis and DNA replication machinery that are essential for S phase entry and transit. In response to mitogenic signals during G1 phase of the cell cycle, RB is phosphorylated and inactivated by cyclin D/CDK (cyclin-dependent kinase) 4/6 complexes, followed by cyclin E/CDK2 and cyclinA/CDK2 complexes, resulting in E2F-target gene expression and S phase transit. Cyclin E/CDK2 regulates a number of other processes involved in the duplication of chromosomes, including the activation of histone gene transcription, as well as promoting the initiation of DNA replication and centrosome duplication.[15,16] Deletion of cyclin E in mice results in defective endoreduplication, while constitutive overexpression of cyclin E has been linked to the generation of polyploidy and chromosomal instability. Thus, the RB pathway integrates intrinsic and external growth signals and is a key mediator of cyclin/CDK complexes that drive cell cycle progression.

CDK inhibitors and phosphatases provide other important mechanisms for counteracting the activity of CDKs and restricting cell cycle progression.[4,11,16] CDK inhibitors fall into two general categories, including specific *in*hibitors of CD*K*4 such as p16[INK4A], and those that target CDK activity more broadly such as p21 or p27. CDK2 is also targeted by inhibitory phosphorylation at its active site by the Wee1 family of protein kinases. Activation of cyclin E(A)/CDK2 during the normal G1/S phase transition thus requires the activity of the CDC25A phosphatase. Phosphorylation of CDC25A itself leads to its subsequent ubiquitin-mediated proteasomal degradation and inhibition of S phase progression. Thus, expression of CDK inhibitors and down-regulation of CDC25A phosphatase activity are means by which checkpoint signals are able to mediate downstream cell cycle arrest. Furthermore, PP2A, a protein phosphatase that is also critical to the process of oncogenic transformation, has been shown to regulate an S phase checkpoint by dephosphorylating pRB and licensing recruitment of pRB to chromatin to suppress DNA replication.[17]

Heralded as the guardian of the genome, *p53* integrates the response to DNA damage, replication stress, hypoxia, telomere dysfunction, and activated oncogenes and mediates downstream checkpoint activation.[4,18–20] Inherited mutations in p53 or its direct upstream activator CHK2 result in the Li Fraumeni cancer predisposition syndrome, and sporadic inactivation of p53 is one of the most frequent events observed in tumor development. Tumors lacking p53 exhibit widespread genomic instability resulting from an inability to arrest the cell cycle or trigger apoptosis in the setting of DNA damage and the cellular stresses previously described. In normal cells, p53 is maintained at low levels in the cytoplasm because of ubiquitination by MDM2 and proteasomal degradation. In response to checkpoint activation and phosphorylation, p53 increases in abundance and translocates to the nucleus, where it activates a transcriptional program that promotes cell cycle arrest, senescence, or apoptosis, depending on the cell type and conditions. The CDK inhibitor p21 is a key transcriptional target of p53 that mediates checkpoint arrest while repair is attempted. In response to a variety of signals p53 can trigger an apoptotic program, in part via transcriptional activation of proapoptotic targets such as NOXA and BAX.[21]

DNA Damage Checkpoints

Activation of cell cycle checkpoints occurs as part of a larger DNA damage response pathway.[22,23] There are three major DNA damage checkpoints, with two of the checkpoints occurring at the boundaries between G1/S and G2/M. The third checkpoint, however, occurs intra-S phase. In addition to promoting cell cycle arrest through the mechanisms described earlier, these pathways coordinate recruitment of repair proteins to the sites of DNA damage, modulation of transcription, activation of subsequent repair, and apoptosis. The signaling network that controls this response is initiated by the key DNA damage sensors, the ataxia-telangiectasia mutated (ATM) and AT and Rad3-related (ATR) protein kinases.[10,11,24,25] ATM is principally activated in response to double-strand breaks, while ATR is activated by replication fork collapse and by bulky DNA lesions. As will be described in more detail later, both proteins phosphorylate multiple targets in coordinating the subsequent DNA damage response. Key signal transducers in this process include CHK2 (activated by ATM) and CHK1 (activated by ATR). p53 is a major substrate for ATM/CHK2 and ATR/CHK1 phosphorylation, and subsequent activation of p53 represents a principal mechanism by which cell cycle checkpoints are activated in response to DNA damage. Replication stress and hypoxia also appear to activate p53 through ATR signaling, while telomere dysfunction contributes to p53 activation through ATM (Fig. 2.1).[18] In addition, a variety of stress responses have been shown to activate p38MAPK, which can promote checkpoint activation through both p53-dependent and -independent pathways.[26,27] CHK2 activation also leads to phosphorylation and degradation of the phosphatase

CDC25A, resulting in activation of an S phase checkpoint.[28]

Spindle Assembly Checkpoint

Errors that occur during mitosis are similarly monitored by a spindle checkpoint, which prevents progression into anaphase when chromosomes are improperly attached to the mitotic spindle.[29] Key sensors of this response include the spindle checkpoint proteins, which assemble onto unattached kinetochores and generate a "wait anaphase" signal that prevents activation of anaphase effector proteins. This pathway is outlined in further detail later.

Cellular Senescence and Crisis

Cellular senescence is another mechanism that limits the progressive accumulation of cells with impaired genomic integrity and oncogenic potential.[4,30–32] Originally described as an irreversible state of cell cycle exit in response to exhausted replicative potential of cultured cells, cellular senescence also occurs as a response to oncogene activation, oxidative stress, suboptimal culture conditions, and chemotherapy. The RB and p53 pathways have been shown to mediate the arrest by replicative senescence, whereby progressive telomere attrition elicits a DNA damage response similar to that induced by other genotoxic stresses (Fig. 2.1). In the setting of RB and p53 pathway inactivation, cells can bypass replicative senescence, but progressive telomere shortening results in the accumulation of massive genetic instability and a state of "crisis." Most cells in crisis will die, but rare malignant clones can emerge. In humans, activation of the enzyme telomerase and subsequent maintenance of telomere length allows such cells to bypass crisis, resulting in cellular immortalization. By contrast, in mice, in which telomeres start out long and seldom shorten to a critical length, a similar but less well understood crisis event occurs that is, at least in part, related to differential sensitivity of mouse cells to oxidative damage in culture.

Senescence induced by oncogene activation, also known as oncogene-induced senescence, results from expression of p16[INK4A] and p14[ARF] (note that p14[ARF] in humans is p19[ARF] in the mouse), which exists in an alternative reading frame within the p16[INK4A] locus.[33,34] p14[ARF] inhibits MDM2 function, in part by sequestering it in the nucleolus, resulting in the accumulation and activation of p53. p16[INK4A] expression is associated with both oncogene activation and genotoxic stress, promoting activation of RB and, in conjunction with HMGA chromatin proteins, the formation of stable heterochromatic foci that envelop and silence E2F target genes.[35] Cellular senescence induced by this latter program is

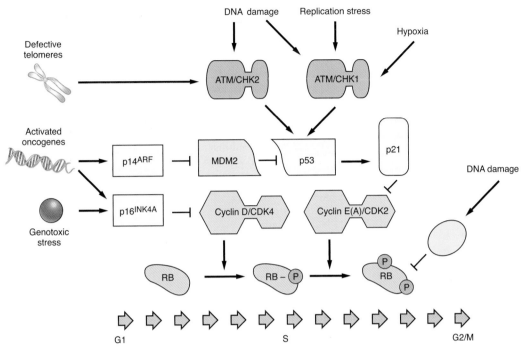

FIGURE 2.1 G1 pathways that can trigger cell cycle arrest, senescence, or apoptosis. A variety of threats to genomic integrity lead to activation of pathways that result in cell cycle arrest. Signaling via ATM/CHK2 and ATR/CHK1 leads to p53 activation, among other effects. One of the principle downstream effects of p53 is activation of p21 expression, with resultant cyclin E(A)/CDK2 inhibition and cell cycle arrest. Senescence, which results in a more sustained cell cycle exit, also involves the up-regulation of p14[ARF] and p16[INK4A]. Both proteins ultimately lead to retinoblastoma protein (RB) activation and G1 arrest via cyclin/CDK inhibition. In response to DNA damage during S phase, activation of PP2A can lead to dephosphorylation of RB and inhibition of DNA synthesis.

refractory to RB and p53 inactivation, although it can be bypassed by inactivation of p16[INK4A] and HMGA proteins. Oncogene-induced senescence is also triggered by DNA replication stress, including prematurely terminated DNA replication forks, DNA double-strand breaks, and DNA hyperreplication.[36,37] In a mouse model, inhibiting the DNA double-strand break response kinase ATM suppressed the induction of senescence and led to increased tumor size and invasiveness.

Oncogene-induced senescence has been shown to occur *in vivo*, limiting tumor progression in models of lung and prostate cancer, melanoma, and lymphoma.[33] Whereas inactivation of the PTEN tumor suppressor and resultant activation of the AKT signaling pathway in prostate epithelial cells appears to promote senescence through p14[ARF], inappropriate activation of RAS signaling in other tissues results in p16[INK4A]-mediated senescence. Nonetheless, targeted activation of oncogenic *K-RAS* alleles in somatic tissues in mice predisposes to a wide variety of tumor types, including early-onset lung cancer, suggesting that this barrier may be readily overcome or that the consequence of RAS expression may vary depending on the context.[38,39] Moreover, expression of endogenous levels of oncogenic K-RAS can pro-

mote proliferation, and it has been demonstrated that oncogene-induced senescence due to RAS activation can be dose-dependent.[40–42]

RAS-induced senescence in lymphocytes depends on heterochromatin formation via the Suv39h1 histone methyltransferase, the disruption of which facilitates lymphoma development in response to RAS activation.[33] Furthermore, disruption of Suv39h1 by itself has been shown to disrupt heterochromatin formation and to promote genetic instability, contributing to lymphomagenesis.[43] This may occur at least in part through cell division failure and the generation of unstable tetraploid cells (see later discussion). These findings confirm the *in vitro* observations that changes in chromatin structure contribute to cell cycle exit by senescence. In addition, they suggest that emerging epigenetic therapies such as histone deacetylase inhibitors and DNA methyltransferase inhibitors that interfere with chromatin silencing may disrupt this senescence barrier, a potential caveat to their use.

MUTATIONS IN CANCER

Despite multiple levels of protection against the development of genomic instability, with age, cells

TABLE 2.1

INHERITED GENOME MAINTENANCE DEFECTS WITH CANCER PREDISPOSITION

Maintenance Mechanism	Syndrome	Gene Defect
Checkpoint response	Li Fraumeni Familial breast cancer	p53, CHK2
	Retinoblastoma	BRCA1, CHK2
	Familial melanoma	RB
		p16^{INK4A}
Mismatch repair	HNPCC/Lynch syndrome	MLH1, MSH2, PMS2, MSH6
Nucleotide excision repair	Xeroderma pigmentosa	XP genes
DSB response/repair	Ataxia telangiectasia	ATM
	AT-like disorder	MRE11
	Nijmegen breakage	NBS1
	Fanconia anemia	Fanc genes
	Familial breast cancer	BRCA1, BRCA2 CHK2, PALB2
	SCID, rare lymphoma	Artemis
	SCID, rare leukemia	Ligase IV
Helicase activity	Bloom	BLM
	Werner	WRN
	Rothmund Thomson	RECQ4
Mitotic checkpoint	Mosaic variegated aneuploidy	BUB1B

HNPCC, hereditary nonpolyposis colorectal cancer; DSB, double-strand break; AT, ataxia telangiectasia; SCID, severe combined immunodeficiency.

can develop genetic alterations that escape detection.[4] One path to genetic instability is inactivation of checkpoint proteins such as those previously described. The subsequent deregulation of the cell cycle and impairment of the response to genomic injury allows the progressive accumulation of lesions that can drive oncogenesis. Additionally, mutations can also occur in genes encoding the proteins that repair DNA damage and protect against the development of chromosome abnormalities. In this setting, accelerated mutation rates and chromosomal instability destabilize the genome and facilitate progression through the steps of oncogenic transformation. The basic types of genetic alterations observed in tumors, and the mechanisms by which genome destabilization can occur, are outlined in the next sections. Cancer predisposition syndromes that result from inherited defects in genome maintenance are highlighted in Table 2.1.

Point Mutations

Changes in the nucleotide sequence can arise from spontaneous mutation, exposure to endogenous or exogenous mutagens, or defects in the ability to detect and/or repair simple sequence errors.[4,21] The spontaneous mutation rate per nucleotide per cell division has been estimated to be on the order of 10^{-9} in somatic cells and 10^{-11} in stem cells.[44] Despite the remarkable fidelity of DNA polymerase and its inherent proofreading capacity, a variety of endogenous and exogenous chemical and radiation exposures can introduce additional DNA lesions, requiring the presence of multiple repair pathways for further protection of genomic integrity. Mutations arise when such errors are not detected and repaired by this machinery, which can occur when repair pathways are overwhelmed or defective. As a result, point mutations are frequently detected via sequencing of both oncogenes and tumor suppressor genes in multiple cancers. Notable examples include activating mutations in oncogenic kinases such as K-RAS in colorectal, pancreatic, and lung cancer, B-RAF in melanoma, and JAK2 in myeloproliferative disorders. In some instances, specific mutations have been linked to epidemiologic features such as tobacco exposure, with oncogenic K-RAS mutations in non–small cell lung cancer (NSCLC) occurring more frequently in smokers and epidermal growth factor receptor (EGFR) mutations in nonsmokers.[45]

Next-generation sequencing technology has ushered in a new era in cancer genomics.[46,47] Massively parallel DNA sequencing platforms now allow for the routine sequencing of billions of bases of DNA per week and the identification of point mutations, insertions and deletions, copy number changes, and genomic rearrangements on a genome-wide basis. Large-scale sequencing of coding sequences from a panel of colorectal and breast tumors, for example, revealed that these cancers harbor approximately 100 mutant genes, with computational methods predicting that 14 to 20 of these mutations will be bona fide tumor suppressor genes or oncogenes.[48] In this unbiased effort, both known and unknown mutations were identified, with each tumor possessing a relatively unique cancer gene mutational signature. In another study, sequencing of coding regions of protein kinases in a large number of cancers identified "driver" mutations in approximately 120 genes across all samples.[49] Although these studies identified a greater number of mutational events associated with oncogenesis than previously thought (the "state" of genome integrity), they do not necessarily imply a high "rate" of mutation, which remains low in most mature tumors.[21]

In two early studies, targeted gene resequencing was also applied to lung adenocarcinoma and glioblastoma multiforme (GBM) tumor samples.[50,51] Both studies integrated the somatic mutation data with other genome-wide characterizations and clinical data. In the lung adenocarcinoma samples, for example, the sequencing data were used to identify multiple pathways, including MAPK signaling, p53 signaling, and the mTOR pathway, that are targeted by a combination of point mutations, copy number amplifications and deletions, and loss of heterozygosity (LOH). In a different study of GBM tumor samples, the sequencing of approximately 20,000 protein coding genes led to the discovery of a variety of genes that were not known to be altered in GBM, including the enzyme isocitrate dehydrogenase (*IDH1*).[52] The cancer-associated *IDH1* mutations result in the novel ability of the enzyme to catalyze the NADPH-dependent reduction of alpha-ketoglutarate to R(-)-2-hydroxyglutarate (2HG), which has been shown to lead to an elevated risk of malignant brain tumors.[53] Subsequently, mutations in *IDH1* have also been identified in acute myeloid leukemia (AML) genomes.[54,55]

More recently, there has been a rapid progression from targeted gene sequencing to targeted whole-genome and whole-transcriptome sequencing. The first sequencing of a whole cancer genome was reported for AML.[56] Acquired mutations in coding sequences of annotated genes were identified in ten genes in the AML genome by comparing the genomic DNA of leukemia cells with normal skin cells obtained from a patient with FAB M1 AML. Two of the identified mutations were in genes previously described to have a role in leukemogenesis, *FLT3* and *NPM1*. The other eight mutations, however, were in genes that were not previously implicated in the pathogenesis of AML. Four of the affected genes (*PTPRT*, *CDH24*, *PCLKC*, and *SLC15A1*), though, are in gene families that are strongly implicated in cancer pathogenesis. Intriguingly, the remaining genes (*KNDC1*, *GPR123*, *EBI2*, and *GRINL1B*) are involved in metabolic pathways.

The genomes of a small cell lung cancer, melanoma, and breast tumor have also been described.[57–59] Interestingly, the mutations in both the lung cancer and melanoma genomes were not distributed evenly throughout the genome—many were present outside the gene-coding regions, suggesting that cells had repaired damaged DNA in those key regions. Sequencing of the melanoma genome, for example, revealed multiple levels of selective DNA repair, including the preferential targeting of repair to transcribed regions compared with nontranscribed regions, to exons compared with introns, to transcribed DNA strands compared with nontranscribed strands, and to the 5' end of genes compared with the 3' end.

Next-generation sequencing has also been applied to RNA ("RNA-Seq") extracted from tumor cells for complete transcriptome characterization.[60,61] This approach is more sensitive than microarrays and also provides data that can be used to evaluate for allele-specific expression, structural and copy-number alterations, alternative splice isoforms, fusion transcripts, and single nucleotide mutations.[60] RNA-Seq, for example, was applied to four granulosa-cell tumors and identified missense point mutations in the *FOXL2* gene, which encodes a transcription factor known to be crucial in granulosa cell development.[62] In a different study, RNA-Seq was used to identify both known and novel fusion transcripts in prostate cancer samples.[63] RNA-Seq has also been used to study the role of microRNAs in the regulation of gene expression in both normal and cancerous cells.

The number of sequenced cancer genomes is likely to expand substantially in coming years. The Cancer Genome Atlas Program of the U.S. National Cancer Institute, for example, initially focused its large-scale genomic analysis on only three tumor types, GBM, ovarian serous cystadenocarcinoma, and lung squamous carcinoma. The scope of the Cancer Genome Atlas Research Network, however, has now expanded to include more than 20 tumor types and thousands of samples. The clinical and translational implications of routine cancer genome sequencing are profound and include the identification of new drug targets, as well as the generation of new insights into the genetic patterns of disease phenotype, prognosis, and therapeutic response. One shortcoming of direct sequencing, though, is its failure to detect epigenetic changes, such as DNA methylation, which may alter gene expression indirectly.

Although the role of 2HG in cancer development remains unclear, the identification of this unexpected class of mutations validates the high-throughput cancer genome sequencing approach. Also, because the mutations in *IDH1* result in a gain of function, there is much excitement about

GENERAL PRINCIPLES

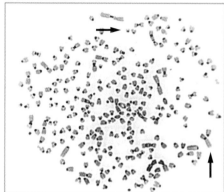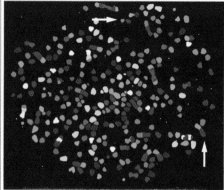

FIGURE 2.2 Common cytogenetic abnormalities. Metaphase spread derived from a mouse tumor model (combined telomerase and p53 deficiency). Individual chromosomes are highlighted by spectral karyotyping (SKY) using fluorescent chromosome probes (**right panel**). Normal mouse cells contain a diploid complement of 40 chromosomes. In this sample, more than 260 chromosomes are observed, with multiple dicentric chromosomes and nonreciprocal translocations.

developing small molecule inhibitors of mutant *IDH1*. Although major clinical impact of large-scale sequencing projects is yet to be realized, the discovery of *IDH1* illustrates the potential of this approach.

Translocations

Unlike point mutations, small insertions, or deletions of nucleotides, larger chromosomal changes such as translocations, amplifications, and deletions may be observed using cytogenetic analysis[4,21] (Fig. 2.2). Chromosome translocation involves juxtaposition of two different chromosome segments, resulting in fusion of two different genes or placement of a gene next to an inappropriate regulatory element. Examples include t(9;22) in chronic myelogenous leukemia, resulting in expression of the growth promoting *BCR-ABL* gene product, and t(14;18) in follicular lymphoma, resulting in overexpression of the antiapoptotic protein BCL2 as a result of its fusion with the immunoglobulin heavy chain promoter. Recent work has also identified a translocation between the immunoglobulin heavy chain and the cytokine receptor CRLF2 in a subset of precursor B-cell acute lymphoblastic leukemia associated with a poor outcome and activating *JAK* mutations.[64,65]

One exciting recent development is that translocations not only create chimeric genes or alter promoter sequences, but can also affect the expression of microRNAs.[66,67] MicroRNAs are short regulatory RNAs that control mRNA stability and/or translation, and changes in microRNA expression have been linked to prognostic factors and progression in diseases such as chronic lymphocytic leukemia.[68]

Although translocations and gene fusions are a hallmark of cancer, the mechanisms underlying their genesis are unclear. Recent work, however, has begun to elucidate the mechanisms of some tissue-specific translocations, such as *TMPRSS2* to *ERG* and *ETV1* in prostate cancer.[69,70] A clever bioinformatics approach, termed *cancer outlier profile analysis*, was used to first identify this recurrent translocation in prostate cancer.[71] This approach was used to successfully identify recurrent gene fusions of *TMPRSS2* to *ERG* or *ETV1* in prostate cancer. Further mechanistic work has shown that this translocation requires two roles of the androgen receptor.[69] First, ligand-dependent binding of the androgen receptor to intronic binding sites near the tumor translocation sites creates specific intra- and interchromosomal interactions that result in the spatial proximity of tumor translocation partners. Second, the intron-bound androgen receptor alters local chromatin architecture and recruits the ligand and genotoxic stress-induced enzymes, including the activation-induced cytidine deaminase and LINE-1 repeat-encoded ORF2 endonuclease, to these regions, which results in the generation of DNA double-stranded breaks (DSB). The DSB are subsequently ligated by the nonhomologous end-joining (NHEJ) machinery to create translocations. Further elucidation of the mechanisms leading to gene- and tissue-specific translocations will advance the understanding of basic mechanisms of cancer, as well as possibly facilitating the development of new therapeutic strategies.

Amplifications and Deletions

Amplifications can be detected cytogenetically as double-minute chromosomes or regions of excess signal intensity using fluorescence *in situ* hybridization. Such "amplicons" may range in size from 0.5 to 10 megabases of DNA, resulting in multiple copies of both oncogenes and their neighboring sequences. Conversely, deletions result in loss of chromosomal regions, and can involve small interstitial segments or entire chromosome arms. Genetic alteration of tumor suppressor genes frequently involves mutation in one allele and deletion of the second allele as part of a larger chromosomal segment, resulting in regions of uniform sequence with LOH.

A recent study reported the high-resolution analysis of somatic copy-number alterations (SCNAs) from 3,131 cancer specimens belonging to 26 histologic types.[72] The most prevalent SCNAs were either very short (focal) or almost the length of a chromosome arm or whole chromosome (arm level). The focal SCNAs occurred at a frequency inversely related to their lengths, with a median length of 1.8 megabases. Arm-level SCNAs occurred approximately 30 times more frequently than expected by the inverse-length distribution associated with focal SCNAs. This observation was seen across all cancer types and applied to both copy gains and losses. The study also identified 158 regions of focal SCNAs that were altered at significant frequency across several cancer types, of which 122 could not be explained by the presence of an oncogene located within the region. Several gene families were enriched among the regions of focal SCNA, including the *BCL2* family of apoptosis regulators and the *NF-kB* pathway. Interestingly, the finding that most of the SCNAs were found in multiple cancer types suggests that the diversity across cancer genomes may reflect the combinations of a limited number of functionally relevant events.

Whole-Chromosome Loss/Gain

Nearly all solid tumor types exhibit whole-chromosome loss or gain, resulting in alterations in chromosome number or aneuploidy.[21,73] As will be described later, such defects are generally the result of chromosomal mis-segregation during mitosis. Glioblastomas, for example, frequently exhibit loss of chromosome 10, inactivating the tumor suppressor *PTEN*, while melanomas often show gain of chromosome 7, from which *B-RAF* is expressed. Monosomy 7 and trisomy 8 are associated with myelodysplasia and AML. Whole-chromosome loss may be underestimated by karyotypic analysis, as loss of one parental chromosome may be accompanied by duplication of the other parental chromosome, resulting in an abnormal "allelotype" with accompanying LOH, or copy neutral loss of heterozygosity (CN-LOH).[74]

CN-LOH, also referred to as uniparental disomy, is common in cancer and has been described in AML, breast cancer, multiple myeloma, basal cell carcinoma, childhood acute lymphoblastic leukemia, chronic lymphocytic lymphoma, myelodysplastic syndrome, and glioblastoma.[75] Furthermore, CN-LOH has been shown to have prognostic significance in a number of these cancer types, including primary and secondary AML.[76] The specific role of CN-LOH in tumorigenesis remains undefined, but possible mechanisms include the duplication of oncogenes, loss of tumor suppressors, or acquisition of improper epigenetic patterns.[77] In mice, it has been demonstrated that Bub1 insufficiency can drive tumor formation through tumor suppressor gene *LOH*.[78] Specifically, Bub1 insufficiency predisposed $p53^{+/-}$ mice to thymic lymphomas and $Apc^{Min/+}$ mice to colonic tumors. These tumors demonstrated CN-LOH and lacked the nonmutated tumor suppressor allele, but had gained a copy of the mutant allele.

Epigenetics

Significant evidence now indicates that epigenetic modifications, or heritable changes in gene expression that are not caused by changes in DNA sequence, are critical factors in the pathogenesis of cancer.[79] Although beyond the scope of this chapter, epigenetic mechanisms controlling the transcription of genes involved in cell differentiation, proliferation, and survival are often targets for deregulation in the development of cancer. These epigenetic alterations include DNA methylation, covalent modifications of histones, and noncovalent changes in nucleosome position. The role of epigenetic modifications in cancer pathogenesis is illustrated by the tumor suppressor *SNF5*, which regulates the epigenome as a member of the SWI/SNF chromatin remodeling complex.[80] Biallelic inactivation of *SNF5* is found in the majority of malignant rhabdoid tumors. Most human *SNF5*-deficient cancers are diploid, lack genomic amplifications/deletions, and are genomically stable.[81] Furthermore, the epigenetically based changes in transcription that occur following loss of *SNF5* correlate with the tumor phenotype.

Recent work with an NSCLC cell line, PC9, has also identified a novel role for epigenetics in acquired drug resistance.[82] Treatment of PC9 cells, which have an activating mutation in the EGFR, with the drug erlotinib results in the death of nearly all of the parental cells. A small percentage of the PC9 cells, however, demonstrate significantly reduced drug sensitivity and remain viable through activation of IGF-1 receptor signaling and an altered chromatin state that requires the histone demethylase RBP2. This drug-tolerant phenotype is transiently acquired at low frequency by individual cells within the population. The drug-tolerant subpopulation can be selectively ablated by treatment with IGF-1 receptor inhibitors or chromatin-modifying agents, such as HDAC inhibitors. There has been much discussion and controversy about the existence of drug-resistant cancer stem cells; the epigenetic effects described in this work provide a potential mechanism for the generation of some "cancer stem cells." Furthermore, this research suggests that the potentially reversible nature of epigenetic changes, unlike genetic mutations, may provide a unique therapeutic avenue in the treatment of cancer.

MECHANISMS OF GENOME DESTABILIZATION IN HUMAN TUMORS

Microsatellite Instability

One of the earliest insights into the contribution of genome destabilization to carcinogenesis came from the study of the familial cancer syndrome HNPCC.[4,11,83] It had been recognized that a subset of sporadic colon cancers and a majority of cancers derived from patients with HNPCC exhibited frequent mutations, particularly in regions of simple repeat sequences known as microsatellites. This type of genetic instability, termed *microsatellite instability* (MIN), had been described in bacteria and yeast mutants defective in mismatch repair. Linkage analysis in kindreds with HNPCC revealed germ line mutations in *hMSH2* and *hMLH1*, which are human homologues of the *mutL* and *mutS* mismatch repair genes in *Escherichia coli*. It is now known that mutations in other components of the human mismatch repair process, *hPMS2*, and *hMSH6*, are also observed in families with HNPCC.

Mismatch repair corrects mispaired bases that can result from errors during DNA replication, as well as mismatched bases occurring in recombination intermediates or occurring as a result of some types of chemical damage to DNA.[84] Mismatched bases are recognized by a complex of MSH2 and MSH6, recruiting MLH1 and PMS2 to the site to initiate the subsequent steps of repair, including excision, DNA synthesis, and ligation (Fig. 2.3). Larger insertion/deletion mispairs due to slippage of the replication machinery in repetitive sequences or recombination errors form a loop structure that is alternatively recognized by a complex of MSH2 and MSH3, with recruitment of an MLH1/MLH3 complex promoting subsequent repair. Cancer cells that exhibit MIN from defects in these components have a nucleotide mutation rate that has been estimated at two to three orders greater than that of normal cells. MLH1 and MSH2 have also been shown to have functions outside mismatch repair, as defects in these proteins have been associated with an impaired G2/M cell cycle checkpoint in response to alkylating agents as well as abnormalities in meiotic recombination in mouse knockout models.[9]

HNPCC is associated with a 60% to 80% lifetime risk of developing colorectal cancer and is responsible for 2% to 5% of all cases of colorectal cancer.[85] Nearly 85% of HNPCC patients have mutations in *MLH1* or *MSH2*, with median age at colon cancer diagnosis being significantly lower in *MLH1* mutation carriers and in males, and with more frequent extracolonic tumors observed in *MSH2* carriers. The MIN phenotype is also observed in 15% of sporadic colon cancers, often due to epigenetic silencing of mismatch

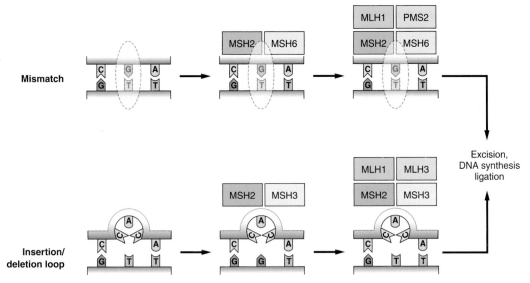

FIGURE 2.3 Mismatch repair pathways. Mispaired bases due to errors in DNA replication or other causes are recognized by the mismatch repair machinery. The initial step involves recognition of simple mismatches by MSH2 and MSH6 (**upper panel**), or recognition of insertion/deletion loops by MSH2 and MSH3 (**lower panel**). Subsequent steps involve recruitment of MLH1 and PMS2 to mismatch sites, or MLH1 and MLH3 to insertion/deletion loop sites. This is followed by excision of the respective lesions, DNA synthesis, and ligation to complete the repair.

repair genes such as *MLH1*. Colorectal cancers exhibiting MIN are typically diploid, in contrast to the remaining 85% of cases, which are associated with chromosomal instability (CIN).[86] Experimental evidence supports the idea that MIN occurs very early in sporadic colorectal cancer formation, prior to anaphase-promoting complex (APC) inactivation, increasing genomic instability and thus obviating the selection pressure to develop another mechanism of genomic instability, CIN. In both sporadic cases and HNPCC, MIN has been associated with more favorable prognosis, lack of *p53* mutation, and a potential resistance to 5-fluorouracil chemotherapy. These observations are in accordance with the hypothesis that the accelerated mutation rate facilitates cancer evolution, but at the same time compromises fitness of cells, presumably by the accumulation of deleterious mutations.

Nucleotide Excision Repair/Base Excision Repair Defects

Whereas the mismatch repair pathway functions primarily in the recognition of and repair of replication errors, the nucleotide excision repair (NER) and base excision repair (BER) pathways respond principally to lesions created by exogenous or endogenous DNA damaging agents.[4,9,84,87] It is becoming apparent that defects in components of these repair pathways have impacts on both cancer pathogenesis and the efficacy of cancer therapy.[88] Ultraviolet radiation or exogenous chemicals such as polycyclic aromatic hydrocarbons and platinum chemotherapeutic drugs can result in bulky, helix-distorting lesions that are recognized by the NER machinery. Components of the NER pathway were in part discovered by mutation in the genetic syndromes xeroderma pigmentosa (*XPA-XPG*) and Cockayne syndrome (*CSA* and *CSB*).[89] Mutation of *XP* genes can also be seen in the related disorder trichothiodystrophy. Whereas all three disorders exhibit dramatic sun sensitivity, only xeroderma pigmentosa is associated with a marked incidence of sun-induced skin cancer.[90] Deletion of *CSB* has been shown to impair tumor formation in cancer-prone mice, and it has been hypothesized that the lack of cancer in Cockayne syndrome may be related to a particular sensitivity of cells to apoptosis or impairment of transcription.[91]

Two separate NER pathways have been identified, one that involves scanning the entire genome for lesions (global genome NER) and another that detects lesions that interfere with elongating RNA polymerases (transcription coupled repair or TCR)[9,87] (Fig. 2.4). *XP* genes are involved in the recognition and repair of lesions in global genome NER, while *CS* genes play a specific role in transcription coupled repair. Subsequent stages of NER are similar and involve ERCC1, an endonuclease involved in excision of the lesion, followed by DNA replication to complete the repair process. Notably, mutant mice defective in NER also accumulate DNA damage, with a more pronounced cancer phenotype and evidence of premature aging. Furthermore, reduced expression of *ERCC1* in NSCLC has been associated with response to cisplatin-based adjuvant chemotherapy.[92] A subgroup analysis of the International Adjuvant Lung Cancer Trial (IALT) demonstrated that *ERCC1* deficiency was observed in tumor samples from 56% of patients and correlated with a significant improvement in survival following cisplatin-based chemotherapy, whereas no benefit was seen in tumors in which normal *ERCC1* expression was maintained. Thus, while reduced *ERCC1* expression may promote genetic instability and facilitate NSCLC development in a significant fraction of patients, the resulting cancers are "stuck" with the deleterious effects of *ERCC1* deficiency and become sensitive to certain therapies. Potentially, this provides a general model for targeted therapy based on fixation of mutations that compromise genomic integrity during tumorigenesis.

BER is primarily involved in the response to damage caused by small chemical alterations and x-rays, as well as spontaneous reactions such as base loss from hydrolysis of glycosyl DNA bonds, which has been estimated to occur on the order of 10^4 times per day per cell.[9,24] Damaged bases are removed by DNA glycosylases, and abasic sites are recognized by a complex that includes the APEX1 endonuclease, poly(ADP-ribose) polymerase (PARP), DNA polymerase and ligase, and XRCC1, a scaffolding protein that interacts with most of the core components (Fig. 2.4). Disruption of any of these genes in the BER pathway results in the cellular accumulation of oxidative DNA damage.

Despite being integrally important to the maintenance of genome stability, human disorders or inherited cancer susceptibility syndromes due to mutation of components of the BER machinery have yet to be described. This may be because of partial redundancy of DNA glycosylases, the fact that mutation of core BER components (in mice) results in embryonic lethality, or simply to the need for additional investigation. As described later, pharmacologic inhibition of PARP may selectively sensitize cancer cells with a pre-existing defect in another repair pathway to death by DNA damage.[93,94]

DNA Damage Response to Double-Strand Breaks

DNA DSBs represent a significant threat to genomic integrity.[4,9] They can occur during DNA replication at sites of stalled replication forks, or after ionizing radiation or oxidative damage.[24] In addition, single-strand nicks can be converted into DSBs by DNA replication. Even a single DSB in budding yeast can trigger a DNA damage response

Nucleotide Excision Repair

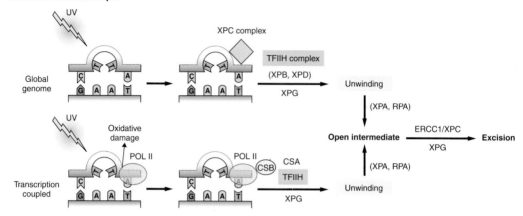

Base Excision Repair

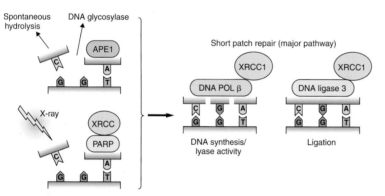

FIGURE 2.4 Nucleotide excision repair and base excision repair. Nucleotide excision repair (NER) is activated in response to bulky lesions that are generated, for example, by UV irradiation (**upper panels**). Global genome (GG) repair involves proteins identified by complementation groups in patients with xeroderma pigmentosa (XP proteins). Initial recognition of lesions occurs by a complex containing xeroderma pigmentosa C (XPC). Transcription coupled repair (TCR) also involves proteins identified by mutation in Cockayne syndrome (CS proteins), and occurs when RNA polymerase II stalls at the site of lesions. Stalled RNA polymerase II recruits Cockayne syndrome B (CSB) to the site of damage. Subsequently, DNA is locally unwound around the injured site by a TFIIH complex containing XPB and XPD. This process also involves XPG, CSA, and other proteins for TCR. Once unwound, XPA and replication protein A (RPA) contribute to stabilization of an open intermediate and recruitment of the ERCC1 and XPF endonucleases that excise the lesion. Subsequent steps involve DNA synthesis and ligation to complete the repair. In base excision repair (BER) (**lower panels**), abasic sites generated by spontaneous hydrolysis, action of DNA glycosylases, or x-ray–induced single-strand breaks are recognized by the APE1 endonuclease, as well as PARP and XRCC1. Subsequent repair is influenced by PARP-mediated ADP ribosylation of histones and other proteins, while XRCC1 serves as a scaffold for recruitment of DNA polymerase β and DNA ligase 3. These latter enzymes catalyze nucleotide reinsertion and ligation into the injured strand as part of the short patch repair pathway (major BER pathway).

checkpoint, a finding that is not surprising as DSBs can promote major cytogenetic abnormalities such as chromosome translocations, amplifications, and deletions. DSBs are detected and repaired by an intricate cascade of proteins, ultimately involving the processes of homologous recombination (HR) or NHEJ. Defects in multiple components of this process have been linked to genomic instability and cancer predisposition.

The initial detection and activation of signal transduction pathways mediating repair of DNA DSBs involves the PI(3)K-like kinases, ATM and ATR.[10,11,24,95] DSBs induced by DNA damage activate ATM, while regions of single-stranded DNA at stalled replication forks recruit and activate ATR. Once activated, ATM and ATR kinase activity results in phosphorylation of multiple targets, including histone H2AX, resulting in the local alteration of chromatin structure. Key downstream targets of ATM and ATR include the checkpoint mediator proteins (CHK), with ATM principally activating CHK2 and ATR activating CHK1. As previously described, ATM/CHK2 as well as ATR/CHK1 can phosphorylate and activate p53, mediating downstream checkpoint activation. ATM/CHK2 and ATR/CHK1 have also been shown to slow progression through S phase by down-regulating CDC25A.[28]

ATM was identified by virtue of its association with the neurodegenerative disorder ataxia telangiectasia, in which patients are also predisposed to malignancies such as acute lymphoblastic leukemia and lymphoma.[9,10] Inactivating mutations in ATR (AT and Rad3-related) result in embryonic lethality in mice and are not observed in familial human cancer syndromes, presumably reflecting the key role of this kinase in normal DNA replication. However, hypomorphic alleles of ATR that result in low levels of expression have been associated with the Seckel syndrome, which results in dwarfism, microcephaly, and chromosome instability in cells treated with mitomycin C.[96] Patients with Seckel syndrome are not significantly predisposed to cancer development, perhaps reflecting the general balancing of fitness effects and oncogenic potential; in Seckel syndrome the disadvantages of compromised ATR for cell viability may outweigh the potential for an increase in cancer-causing mutations. As previously described, the important caretaker function of *CHK2* is evidenced by its mutation in a subset of patients with Li Fraumeni syndrome. *CHK2* mutation has also been observed in familial breast cancer, and in multiple sporadic tumor types.[97] Mutation of *CHK1* is observed less frequently in tumors, which, similar to ATR, could reflect strongly disadvantageous effects of *CHK1* loss on viability.

The initiation of the repair process itself involves recruitment of multiple other proteins to sites of DSBs in conjunction with ATM and ATR.[4,9] DSBs are recognized by the MRN complex, consisting of MRE11 (meiotic recombination 11)/RAD50/NBS1 (Nimjen breakage syndrome 1).[98] Mutations in MRE11 result in an ataxia telangiectasia-like disorder, while NBS1 is mutated in the Nijmegen breakage syndrome, and both diseases are characterized by immunodeficiency, cellular sensitivity to ionizing radiation, chromosomal instability, and a high frequency of malignancies. In addition to their role in DSB repair by HR, the MRN proteins have important roles in telomere maintenance, and, at least in yeast, in NHEJ. ATR/CHK1 signaling is linked with activation of the Fanconi anemia pathway and *BRCA2*.

DNA Repair of Insterstrand DNA Crosslinks

Fanconi anemia is another autosomal recessive human disease characterized by bone marrow failure, congenital abnormalities, cellular hypersensitivity to DNA cross-linking agents such as mitomycin C and cisplatin, and predisposition to malignancies such as acute leukemia and squamous cell carcinomas.[99,100] There are 13 known FA genes,

and the encoded FA proteins cooperate in a common DNA repair pathway. Eight of the FA proteins are assembled in a multisubunit ubiquitin ligase complex. In response to DNA damage, or during normal S phase progression, this ligase monoubiquitinates two additional FA proteins, FANCD2 and FANCI. Monoubiquitination is activated by the ATR/CHK1 pathway.[101] Monoubiquitinated FANCD2 and FANCI are required for normal homologous recombination repair, and these proteins further interact with the downstream FA proteins, FANCD1, FANCJ, and FANCN/PALB2.[102,103] Interestingly, FANCD1 is identical to the *BRCA2* gene.[104]

The three downstream FA genes are breast/ovarian cancer susceptibility genes, and heterozygote carriers, with mutations in a single copy of FANCJ, FANCD1, or FANCN have an increased cancer risk. Biochemical functions of monoubiquitinated FANCD2/FANCI were recently elucidated. In a cell-free system, this complex was required for nucleolytic incisions near an interstrand cross-link and for translesion DNA synthesis past the cross-link. Thus, the FA pathway was shown to be required for the generation of a new, partially processed DNA substrate that can be further repaired by the downstream homologous recombination machinery.[105]

Homologous Recombination

In repair by HR, sequences from a homologous DNA duplex are used to provide a template for reconstruction of the damaged DNA segment.[4,9] The template for repair can either be the identical sister chromatid (the preferred substrate in mitotic cells) or the homologous chromosome (the preferred substrate during meiosis). The classic HR pathway involves the following basic steps (Fig. 2.5). DSBs are recognized by the MRN complex and by checkpoint proteins as previously described. A 5′-3 exonuclease generates 3′ overhangs, which are then coated with replication protein A (RPA). "Mediator" proteins such as BRCA2 or Rad52 then facilitate the recruitment of Rad51-related proteins, which form filaments on the single-stranded DNA, replacing RPA. A homology search ensues, followed by strand invasion and DNA synthesis. The links between DNA strands (double Holliday junctions) can be resolved to produce exchange between chromosomes (crossovers) or no exchange (non-crossovers). Enzymes such as the RecQ helicase BLM, in conjunction with topoisomerase IIIα can resolve these double Holliday junctions.[106]

Several other HR pathways also exist. A potentially important mechanism for cancer development is break-induced replication (BIR).[107] During BIR a broken chromosome end invades a homologous site and replication proceeds to copy the entire sequence of the template chromosome. This

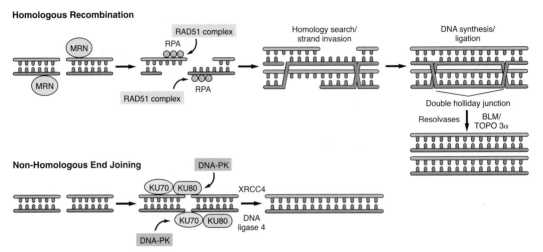

FIGURE 2.5 Double-strand break (DSB) repair by homologous recombination and nonhomologous end-joining (NHEJ). In homologous recombination (HR), DSBs are recognized by the MRN complex, among other proteins. 5′-3′ exonuclease activity results in the generation of single-strand overhangs that are coated with RPA. Mediator proteins such as BRCA2 and RAD52 stimulate assembly of a RAD51 nucleoprotein filament complex that guides subsequent homology search and strand invasion into the homologous strand (e.g., the identical sister chromatid in late S/G2 phase and mitosis). Subsequent DNA synthesis and ligation results in the formation of recombination intermediates that contain double Holliday junctions. These are resolved by resolving enzymes such as the RecQ helicase BLM, in conjunction with topoisomerase 3α. The process of NHEJ involves recognition of DSB ends by the Ku70-Ku80 heterodimer, with subsequent recruitment of DNA-dependent protein kinase. DNA ends are then ligated following recruitment of XRCC4 and DNA ligase 4.

is relevant to cancer because it can result in large-scale LOH. Furthermore, BIR is an important mechanism for healing breaks at chromosome ends resulting from telomere attrition.[108] Finally, in yeast, aging is accompanied by a switchlike increase in mutagenesis and BIR after a certain number of generations.[109]

Disruption of recombination pathways produces complex effects that pose the danger of chromosomal rearrangement due to the accumulation of recombination intermediates.[4,9] These are then channeled into alternate, often suboptimal, repair pathways, increasing the potential for errors and rearrangements. Cancer-causing mutations have been associated with multiple steps in HR. Given that RecQ helicases are particularly important resolving enzymes in this process, their inactivation results in widespread accumulation of recombination intermediates.[106,110,111] Mutation of BLM results in Bloom syndrome, a disease characterized by immunodeficiency, male sterility, dwarfism, skin disorders, and a high incidence of both leukemia and solid tumors. In addition, the WRN helicase was identified by virtue of its mutation in Werner syndrome, a disorder characterized by premature aging, with early atherosclerosis, type 2 diabetes, osteoporosis, and age-associated malignancies. Rothmund-Thomson syndrome is associated with mutation in the related RecQ helicase RECQ4, and affected patients exhibit characteristic photosensitivity with poikiloderma-

tous skin changes, early alopecia and hair graying, juvenile cataracts, growth deficiency, and an elevated frequency of malignancies such as osteogenic sarcomas. RecQ helicases have also been shown to facilitate NHEJ, interact with components of the MMR and BER machinery, and play an important role in telomere maintenance. The combination of aging and cancer predisposition phenotypes associated with RecQ lesions provides yet another example of the balance between the deleterious and growth-promoting effects of genomic instability on developing cancer cells.

BRCA1 and *BRCA2* are perhaps the most extensively studied cancer susceptibility genes required for HR. They are mutated in familial breast and ovarian cancer syndromes and represent key components of the response to DSBs and subsequent repair by HR.[112–114] BRCA1 forms a heterodimer with the structurally related protein BARD1, and as previously described, forms a complex together with BRCA2, RAD51, and other proteins involved in the regulation of repair by HR. Another large, multiprotein complex termed BASC (*BRCA1*-associated genome surveillance complex) has been identified, containing tumor suppressors, mismatch repair proteins, ATM, MRN, and BLM, with a presumed role in the global sensing and coordinated response to DNA damage. *BRCA1* has also been implicated in S phase and G2/M checkpoint control, and in the organization of heterochromatin.

Mutations in *BRCA1* and *BRCA2* are associated with a 60% to 85% lifetime risk of developing breast cancer and a 15% to 40% lifetime risk of developing ovarian cancer, although only 2% to 3% of all breast cancer cases are associated with mutation in one of these genes.[113] They account for approximately 40% of cases of familial breast cancer, with mutations in *CHK2* and *p53* responsible for an additional 5% and 1% of cases, respectively. Recently, mutation in *PALB2*, which encodes a BRCA2-binding partner, has also been described in familial breast cancer, and may contribute to inherited prostate cancer as well.[115] *PALB2* is also identical to the Fanconi anemia gene *FANCN*.[116] Germ line biallelic mutations in *PALB2* or *BRCA2* (*FANCD1*) result in Fanconi anemia.[117]

Although it is clear that mutations in *BRCA1* and *BRCA2* can destabilize the genome and promote cancer susceptibility, it remains poorly understood which roles of these proteins are specifically involved in tumor suppression and why patients with germ line defects primarily develop breast and ovarian cancer. Somatic inactivation of *BRCA1* and *BRCA2* has been reported in other tumor types such as colorectal cancer, as have defects in other components of DSB repair such as *ATM* and *FANC* genes. A subset of sporadic breast cancer, defined by lack of expression of the estrogen and progesterone receptors and absence of *HER2* amplification (termed *triple-negative breast cancer*) and a "basal-like" phenotype shares strong similarities with the tumors that develop in patients with germ line *BRCA1* and *BRCA2* mutations. These sporadic basal-like cancers also exhibit defects in X chromosome inactivation,[118] and co-cluster with *BRCA10*-deficient breast cancers on transcriptional arrays. Although these sporadic triple-negative breast cancers appear to have normal *BRCA1*, these similarities have led to the suggestion that they may be defective at another point within the *BRCA1* pathway. Another possibility is that breast tissue selectively accumulates genotoxins that induce a heightened requirement for *BRCA1* and *BRCA2*. Further study is needed to elucidate the mechanism behind the tissue-specific nature of *BRCA1* and *BRCA2* mutant cancer.

Nonhomologous End-Joining

Given that HR uses an identical sister chromatid as template to guide repair, in principle it should be error-free.[4,95,119,120] In yeast, where the genome lacks extensive repetitive sequences, HR is indeed mostly error-free. However, in humans, where the genome contains extensive repetitive sequences, HR poses the danger of repeat sequence recombination resulting in gross chromosomal rearrangements. One factor that prevents this type of error is that repair by HR is limited to late S and G2 phases of the cell cycle, after DNA replication. Thus, HR predominantly occurs when a homologous template sequence is held in close physical proximity to the break by the cohesion between sister chromatids. In humans and other higher eukaryotes it appears that NHEJ is relatively more important than in other organisms such as fungi. It seems that, at least in G1 cells, the small-scale errors generated by NHEJ are less detrimental than the potential large-scale errors (deletions or translocations) that could arise from HR. NHEJ involves direct end-joining of the broken double-strand DNA ends, without a template for repair. Thus, NHEJ can occur during any phase of the cell cycle, although it primarily occurs during G1 phase.

In the process of NHEJ, broken DNA ends are recognized by a heterodimer of Ku70/Ku80, which recruits the catalytic subunit of DNA-dependent protein kinase (DNA-PK) and the Artemis nuclease[120–122] (Fig. 2.5). DNA-PK–mediated phosphorylation of Artemis facilitates its activation and results in the processing of DNA ends in a subset of DSBs, contributing to the error-prone nature of NHEJ. DNA ligation is subsequently mediated by a complex that contains XRCC4 and DNA ligase IV. NHEJ is integrally involved in the V(D)J recombination and class switching that occurs during normal lymphocyte maturation. During V(D)J recombination and certain other physiologic settings, cleavage induced by the RAG nuclease may generate regions of microhomology that allow for relatively precise end-joining.

While mutations in these core NHEJ components in mice cause severe immunologic defects, apoptosis, and premature senescence of cultured fibroblasts, concomitant p53 inactivation results in a high frequency of lymphomas with recurrent, clonal rearrangements.[123] Certain chromosome regions, such as the *c-myc* and the immunoglobulin heavy chain (IgH) loci, are targeted in a recurrent fashion in these lymphomas, similar to common translocations observed human lymphomas. These regions may contain specific sites that are recognized by the RAG nuclease, and the initial cleavage combined with defective NHEJ may be responsible for these aberrant chromosome fusions. Alternatively, NHEJ deficiency has been linked to impaired telomere capping and end-to-end fusions, with so-called breakage-fusion-bridge cycles (see later discussion) promoting translocations and gene amplifications. It is also possible that fragile sites within these chromosomal loci and elsewhere throughout the genome may account for the particular susceptibility of certain chromosome regions to breakage and rearrangement.

Although there is abundant evidence that NHEJ defects can promote tumorigenesis in mouse models—at least in the setting of concomitant *p53* deficiency—there are few reports that implicate NHEJ deficiency in human cancer. The reasons for this are unclear. Loss of NHEJ may be cell-lethal in humans. Consistent with this idea, Artemis deficiency, which results in a very restricted NHEJ defect, is observed in rare lymphoma-prone patients. Similarly, there is a report of a ligase IV mutation in a leukemia patient.[124] However, it may also be the case that more human tumors need to be carefully characterized for subtle mutations, haploinsufficiency, and epigenetic silencing.

Telomere Maintenance

Telomeres, the structures at the ends of chromosomes composed of repetitive sequences and a 3' G-strand overhang, are key mediators of genomic instability.[125] In humans, telomerase is expressed at low to undetectable levels in somatic tissues, leading to an age-dependent compromise of telomere integrity and resultant telomere dysfunction. By contrast, telomerase is expressed in many tumors, resulting in stabilization of telomere length and restoration of capping function. The activation of telomerase expression during cancer progression supports the idea that telomere dysfunction contributes to chromosome instability during a specific window in oncogenesis.[126,127] For example, telomerase activity is low in small and intermediate-sized colon polyps, and high in late adenomas and colorectal carcinomas, consistent with the observation that CIN arises early during colorectal tumorigenesis, at a time of short telomere length. Furthermore, telomere shortening as a consequence of cell turnover in the setting of chronic inflammatory states such as hepatocellular cirrhosis may contribute to chromosome instability and carcinogenesis in these settings. Conversely, the lack of complex karyotypes in many lymphomas may be related to early activation of telomerase in the setting of the frequent dysregulation of *Myc*, a positive regulator of telomerase expression.[128]

Studies of mice deficient in telomerase activity have yielded powerful evidence that telomere dysfunction can drive chromosomal instability and epithelial carcinogenesis. Strongly reminiscent of the shift in tumor spectrum to epithelial malignancies on aging humans, aging mice deficient in telomerase and heterozygous for mutant *p53* exhibit carcinomas of the breast, colon, and skin.[128] Such tumors are exceedingly rare in wild type mice, which primarily develop sarcomas and hematopoietic malignancies. Moreover, the presence of cytogenetic profiles similar to human carcinomas supports a role for telomere dysfunction in epithelial carcinogenesis. A breakage-fusion-bridge cycle is believed to be responsible for chromosomal fragmentation and the nonreciprocal translocations observed in such tumors (Fig. 2.6). With progressive erosion of telomeres, unprotected chromatid ends can undergo end-to-end fusion, with the formation of a dicentric chromosome. During mitosis, the fused chromosome ends form anaphase bridges as sister centromeres are pulled to opposite centrosomes, resulting in chromosome breakage. The further generation of atelomeric chromosomes by this process can result in propagation of breakage-fusion-bridge mechanisms and continued chromosome instability. In addition to generating translocations, this form of genetic instability can also result in amplifications and deletions.[129,130] The observation that mouse epithelial tumors in this model exhibit amplified and deleted regions syntenic to those seen in human carcinomas lends further support to the notion of chromosomal fragile sites that may be conserved between species.

More recently, key regulatory elements of telomere structure have been implicated in genomic instability and tumorigenesis.[131,132] TRF2, an important regulator of telomere protection and telomere length, is overexpressed in a variety of epithelial malignancies, including lung, skin, and breast cancer, and has been shown to interact with a number of DNA repair proteins, such as the MRN complex, the WRN and BLM helicases, DNA-PK, PARP, and ERCC1/XPF. Moreover, mice develop an XP-like syndrome when TRF2 is expressed in the skin at high levels, with UV-induced skin cancer, severe telomere shortening, and chromosomal instability.[133] Concomitant telomerase inactivation in these mice dramatically accelerates carcinogenesis, with TRF2 promoting recombination at telomeres and de-repression of pathways that lead to alternative lengthening of telomeres (ALT).[131] ALT involves recombination between telomeres as an alternative means of telomere extension and is operative in a small minority of tumors that are telomerase-negative. Taken together, these studies identify a fundamental role for telomeres and their regulatory proteins in the genesis of chromosome abnormalities and epithelial malignancies.

Telomerase may also play important roles beyond telomere maintenance in the regulation of genome stability.[134] It is expressed at low levels during S phase in normal cells, and targeted disruption of hTERT, the catalytic subunit of telomerase, has been shown to impair heterochromatin formation on a global level and to disrupt the response to DNA damage in normal human fibroblasts.[134,135] These results are consistent with the emerging ties between regulators of telomere maintenance, heterochromatin structure, and components of DNA damage response.[136–138] In addition, they lend further support to the idea that stem cells, which express higher levels of telomerase than their differentiated progeny, are protected from genomic injury. It is important to note, however, that telomerase-deficient mice are viable and do not exhibit significant phenotypic defects until later generations. The specific role of telomerase in chromatin maintenance and the DNA damage response remains to be elucidated, and the reason it is down-regulated in association with cell differentiation remains to be determined.

Breakage – Fusion – Bridge Cycle

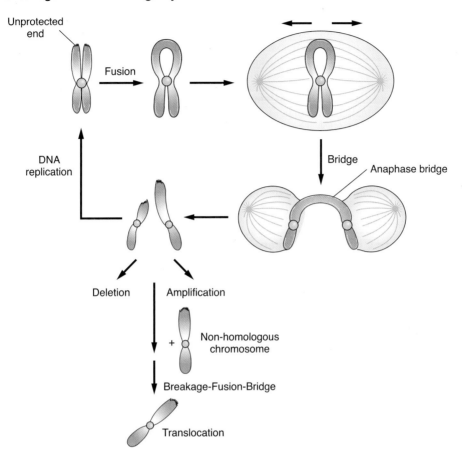

FIGURE 2.6 Breakage-fusion-bridge cycle. In the setting of telomere dysfunction and uncapping of chromosome ends, telomeric fusions may occur between identical sister chromatids or between different chromosomes (dicentrics). During anaphase, as sister chromatids are pulled to opposite poles, the fused chromosome ends are placed under tension and form anaphase bridges. These pulling forces result in chromosome breaks that contribute to deletions, amplifications, and translocations. In addition, because of the further generation of unprotected chromosome ends, the cycle may be repeated.

The role of telomere dysfunction in promoting cancer is further supported by findings in a rare genetic disorder, dyskeratosis congenita (DC). DC is a progressive bone marrow failure syndrome that is classically associated with the clinical triad of abnormal skin pigmentation, leukoplakia, and nail dystrophy. X-linked DC is caused by mutations in dyskerin, which leads to reduced levels of TERC and telomerase activity. Autosomal dominant DC can be caused by mutations in *TERT*, *TERC*, or the telomere binding protein TRF1-interacting nuclear factor 2. Autosomal recessive DC can be caused by mutations in the dyskerin-associated proteins NHP2 and NOP10. In all cases, patients have very short germ line telomeres. In addition to bone marrow failure, patients with DC are also prone to develop myelodysplastic syndrome, leukemia, and solid tumors. Thus, telomere-shortening syndromes in humans recapitulate the impaired maintenance of proliferative tissues and the tumor predisposition seen in telomerase-knockout mice.

WHAT CAUSES CHROMOSOMAL INSTABILITY AND WHOLE-CHROMOSOME ANEUPLOIDY?

Chromosomal instability (CIN), defined as a persistently high rate of loss and gain of whole chromosomes, is a common characteristic of many cancers. CIN, or the "rate" of karyotypic change, should be distinguished from aneuploidy, or the "state" of the karyotype. Although CIN leads to aneuploidy, not all aneuploid tumors exhibit CIN; some tumors are aneuploid with a uniform, stable karyotype. The first breakthrough in understanding the mechanisms of CIN came from studying different colon cancer cell lines that exhibited either a CIN or MIN phenotype.[139] In a single-cell cloning assay, the colon cancer cell lines with MIN maintained a stable chromosome content, but the aneuploid colon carcinoma cells exhibited deviations from the modal chromosome number, indicating the presence of CIN. The fusion of MIN and CIN cells resulted in hybrid cells that retained the CIN phenotype, suggesting that the mechanisms that cause CIN act in dominant fashion. Subsequent work demonstrated that a compromised spindle assembly checkpoint could result in CIN.[140]

Chromosome Cohesion Defects

Accurate chromosome segregation is achieved through carefully orchestrated interactions between the mitotic spindle, kinetochores, and cohesin.[11,29] Replicated chromosomes attach to the spindle microtubules via the kinetochore, an organelle that is assembled onto centromeric chromatin. Prior to anaphase, replicated sister chromatids are held together by cohesin, a protein ring that physically links the sisters.[141,142] The detailed molecular mechanism of how cohesin holds sisters together is a topic of much current research.[143] Most cohesin is lost from chromosome arms prior to metaphase in a manner that requires the Polo and Aurora B kinase. Centromere cohesion is then lost after anaphase onset, a direct consequence of the protease separase cleaving a cohesin subunit (Fig. 2.7). Recently, mutations in genes involved in sister chromatid cohesion, including subunits of the cohesion complex, were identified in colorectal tumors through the sequencing of human homologues of genes known to cause CIN in budding yeast.[144] The frequency and functional consequences of these mutations has not yet been tested experimentally. Additional evidence suggesting a role for the disruption of cohesion in the development of CIN comes from data demonstrating that some breast cancer tumors, as well as osteosarcoma and prostate tumors, express high levels of separase.[145–147] Although, in theory, excessive separase could cause premature chromatid disjunction and subsequent chromosome mis-segregation events, the significance of this mechanism in generation of CIN has not been definitively established.

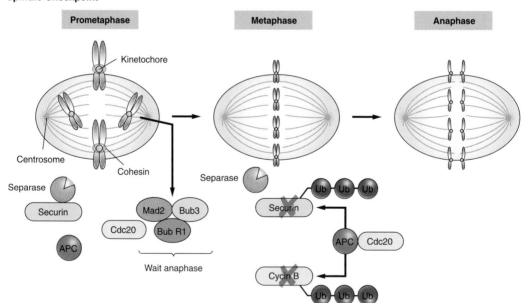

FIGURE 2.7 Spindle checkpoint. During metaphase, paired sister chromatids attach to the bipolar mitotic spindle apparatus at kinetochores, organelles that are assembled onto centromeric chromatin. Sister chromatids are held together by a cohesin, a protein ring that physically links them together. Kinetochores that remain unattached to the spindle catalyze the formation of an active MAD2 complex ("wait" anaphase signal) that binds and inhibits CDC20. Once the final kinetochore is occupied by the spindle, the wait anaphase signal is lost, and CDC20 activates the anaphase-promoting complex to ubiquitinate substrates such as cyclin B and securin. The resultant proteasomal degradation of securin releases the enzyme separase to cleave cohesin and allow for sister chromatid separation under the tension of the mitotic spindle.

Spindle Assembly Checkpoint Defects

Attachment of kinetochores to microtubules is monitored by the spindle checkpoint (Fig. 2.7).[29,148,149] A number of spindle checkpoint proteins have been identified, initially via screens in budding yeast, and include MAD1, MAD2, BUB1, BUBR1, BUB3, and a BUB3-related protein RAE1. Although mutations in these spindle assembly checkpoint proteins do occur in human tumors it appears to be a relatively rare event, as discussed in the next section.[150] To prevent chromosome mis-segregation, the spindle checkpoint proteins bind to kinetochores that are improperly attached to the spindle and form a "stop" or "wait" anaphase signal. Ultimately the wait anaphase signal prevents cleavage of cohesin by separase. This involves a cascade of events that include activation of spindle checkpoint proteins at the kinetochore, diffusion of the activated signal throughout the cell, and binding of spindle checkpoint proteins to CDC20, which is the key activator of the E3 ubiquitin ligase complex, the APC. Once all kinetochores are attached to the spindle, the wait anaphase signal is lost and CDC20 is released. Activated APC then triggers mitotic cyclin degradation, separase activation, and cohesin cleavage. How this checkpoint signal is rapidly reversed is poorly understood.

It is important to note that although some CIN cell lines have a defective spindle assembly checkpoint (SAC), several live-cell imaging studies have demonstrated that most CIN cells actually have an intact and functional checkpoint.[151–153] Likewise, in another study, both diploid and CIN cells underwent mitotic arrest in response to spindle poisons with equal efficiency.[151]

Kinetochore-Microtubule Attachment Defects

Attachment of kinetochores to microtubules is necessary but not sufficient for proper chromosome segregation. The spindle checkpoint is also activated if kinetochores are attached but not under proper tension, an indication of successful biorientation.[154] Improper kinetochore-microtubule attachments that are not under normal tension are disassembled by a mechanism involving phosphorylation of kinetochore proteins by the Aurora B kinase.[155,156] Recent work has shown that phosphorylation of an Aurora B substrate at the kinetochore depends on its distance from the kinase at the inner centromere. Repositioning Aurora B closer to the kinetochore prevents stabilization of bioriented attachments and activates the spindle checkpoint. Thus, centromere tension can be sensed by increased spatial separation of Aurora B from kinetochore substrates, which reduces phosphorylation and stabilizes kinetochore microtubules.[157]

The efficient correction of microtubule-kinetochore attachment errors requires the release of incorrectly attached microtubules. Thus, interactions that inappropriately stabilize microtubule attachments might be expected to increase chromosome mis-segregation errors and generate CIN. In fact, recent work demonstrated that kinetochore-microtubule attachments were more stable in cancer cells with CIN than in a noncancerous, diploid cell line.[158] Furthermore, increasing the stability of kinetochore-microtubule attachments in the diploid cell line was sufficient to cause chromosome segregation defects at levels comparable to those in cancer cells with CIN. Conversely, overexpression of proteins that cause increased kinetochore-microtubule dynamics was sufficient to restore stability to chromosomally unstable tumor cell lines.[159] This work demonstrates that the temporal control of microtubule attachments to chromosomes during mitosis is central to genome stability in human cells.

Supernumerary Centrosomes

CIN is also known to be correlated with extra centrosomes. Although this relationship was long-standing, it was not until recently that a mechanism was proposed to link these two common characteristics of cancer cells. Early theories hypothesized that extra centrosomes generate CIN by promoting a multipolar anaphase, which results in three or more aneuploid daughter cells. Recent long-term, live-cell imaging experiments, however, revealed that cells with extra chromosomes typically cluster the extra chromosomes during mitosis to ensure that anaphase occurs with a bipolar spindle.[160–164] The imaging also demonstrated, though, that these cells with extra centrosomes had a significantly increased frequency of lagging chromosomes during anaphase. Further analysis revealed that these segregation errors were a result of the cells with supernumerary centrosomes passing through a transient "multipolar spindle intermediate" in which merotelic kinetochore-microtubule attachment errors accumulated before centrosome clustering and anaphase (Fig. 2.8). Merotely, a conformation where a single kinetochore is attached to microtubules arising from opposite spindle poles, was previously known to generate lagging chromosomes during anaphase and cause chromosome segregation errors.[165,166] The results of these live-cell imaging experiments, consequently, provide a direct mechanistic link between extra centrosomes and CIN, two common characteristics of solid tumors. Thus, for chromosome segregation, "CIN geometry" may be as important as "CIN genes."

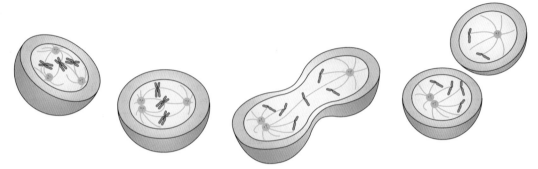

FIGURE 2.8 A mechanism linking extra centrosomes to chromosomal instability. The first cell illustrates a cancer cell with extra centrosomes undergoing a multipolar metaphase. Note that the geometry predisposes to "merotelic" attachments (see chromosome in the middle) where a single chromatid forms attachments to different spindle poles. The second cell illustrates the clustering of centrosomes, which is required for cancer cell survival. Note that the merotelic attachment persists and does not activate the spindle assembly checkpoint. Cell three has undergone anaphase and the merotelic attachment results in a lagging chromosome. Lastly, daughter cells are illustrated with resulting aneuploidy. (Figure provided by L. Kelley and J. DiGianni.)

DOES WHOLE-CHROMOSOME ANEUPLOIDY CAUSE CANCER?

Whole chromosome losses or gains are very common in human cancer.[73] Although the specific gains or losses vary from tumor to tumor, some changes are recurrent in a given tumor type. For example, the gain of chromosome 3 or 3q is reportedly as common in cervical cancer as the Philadelphia chromosome is in chronic myelogenous leukemia.[167] Likewise, glioblastomas frequently exhibit loss of chromosome 10 and melanomas often show gain of chromosome 7. Despite the fact that whole chromosome loss or gain is frequently observed in both solid and hematologic malignancies, a causal role for aneuploidy in cancer progression has been controversial.[168,169]

The identification of germ line mutations in the gene encoding BUBR1 in the disease mosaic variegated aneuploidy has provided the strongest evidence for a causal link between aneuploidy and cancer in humans because patients with this disorder exhibit growth retardation, microcephaly, and multiple childhood malignancies. Premature chromatid separation is frequently seen in more than 50% of lymphocytes from patients with mosaic variegated aneuploidy and many tissues exhibit more than 25% aneuploid cells. Mutations in other components of the spindle assembly checkpoint, including MAD1 and MAD2, have also been described in sporadic cancers and cell lines. Deregulated expression of spindle checkpoint proteins is potentially more common in tumors, but it is always difficult to know which cells to compare with the tumor cells.

Mouse models support the notion that spindle checkpoint misregulation can contribute to tumorigenesis.[150,170–172] However, they also illustrate that there is no simple one-to-one correspondence between checkpoint defects and cancer. Homozygous null mutations in spindle checkpoint genes are early embryonic-lethal. Heterozygous wild type/null animals are viable, but display increased aneuploidy. This illustrates an important point that partial loss of spindle checkpoint function is biologically significant. Although heterozygous checkpoint mouse models do not display a dramatic increase in spontaneous tumors, many models display an increase in tumors after carcinogen exposure. Overexpression of MAD2, which is commonly observed in sporadic tumors and can result from RB inactivation, causes extensive chromosomal abnormalities associated with a wide variety of tumors in mice.[173,174] Over 50% of mice engineered to overexpress MAD2 exhibit tumors including hepatocellular carcinomas, lung adenomas, fibrosarcomas, and lymphomas. Furthermore, MAD2 is not required for tumor maintenance in this setting, as restoration of normal MAD2 levels had no effect on subsequent tumor progression. This observation is consistent with the idea that MAD2 overexpression triggers genetic instability during an early phase of tumor development, promoting subsequent self-sufficiency in tumor growth.

However, at least in theory, spindle checkpoint genes, including MAD2, may have additional functions outside mitosis, making it difficult to isolate a primary mitotic defect as the cause of tumor formation in these mice. This issue has been addressed by targeted deletion of CENP-E, a kinetochore-associated motor protein that is specifically expressed during mitosis. Heterozygous loss of CENP-E results in an age-dependent increase in aneuploidy in mice, with associated formation of splenic lymphomas and benign lung tumors.[175] Nonetheless, CENP-E heterozygosity also inhibits tumor formation in the setting of p19[ARF] loss, suggesting that aneuploidy can act both oncogenically and as a tumor suppressor depending on the genetic context. The tumor-suppressing effect of aneuploidy likely reflects the fitness cost from gene expression imbalance.[176,177] Consistent with this idea, mice with significantly reduced BUBR1 display an array of early aging phenotypes: reduced lifespan, cachectic dwarfism, muscle atrophy, cataracts, and infertility.[170]

An additional, facile way to accumulate whole-chromosome aneuploidy is via a tetraploid intermediate.[178–180] Interestingly, many studies have linked tetraploidy to tumorigenesis. A number of cell-division defects can lead to cytokinesis failure and tetraploidy: errors in DNA replication or repair, or errors in spindle function and chromosome segregation. Mitotic defects lead to spindle checkpoint activation, but cells eventually recover and fail cytokinesis in the face of persistent chromosome segregation errors. This phenomenon is known as *mitotic slippage*. Recent work has also identified a pathway linking telomere damage to tetraploidy.[181] Persistent telomere dysfunction in *p53*-deficient cells activates an ATM/ATR and Chk1/Chk2 signaling cascade that blocks entry into mitosis and extends G2. Eventually, the cells switch to a state resembling G1 in which the DNA replication inhibitor geminin, which prevents re-replication in G2, is degraded and Cdt1, which is required for origin licensing, is re-expressed. Thus, in the face of persistent telomere or other DNA damage, cells skip mitosis entirely and "endocycle" between G1 and S phase, producing tetraploid cells. Cell fusion is also an additional mechanism by which tetraploidy is generated.

It has been hypothesized that the presence of an additional complement of normal chromosomes may enhance fitness by buffering against the effects of deleterious mutations. In addition, tetraploidy itself may enhance genomic instability by the presence of extra centrosomes. As previously described, work has shown that extra centrosomes promote CIN and chromosome mis-segregation through a transient multipolar spindle intermediate.[161,162] Further evidence for this tetraploid intermediate model has also come from the study of progressive dysplasia in Barrett's esophagus, which reveals that early loss of *p53* is correlated with the development of tetraploidy and subsequent aneuploidy.[182] Moreover, experimental inhibition of cytokinesis in *p53*-null cells results in the generation of whole-chromosome aneuploidy, chromosome rearrangements, and rapid tumor formation in a mouse breast cancer model.[179] Finally, recent studies suggest that genetic inhibition of cytokinesis or viral induction of cell fusion can promote tumorigenesis.

Finally, aneuploidy associated with APC loss has been shown to result from a combination of defects in mitosis and apoptosis that results in an early stage of tetraploidy and polyploidy.[183,184] Given that APC loss occurs early in colorectal cancer development and is associated with the majority of the 85% of sporadic cancers with CIN, it is possible that genomic instability in this setting is related to the formation of a tetraploid intermediates.[86] However, this remains an open issue because little genomic instability has been detected at early stages in APC-deficient mouse models.[185] Finally, the mechanism by which *MAD2* overexpression generates aneuploidy appears to involve mitotic slippage, resulting in the formation of tetraploid cells.[173] Because RB pathway inactivation is fundamental to tumorigenesis, it is possible that associated up-regulation of *MAD2* promotes aneuploidy more generally in cancer cells via the production of unstable tetraploid cells.

What is the Mechanism of Tumorigenesis?

There are multiple theories of how whole-chromosome aneuploidy could promote tumorigenesis. Extra copies of chromosomes could provide an advantage under certain selective pressures by increasing the expression of a single gene, or a combination of multiple genes on the aneuploid chromosome. This type of mechanism has been described for budding yeast to adapt to defects in cytokinesis, as well as the acquisition of drug resistance by *Candida albicans*.[186,187] An alternative explanation for the tumor-promoting activity of aneuploidy is that the extra chromosomes buffer cancer cells against the effects of deleterious mutations in essential and haploinsufficient genes.

Another theory proposes that the driving force of tumorigenesis is the inherent instability of aneuploid karyotypes.[169] According to this theory, a chromosome mis-segregation event, which is initiated by either a carcinogen or spontaneously, generates additional karyotypic evolution by destabilizing the proteins that segregate, synthesize, and repair chromosomes. Sporadically, such evolutions generate new cancer-causing karyotypes, which are stabilized by selection for their oncogenic function. Thus, in this model, CIN is generated in an autocatalytic fashion. A variation on this theme suggests that aneuploidy can cause protein imbalances that generate additional, non–whole-chromosome genomic instability, such as the acquisition of transforming mutations. In support of this model, structural chromosome abnormalities, such as nonreciprocal translocations, dicentric chromosomes, and double-minute chromosomes, are often noted alongside numerical chromosome abnormalities.[179] It is unclear, though, whether these structural rearrangements are directly linked to the mis-segregation events.

Aneuploidy may also contribute to tumorigenesis through loss of heterozygosity. The possible roles for LOH in tumorigenesis include the duplication of oncogenes, loss of tumor suppressors, or acquisition of improper epigenetic patterns.[77] As discussed earlier, it has been demonstrated in mice that Bub1 insufficiency can drive tumor formation through tumor suppressor gene *LOH*.[78]

PERSPECTIVES AND IMPLICATIONS FOR CANCER THERAPEUTICS

Oncogenesis represents an evolutionary process by which cells acquire successive genetic alterations that facilitate growth, survival, and ultimately properties that allow for dissemination to distant sites. Genomic instability can facilitate tumor development by accelerating the accumulation of such growth-promoting mutations, but this potentially comes with the cost of acquiring deleterious mutations that can impair fitness. Thus, the outcome of genomic instability can be cancer, but it can also be tissue degeneration, cell death, and aging. As detailed in this chapter, a wide variety of mechanisms can result in the generation of genomic instability. At one end of the spectrum, mutations in proteins such as the RecQ helicases, which play critical roles in normal genome maintenance, result in predominantly degenerative disease, manifesting premature aging phenotypes in addition to cancer development. On the other hand, mutations in mismatch repair genes, such as *MLH1, MSH2,* and *BRCA*, which have more limited and overlapping roles in the DNA damage response, result in normal development but a tissue-specific predisposition to cancer. Thus, destabilization of the genome can vary in the degree to which cancer promotion or tissue degeneration is favored. A major challenge for the field now is to elucidate the specific mechanisms and genetic interactions that tip the balance in one direction or the other.

Another important consideration is whether conditions leading to genomic instability are present in cancers at diagnosis or are transient, hit-and-run events. For example, inherited cancer syndrome mutations such as mismatch repair gene defects in HNPCC can speed up the acquisition of critical growth-promoting mutations, but, once transformed, the fitness of the tumor cells may be compromised by the ongoing mutator phenotype. Likewise, in sporadic tumors, loss of repair proteins such as ERCC1 in NSCLC may initially promote tumorigenesis, but the presence of these defects in mature tumors may provide a point of attack for certain chemotherapeutic agents. For instance, recent studies suggest the ERCC1-deficient lung tumors are more sensitive to the cytotoxic agent cisplatin.[92] However, some genome-destabilizing events are transient. For instance, some *FANC* genes are methylated and silenced early in cancer progression, leading to genomic instability.[188] However, later in tumorigenesis, these genes may be reactivated, resulting in a tumor with a stable genome. Also, although short telomeres can produce a crisis accompanied by gross chromosomal rearrangements, rampant aneuploidy is suppressed by telomerase re-expression. Similarly, cytokinesis failure and tetraploidy may be transient early events. If the major genome destabilization is transient, cancer cells may be aneuploid, but stably aneuploid. Indeed, it is fairly common for every cell in an aneuploid tumor to have the same abnormal karyotype; metastases and recurrences can have the same abnormal karyotype as the primary tumor. Ill-defined adaptations may enable many tumors to tolerate their altered genomes.

Understanding the mechanisms of genome destabilization that are operative in specific tumors will likely have important consequences for cancer therapeutics. Traditional cytotoxic chemotherapy combinations have largely been derived empirically. Many cytotoxic agents, such as platinum chemotherapies, induce cancer cell killing through DNA damage, with a therapeutic window that is relatively narrow. Tumor cell killing is at least in part correlated with *p53* expression and the ability of cancer cells to undergo apoptosis in response to damaging agents. Indeed, the recent observation that restoration of wild type *p53* function in mouse models of oncogenesis induces spontaneous tumor regression highlights the fact that some tumors become "addicted" to *p53* loss.[18,189] However, the heterogeneity of response within tumor types also suggests that genome-destabilizing mutations present in the cancer genome may sensitize certain subtypes to specific cytotoxic agents. The apparent sensitivity of ERCC1-deficient NSCLC to platinum-based chemotherapy highlights this point.[92] Moreover, topoisomerase I inhibitors such as the camptothecins have been shown to have enhanced sensitivity in the setting of defects in the multiple protein components that respond to DSBs.[190] Similarly, spindle checkpoint defects, if they become fixed in cancer cell populations, may modulate the response to microtubule-based agents such as taxanes and vinca alkaloids.[191,192]

This idea, in which defects in one pathway facilitate sensitivity to DNA-damaging agents, or alternatively, predispose to cell death in response to targeted inhibition of another pathway, relates to the concept of synthetic lethality.[193,194] Originally defined in yeast, extension of this concept to targeted cancer therapy may ultimately result in improved selective cancer cell killing with a wider therapeutic window. An elegant example of this approach has been demonstrated *in vitro* for *BRCA1*- and *BRCA2*-deficient cells.[93,94] Deficiency or inhibition of PARP1 in normal cells results in impairment of the BER response, causing lesions that would normally be repaired by

BER to be channeled into the HR pathway. Exposure of cells lacking *BRCA1* and *BRCA2* to PARP inhibition results in the lethal accumulation of DNA damage. Thus, PARP inhibition appears to be selectively toxic for *BRCA*-deficient cancer cells, with potential efficacy in other contexts in which HR or even other types of DNA damage responses are impaired.

The profound sensitivity of *BRCA* mutant cells to PARP inhibition has led to the development of a number of clinical trials to test the efficiency of this approach.[195] A recent phase 1 study reported that the orally active PARP inhibitor olaparib (AZD2281) is well tolerated and has few of the adverse effects associated with conventional chemotherapy.[196] Furthermore, objective antitumor activity was reported in patients with *BRCA1* or *BRCA2* mutations, all of whom had ovarian, breast, or prostate cancer. PARP inhibitors are also being used in combination regimens, as inhibition of PARP can potentiate the effects of numerous DNA-damaging agents, such as temozolomide and irinotecan.

The concept of synthetic lethality has also been applied to tumors harboring mutations in PTEN, MSH2, VHL, and RAS.[197–201] The work with RAS, for example, suggests that targeting the NF-κB signaling pathway might be one strategy to treat K-RAS mutant tumors.[200] Furthermore, this concept might be further generalizable. For example, certain genes in yeast are required for the survival of polyploid cells, with deletion of these genes resulting in so-called ploidy-specific lethality.[202] Identification of similar targets in human cancer cells may facilitate the design of targeted agents that selectively impair the growth of tumors with increased numbers of chromosomes or centrosomes.[203]

Finally, the advent of genomic technologies and large-scale characterization of cancer genomes will allow for a more refined view of carcinogenesis and enhanced subclassification of tumors. Knowledge of genome-destabilizing pathways that promote oncogenesis but impair fitness in specific tumors may eventually allow better tailoring of therapies in individual patients.

Selected References

The full list of references for this chapter appears in the online version.

1. Hanahan D, Weinberg RA. The hallmarks of cancer. *Cell* 2000;100:57.
4. Weinberg R. *The Biology of Cancer*. New York: Garland Science; 2006.
10. Kastan MB, Bartek J. Cell-cycle checkpoints and cancer. *Nature* 2004;432:316–323.
16. Malumbres M, Barbacid M. Cell cycle, CDKs and cancer: a changing paradigm. *Nat Rev Cancer* 2009;9:153–166.
23. Jackson SP, Bartek J. The DNA-damage response in human biology and disease. *Nature* 2009;461:1071–1078.
32. Collado M, Serrano M. Senescence in tumours: evidence from mice and humans. *Nat Rev Cancer* 2010;10:51–57.
36. Bartkova J, Rezaei N, Liontos M, et al. Oncogene-induced senescence is part of the tumorigenesis barrier imposed by DNA damage checkpoints. *Nature* 2006;444: 633–637.
38. Johnson L, Mercer K, Greenbaum D, et al. Somatic activation of the K-ras oncogene causes early onset lung cancer in mice. *Nature* 2001;410:1111–1116.
46. Stratton MR, Campbell PJ, Futreal PA. The cancer genome. *Nature* 2009;458:719–724.
49. Greenman C, Stephens P, Smith R, et al. Patterns of somatic mutation in human cancer genomes. *Nature* 2007; 446:153–158.
50. Comprehensive genomic characterization defines human glioblastoma genes and core pathways. *Nature* 2008;455: 1061–1068.
53. Dang L, White DW, Gross S, et al. Cancer-associated IDH1 mutations produce 2-hydroxyglutarate. *Nature* 2009;462: 739–744.
55. Ward PS, Patel J, Wise DR, et al. The common feature of leukemia-associated IDH1 and IDH2 mutations is a neomorphic enzyme activity converting alpha-ketoglutarate to 2-hydroxyglutarate. *Cancer Cell* 2010;17:225–234.
56. Ley TJ, Mardis ER, Ding L, et al. DNA sequencing of a cytogenetically normal acute myeloid leukaemia genome. *Nature* 2008;456:66–72.
59. Pleasance ED, Cheetham RK, Stephens PJ, et al. A comprehensive catalogue of somatic mutations from a human cancer genome. *Nature* 2010;463:191–196.

60. Wang Z, Gerstein M, Snyder M. RNA-Seq: a revolutionary tool for transcriptomics. *Nat Rev Genet* 2009;10:57–63.
63. Maher CA, Kumar-Sinha C, Cao X, et al. Transcriptome sequencing to detect gene fusions in cancer. *Nature* 2009; 458:97–101.
68. Garzon R, Calin GA, Croce CM. MicroRNAs in Cancer. *Annu Rev Med* 2009;60:167–179.
69. Lin C, Yang L, Tanasa B, et al. Nuclear receptor-induced chromosomal proximity and DNA breaks underlie specific translocations in cancer. *Cell* 2009;139:1069–1083.
72. Beroukhim R, Mermel CH, Porter D, et al. The landscape of somatic copy-number alteration across human cancers. *Nature* 2010;463:899–905.
75. Tuna M, Knuutila S, Mills GB. Uniparental disomy in cancer. *Trends Mol Med* 2009;15:120–128.
78. Baker DJ, Jin F, Jeganathan KB, van Deursen JM. Whole chromosome instability caused by Bub1 insufficiency drives tumorigenesis through tumor suppressor gene loss of heterozygosity. *Cancer Cell* 2009;16:475–486.
80. McKenna ES, Roberts CW. Epigenetics and cancer without genomic instability. *Cell Cycle* 2009;8:23–26.
82. Sharma SV, Lee DY, Li B, et al. A chromatin-mediated reversible drug-tolerant state in cancer cell subpopulations. *Cell* 2010;141:69–80.
89. Cleaver JE, Lam ET, Revet I. Disorders of nucleotide excision repair: the genetic and molecular basis of heterogeneity. *Nat Rev Genet* 2009;10:756–768.
92. Olaussen KA, Dunant A, Fouret P, et al. DNA repair by ERCC1 in non-small-cell lung cancer and cisplatin-based adjuvant chemotherapy. *N Engl J Med* 2006;355:983–991.
94. Bryant HE, Schultz N, Thomas HD, et al. Specific killing of BRCA2-deficient tumours with inhibitors of poly(ADP-ribose) polymerase. *Nature* 2005;434:913–917.
100. Moldovan GL, D'Andrea AD. How the Fanconi anemia pathway guards the genome. *Annu Rev Genet* 2009;43: 223–249.
105. Knipscheer P, Raschle M, Smogorzewska A, et al. The Fanconi anemia pathway promotes replication-dependent DNA interstrand cross-link repair. *Science* 2009;326:1698–1701.
110. Chu WK, Hickson ID. RecQ helicases: multifunctional genome caretakers. *Nat Rev Cancer* 2009;9:644–654.

121. Lieber MR, Ma Y, Pannicke U, Schwarz K. Mechanism and regulation of human non-homologous DNA end-joining. *Nat Rev Mol Cell Biol* 2003;4:712–720.

127. Artandi SE, DePinho RA. Telomeres and telomerase in cancer. *Carcinogenesis* 2010;31:9–18.

128. Artandi SE, Chang S, Lee SL, et al. Telomere dysfunction promotes non-reciprocal translocations and epithelial cancers in mice. *Nature* 2000;406:641–645.

130. Maser RS, Choudhury B, Campbell PJ, et al. Chromosomally unstable mouse tumours have genomic alterations similar to diverse human cancers. *Nature* 2007;447:966–971.

139. Lengauer C, Kinzler KW, Vogelstein B. Genetic instability in colorectal cancers. *Nature* 1997;386:623–627.

150. Schvartzman JM, Sotillo R, Benezra R. Mitotic chromosomal instability and cancer: mouse modelling of the human disease. *Nat Rev Cancer* 2010;10:102.

151. Gascoigne KE, Taylor SS. Cancer cells display profound intra- and interline variation following prolonged exposure to antimitotic drugs. *Cancer Cell* 2008;14:111–122.

157. Liu D, Vader G, Vromans MJ, et al. Sensing chromosome bi-orientation by spatial separation of aurora B kinase from kinetochore substrates. *Science* 2009;323:1350–1353.

161. Ganem NJ, Godinho SA, Pellman D. A mechanism linking extra centrosomes to chromosomal instability. *Nature* 2009;460:278–282.

162. Silkworth WT, Nardi IK, Scholl LM, Cimini D. Multipolar spindle pole coalescence is a major source of kinetochore mis-attachment and chromosome missegregation in cancer cells. *PLoS One* 2009;4:e6564.

165. Cimini D, Howell B, Maddox P, et al. Merotelic kinetochore orientation is a major mechanism of aneuploidy in mitotic mammalian tissue cells. *J Cell Biol* 2001;153:517–527.

175. Weaver BA, Silk AD, Montagna C, et al. Aneuploidy acts both oncogenically and as a tumor suppressor. *Cancer Cell* 2007;11:25–36.

177. Williams BR, Prabhu VR, Hunter KE, et al. Aneuploidy affects proliferation and spontaneous immortalization in mammalian cells. *Science* 2008;322:703–709.

179. Fujiwara T, Bandi M, Nitta M, et al. Cytokinesis failure generating tetraploids promotes tumorigenesis in p53-null cells. *Nature* 2005;437:1043–1047.

189. Luo J, Solimini NL, Elledge SJ. Principles of cancer therapy: oncogene and non-oncogene addiction. *Cell* 2009;136:823–837.

193. Kaelin WG Jr. The concept of synthetic lethality in the context of anticancer therapy. *Nat Rev Cancer* 2005;5:689–698.

195. Ashworth A. A synthetic lethal therapeutic approach: poly(ADP) ribose polymerase inhibitors for the treatment of cancers deficient in DNA double-strand break repair. *J Clin Oncol* 2008;26:3785–3790.

200. Barbie DA, Tamayo P, Boehm JS, et al. Systematic RNA interference reveals that oncogenic KRAS-driven cancers require TBK1. *Nature* 2009;462:108–112.

201. Scholl C, Frohling S, Dunn IF, et al. Synthetic lethal interaction between oncogenic KRAS dependency and STK33 suppression in human cancer cells. *Cell* 2009;137:821–834.

202. Storchova Z, Breneman A, Cande J, et al. Genome-wide genetic analysis of polyploidy in yeast. *Nature* 2006;443:541–547.

CHAPTER 3 EPIGENETICS OF CANCER

PETER A. JONES AND KARIN B. MICHELS

Cancer is a disease involving the failure of function of regulatory genes that control normal cellular homeostasis. The key roles of mutational processes in the generation of human cancer have been identified in the past decades. More recently the potential for epigenetic processes to complement genetic changes has been realized. In addition to multiple mutations, almost all human cancers contain substantial epigenetic abnormalities that cooperate with genetic lesions to generate the cancer phenotype. Epigenetic aberrations arise early in carcinogenesis preceding gene mutations and therefore provide targets for early detection. Epimutations may be reversed by drug treatments, providing the opportunity to design epigenetic therapies. This chapter will describe the role of epigenetic processes in cancer etiology and discuss their potential as biomarkers for early detection of cancer and precancerous lesions and their promise for drug development.

EPIGENETIC PROCESSES

Epigenetic processes are essential to ensure the appropriate packaging of the genome to fit within the confines of the mammalian nucleus, while maintaining its functionality. DNA is not found as a naked molecule in the nucleus but is wrapped up in nucleosomes composed of histone octamers and 146 base pairs (bp) of DNA, which are the fundamental building blocks of chromatin. Epigenetics is fundamental to organismal development: pluripotent cells arising at fertilization progressively lose their plasticity as they move through the consecutive differentiation steps necessary for embryogenesis. The recent development of whole epigenome approaches allows for the appreciation of the plethora of epigenomic processes that occur during development and the understanding of their role in activation and silencing of regulatory pathways.

The development of "next generation" sequencing approaches coupled with chromatin immunoprecipitation permits assessment of the distribution of the chemical "marks" imparted on the chromatin proteins and DNA. These epigenetic marks include DNA methylation and histone modifications (Table 3.1) and allow the orchestration of activation and silencing pathways. The marks or chemical modifications are placed on the chromatin components by enzymes such as methyltransferases and some of them can be removed by other enzymes (Table 3.1). While we are just beginning to understand the potential roles of specific chemical marks in ensuring the mitotically heritable variation in cell metabolism, which does not involve direct changes in the DNA sequence itself, the key role of a subset of these marks in controlling the potential for gene expression is becoming apparent (Table 3.1).

The fundamental process of DNA methylation applies methyl groups to cytosine residues in CpG dinucleotides to form 5-methylcytosine catalyzed by three DNA methyltransferase enzymes (DNMT1, DNMT3a, DNMT3b).[1] Methylation patterns, once established, can be faithfully copied over a protracted period of time. The CpG dinucleotide is asymmetrically distributed in human DNA with about half of human genes containing CpG-rich regions termed "CpG islands" at their transcriptional start sites (TSS). Mostly, CpG islands are not methylated and genes are switched on or off without changing the methylation status of the CpG sites within islands. However, in certain physiologic situations such as X-chromosome inactivation or genomic imprinting, the CpG islands do become methylated in a manner that ensures permanent silencing due to the inherent mitotic heritability of the DNA methylation patterns. In contrast, embryonic stem cells keep genes quiet but poised for later expression during differentiation by using histone marks that are easier to reverse than DNA methylation to accomplish this purpose.[2]

The histone tails that protrude from the histone octamer, containing 146 bp of DNA in the nucleosome, are also modulated by enzymes and have functional significance for gene expression.[3] Acetylation of the lysine residues (particularly lysines 9 and 14) is strongly associated with gene expression and is highly localized to the TSS of genes. The overall level of lysine modification in chromatin is dictated by opposing enzyme functions involving histone acetyltransferases (HATs) and histone deacetylases (HDACs), which apply

TABLE 3.1

SOME EPIGENETIC MODIFICATIONS AND THEIR ROLES IN GENE ACTIVITIES

Macromolecule	Modification	Enzymes	Function	Drug
DNA	Cytosine methylation	DNMT1 DNMT3A DNMT3B	Gene silencing	5-azacytidine (5-Aza-CR) 5-aza-2'-deoxycytidine (5-Aza-CdR)
Histone H3/H4	Lysine 9 acetylation (H3K9ac) Lysine 16 acetylation (H4K16ac)	HAT HDAC	Gene activation Gene repression	None Histone deacetylase inhibitors (SAHA, depsipeptide) and many others
Histone H3	Lysine 4 methylation (H3K4me3)	MLL and several others	Gene activation	None
Histone H3	Lysine 9 methylation (H3K9me3)	G9a SUV39h	Gene repression	BIX-01294
Histone H3	Lysine 27 methylation (H3K27me3)	EZH2	Gene repression	3-deazaneplanocin A (DZNep)
Histone H2AZ	Replacement histone		Gene activation	None

The macromolecules that constitute chromatin undergo various covalent modifications, which result in cellular memory of transcriptional competency. The table lists only a subset of these marks and covalent modifications and focuses on those that are mainly localized to the start sites of human genes. The table also lists drugs that are currently in the clinic or are known to modify these processes, thus providing avenues for epigenetic therapies. DNMT, DNA methyltransferase; HAT, histone acetyltransferase; DHAC, histone deacetylases; SAHA, suberoylanilide hydroxamic acid; SUV39h, histone 3 lysine 9 trimethyltransferase; MLL, histone 3 lysine 4 trimethyltransferase; G9a, histone 3 lysine 9 trimethyltransferase, EZH2, histone 3 lysine 27 trimethyltransferase.

or remove acetyl groups on lysine residues, respectively. The level of acetylation correlates with the level of expression, and HDACs have received considerable attention as potential drug targets. The TSS of human genes are also marked by the presence of three methyl groups on the lysine 4 residue of histone H3 (H3K4me3). Overexpression of enzymes that attach the methyl groups to this residue has profound implications for human cancer development. Trimethylation of histone H3 lysine 9 (H3K9me3) or lysine 27 (H3K27me3) is associated with gene repression (Table 3.1). The H3K9me3 is applied by several different methyltransferases, including G9a, and is associated with abnormally silenced methylated CpG islands. The H3K27me3 mark is applied by an enzyme of the polycomb repression complex 2, histone-lysine N-methyltransferase (EZH2), and aberrant activity of this enzyme is associated with human cancer development.

Figure 3.1 depicts the positions of a small subset of the possible modifications on the histone H3 protein in the context of nucleosomes. Although there are other modifications such as phosphorylation, ubiquitination, and sumolation of this and other histones, the discussion here is restricted to methylation and acetylation, since their function and potential for drug development is currently

best understood. The various modifications can be interpreted by other proteins (not shown) sometimes called "readers," which modify local chromatin structure to either stimulate or repress gene expression. Still other proteins (also not shown), such as histone deacetylases or histone demethylases, can remove the modifications in response to cellular and environmental signals, resulting in a dynamic state.

The positioning of the modifications relative to the TSS of genes is also critical for their function: Figure 3.2 shows the start site of a hypothetical gene with a CpG island in its promoter, which is normally free of DNA cytosine methylation. Active genes attach the activating H3K4me3 and H3K9ac modifications to the nucleosomes flanking the TSS. These may serve as "beacons," allowing the transcriptional apparatus to "find" the start site and begin producing mRNA.

The silencing of the gene can be brought about in several ways, such as the removal of the activating H3K4me3 and H3K9ac modifications and application of the H3K27me3 mark (Fig. 3.2). Insertion of a nucleosome into the nucleosome-free region characteristic for CpG island–containing genes may also facilitate the silencing process. Genes silenced through DNA cytosine methylation also have nucleosomes at the start site of the

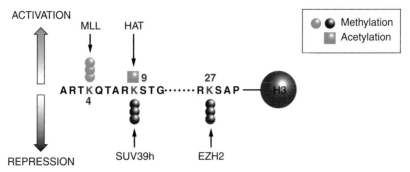

FIGURE 3.1 Covalent modifications of histones can regulate gene activity. The location of activating and repressive marks on histone H3 are shown as an example. These covalent modifications, including trimethylation of lysine 4 (K4me3) and acetylation of lysine 9 (K9ac), are highly localized in start sites of genes and associated with active gene transcription. Conversely, methylation of lysine 9 (K9me3) or lysine 27 (K27me3) is associated with gene inactivity. It is the balance between these marks that define the transcriptional competence of a given gene. Unlike the two activating marks shown (*green*), the two repressive marks (*red*) tend to be more widely distributed on chromatin and potential drug targets. The figure is not intended to be comprehensive, and many additional modifications on histone H3 and other histones are known to participate in the structure of the epigenome. MLL, histone 3 lysine 4 trimethyltransferase; HAT, histone acetyltransferase; SUV39h, histone 3 lysine 9 trimethyltransferase; EZH2, histone 3 lysine 27 trimethyltransferase.

gene but include the H3K9me3 modification rather than the H3K27me3 modification as a distinguishing feature.[4] This more permanent mitotically heritable silencing process is used to ensure the long-term silencing of X-chromosome–linked genes and other important genes such as imprinted genes throughout the life of a human. These silencing mechanisms are all essential for mammalian development and maintenance of normal physiologic functions and can become pathologically altered in cancer and precancerous conditions, leading to widespread mitotically heritable

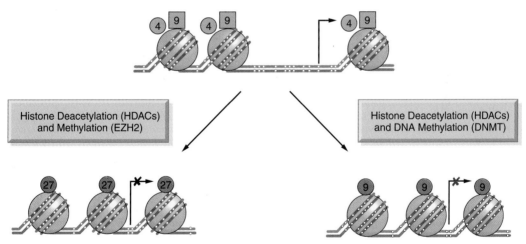

FIGURE 3.2 DNA methylation, histone modifications, and nucleosome occupancy define active and silenced states. The figure depicts a hypothetical CpG island that is active in gene expression and contains unmethylated CpG sites (*white dots*) within the CpG island and the presence of active histone H3 marks, including lysine 4 methylation (H3K4me3) (*green circles*) and lysine 9 acetylation (H3K9Ac) (*green squares*). Genes repressed by histone deacetylation and methylation by EZH2 show the insertion of a nucleosome (*large orange circles*) into the transcriptional start site and the application of lysine 27 trimethylation (H3K27me3) (*red circles*). This state is commonly observed in embryonic stem cells and holds genes in a poised silent state so that they can be called upon later for expression during embryogenesis and cell differentiation. The CpG island can also become silenced in a more permanent manner by histone deacetylation and DNA methylation, resulting in the presence of 5-methylcytosine (*red dots*) near the transcriptional start site. The histone mark associated with this state is often (but not exclusively) lysine 9 methylation (*red circles*). Genes silenced by this mechanism tend to be permanently silenced, and examples include genes on the inactive X-chromosome in mammalian cells.

aberrations in gene expression that characterize the cancer state.

Epigenetic processes such as those discussed above not only play important roles during development, but also are involved in maintaining tissue-specific patterns of gene expression in differentiated cells. In particular, DNA methylation patterns vary in different cell types, particularly at the transcription start sites of genes that do not contain CpG islands. Although the exact relations between these methylation patterns and control of gene expression have not been completely worked out, they probably assist in mitotic maintenance of differentiated states.

EPIGENOMIC CHANGES IN CANCER

DNA methylation patterns and histone modifications are essential for physiologic processes yet their dysregulation contributes to the cancer process. Epigenomic changes tend to be self-reinforcing and progressive and arise in normal cellular processes such as aging, which is one of the strongest risk factors for cancer. Several elements such as key genes that control the integrity of the genome (e.g., tumor suppressor genes, the adhesiveness of cells, the regulation of cell division, and the execution of apoptotic pathways) are all subject to inappropriate epigenetic silencing in cancer cells.

The field of cancer epigenetics started more than three decades ago with the observation that DNA methylation levels were profoundly altered in cancer cells relative to their normal counterparts.[5] Subsequently, it became clear that the overall hypomethylation of the genome observed in cancer relative to normal cells was accompanied by focal hypermethylation near the TSS of key regulatory genes such as tumor suppressor genes.[6] This focal hypermethylation of the CpG island regions at the TSS of the genes is associated with mitotically heritable silencing. Because of the inherent ability of DNA methylation patterns to be copied over a protracted time period, it was soon realized that these methylation changes could result in a molecular pathway that satisfies Knudson's hypothesis for the inactivation of tumor suppressor genes. Knudson hypothesized that at least two hits were required for the inactivation of tumor suppressor genes in familial cancers such as retinoblastoma (RB).[7] He proposed that mutations in the coding regions of genes such as the *RB* gene, followed by a loss of the wild-type copy through various pathways, could give rise to the cancer phenotype. However, we now know that inappropriate methylation of the TSS of a gene can also result in its mitotically heritable silencing and give rise to the cancer phenotype.[6] This hypothesis has been confirmed in several human cancers, including gastric cancers in Pacific Islanders. In these cases, families bearing a germline mutation in one allele of the E-cadherin gene show a high propensity for developing gastric cancer at later stages in their lives.[8] In many cases, the wild-type allele of the gene had become inappropriately silenced by aberrant DNA methylation, therefore leading to the initiation of the carcinogenic process in the stomach epithelium.

Widespread alterations in DNA methylation patterns in specific genes known to participate in human carcinogenesis have been identified in numerous studies. In addition, methylation-induced dysregulation of genomic imprinting is also found in cancer. Loss of imprinting of *IGF2* and other imprinted genes have been associated with various childhood and adult cancers. The development of new high-throughput sequencing technologies has resulted in the discovery of even more loci that undergo epigenetic changes, some of which are relevant to the cancer phenotype. This has allowed identification of specific epigenetic cancer signatures such as the CpG island methylator phenotype (CIMP) in sporadic colorectal cancer.[9] Many of these changes occur as a function of aging, which may explain the increased risk of various cancers in older individuals.[10] Epidemiologic studies are beginning to reveal the influence of environmental factors on the epigenome[11] and have identified epigenetic alterations as contributing mechanisms, linking lifestyle factors and cancer incidence and prognosis.[12,13] Future studies with improved design, including larger sample sizes, defined study populations, and control for confounding variables, will allow identification of the key loci affected by aberrant methylation in a substantial proportion of individuals affected by specific cancer types.[14]

Substantial alterations in DNA methylation pattern have also been found in the apparently normal tissues of individuals with infections. Perhaps the best characterized example is the gastric epithelium of patients infected by *Helicobacter pylori*. The infection leads to hypermethylation of the TSS of specific genes that are lost when the infection is cured by suitable antibiotic intervention.[15] Since the antibiotics do not cause demethylation directly, the loss of hypermethylation in these individuals is probably due to the loss of chronic inflammation. Since infections such as *H. pylori*, human papilloma virus, and other viral infections are causal players in carcinogenesis, these changes suggest that epigenetic alterations may play pivotal roles in the formation of cancers in infected individuals.

More recently with the development of chromatin immunoprecipitation (ChIP), coupled with high-throughput sequencing (ChIP-Seq), it has been realized that changes in DNA methylation are only part of the epigenomic alterations in cancer cells. Widespread alterations in the chromatin of cancer cells include genes that, although not silenced by DNA methylation, are repressed by histone modifications such as the application of aberrant patterns of H3K27me3 by the enzyme EZH2.[16] Although these changes may not be as mitotically stable as those induced by DNA hypermethylation, they nevertheless represent important therapeutic targets. Likewise, genes silenced by histone acetylation can be reactivated by treatment with histone deacetylase drugs. Thus, the field of cancer epigenetics is moving into a more holistic appreciation of epigenome-wide changes that occur in human cancer and an understanding of how these dysregulations contribute to cancer pathology.

THE TIMING OF EPIGENETIC ALTERATIONS

Aberrant epigenetic gene silencing probably occurs at a very early stage in neoplastic development. Epimutations may therefore be initiators in carcinogenesis, allowing for the early clonal expansion of cells subsequently at risk for additional alterations. The abnormal silencing of epigenetic "gatekeepers" might be induced by risk factors such as aging and inflammation.[17] Such gatekeepers normally restrict the division potential of stem cells to balance stem or precursor cell hierarchies. Silencing of genes such as p16, SFRPs, GATA4 and GATA5, and APC in the colon, for example, may lock these cells into a proliferative state, thus creating a population of cells at increased risk for additional epigenetic and genetic aberrations.

Recent epigenomic analyses have suggested that genes that control the growth and differentiation of stem cells are often suppressed by the polycomb repressive complex and that their activation results in the cessation of growth in stem cell populations. An early epigenetic alteration that could involve a switch from one type of silencing mechanism to another may be pivotal in moving the genes from a repressed but reversible configuration into a permanently locked state. Indeed, genes silenced by the polycomb repressive complex that involves H3K27me3 are at a much increased risk of switching to a DNA methylation state.[16] Locking these genes may make it difficult for cells to express them at key developmental times in order to undergo differentiation. The change in silencing mechanism, however, makes genes sensitive to drugs that can unlock them and potentially restore normal cell regulation. If these epigenetic gatekeeper genes are at the root of the disruption of normal stem cell homeostasis in epithelia, epigenetic drugs may be able to reverse the early steps of carcinogenesis.

Despite the fact that we now know of many classes of genes that become inappropriately silenced during the formation of human cancer, we still do not fully understand the mechanisms. As mentioned above, genes subject to polycomb silencing in embryonic stem cells and other stem cell types seem to be particularly disposed to switch to DNA methylation silencing in cancer. Conversely, many of the genes that become silenced are not regulated by the polycomb system yet become methylated in cancer. Although some types of genes seem predisposed to silencing by DNA methylation, natural selection may play a role in the evolution of tumors in cells that have undergone epigenetic alterations. For example, epigenetic silencing of a gene (such as p16) that restricts cellular growth might allow for the progressive selection of cells that have gradually begun to silence the gene. Evidence for the role of selection comes from studies in which tumors harboring p16 gene mutations show expression of the mutant but not the wild-type allele.[18] Since the promoters of both the wild-type and mutant allele are identical, yet only one undergoes DNA methylation silencing, epigenetic processes in cancer cells may be selected for in the host by giving a cell a growth advantage in an evolving process.[19]

The role of the polycomb repressive complex 2 (PRC2) in preventing cellular differentiation in embryonic stem cells and its subsequent dysregulation in cancer provides a basis for understanding these two processes. Levels of the histone methyltransferase (EZH2), which is part of the polycomb complex and another protein BMI1, are significantly up-regulated in cancer.[20] The normal function of PRC2 is to control genes in embryonic stem cells and differentiated cells; up-regulation of these proteins may repress genes controlling cell division. The mechanisms responsible for the up-regulation of EZH2 have remained obscure; however, a particular miRNA (mir101) has recently been found to down-regulate the level of EZH2 in physiologic states.[21] Since mir101 is commonly down-regulated in cancer, this may lead to an increase in the EZH2 protein followed by down-regulation of genes, decreasing differentiation and increasing cell growth. This type of dysregulation may be important in the regulation of stem cells and possibly cancer progenitor cells and thus represent an excellent drug target.

Inappropriate gene activation is also a hallmark of cancer, and this process can have an epigenetic basis as well. Hypomethylation of the genome is common in most human neoplasms and leads to demethylation of repetitive elements such as Alus and long interspersed nuclear elements (LINEs), resulting in genome instability. Alternatively it might lead to ectopic gene expression if it occurs in a potentially functional Alu or LINE promoter.[22] Hypomethylation of CpG-poor promoters may also activate cancer-related genes such as oncogenes. Translocations may also reprogram epigenetic modifiers such as in the MLL fusion gene, which is a histone methyltransfease resulting in decreased levels of H3K4me3 (Table 3.1, Fig. 3.1) and decreased gene expression.

EPIGENETIC BIOMARKERS FOR EARLY DETECTION OF CANCER

Since aberrant DNA hypermethylation is among the most common molecular alterations in human neoplasia and involved in the early stages of tumorigenesis, it lends itself as a biomarker for early detection with the ultimate goal of preventing advanced stages of cancer and death. Attributes of a good biomarker include high sensitivity and specificity. DNA hypermethylation of gatekeeper genes such as tumor-suppressor genes is highly specific to neoplastic cells, and methylation microarrays have revealed tissue- and tumor-type-specific patterns. A panel of genes with a high frequency of hypermethylation in cancer can probably be identified,[23] and sensitive methods for the detection of DNA methylation are available. Easy accessibility of DNA from tumor cells is essential for the successful population-based application. As tumor tissue cannot always be easily obtained, sophisticated techniques are available to capture circulating tumor cells in blood, urine, and other bodily fluids[24] may be coupled with highly sensitive DNA methylation methods. Alternatively, DNA from peripheral blood lymphocytes or whole blood cells has shown aberrant methylation correlated with patterns found in tumor tissues and is easily accessible.[25]

A number of studies support the potential of DNA methylation markers for the early detection of various cancers, including prostate,[26] bladder,[27] breast,[28] lung,[29] and others. Some of these studies have demonstrated that aberrant methylation changes can be observed several years prior to cancer diagnosis. Additional studies with improved design, including larger samples size, appropriate selection of the case and control population with prediagnostic samples, adjustment for confounding variables, and use of standardized DNA methylation techniques, will be necessary to establish and validate reference panels of characteristically methylated genes.[30,31]

EPIGENETIC THERAPIES

The occurrence of widespread epigenetic alterations, particularly aberrant DNA methylation in human cancers, has encouraged the development of drugs that can reverse these epimutations and restore normal gene expression patterns to cancer cells. The fact that epigenetic alterations can be observed early in the process of carcinogenesis makes this process an attractive target for chemoprevention. Currently there are four drugs that have been approved by the U.S. Food and Drug Administration (FDA) for the treatment of hematologic malignancies (Fig. 3.3). The nucleoside analogues 5-azacytidine (5-aza-CR) and 5-aza-2'-deoxycytidine (5-aza-CdR) were initially developed in Czechoslovakia in the 1960s as cancer chemotherapy agents.[32] These drugs have unstable pyrimidine rings and it was thought that they might be effective cytotoxins following incorporation into DNA and the subsequent hydrolysis of the azanucleoside ring. The azanucleoside ring, however, is quite stable once incorporated into the DNA helix and acts as a powerful mechanism-based inhibitor of DNMTs.[33] These enzymes, responsible for epigenetic maintenance of transcriptional memory, extract the cytosine ring from the DNA molecule, form a covalent bond with the six position of the pyrimidine, and reinsert the base into the helix following the transfer of a methyl group to the five position of the cytosine. DNMTs become attached to DNA containing 5-azacytosine, which leads to proteolytic destruction of the enzymes and a pharmacologic knockdown of DNMT activity.[34] Thus, both drugs require incorporation into DNA, and the ribose analogue (5-aza-CR) needs to be reduced by ribonucleotide reductase in order to enter the DNA during DNA synthesis. Although both drugs are cytotoxic at high doses, their optimal biological effects in inducing gene expression are at lower concentrations. They are both extraordinarily effective at removing DNA methylation from newly synthesized DNA resulting in gene reactivation. Once a hypomethylation pattern has been induced, it can be carried over through subsequent cell divisions, resulting in prolonged alterations of gene expression. Unfortunately, cells show a tendency to remethylate DNA sequences that have been demethylated by drug treatment, resulting in the gradual blunting of the cellular response.[35] This problem requires understanding of what triggers remethylation and the development of a new generation of therapeutics that can be repeatedly administered in order to prevent the remethylation process.

Although the causal relation between the chemically induced DNA hypomethylation and gene expression has been well established in cell culture models, it has been more difficult to demonstrate this causality in patients. The 5-Aza-CR prolonged life expectancy of myeloid dysplastic syndrome (MDS) patients in a phase 3 clinical trial[36] and this hypomethylating agent has now become the standard of care for this type of premalignant condition. Global demethylation occurs in the cells of treated patients; however, the relation between the demethylation and a clinical response remains to be demonstrated.[37] The deoxy analogue 5-aza-CdR (decitabine) has also shown good responses in a variety of small clinical trials; however, a large trial failed to show a survival benefit for patients.[38] This result was surprising, since the deoxy analogue is more directly incorporated into DNA without concomitant incorporation into RNA and would therefore be expected to be more effective

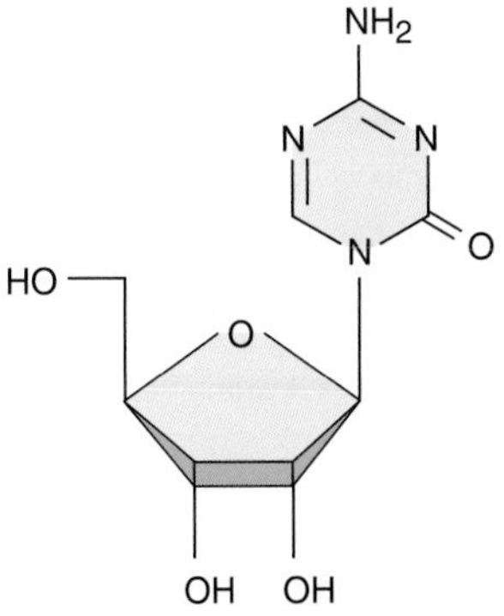

5-Azacytidine

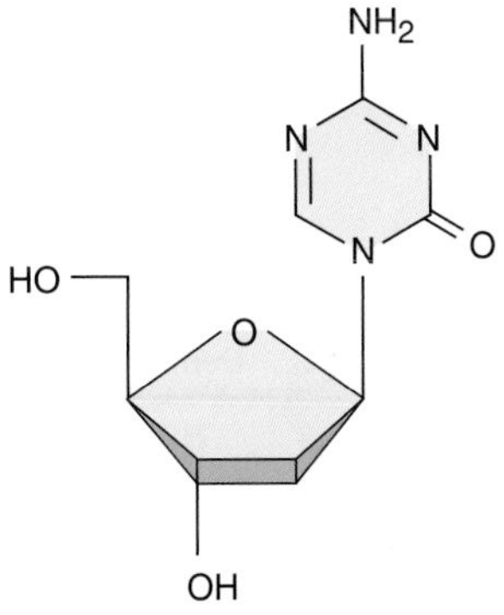

5-Aza-2′-deoxycytidine

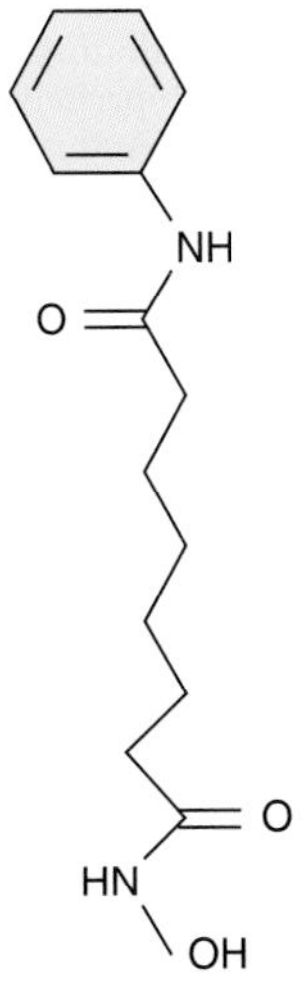

SAHA

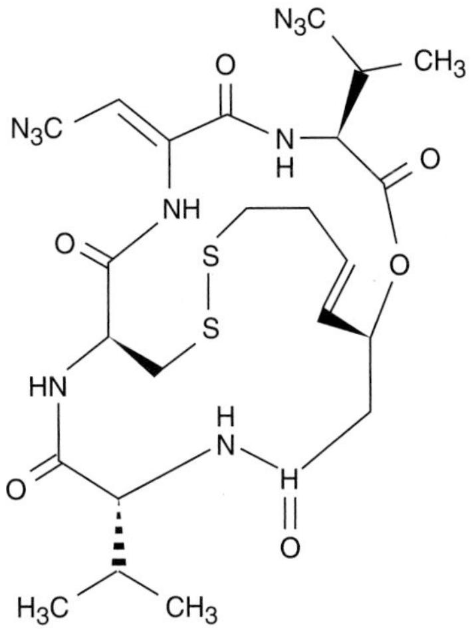

Depsipeptide

FIGURE 3.3 Structures of epigenetic drugs currently approved for use in humans by the U.S. Food and Drug Administration. The DNA methylation inhibitors (5-aza-CR and 5-aza-CdR) are both approved for use with myeloid dysplastic syndrome (MDS), and the two histone deacetylase inhibitors, suberoylanilide hydroxamic acid (SAHA) and depsipeptide, are approved for use in cutaneous T-cell lymphoma.

in the clinic. Possible explanations include a suboptimal study design regarding drug dosing and scheduling, and future trials will directly compare the efficacies of the two analogues.

The two histone deacetylase inhibitors suberoylanilide hydroxamic acid (SAHA) and depsipeptide have been found effective in the treatment of cutaneous T-cell lymphomas.[39] These agents are relatively nonspecific inhibitors of histone deacetylase enzymes. As with the DNA demethylation agents, the clinical efficacy of the drugs have been demonstrated, yet the causal relation between histone acetylation and patient outcome remains to be shown.

Because epigenetic processes are highly interactive and reinforce one another, there is considerable interest in the development of combination therapies, in particular combinations between DNA demethylation and histone deacetylase inhibitors. Since gene expression requires both demethylation and histone acetylation, combinations of drugs that alter both processes may be more effective in treating cancer. Several clinical trials have been designed to test this hypothesis in an attempt to increase the reach of epigenetic therapies beyond the hematological arena into the treatment of solid tumors. Since many pathways relevant to cancer development are silenced simultaneously by epigenetic mechanisms, epigenetic therapy has the potential to reactivate them all at once (Fig. 3.4). The efficacy of epigenetic therapy may also be enhanced through combination with other treatment modalities (e.g., immunotherapy or chemotherapy).

GENERAL PRINCIPLES

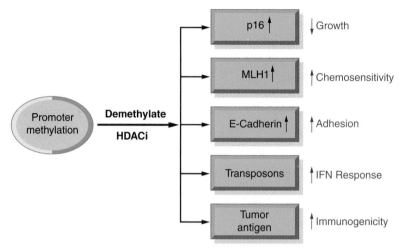

FIGURE 3.4 Combination therapies with DNA methylation inhibitors and histone deacetylase inhibitors can lead to the activation of genes inappropriately silenced in multiple pathways relevant for the generation of human cancer. Activation of these pathways by a drug regimen can result in many properties relevant to normal cell function such as decreased growth rate, increase in chemosensitivity, increased adhesion, and increased response to immunologic activities.

PROBLEMS WITH EPIGENETIC THERAPIES

Although epigenetic therapies have been clinically effective in randomized trials, problems remain with the widespread application to cancer care. One concern relates to the relative nonspecificity of the drugs in inhibiting epigenetic processes. For example, the DNMT inhibitors require incorporation into DNA where they are effective inhibitors of all three known DNMTs. Also, few specific histone deacetylase inhibitors are currently available. There is much interest in the development of more targeted drugs that may not require incorporation into DNA and be more specific in the enzymes they affect. Currently there are few inhibitors of other histone modifications such as H3K27me3, which is likely to be a critical target in cancer cells.

Another problem with current epigenetic therapies is their potential effects on normal cells and collateral damage to regular epigenetic processes within them, resulting in ectopic gene activation.

However, since the DNA methylation inhibitors require incorporation into DNA to be effective, they have no measureable effects on noncycling cells, which constitute the bulk of the cell population within the patient. Conversely, cancer cells tend to scavenge nucleosides more effectively than normal cells, incorporating more drug into the DNA of cancer cells than normal cells, which mitigates some of the concern.[40] There are also concerns related to the potential activation of oncogenic pathways in normal cells, although this does not appear to be as serious as initially imagined. However, patients currently receiving these drugs unfortunately do not have their lives extended to the point where secondary carcinogenic effects might become manifest. The remaining uncertainty makes it unlikely for these agents to find application in diseases that are not life-threatening. In the future, nonnucleoside inhibitors of DNA methylation that can be repeatedly administered may have the potential to reverse epimutations and significantly decrease the manifestation of cancer.

References

1. Jones PA, Liang G. Rethinking how DNA methylation patterns are maintained. *Nat Rev Genet* 2009;10:805.
2. Bernstein BE, Mikkelsen TS, Xie X, et al. A bivalent chromatin structure marks key developmental genes in embryonic stem cells. *Cell* 2006;125:315.
3. Campos EI, Reinberg D. Histones: annotating chromatin. *Annu Rev Genet* 2009;43:559.
4. Lin JC, Jeong S, Liang G, et al. Role of nucleosomal occupancy in the epigenetic silencing of the MLH1 CpG island. *Cancer Cell* 2007;12:432.
5. Riggs AD, Jones PA. 5-methylcytosine, gene regulation, and cancer. *Adv Cancer Res* 1983;40:1.
6. Jones PA, Laird PW. Cancer epigenetics comes of age. *Nat Genet* 1999;21:163.
7. Knudson AG Jr. Mutation and cancer: statistical study of retinoblastoma. *Proc Natl Acad Sci U S A* 1971;68:820.
8. Grady WM, Willis J, Guilford PJ, et al. Methylation of the CDH1 promoter as the second genetic hit in hereditary diffuse gastric cancer. *Nat Genet* 2000;26:16.
9. Toyota M, Ahuja N, Ohe-Toyota M, et al. CpG island methylator phenotype in colorectal cancer. *Proc Natl Acad Sci U S A* 1999;96:8681.
10. Issa JP. Epigenetic variation and human disease. *J Nutr* 2002;132:2388S.

11. Christensen BC, Houseman EA, Marsit CJ, et al. Aging and environmental exposures alter tissue-specific DNA methylation dependent upon CpG island context. *PLoS Genet* 2009;5:e1000602.

12. Waterland RA, Michels KB. Epigenetic epidemiology of the developmental origins hypothesis. *Annu Rev Nutr* 2007; 27:363.

13. Marsit CJ, Houseman EA, Schned AR, et al. Promoter hypermethylation is associated with current smoking, age, gender and survival in bladder cancer. *Carcinogenesis* 2007;28:1745.

14. Michels KB. The promises and challenges of epigenetic epidemiology. *Exp Gerontol* 2010;45:297.

15. Niwa T, Tsukamoto T, Toyoda T, et al. Inflammatory processes triggered by Helicobacter pylori infection cause aberrant DNA methylation in gastric epithelial cells. *Cancer Res* 2010;70:1430.

16. Gal-Yam EN, Egger G, Iniguez L, et al. Frequent switching of polycomb repressive marks and DNA hypermethylation in the PC3 prostate cancer cell line. *Proc Natl Acad Sci U S A* 2008;105:12979.

17. Jones PA, Baylin SB. The fundamental role of epigenetic events in cancer. *Nat Rev Genet* 2002;3:415.

18. Myohanen SK, Baylin SB, Herman JG. Hypermethylation can selectively silence individual p16ink4A alleles in neoplasia. *Cancer Res* 1998;58:591.

19. Varambally S, Cao Q, Mani RS, et al. Genomic loss of microRNA-101 leads to overexpression of histone methyltransferase EZH2 in cancer. *Science* 2008;322:1695.

20. Varambally S, Dhanasekaran SM, Zhou M, et al. The polycomb group protein EZH2 is involved in progression of prostate cancer. *Nature* 2002;419:624.

21. Friedman JM, Liang G, Liu CC, et al. The putative tumor suppressor microRNA-101 modulates the cancer epigenome by repressing the polycomb group protein EZH2. *Cancer Res* 2009;69:2623.

22. Wolff EM, Byun HM, Han HF, et al. Hypomethylation of a LINE-1 promoter activates an alternate transcript of the MET oncogene in bladders with cancer. *PLoS Genet* 2010;6 (4):e1000917.

23. Laird PW. The power and the promise of DNA methylation markers. *Nat Rev Cancer* 2003;3:253.

24. Nagrath S, Sequist LV, Maheswaran S, et al. Isolation of rare circulating tumour cells in cancer patients by microchip technology. *Nature* 2007;450:1235.

25. Sharma G, Mirza S, Prasad CP, et al. Promoter hypermethylation of p16INK4A, p14ARF, CyclinD2 and Slit2 in serum and tumor DNA from breast cancer patients. *Life Sci* 2007; 80:1873.

26. Cairns P, Esteller M, Herman JG, et al. Molecular detection of prostate cancer in urine by GSTP1 hypermethylation. *Clin Cancer Res* 2001;7:2727.

27. Hoque MO, Begum S, Topaloglu O, et al. Quantitation of promoter methylation of multiple genes in urine DNA and bladder cancer detection. *J Natl Cancer Inst* 2006;98: 996.

28. Novak P, Jensen TJ, Garbe JC, et al. Stepwise DNA methylation changes are linked to escape from defined proliferation barriers and mammary epithelial cell immortalization. *Cancer Res* 2009;69:5251.

29. Palmisano WA, Divine KK, Saccomanno G, et al. Predicting lung cancer by detecting aberrant promoter methylation in sputum. *Cancer Res* 2000;60:5954.

30. Brooks J, Cairns P, Zeleniuch-Jacquotte A. Promoter methylation and the detection of breast cancer. *Cancer Causes Control* 2009;20:1539.

31. Cairns P. Gene methylation and early detection of genitourinary cancer: the road ahead. *Nat Rev Cancer* 2007;7:531.

32. Vesely J, Cihak A. 5-Azacytidine: mechanism of action and biological effects in mammalian cells. *Pharmac Ther A* 1978; 2:813.

33. Jones PA, Taylor SM. Cellular differentiation, cytidine analogs and DNA methylation. *Cell* 1980;20:85.

34. Ghoshal K, Datta J, Majumder S, et al. 5-Aza-deoxycytidine induces selective degradation of DNA methyltransferase 1 by a proteasomal pathway that requires the KEN box, bromo-adjacent homology domain, and nuclear localization signal. *Mol Cell Biol* 2005;25:4727.

35. Bender CM, Gonzalgo ML, Gonzales FA, et al. Roles of cell division and gene transcription in the methylation of CpG islands. *Mol Cell Biol* 1999;19:6690.

36. Fenaux P, Mufti GJ, Hellstrom-Lindberg E, et al. Efficacy of azacitidine compared with that of conventional care regimens in the treatment of higher-risk myelodysplastic syndromes: a randomised, open-label, phase III study. *Lancet Oncol* 2009;10:223.

37. Yang AS, Doshi KD, Choi SW, et al. DNA methylation changes after 5-aza-2'-deoxycytidine therapy in patients with leukemia. *Cancer Res* 2006;66:5495.

38. Lübbert M. Epigenetic therapy for myelodysplastic syndromes has entered center stage. *Leuk Res* 2009;33(Suppl 2):S27.

39. Marks PA, Xu WS. Histone deacetylase inhibitors: potential in cancer therapy. *J Cell Biochem* 2009;107:600.

40. Cheng JC, Yoo CB, Weisenberger DJ, et al. Preferential response of cancer cells to zebularine. *Cancer Cell* 2004;6: 151.

GENERAL PRINCIPLES

CHAPTER 4 TELOMERES, TELOMERASE, AND CANCER

KWOK-KIN WONG, NORMAN E. SHARPLESS, AND RONALD A. DEPINHO

Maintenance of most adult organ systems requires extensive cell renewal, typified most strikingly by the replacement of the intestinal lining on a weekly basis and the production of trillions of new blood cells daily. Yet a lifetime of factors including continual telomere erosion, errors in DNA replication, intrinsic and carcinogen-induced somatic mutations, cancer-relevant germline variants, and epigenetic insults conspire to endow cells with the large number of changes needed for malignant transformation. How is it that replicating tissues, showered with myriad cancer-relevant somatic alterations, resist malignant transformation? That these mutations are indeed present in normal human tissues is reflected by the remarkable observations that roughly 1% of neonatal cord blood collections contain significant numbers of myeloid clones harboring oncogenic fusions such as the AML1-ETO fusion associated with acute leukemia,[1] and that approximately one-third of adults possess the *IgH-BCL2* translocation associated with follicular lymphomagenesis.[2] As the prevalence of these cancers is far lower in the general population, these observations imply that potent tumor suppressor mechanisms must be operating to constrain the growth and survival of these aspiring cancer cells.

The most prominent biologic manifestations of an activated tumor suppressor response are apoptosis (cell death) and senescence (permanent cell cycle arrest). These biologic processes are linked to powerful checkpoint effector molecules involving the p16^{INK4a}-Rb pathway, the ARF-p53 pathway, and specialized chromosomal DNA ends termed *telomeres*. These genetic elements comprise powerful tumor suppressor barriers and act cooperatively to eliminate or to place a limit on the replicative lifespan of rogue would-be cells. The importance of apoptosis in preventing cancer is further discussed in Chapter 7. The focus of this chapter will be on the role of telomere dynamics and associated telomere-related cellular checkpoint processes, particularly senescence, in the regulation of neoplastic transformation. A significant body of clinical and translational science now supports such a role for telomeres and cellular

senescence, and in this chapter, we present rapidly increasing clinical data pointing to the relevance of these processes in human disease, particularly cancer. Indeed, it is worth noting that the Nobel Prize for physiology or medicine in 2009 was awarded to Blackburn, Greider, and Szostak for their pioneering and seminal work in telomere biology that advanced our present understanding of aging and cancer.

TELOMERES AND TELOMERASE

Telomere dysfunction is a principal tumor suppressor mechanism manifesting most prominently as apoptosis and senescence. At the same time, when accompanied by functional p53 loss, the genome-destabilizing impact of telomere dysfunction can cause widespread mutations that propel normal cells toward malignant transformation. Thus, the telomere-based anticancer mechanism can actually fuel tumorigenesis in certain contexts. The knowledge of the basic biology of telomeres and telomerase has yielded fundamental insights into both cancer prevention and cancer promotion. The powerful and complex impact of telomere dynamics in model organisms and humans reflects the crucial role of telomere function in processes of genomic instability, organ homeostasis, chronic diseases, aging, and tumorigenesis. With respect to tumorigenesis, the study of telomeres in the mouse has provided insight into how advancing age in humans fuels the development of epithelial cancers as well as how chronic inflammation and degeneration may engender increased cancer risk in affected organs. These advances in the basic understanding of telomere maintenance are now being translated into clinically relevant applications that may have an impact on the diagnosis and management of a broad spectrum of cancers as well as aging, age-related disorders, and degenerative conditions. The important role of telomere biology in aging and degenerative diseases has been reviewed elsewhere.[3,4]

Telomeres

Telomeres are specialized nucleoprotein complexes at the ends of linear chromosomes consisting of long arrays of double-stranded TTAGGG repeats, a G-rich 3′ single-strand overhang, and associated telomeric repeat binding[5–7] (Fig. 4.1). The work of Muller and McClintock in the 1930s led to the concept that telomeres function to "cap" chromosomal termini and prevent end-to-end recombination, thereby maintaining chromosomal integrity. Subsequent work has substantiated this model across the animal and plant kingdom, underscoring the critical roles served by the telomere complex.

Telomere structure and function have been studied extensively in mammals. Although the overall structural features of telomeres are preserved among different mammalian organisms, lengths can vary considerably from species to species: for example, 5 to 15 kb for humans versus 20 to 80 kb for the laboratory mouse. On the structural level, electron microscopy and other studies have shown that telomeres form complex secondary and tertiary structures via DNA-DNA

interactions between the telomeric repeats, DNA-protein interactions between the telomeric DNA and the telomeric repeat binding proteins (shelterins or telosomes[8,9]), and protein-protein interactions between the telomeric repeat binding proteins themselves and other associated proteins (Fig. 4.1). The formation of this well-documented, higher-order DNA-protein complex has provided a working model of how the telomere functions as a capping structure, preventing the ends of linear chromosomal DNA from being recognized as either a DNA double-strand break (DSB) or DNA single-strand break, thereby avoiding activation of the DNA damage response and the formation of chromosomal end-to-end fusions through the DNA repair machinery.[7]

Many proteins involved in DNA DSB repair, including nonhomologous end-joining and homologous recombination processes, have been found to be physically associated with the telomeres.[7–10] These findings have fueled speculation that DSB repair proteins provide a protective role at the telomere; for example, by sequestering the telomere end from the DNA damage surveillance/repair machinery. Experimental support for

GENERAL PRINCIPLES

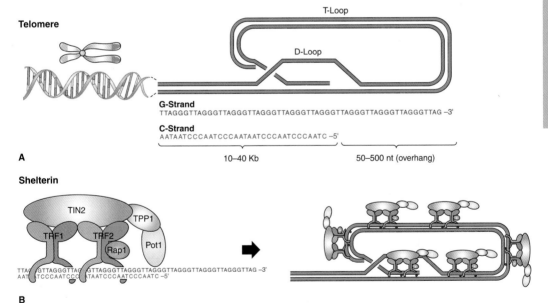

FIGURE 4.1 Human telomere structure. **A:** Human telomeres form telomere loop (T loop) and displacement loop (D loop) secondary structures. Long stretches of telomeric repeats create a loop-back structure (T loop), completed by the invasion of the single GT-rich 3′ overhang into the double-stranded DNA molecule (D loop), thus protecting the chromosome terminus. **B:** In human cells, double-stranded telomeric repeats are bound directly by two proteins, TRF1 (TTAGG repeat binding factor 1) and TRF2. Cell culture studies have suggested that the main function of TRF1 is to regulate telomere length, whereas TRF2 functions to protect telomeres from activating nonhomologous end-joining (NHEJ) and other DNA repair or DNA damage response pathways. TRF2 also interacts with the human Rap1 protein (hRap). Biochemical studies also suggest that the formation of the T loop depends on TRF2. Another protein, POT1 (protection of telomere 1), has been shown to bind to the single-stranded human telomeric 3′ overhang. Two shelterin proteins, TIN2 and TPP1, connect POT1 to TRF1 and TRF2. POT1 has been proposed to interact with TRF1 complexes to regulate telomere length. Thus, there is significant interplay between telomeric binding proteins and the formation of the secondary/tertiary structures that protect the ends of chromosomes.

this hypothesis has emerged from the mouse, in which germ line inactivation of various repair proteins (e.g., Ku and DNA-PK) results in reduced telomere length or loss of capping function, or both, leading to increased end-to-end fusions.[11] Correspondingly, in cultured human cells, experimental disruption of telomere-binding proteins results in the unraveling of higher-order nucleoprotein structure and telomere localization of DNA DSB surveillance/repair proteins (e.g., 53BP1, gamma-H2AX, Rad17, ATM, and Mre11), establishing that dysfunctional telomeres can indeed serve as substrates for the classic DNA repair machinery.[12] Recently, elegant *in vitro* and mouse genetic experiments have shown that subunits of the shelterin complex actively repress the ATM and ATR DNA damage signaling pathways.[7,13]

A further understanding of the molecular mechanisms governing the repression versus activation of the DNA DSB surveillance/repair apparatus at the telomere could lead to the development of novel cancer therapeutic options. For example, the design of agents that can uncap telomeres while preserving the DNA damage checkpoint response yet neutralize the actual DNA damage repair process would be ideal because they would produce unrepaired DSBs and elicit cell-cycle arrest or apoptosis responses. Lastly, in the near future, agents designed to uncap the telomeres could be used in combination with conventional chemotherapeutic agents that create DSB for cancer treatment, thereby simultaneously targeting these intertwined pathways.

Telomerase

Conventional DNA polymerases operating in the S phase of the cell cycle require an RNA primer for reverse-strand synthesis, resulting in incomplete DNA replication of telomeres during each cell division. The solution to this "end-replication problem" is the telomere-synthesizing telomerase enzyme, a specialized ribonucleoprotein complex with reverse transcriptase activity. The functional telomerase holoenzyme is a large multisubunit complex that includes an essential telomerase RNA (hTERC) component serving as a template for the addition of telomere repeats and a telomerase reverse transcriptase (hTERT) catalytic subunit.[14] In some normal human somatic cells, telomerase levels are insufficient to maintain telomere length, resulting in progressive attrition with each cell division. This forms the basis for the theory that the metered loss of telomeres can serve as a cellular mitotic clock that ultimately limits the number of cell divisions and cellular lifespan. In support of this view, shortening of telomere length with aging can be demonstrated in human peripheral blood cells,[15–17] and the rate of shortening can be associated with conditions of increased hematopoietic

stem cell turnover (e.g., in paroxysmal nocturnal hemoglobinuria).[18]

Many normal somatic human cells and differentiated tissues express readily detectable levels of the hTERC component. In contrast, hTERT expression and activity are more restricted because of stringent regulation on the levels of transcriptional initiation, alternative RNA processing, posttranslational modification, and subcellular localization. With the identification of an increasing number of TERT-associated proteins, it is likely that additional regulatory mechanisms will surface, such as those governing the accessibility of the telomerase holoenzyme onto the telomere end.[19] Here again, a more complete elucidation of these regulatory mechanisms may provide additional therapeutic strategies that can preferentially target telomerase-mediated telomere maintenance in cancer cells. Indeed, the development of such selective strategies may become paramount and more challenging as recent studies have revealed low telomerase levels in cycling somatic human cells that were previously thought to have no telomerase activity.[20] Eradication of residual telomerase function in these primary cells alters the maintenance of the 3' single-strand telomeric overhang without changing the rate of overall telomere shortening, resulting in diminished proliferation rates and overall reduction in proliferative capacity. These studies support an additional protective function of telomerase at the telomeres[21] and raise concerns that generalized antitelomerase therapy could lead to the immediate uncapping of telomeres in normal cells, thus limiting the use of antitelomerase therapy in cancer patients.

Lastly, in addition to forming the telomerase holoenzyme complex with TERC, TERT was recently shown to be able to interact with the RNA component of mitochondrial RNA processing endoribonuclease (RMRP). This distinct TERT/RMRP ribonucleoprotein complex has RNA-dependent RNA polymerase activity and produces double-stranded RNAs that can be processed into small interfering RNAs.[22] Also, there is compelling experimental evidence that TERT can interact and engage the Wnt signaling pathway.[23,24] These results suggest that TERT contributes to cell physiology independently of its ability to elongate telomeres, a fact that further complicates efforts to specifically target telomerase enzymatic activity as an anticancer therapy.

SENESCENCE

Primary human cells, even when cultured under optimal conditions, will eventually encounter a cell division barrier, termed *cellular senescence*, triggered by critically shortened telomeres. Senescence is a specific cell biologic phenotype composed of a permanent and durable growth arrest, alterations in cellular morphology, expression of characteristic markers of senescence such as senescence-associated (SA) β-galactosidase activity, and alterations of chromatin structure to a growth-repressive state.[25] Induction of senescence is intimately associated with p16^{INK4a} and p53 activation, and when induced *in vitro* as a result of telomere dysfunction, this barrier is termed the *Hayflick limit* (M1) in honor of the discoverer of senescence.[26] Because loss of p16^{INK4a}-RB and/or p53 pathway function in primary human cells permits additional cell divisions beyond the Hayflick limit, these pathways appear to be involved in the activation of this senescence program brought about by the "shortened telomere" signal.

Beyond the connection with telomeres, cellular senescence appears to be a general anticancer mechanism, induced by a variety of oncogenic stresses. In addition to telomere erosion or structural uncapping (see later discussion), senescence is also induced by forms of DNA damage, oxidative stress, suboptimal growth conditions, and activation of certain oncogenes (reviewed in refs. 8 and 13). Senescence requires activation of the Rb and/or p53 protein; and expression of their regulators such as p16^{INK4a}, p21^{CIP}, and ARF (Fig. 4.2).[27-30] An important form of senescence is induced by p53, which has several antiproliferative activities including stimulation of the expression of p21^{CIP}, a cyclin-dependent kinase inhibitor. These inhibit progression through the cell cycle by inhibiting cyclin-dependent kinases that phosphorylate and thereby inactivate Rb and related proteins p107 and p130.[31] The activation of p53 is predominantly effected by specific posttranslational modifications and its stabilization, which are prompted by the same stimuli that induce its expression, including telomere dysfunction, DNA damage, and oncogene activation (reviewed in refs. 18 through 20), as well as inappropriate cell cycle entry.[32,33] A major sensor of oncogene activation and inappropriate cell cycle entry is ARF (also designated p14^{ARF} in the human or p19^{ARF} in the mouse), which binds to and blocks MDM2-mediated degradation of p53.[33-36]

Another prominent molecular correlate of senescence is up-regulation of the cyclin-dependent kinase inhibitor, p16^{INK4a}, which increases markedly in senescent cells on passage in culture or advancing age in tissues.[37] Correspondingly, ectopic expression of p16^{INK4a} is sufficient to induce senescence in some cell types,[38] and senescence can be delayed or prevented in some cell types by p16^{INK4a} silencing or neutralization by antisense or siRNA.[39-43] The regulation of p16^{INK4a} is not as well understood as that of p53, although it appears to be induced by several stimuli, including oncogene activation and growth in culture.[37] Activation of p53 (and hence p21^{CIP1}) and/or accumulating levels of p16^{INK4a} is able to produce Rb-family member protein hypophosphorylation

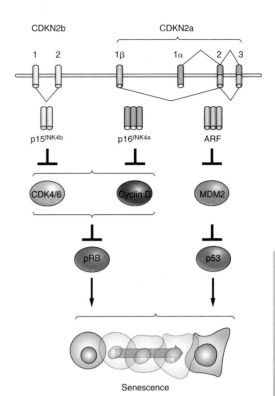

FIGURE 4.2 The *INK4a/ARF/INK4b* locus (also called *CDKN2a* and *CDKN2b*) and downstream pathways. The locus contains three open reading frames encoding the ARF, p15^{INK4b}, and p16^{INK4a} tumor suppressor proteins. p16^{INK4a} and p15^{INK4b} inhibit the activity of the proliferative kinases CDK4/6, which phosphorylate RB and related proteins p107 and p130. Therefore, *INK4* expression induces RB-family hypophosphorylation, which in turn represses E2F-regulated transcription and cell-cycle arrest. ARF inhibits the MDM2-mediated degradation of p53; and p53 stabilization in turn induces a number of targets including many proteins involved in cell-cycle arrest or apoptosis. The entire locus spans a mere 35 kb in the human genome, and inactivation of all three genes by a single genetic deletion is common in many human and murine cancers.

and activation, which leads to repression of cell-cycle progression,[27,30] enabling initiation of the senescence process. Recent data have suggested that Rb may be of particular importance in the promotion of senescence compared with its related family members p107 and p130, likely explaining the frequent inactivation of Rb in human cancers relative to the other Rb-family members.[44]

Senescence as a Cancer Prevention Mechanism

Several lines of evidence have suggested an important role for senescence in the prevention of cancer *in vivo*. It is important to note that the field has been limited by the lack of robust *in vivo* biomarkers of senescence. Although (SA)-β-galactosidase and p16^{INK4a} expression have been used as markers of *in vivo* senescence, both have certain limitations and neither can be considered unequivocal proof of senescent state *in vivo*. These technical shortcomings notwithstanding, a growth arrest important for the prevention of tumorigenesis with characteristic features of senescence (p16^{INK4a} expression and (SA)-β-galactosidase expression) has been noted in several murine and human *in vivo* tumor systems, and we believe the data suggest bona fide senescence occurs in the intact organism.

The lines of evidence for senescence as a tumor suppressor mechanism are quite strong. First, the aforementioned minimal residual disease data showing frequent oncogenic translocations and other mutagenic events demonstrate a constant need for tumor suppression, even in young animals. Additionally, several of the initially described "tumor suppressor" proteins that are mutated in familial cancer syndromes (e.g., p16^{INK4a}, p53, Rb) are intimately involved in the induction of senescence. Mice lacking p16^{INK4a} or p53 are prone to spontaneous cancers,[45–47] and mice with severe compromise of the senescence pathway due to combined p16^{INK4a} and p53 inactivation die of cancer, often harboring multiple synchronous primary tumors, with a median age of 8 weeks (compared with a normal murine lifespan of more than 100 weeks).[19] Importantly, mice and humans with impaired p16^{INK4a} and/or p53 function develop with only modest phenotypic alterations other than an age-dependent increase in cancer and an increased susceptibility to cancer following carcinogen exposure. Several groups have demonstrated a senescencelike growth arrest in murine and human tissues in association with somatic oncogenic events.[48–54] For example, some forms of benign cutaneous nevi appear to be collections of senescent melanocytes, suggesting that these common benign neoplasms would transform into melanomas were it not for the successful interdiction of this process by the senescence tumor suppressor mechanism. In aggregate, these data establish that senescence-promoting molecules are critical to the prevention of mammalian cancer with advancing age.

Lastly, although the concept of "tumor maintenance" is becoming well established with regard to oncogene-activation,[55] a similarly important role for the persistent inactivation of the senescence checkpoint has been established in cancer. Several groups have established in genetically engineered murine models, for example, that persistent p53 inactivation is required for tumor maintenance.[51,52,56] Therefore, just as the finding that tumors in murine models require persistent RAS activation presaged the successful development of therapeutic compounds such as epidermal growth factor receptor inhibitors that target pathways required for tumor maintenance *in vivo*,

similarly, these data support the notion that reactivation of senescence-promoting mechanisms such as p53 could be of therapeutic benefit in some cancers. In fact, it is likely that certain chemotherapeutics exert their therapeutic effects through the promotion of senescence by activating p53 and related senescence-inducing pathways.[57]

Dysfunction of self-renewing somatic stem cell compartments has also been suggested to play a role in organismal aging.[25,58] In this model, the activation of p16^{INK4a} and p53 in response to cellular stresses including telomere dysfunction causes a decline in tissue-regenerative capacity (Fig. 4.3). This model is supported by murine studies[59–63] and makes several predictions relevant to human disease. For example, this hypothesis suggests that heritable differences in regulation of the senescence-promoting machinery should alter individual susceptibility to human age-associated diseases, a concept that has been supported by a plethora of recent genomewide association studies.[64] With regard to oncology, this model predicts that some agents and ionizing radiation used to treat cancer,

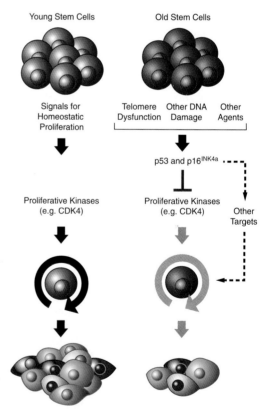

FIGURE 4.3 Senescence and aging. Activation of p53- and/or p16^{INK4a}-mediated senescence pathways in stem cell compartments in response to DNA damage, telomere dysfunction, or other unknown stimuli leads to attrition of tissue-specific stem cells (e.g., hematopoietic stem cell and pancreatic β-cells) with attendant compromise of organ function and aging.

for example, by inducing DNA damage, also can potentially induce senescence of important self-renewing cells of nonmalignant tissues such as the bone marrow. Studies in irradiated or chemotherapy-treated mice support such a role of senescence in the long-term hematopoietic toxicities of these therapeutic approaches.[65,66] Likewise, somatic attrition of regenerative self-renewing cells as a result of senescence activation may place an increased replicative demand on the remaining functional cells of a given tissue, which may increase the rate of telomere dysfunction and speed transformation in other stem cells of a tissue in a cell nonautonomous manner (see later discussion).

In aggregate, these genetic and *in vivo* data support the view that senescence prevents cancer in the intact organism on a near-daily basis and that reactivation of this mechanism in fully established cancers can effect dramatically beneficial responses, but also has the potential to produce long-term toxicity in nonmalignant tissues. It stands to reason that an improved understanding of the molecular basis of senescence could lead to therapeutic approaches designed to beneficially reawaken this potent tumor suppressor mechanism.

The *INK4a/ARF/INK4b* Senescence-Promoting Locus

Senescence is intimately associated with activation of the *INK4a/ARF* locus (also known as *CDKN2a*). This locus possesses an unusual gene structure that dually encodes p16[INK4a] and ARF (or p14[ARF] in humans and p19[ARF] in mice) in nonoverlapping open reading frames (Fig. 4.2). The locus also harbors the neighboring *CDKN2b* gene, which encodes p15[INK4b], a protein highly related to p16[INK4a] that also activates Rb, which is located a short physical distance (10 kb) from the first exon of ARF. In addition to the links of p15[INK4b]/p16[INK4a] and ARF to Rb and p53 pathways, respectively, data showing that these proteins play prominent roles in the prevention of human cancer are strong. Activation of the locus in response to stimuli, which may be both independent and dependent on telomere dysfunction, is thought to promote tumor suppression through induction of senescence.

As the *INK4a/ARF/INK4b* locus at chromosome 9p21 is the most frequent site of single copy or homozygous deletion in human cancers,[67,68] extensive analysis of this cytogenetic region has been performed. As somatic deletions in cancer frequently abrogate expression of all three *INK4a/ARF/INK4b* proteins (p15[INK4b], p16[INK4a], and ARF), debate has focused on which member or members of the locus represents the principal tumor suppressor activity located at human chromosome 9p21. A substantial body of human and murine data has now unequivocally shown that all three proteins are human tumor suppressors.[37] For example, p15[INK4b] appears mainly important

in the suppression of hematopoietic malignancies, whereas p16[INK4a] and ARF appear to play more general anticancer roles in several tumor types. Elegant murine studies[69] have further shown that these tumor suppressor genes can play "back-up" roles to each other, suggesting that combined inactivation of the locus is more oncogenic than deletion of any single member. Therefore, although the human and murine genetic data considered as a whole establish that the *INK4a/ARF/INK4b* locus encodes three major human tumor suppressor proteins, their relative and combinatorial importance in a particular tumor type is a subject of ongoing study.

Crisis, Telomerase Reactivation, and Alternative Lengthening of Telomeres

Under circumstances of extended cell divisions beyond the Hayflick limit with inactivation of the p16[INK4a] and p53 pathway, progressive telomere erosion ultimately leads to loss of telomere capping function, resulting in increasing chromosomal instability. This leads to progressive loss of cell viability and proliferative capacity across the cell population, ultimately resulting in "cellular crisis." The cellular phenotypes of massive cell death and growth arrest are likely by-products of DNA damage checkpoint responses and rampant chromosomal instability with associated loss of essential genetic material. Emergence from crisis is a rare event in human cell culture and requires restoration of telomere function either by up-regulation of telomerase activity or activation of the alternative lengthening of telomeres (ALT) mechanism.[70] The restoration of functional telomeres serves to quell DNA damage signaling and high levels of chromosomal instability, thereby enhancing the viability of cells with procancer genotypes. Finally, the extent to which normal tissues experience telomere-associated Hayflick and crisis transitions continues to be an area of ongoing investigation. Nevertheless, although clear evidence of the presence of these events is still lacking, strong support is mounting for telomere-based crisis, particularly during early stages of neoplastic development.

Transcriptional up-regulation of the *TERT* gene seems to be a key rate-limiting step in telomerase reactivation, whereas the telomerase-independent ALT pathway appears to be executed via a poorly understood process involving activation of the homologous recombination pathway.[71,72] The analysis of pathways regulating *TERT* gene transcription has forged links to well-known oncoproteins and tumor suppressors including Myc, Mad, and Menin, among others, demonstrating the capacity of these proteins to engage the *TERT* gene promoter directly.[73–75] In contrast, the enigmatic ALT process has been variously

GENERAL PRINCIPLES

associated with p53 deficiency and with tumors of mesenchymal origin.[76]

Studies in yeast have also shown that ALT is enhanced in mismatch repair-deficient cells, owing to increased homologous recombination between chromosomes. The rare use of ALT by epithelial-derived tumors, coupled with functional comparisons of telomerase versus ALT-mediated telomere maintenance, has shown that ALT may not be as biologically robust in advancing malignancy, a finding that diminishes the theoretical concern that ALT may provide a robust resistance mechanism to antitelomerase therapy in advanced malignancy.[77] The idea that ALT may be a less effective telomere maintenance mechanism derives additional support from studies in human cell culture and the mouse revealing that telomerase per se is needed for full malignant transformation, including metastatic potential.[78] The fundamental mechanistic differences between ALT and telomerase reactivation in telomere maintenance may provide an explanation for the report of more favorable clinical outcomes for ALT-positive compared with telomerase-positive glioblastomas,[79] although analysis of 71 human osteosarcoma cases failed to show a more favorable clinical outcome for the ALT-positive subset.[80] However, it should be noted that, in the latter, the absence of any telomere maintenance mechanism was more associated with improved survival than stage or response to chemotherapy, further emphasizing the general importance of telomere maintenance in cancer.

TELOMERE MAINTENANCE AND CANCER

Robust telomerase activity is observed in more than 80% of all human cancers,[81] a profile consistent with its role in promoting malignant progression. However, another side to the telomerase-cancer connection has emerged from mouse models and correlative data in staged human tumors. These data have indicated that a lack of telomerase and associated telomere attrition during the early stages of neoplastic growth provides a potent mutator mechanism that enables would-be cancer cells to achieve the high threshold of cancer-promoting changes required to traverse the benign to malignant transition.

Indeed, telomeres of human cancer cells are often significantly shorter than their normal tissue counterparts, suggesting that telomere attrition has occurred during the life history of these cancer cells, apparently at very early phases of the transformation process when telomerase activity is low. The subsequent reactivation of telomerase restores telomere function, albeit at a shorter set length. Thus, although reactivation of telomerase is critical to the emergence of immortal human cells, this preceding and transient period of telomere shortening and dysfunction promotes the carcinogenic process through the generation of chromosomal rearrangements. These chromosomal rearrangements are brought about through breakage-fusion-bridge (BFB) cycles (Fig. 4.4). A DSB created by these BFB cycles is now known to provide a nidus for amplification and/or deletion at the site of breakage for the resulting daughter cells. The broken chromosome may become fused to another chromosome, generating a second dicentric chromosome and perpetuating the BFB cycle. The accumulation of wholesale genetic changes via aneuploidy, nonreciprocal translocations, amplifications, and deletions by the BFB cycles coupled with the reactivation of telomerase enables rare cells incurring a threshold number of carcinogenic changes needed to initiate the transformation process.

Although at first glance the cancer-promoting effects of telomere-based crisis seem to counter the established role of telomerase activation in cancer progression, this mechanism is less paradoxical if one considers that many early-stage cancers deactivate pathways essential for telomere checkpoint responses, thus increasing the survival and proliferation of cells experiencing increasing chromosomal instability.[75,82] This hypothesis of "episodic instability" derives additional support from genetic studies in the mouse showing that telomere-based crisis coupled with loss of the p53-dependent DNA damage response can act cooperatively to effect malignant transformation. In humans, the accumulation of oncogenic lesions during normal aging or accelerated accumulation of DNA damage (e.g., environmental carcinogen exposure or oxidative damage) may deactivate the telomere checkpoint response, accelerate telomere attrition, and drive the affected premalignant cells into crisis. It is the rare transformed cell that emerges from this process, often with reactivated telomerase. Thus, telomeric shortening can be viewed as a barrier to cancer development in the presence of intact checkpoint response and as a facilitator for numerous genetic changes necessary for the emergence of nascent cancer cells in the absence of the checkpoint response pathways.

It has also been suggested that telomere dysfunction can be oncogenic in a cell nonautonomous process.[83] Murine data in the hematopoietic system suggest that telomere dysfunction leads to stem cell dysfunction.[84,85] Therefore, telomere dysfunction could induce premature loss of stem cells (as described in Fig. 4.3), which might induce a compensatory hyperproliferation of remaining functional stem cells. This increased proliferative drive might facilitate mutagenesis in the remaining functional self-renewing cells, and in turn select for clones with damaged genomes, in particular those harboring defects in the senescence-promoting machinery.

Several recent lines of evidence have suggested that the oncogenic effects of telomere dysfunction

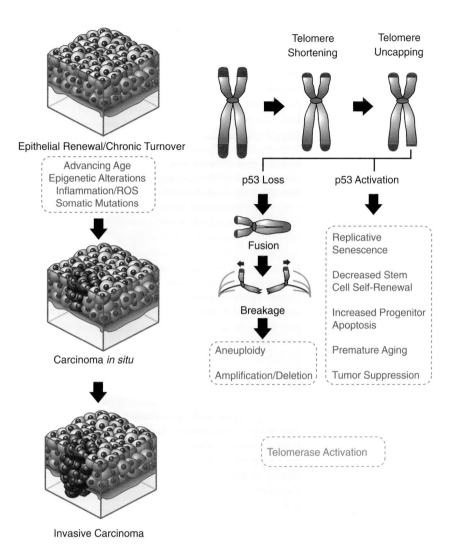

Epithelial Renewal/Chronic Turnover

Advancing Age
Epigenetic Alterations
Inflammation/ROS
Somatic Mutations

Carcinoma *in situ*

Invasive Carcinoma

Telomere Shortening   Telomere Uncapping

p53 Loss   p53 Activation

Fusion

Breakage

Aneuploidy

Amplification/Deletion

Replicative Senescence

Decreased Stem Cell Self-Renewal

Increased Progenitor Apoptosis

Premature Aging

Tumor Suppression

Telomerase Activation

FIGURE 4.4 Dysfunctional telomere-induced genomic instability model of epithelial carcinogenesis. Continuous epithelial turnover during aging coupled with somatic mutations inactivating checkpoint responses is thought to lead to critical telomere erosion, resulting in telomere uncapping and the initiation of breakage-fusion-bridge (BFB) cycles. The double-strand breaks created by the BFB cycles are nidi for amplifications and deletions for the resulting daughter cells. The broken chromosome may become fused to another chromosome, generating a second dicentric chromosome and perpetuating the BFB cycle. This facilitation of the accumulation of genetic changes (via aneuploidy, nonreciprocal translocations, amplifications, and deletions) by the BFB cycles coupled with the reactivation of telomerase enables cells to emerge from crisis and proceed to malignancy.

are an important determinant of susceptibility to human cancer. For example, several human kindreds have been identified with congenital telomerase deficiency syndromes due to inactivating mutations of *TERT* or other members of the shelterin complex.[4] Such patients exhibit age-associated pathologies such as bone marrow failure and pulmonary fibrosis, but also appear to be at increased risk for several cancers including acute myelogenous leukemia and cutaneous carcinomas.[4,83,86–88] Likewise, human genomewide association studies of large human cohorts have pointed to sequence variants in the chromosome 5p15.33 locus as a susceptibility locus for many types of cancer, including tumors of the skin, lung, bladder, prostate, and cervix.[89] The single nucleotide polymorphisms associated with these cancers are near to both the *CLPTM1L* (cisplatin resistance-related protein CRRP9) gene and the *TERT* gene. It is unclear whether one or both of these genes are responsible for the association as there is limited functional biological validation.

These human data suggest that telomere dysfunction could be oncogenic, and that hypomorphic alleles of TERT could contribute to human cancer susceptibility on a population basis.

Telomere-Induced Chromosomal Instability

The study of senescence and telomeres has provided some insights into the link between advancing age and increased cancer risk. In humans, there is a dramatic escalation in cancer risk between the ages of 40 and 80, resulting primarily from a marked increase in epithelial malignancies such as carcinomas of the breast, lung, colon, and prostate. A conventional view is that the cancer-prone phenotype of older humans reflects the combined effects of cumulative mutational load, decreased DNA repair capabilities, increased epigenetic gene silencing, and altered hormonal and stromal milieus. Although these factors are almost certain to contribute to increasing cancer incidence in aged humans, it is less evident why such processes would spur the preferential development of epithelial cancers. Moreover, these mechanisms do not readily explain one of the cardinal features of adult epithelial carcinomas—namely, a radically altered genome typified by marked aneuploidy and complex nonreciprocal chromosomal translocations.

The study of telomere dynamics in normal and neoplastic cells of the mouse has provided a potential explanation for the observed tumor spectrum and associated cytogenetic profiles in aged humans. In *Terc p53* compound mutant mice, the presence of telomere dysfunction results in a dramatic shift in the tumor spectrum toward epithelial cancers, including those of the lung, colon, and skin.[90] Moreover, in contrast to the largely normal cytogenetic profiles of cancers arising in mice with intact telomeres, the cancers generated in the *Terc p53* compound mutant mice had highly complex cytogenetic profiles with a striking resemblance to human epithelial cancer genomes.

In attempting to assign relevance of these murine studies to humans, it is worth considering that the typical adult cancer, an epithelial carcinoma, derives from a compartment that has undergone continued renewal throughout the human lifespan. Against this backdrop of physiologic cell turnover, combined with the occasional pro-proliferative oncogenic mutation, telomere lengths would shorten in self-renewing progenitor cells of these epithelial tissues. If somatic mutations also neutralize Rb/p16^{INK4a}/p53-dependent senescence checkpoints, continued growth beyond the Hayflick limit further drives telomere erosion and loss of the capping function, culminating in cellular crisis with attendant genomic instability. In this manner, telomere-based crisis provides the means to generate many additional mutations

required to reach the early stages of malignant transformation. The subsequent reactivation of telomerase in transformed clones would serve to stabilize the genome to a level compatible with cell viability, allowing these initiated neoplasms to mature further.[91] It is unclear whether additional somatic mutations, beyond telomerase activation, would be needed to produce a fully malignant phenotype that includes invasive and metastatic potential. Thus, a transient period of explosive chromosomal instability before telomerase reactivation appears to be required for the stochastic acquisition of the relatively high number of mutations thought to be required for adult epithelial carcinogenesis. Another line of support is the fact that a proportion of early-stage epithelial cancers are hardwired for lethal metastatic progression, suggesting that many cancers acquire a full profile of genome change early in their life history.

The episodic instability model of epithelial carcinogenesis fits well with current knowledge regarding the timing of telomerase activation and evolving genomic changes during various stages of human carcinoma development, particularly those of the breast, esophagus, and colon. Comparative genome hybridization has demonstrated that dysplastic human breast, esophageal, and colon lesions sustain widespread gains and losses of regions of chromosomes early in their development, often well before these tissues exhibit carcinoma *in situ* or invasive growth.[92–94] The ploidy changes detected by comparative genome hybridization appear to correlate tightly with the presence of complex chromosomal rearrangements, and these markers of genomic instability are evident in the stages of advanced dysplasia of these tissues (e.g., ductal carcinoma *in situ*, Barrett's esophagus). As these cancers progress through invasive and metastatic stages, genomic instability continues, apparently at a moderate rate, but further mutations would be predicted to derive from non–telomere-based mechanisms. Correspondingly, the measurement of telomerase activity in adenomatous polyps and colorectal cancers has established that telomerase activity is low or undetectable in small and intermediate-sized polyps, reflecting less intact telomere function. In contrast, telomerase increases markedly in large adenomas and colorectal carcinomas, reflecting stabilization of telomere function.[95] Therefore, it appears that widespread and severe chromosomal instability is present early on during human tumorigenesis at a time when telomerase activity is low.

Additional support for this episodic instability model derives from the documentation of anaphase bridging (a correlate of telomere-based crisis) in evolving human colorectal cancers and in genomically unstable pancreatic cancers.[96,97] This suggests that the DSB-induced conditions (including but not limited to telomere dysfunction), coupled with mutations that allow survival in the face of a DSB, could provide amplification/deletion mechanisms across the genome. Biologic selection forces would in turn lead to the emergence of clones with the amplifications and deletions that target cancer-relevant loci. Studies in the telomerase mutant mouse have begun to provide mechanistic insight into how BFB leads to cancer-relevant changes. In particular, telomerase-p53 compound mutant mice with telomere dysfunction have increased end-to-end fusions, and the ensuing BFB process is associated with chromosomal regional gains and losses that appear linked to nonreciprocal translocations.[55,75]

In future human studies, it will be important to document telomere attrition in renewing epithelial stem cells and to perform a simultaneous comparison of telomere status, telomerase activity, and chromosomal instability in the same tumor samples, particularly during the earliest stages of human epithelial cell transformation. Defining the temporal point at which telomerase is reactivated in the genesis and progression of the different cancers may also lead to the development of biomarkers for diagnosis, prognosis, and outcomes prediction. Such studies are needed to more firmly establish a causal link between telomere dysfunction and early chromosomal instability in human neoplasms.

Telomere Dynamics, Inflammatory Diseases, and Cancer

The telomere dysfunction-induced genomic instability model also suggests some unanticipated opportunities for the therapies of other human diseases. For example, this model provides a potential explanation for the high cancer incidence associated with diseases characterized by chronic cell destruction and renewal as well as inflammation. One of the most notable examples of this tight link is the high incidence of hepatocellular carcinoma in late-stage cirrhotic livers. Cirrhosis is the phenotypic end point of prolonged cycles of hepatocyte destruction and regeneration, and cirrhotic livers show a documented reduction in telomere length over time. Humans with congenital telomerase deficiency may be predisposed to fibrotic liver disease, including cirrhosis.[87] Mouse models involving the telomerase-deficient mouse have shown that critical reductions in telomere length and function can accelerate the development of cirrhosis and hepatocellular carcinoma in chronic liver injury experiments.[98–100] Another example of a telomere-based pathogenic relationship between chronic tissue turnover, telomere-based crisis, and increased cancer risk is ulcerative colitis, a condition characterized by rapid cell turnover and oxidative injury to the intestines, and a high incidence of intestinal dysplasia or cancer.[97] In addition to the progressive telomere attrition resulting from the cell turnover, accelerated telomere attrition might occur via increased oxidative stress and from the altered inflammatory microenvironment milieu. Together, such observations suggest the intriguing possibility that early somatic reconstitution of telomerase could attenuate telomere attrition and paradoxically reduce the occurrence of cancers in these high-turnover disease states, a theory that requires additional preclinical studies. In addition, serial analyses of telomere length from these tissues may provide prognostic information regarding the rising risk of cancer development. Thus, progress in our understanding of telomere biology has mechanistically connected diverse fields in medicine involving chronic inflammatory diseases, degenerative diseases, geriatrics, and oncology.

Telomerase and Telomere Maintenance as Therapeutic Targets

Some evidence supports the view that telomerase-mediated telomere maintenance represents a near-universal therapeutic target for cancer. Indeed, cell culture–based studies of human cancer cells have established that inhibition of telomerase culminates in cell death after extended cell divisions. The past few years have witnessed intense efforts to design therapeutic strategies capable of targeting telomere structure and the telomerase holoenzyme function.[14,101,102] Unfortunately, most of these compounds and agents are still in preclinical and early clinical development and thus their safety and efficacy profiles in human patients are not fully known.

Presently, the only clinically advanced telomerase-related cancer treatment strategy is immunotherapy, targeting immune recognition and the destruction of cells that express telomerase. Immune responses, specifically cytotoxic T-cell responses, have been generated against peptide sequences of the hTERT protein, and it has been demonstrated that these cytotoxic T cells are capable of selectively lysing target cells that express TERT peptides presented on the cell surface in the context of major histocompatibility complex class I molecules. There have been several promising completed phase 1/2 trials using peptides from telomerase as vaccines.[103,104] A large randomized phase 3 trial comparing gemcitabine alone versus gemcitabine with a telomerase peptide vaccine (GV1001) showed no difference in survival benefit in the first 360 enrolled patients, and the trial was stopped. A second large 1,110 pancreatic cancer patient trial comparing gemcitabine/capecitabine combination therapy with concurrent and sequential gemcitabine/capecitabine therapy with GV1001 is still ongoing. Lastly, other TERT-based immune approaches, such as infusion of patient's primed antigen-presenting dendritic cells *ex vivo* with TERT mRNA, are also currently in early clinical trials.[105]

As for the ongoing design of rational clinical trials of telomere-based therapeutics, such efforts will be informed by the considerable body of knowledge accumulated in telomere biology. Experience with the telomerase mutant mouse model and human cell culture systems should serve to guide the design of human clinical trials. These studies suggest that inhibitors of telomerase activity might be expected to exhibit a long lag time and might promote malignancy in some circumstances, but also may be particularly useful in the setting of minimal residual disease after the administration of standard chemotherapeutic agents and surgery. In addition, pharmacodynamic assays capable of assessing inhibition of telomerase activity in individual patients are needed. Moreover, given that the activation of senescence-promoting mechanisms such as p53 and p16[INK4a] has been associated with aging-like pathologies in several tissues,[59–63] some caution is warranted regarding the toxicity resulting from the induction of premature senescence in nondiseased tissues. This potential is underlined by evidence of germ cell defects, defects in proliferative homeostasis of certain tissues, and an increased rate of spontaneous malignancy in mice with telomere dysfunction, suggesting that clinical trials of such agents will need to be actively monitoring patients for these sequelae.

Furthermore, it seems prudent that the genetic profile of tumors enlisted into clinical trials should be determined to assess the integrity of p53. This caution relates to mouse models showing that the combination of p53 deficiency and telomere dysfunction drives greater genomic instability and thus potential for emergence of therapeutic resistance. In contrast, when p53 responses are intact, critical telomere shortening should induce p53-dependent senescence and apoptosis. The final answers to these safety questions reside in the analyses of current and future clinical trials with humans.

Conversely, the telomerase-deficient mouse model has also informed that cells and animals with telomere dysfunction are more sensitive to ionizing radiation and DNA DSB chemotherapeutic agents; thus, telomerase activity inhibitors may be more effective when paired with radiation or certain classes of chemotherapy that produce DSBs, as they might produce synergistic cytogenetic catastrophe. Again, however, particular care is warranted here as the combination of increased DNA damage with reduced capacity for normal repair may also produce marked increases in the toxicity of chemoradiotherapy.

Recent years have witnessed significant progress in the telomere biology field that is now maturing into new opportunities for improved diagnostics and novel therapeutic applications in human diseases, including cancer. Discoveries in telomere biology, rewarded with the 2009 Nobel Prize, have provided new mechanistic insights into the pathogenesis of human cancer and of inherited and acquired degenerative disorders. The role of telomere dysfunction driving episodic genomic instability in epithelial cancers—first seen in the telomerase-deficient mouse—has now been substantiated in the study of several human cancer types, with further support from genomewide association studies and kindreds with congenital telomerase deficiency. The pivotal role of telomere attrition in the pathogenesis of cancer and tissue aging provides potential avenues for the development of cancer risk biomarkers, diagnostics, and rationally designed therapeutics.

Selected References

The full list of references for this chapter appears in the online version.

3. Sahin E, Depinho RA. Linking functional decline of telomeres, mitochondria and stem cells during ageing. *Nature* 2010;464:520.
4. Calado RT, Young NS. Telomere diseases. *N Engl J Med* 2009;361:2353.
6. O'Sullivan RJ, Karlseder J. Telomeres: protecting chromosomes against genome instability. *Nature Rev* 2010;11:171.
7. de Lange T. How telomeres solve the end-protection problem. *Science* 2009;326:948.
8. de Lange T. Shelterin: the protein complex that shapes and safeguards human telomeres. *Genes Dev* 2005;19:2100.
10. Zhu XD, Kuster B, Mann M, Petrini JH, de Lange T. Cell-cycle-regulated association of RAD50/MRE11/NBS1 with TRF2 and human telomeres. *Nat Genet* 2000;25:347.
12. Takai H, Smogorzewska A, de Lange T. DNA damage foci at dysfunctional telomeres. *Curr Biol* 2003;13:1549.
13. Deng Y, Chan SS, Chang S. Telomere dysfunction and tumour suppression: the senescence connection. *Nat Rev Cancer* 2008;8:450.

16. Valdes AM, Andrew T, Gardner JP, et al. Obesity, cigarette smoking, and telomere length in women. *Lancet* 2005;366:662.
19. Artandi SE, DePinho RA. Telomeres and telomerase in cancer. *Carcinogenesis* 2010;31:9.
20. Masutomi K, Yu EY, Khurts S, et al. Telomerase maintains telomere structure in normal human cells. *Cell* 2003;114:241.
22. Maida Y, Yasukawa M, Furuuchi M, et al. An RNA-dependent RNA polymerase formed by TERT and the RMRP RNA. *Nature* 2009;461:230.
24. Park JI, Venteicher AS, Hong JY, et al. Telomerase modulates Wnt signalling by association with target gene chromatin. *Nature* 2009;460:66.
25. Sharpless NE, DePinho RA. Telomeres, stem cells, senescence, and cancer. *J Clin Invest* 2004;113:160.
26. Hayflick L, Moorhead P. The serial cultivation of human diploid cell strains. *Exp Cell Res* 1961;25:585.
28. Kamijo T, Zindy F, Roussel MF, et al. Tumor suppression at the mouse INK4a locus mediated by the alternative reading frame product p19ARF. *Cell* 1997;91:649.
29. Sage J, Miller AL, Perez-Mancera PA, Wysocki JM, Jacks T. Acute mutation of retinoblastoma gene function is sufficient for cell cycle re-entry. *Nature* 2003;424:223.

31. Classon M, Harlow E. The retinoblastoma tumour suppressor in development and cancer. *Nat Rev Cancer* 2002; 2:910.

36. Zhang Y, Xiong Y, Yarbrough WG. ARF promotes MDM2 degradation and stabilizes p53: ARF-INK4a locus deletion impairs both the Rb and p53 tumor suppression pathways. *Cell* 1998;92:725.

37. Kim WY, Sharpless NE. The regulation of INK4/ARF in cancer and aging. *Cell* 2006;127:265.

43. Jacobs JJ, de Lange T. Significant role for p16INK4a in p53-independent telomere-directed senescence. *Curr Biol* 2004;14:2302.

44. Chicas A, Wang X, Zhang C, et al. Dissecting the unique role of the retinoblastoma tumor suppressor during cellular senescence. *Cancer Cell* 2010;17:376.

45. Donehower LA, Harvey M, Slagle BL, et al. Mice deficient for p53 are developmentally normal but susceptible to spontaneous tumours. *Nature* 1992;356:215.

47. Sharpless NE, Bardeesy N, Lee KH, et al. Loss of p16Ink4a with retention of p19Arf predisposes mice to tumorigenesis. *Nature* 2001;413:86.

48. Braig M, Lee S, Loddenkemper C, et al. Oncogene-induced senescence as an initial barrier in lymphoma development. *Nature* 2005;436:660.

49. Collado M, Gil J, Efeyan A, et al. Tumour biology: senescence in premalignant tumours. *Nature* 2005;436: 642.

50. Chen Z, Trotman LC, Shaffer D, et al. Crucial role of p53-dependent cellular senescence in suppression of Pten-deficient tumorigenesis. *Nature* 2005;436:725.

51. Ventura A, Kirsch DG, McLaughlin ME, et al. Restoration of p53 function leads to tumour regression in vivo. *Nature* 2007;445:661.

52. Xue W, Zender L, Miething C, et al. Senescence and tumour clearance is triggered by p53 restoration in murine liver carcinomas. *Nature* 2007;445:656.

53. Michaloglou C, Vredeveld LC, Soengas MS, et al. BRAFE600-associated senescence-like cell cycle arrest of human naevi. *Nature* 2005;436:720.

55. Chin L, Artandi SE, Shen Q, et al. p53 deficiency rescues the adverse effects of telomere loss and cooperates with telomere dysfunction to accelerate carcinogenesis. *Cell* 1999;97:527.

56. Martins CP, Brown-Swigart L, Evan GI. Modeling the therapeutic efficacy of p53 restoration in tumors. *Cell* 2006; 127:1323.

57. Schmitt CA, Fridman JS, Yang M, Baranov E, Hoffman RM, Lowe SW. Dissecting p53 tumor suppressor functions in vivo. *Cancer Cell* 2002;1:289.

58. Campisi J. Suppressing cancer: the importance of being senescent. *Science* 2005;309:886.

61. Krishnamurthy J, Ramsey MR, Ligon KL, et al. p16INK4a induces an age-dependent decline in islet regenerative potential. *Nature* 2006;443:453.

64. Sharpless NE, DePinho RA. How stem cells age and why this makes us grow old. *Nature Rev* 2007;8:703.

68. Beroukhim R, Mermel CH, Porter D, et al. The landscape of somatic copy-number alteration across human cancers. *Nature* 2010;463:899.

69. Krimpenfort P, Ijpenberg A, Song JY, et al. p15Ink4b is a critical tumour suppressor in the absence of p16Ink4a. *Nature* 2007;448:943.

73. Blasco MA. Telomerase beyond telomeres. *Nat Rev Cancer* 2002;2:627.

74. Lin SY, Elledge SJ. Multiple tumor suppressor pathways negatively regulate telomerase. *Cell* 2003;113:881.

75. O'Hagan RC, Chang S, Maser RS, et al. Telomere dysfunction provokes regional amplification and deletion in cancer genomes. *Cancer Cell* 2002;2:149.

78. Chang S, Khoo CM, Naylor ML, Maser RS, DePinho RA. Telomere-based crisis: functional differences between telomerase activation and ALT in tumor progression. *Genes Dev* 2003;17:88.

81. Shay JW, Bacchetti S. A survey of telomerase activity in human cancer. *Eur J Cancer* 1997;33:787.

85. Rossi DJ, Bryder D, Seita J, Nussenzweig A, Hoeijmakers J, Weissman IL. Deficiencies in DNA damage repair limit the function of haematopoietic stem cells with age. *Nature* 2007;447:725.

89. Rafnar T, Sulem P, Stacey SN, et al. Sequence variants at the TERT-CLPTM1L locus associate with many cancer types. *Nat Genet* 2009;41:221.

90. Artandi SE, Chang S, Lee SL, et al. Telomere dysfunction promotes non-reciprocal translocations and epithelial cancers in mice. *Nature* 2000;406:641.

97. O'Sullivan JN, Bronner MP, Brentnall TA, et al. Chromosomal instability in ulcerative colitis is related to telomere shortening. *Nat Genet* 2002;32:280.

99. Farazi PA, Glickman J, Jiang S, Yu A, Rudolph KL, DePinho RA. Differential impact of experimental telomere dysfunction on initiation and progression of hepatocellular carcinoma. *Cancer Res* 2003;63:5021.

100. Rudolph KL, Chang S, Millard M, Schreiber-Agus N, DePinho RA. Inhibition of experimental liver cirrhosis in mice by telomerase gene delivery. *Science* 2000;287:1253.

102. Shay JW, Wright WE. Telomerase therapeutics for cancer: challenges and new directions. *Nat Rev Drug Discov* 2006; 5:577.

GENERAL PRINCIPLES

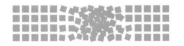

CHAPTER 5 CELL SIGNALING, GROWTH FACTORS AND THEIR RECEPTORS

LEWIS C. CANTLEY, CHRIS L. CARPENTER, WILLIAM C. HAHN, AND MATTHEW MEYERSON

SIGNAL TRANSDUCTION SYSTEMS

Signal transduction is the chemistry that allows communication at the cellular level. Cells sense signals from the extracellular and intracellular environments, as well as directly from other cells. Cells respond to these signals in a variety of ways, primarily by modifying protein levels, activities, and locations. Protein levels are controlled by rates of transcription, translation, and proteolysis, whereas protein activities are affected by covalent modifications and noncovalent interactions with other proteins and small molecules. Signal transduction pathways regulate differentiation, division, and death in the mature and developing organisms. Some pathways are common to all cells, but others are specific to specialized cells (e.g., synthesis and secretion of insulin by the pancreas, migration and phagocytosis by neutrophils). Disruption or alterations of signal transduction pathways plays a key causative role in disease. Indeed, mutations in nearly all of these signaling pathways are found in a wide range of cancers.

To emphasize the essentials of signal transduction, the focus in this chapter is on the variety of solutions to the two common problems faced by cells and organisms in signal transduction:

1. How is a signal sensed?
2. How are the levels, activities, and locations of proteins modified in response to the signal?

Most signals are initiated by ligands and are sensed by the receptors to which they bind. Binding of a ligand to a receptor stimulates the activities of proteins necessary to continue the transmission of the signal through the formation of multiprotein complexes and the generation of small-molecule second messengers. Integration of signals from multiple pathways determines the cell's ultimate response to competing and complementary signals. In addition, cell signaling pathways are highly interconnected to permit dynamic regulation of the strength, duration, and timing of cell responses.

SENSORY MACHINERY: LIGANDS AND RECEPTORS

Signals

Signal transduction pathways have evolved to respond to an enormous variety of stimuli. Molecules that initiate signaling cascades include proteins, amino acids, lipids, nucleotides, gases, and light (Table 5.1). Most extracellular signals, such as growth factors, bind to receptors on the plasma membrane, but others such as androgens or estrogen, diffuse into the cell and bind to receptors in the cytoplasm and nucleus. Some signals are continuous, such as those sent by the extracellular matrix, whereas others are episodic, like the secretion of insulin by pancreatic β cells in response to increases in blood glucose. Signaling molecules originate from a variety of sources. Some, such as neurotransmitters, are stored in the cell and are released to provide communication with other cells under specific conditions. Other ligands are stored outside the cell (e.g., in the extracellular matrix) and become accessible in response to tissue damage or remodeling. Traditionally, signals have been divided based on the cell of origin into those that affect distant cells (endocrine), nearby cells (paracrine), or the same cell (autocrine). Cells also respond to signals that arise from within. Important examples include the checkpoint pathways that ensure the orderly progression of the cell cycle and the pathways that sense and repair damaged DNA.[1]

Receptors

The plasma membrane of eukaryotic cells serves to insulate the cell from the outside environment, but this barrier must be breached to transmit signals of extracellular origin. This fundamental

TABLE 5.1

LIGANDS THAT STIMULATE SIGNAL TRANSDUCTION PATHWAYS

Types of Ligands	Examples
PROTEIN	
Soluble	Insulin
Matrix	Fibronectin
Bound to other cells	Ephrines
AMINO ACIDS	
Nucleotides	
Soluble	Adenosine triphosphate
DNA	Double-strand breaks
LIPIDS	Prostaglandins
GASES	Nitric oxide
LIGHT	Rhodopsin, visual system

problem of transmitting extracellular signals is solved in two ways. Signals cross the plasma membrane either by activating transmembrane receptors or by using ligands that are membrane permeable (Table 5.2). Cells are exquisitely sensitive to most ligands. The affinity of receptors for ligands generally is in the picomolar to nanomolar range, and very few receptors need to be occupied to transmit a signal. For example, it has been estimated that activation of ten T-cell receptors is sufficient to send a maximal signal. Cytokine-responsive cells may express only a few hundred receptors on the cell surface. Given the small number of receptors that are activated, amplification of most signals is necessary for cellular responses. A requirement for signal amplification also allows opposing or complementary pathways to affect

signal strength more efficiently.[2] As a result of ligand binding, receptors undergo conformational changes or oligomerization, or both, and the intrinsic activity of the receptor or of associated proteins is stimulated. Receptors may bind and respond to more than one ligand. For example, the epidermal growth factor (EGF) receptor binds to transforming growth factor-alpha (TGF-α), EGF, heparin-binding EGF (HB-EGF), beta-cellulin, epiregulin, epigen, and amphiregulin. The stimulation of most receptors leads to the activation of several downstream pathways that either function cooperatively to activate a common target or stimulate distinct targets. Generally, some of the pathways activated are counter-regulatory and serve to attenuate the signal. Receptors may also activate other receptors. A well-studied example is the activation of the EGF receptor by G protein-coupled receptors (GPCR), which occurs as a result of protease cleavage and activation of HB-EGF.

There are a number of transmembrane receptor families. This chapter will discuss several of them to illustrate distinct signaling mechanisms.

Receptor Tyrosine Kinases

Receptor tyrosine kinases are transmembrane proteins that have an extracellular ligand-binding domain, a transmembrane domain, and a cytoplasmic tyrosine kinase domain.[3] The ligands for these receptors are proteins or peptides. Most receptor tyrosine kinases are monomeric, but members of the insulin-receptor family are heterotetramers in which the subunits are linked by disulfide bonds. Receptor tyrosine kinases have been divided into six classes, primarily on the basis of the sequence of the extracytoplasmic domain. Examples of tyrosine kinase receptors include the insulin receptor, the platelet-derived growth factor (PDGF)

TABLE 5.2

RECEPTORS IN SIGNAL TRANSDUCTION

Types of Receptors	Examples	Types of Ligands
Tyrosine kinase	PDGF, EGF, FGF, and insulin receptors	Peptide growth factors
Serine kinase	TGF-β receptor	Activin
Heterotrimeric G protein	Thrombin, smell receptors	Thrombin
Receptors bound to tyrosine kinases	IL-2, interferon receptors	IL-2
TNF family	Fas receptor	Fas
Notch	Notch	Delta-Serrate-LAG-2
Guanylate cyclase	Atrial naturic factor receptor	Atrial natriuretic factor
Tyrosine phosphatase	CD45, LAR	Contactin
Nuclear receptors	Estrogen, androgen receptors	Estrogen
Adhesion receptors	Integrins, CD44	Fibronectin, hyaluronic acid

PDGF, platelet-derived growth factor; EGF, epidermal growth factor; FGF, fibroblast growth factor; TGF-β, transforming growth factor-β; IL-2, interleukin-2; TNF, tumor necrosis factor.

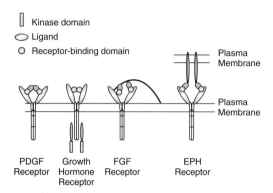

FIGURE 5.1 Dimerization of tyrosine kinase receptors. Most tyrosine kinase receptors are activated by ligand-induced dimerization. Some ligands, such as platelet-derived growth factor (PDGF), are dimeric and induce dimerization using the two receptor-binding domains. Other ligands, such as growth hormone, contain two receptor-binding domains in the same molecule. The fibroblast growth factors (FGFs) relay on proteoglycans to aid the formation of ligand dimmers. Some ligands, such as the ephrins (EPHs), are present on nearby cells and, when the cells come into contact, bind to the receptors and promote clustering.

receptor, the EGF receptor family, and the fibroblast growth factor (FGF) receptor family.

Activation of receptor tyrosine kinases is generally believed to require tyrosine phosphorylation of the receptor. In the case of the insulin receptor, an insulin-stimulated conformational change activates the kinase. Most of the tyrosine kinases are activated by oligomerization, which brings the kinase domains of distinct molecules into close proximity so that they cross-phosphorylate. Autotransphosphorylation of tyrosine in the activation loop of the kinase domain locks the kinase into a high-activity conformation, stimulating phosphorylation of other sites on the receptor, as well as other substrates. However, cancer-derived mutants of the EGF receptor may be activated without receptor autophosphorylation.[4]

Ligands stimulate receptor oligomerization in a variety of ways (Fig. 5.1). Some ligands, such as PDGF, are dimeric, so that the ligand is able to bind two receptors simultaneously.[5] Other ligands, such as growth hormone, are monomeric but have two receptor-binding sites that allow them to induce receptor dimerization.[6] FGFs are also monomeric but have only a single receptor-building site. FGF molecules bind to heparin sulfate proteoglycans, which concentrates FGF and facilitates dimerization of the FGF receptor.[7] EGF is also monomeric, but binding of EGF to the receptor changes the receptor conformation and promotes interaction with a second ligand or receptor dimmer, leading to activation.[8] Some ligand-receptor interactions result in signaling by the ligand, in addition to the receptor. Ephrins are ligands for EPH tyrosine kinase activity in the target cell, but they also stimulate signaling by ephrins in the ephrin-presenting cell.[9]

Studies of the EGF receptor-family illustrate some important concepts. The EGF-signaling pathways involve four receptors (EGF receptor, ERB2, ERB3, and ERB4) and many ligands.[10] EGF stimulates homodimerization of the EGF receptor, but, under certain conditions, heterodimerization with other family members also occurs. Activation of EGFR proceeds via asymmetric dimerization of the receptor. Ligand causes extracellular dimerization, which then causes the kinase domains to form an intracellular head-to-tail dimer, which activates the receptor.[11,12]

Receptors that Activate Tyrosine Kinases

A number of receptors do not have intrinsic enzymatic activity but stimulate associated tyrosine kinases. Important examples of this type of receptor include the cytokine and interferon receptors that associate constitutively with members of the Jak family of tyrosine kinases[13] and the multichain immune recognition receptors that activate SKF and Syk family tyrosine kinases.[14,15] The kinase appears to be inactive in the absence of ligand, but, as happens in receptors with intrinsic tyrosine kinase activity, signaling is initiated by ligand-stimulated heterodimerization and conformational changes of the receptors.

Serine-Threonine Kinase Receptors

The TGF-β family of receptors are transmembrane proteins with intrinsic serine-threonine kinase activity.[16] TGF-β ligands are dimmers that bind to and oligomerize type I and type II receptors. The type I and type II receptors homologous but distinctly regulated. The type II receptors seem to be constitutively active but do not normally phosphorylate substrates, whereas the type I receptors are normally inactive. Ligand-mediated dimerization of the type I and type II receptors causes the type II receptor to phosphorylate the type I receptor, converting it to an active kinase. Subsequent signal propagation is dependent on the kinase activity of the type I receptor and the phosphorylation of downstream substrates.

Receptor Phosphotyrosine Phosphatases

Receptor protein tyrosine phosphatases (RPTPs) have an extracellular domain, a single transmembrane-spanning domain, and cytoplasmic catalytic domains.[17] The extracellular domains of some receptor tyrosine phosphatases contain fibronectin and immunoglobulin repeats, suggesting that these receptors may recognize adhesion molecules as ligands. Several RPTPs are capable of homotypic interaction, but no true ligands are yet known for RPTPs. Most receptor tyrosine phosphatases have two catalytic domains, and both are active in at least some receptors. Functional and structural evidence suggests that the phosphatase activity of some of these receptors is inhibited by dimerization. Ligand-dependent dimerization could cause constitutively active tyrosine phosphatases to lose activity, enhancing signals emanating from tyrosine kinases. RPTPs do not always function in strict opposition to tyrosine kinases, however. For example, CD45 is necessary for signaling by the B-cell receptor, which also requires tyrosine kinase activity.[18] Since some Tyr-phosphorylation events, such as phosphorylation of a Tyr near the C-terminus of src-family protein-Tyr kinases, can be inhibitory to the Tyr kinase activity, activation of certain phospho-Tyr phosphatases can paradoxically cause an increase in global tyrosine phosphorylation (discussed in more detail below).

G Protein-Coupled Receptors

GPCRs are by far the most numerous receptors.[19] Almost 700 GPCRs are present in the human genome.[20] The number of GPCRs is so high because they encode the light, smell, and taste receptors, all of which require great diversity. These receptors have seven membrane-spanning domains: The N-terminus and three of the loops are extracellular, whereas the other three loops and the C-terminus are cytoplasmic. A wide variety of ligands bind GPCRs, including proteins and peptides, lipids, amino acids, and nucleotides. No common binding domain exists for all ligands, and interactions of ligands with GPCRs are fairly distinct.[21] In the case of the thrombin receptor, thrombin cleaves the N-terminus of the receptor, freeing a new N-terminus that self-associates with the ligand pocket, leading to activation. Amines and eicosanioids bind to the transmembrane domains of their GPCRs, whereas peptide ligands bind to the transmembrane domains of their GPCRs, and peptide ligands bind to the transmembrane domains and the extracellular loops of their GPCRs. Neurotransmitters and some peptide hormones require the N-terminus for binding and activation.

Intramolecular bonds that involve residues in the transmembrane or juxtamembrane regions keep GPCRs in an inactive conformation.[22] In the inactive state, the receptor is bound to a heterotrimeric G protein, which is also inactive. Agonist binding causes a conformational change that stimulates the guanine nucleotide exchange activity of the receptor. Exchange of guanosine triphosphate (GTP) for guanosine diphosphate (GDP) on the α-subunit of the heterotrimeric G proteins initiates signaling. Ultimately, GPCRs stimulate the same downstream pathways as other receptor types, including ion channels, cytosolic protein tyrosine and serine kinases, and enzymes that phosphorylate or hydrolyze membrane lipids.[19] Certain GPCRs also activate receptor tyrosine kinases. As mentioned earlier, GPCR-dependent cleavage of HB-EGF stimulates the EGF receptor, which is necessary for the GPCR to activate the mitogen-activated protein kinase (MAP kinase) pathway.

Notch Family of Receptors

The Notch receptor has a large extracellular domain, a single transmembrane domain, and a cytoplasmic domain.[23] Ligands for the Notch receptor are proteins expressed on the surface of adjacent cells, and activation results in two proteolytic cleavages of Notch. Initial cleavage by ADAM family proteases removes the extracellular domain and causes endocytosis. Subsequent proteolysis by the preselinin protease family releases the cytoplasmic region of Notch as a soluble signal. This fragment moves to the nucleus, where it complexes with the transcriptional repressor CBFI, relieving its inhibitory effects and stimulating transcription.

Guanylate Cyclases

Guanylate cyclases (GCs) convert guanosine triphosphate to cyclic guanosine monophosphate (cGMP) upon activation.[24] There are both transmembrane and soluble forms of GCs. The membrane GCs are receptors for atrial natriuretic hormone, peptides that regulate intestinal secretion and are necessary for regulating cGMP levels for vision. In addition to the catalytic domain, the cytoplasmic tail includes a protein kinase homology domain that lacks kinase activity. Soluble GCs are activated by nitrous oxide. These receptors are widely expressed and regulate vascular tone and neuron function. They are heterodimers and each subunit has catalytic activity.

Tumor Necrosis Factor Receptor Family

The tumor necrosis factor family of receptors has a conserved cysteine-rich region in the extracellular domain, a transmembrane domain, and a domain called the *death domain* in the cytoplasmic tail.[25] The receptors undergo oligomerization after ligand binding, which is necessary for signaling. These receptors are distinct in several respects. Stimulation of the receptor leads to recruitment of cytoplasmic proteins that bind to each other and the receptor through death domains, thereby activating a protease, caspase 8, that initiates apoptosis. Under some conditions, however, tumor necrosis factor receptors (TNFRs) stimulate antiapoptotic signals. This family of receptors also includes "decoys" or receptors that are missing all or part of the cytoplasmic tail and thus cannot transmit a signal. This feature provides a unique mechanism for inhibiting and further regulating signaling. A second class of TNFRs lack death domains but bind to TNFR-associated factors.

WNT Receptors

The Wnt family of growth and differentiation factors are small proteins that bind to cell surface receptors of the Frizzled family.[26] These receptors resemble GPCRs but utilize a unique mechanism

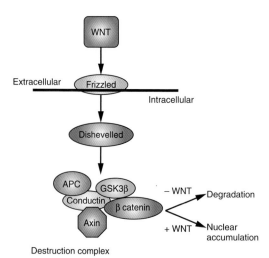

FIGURE 5.2 Wingless (Wnt)/β catenin signaling. Wnt extracellular ligands bind Frizzled receptors and regulate the phosphorylation status of axin. Axin functions as part of the destruction complex that regulates the stability of β-catenin, a transcriptional regulator.

of signal transduction (Fig. 5.2). Binding of Wnt to the receptor suppresses a kinase cascade involving the protein Ser/Thr kinases casein kinase I (CK I) and glycogen synthase kinase 3 (GSK3) and the low-density lipoprotein-related protein (LRP). Active Wnt signaling requires inactivation of Axin and the adenomatous polyposis coli (APC) protein. This complex mediates phosphorylation and ultimately proteosome-dependent degradation of β-catenin. Suppression of β-catenin degradation in response to Wnt allows β-catenin to accumulate to higher levels in the cell and to migrate into the nucleus where it regulates genes involved in cell growth regulation, acting as a heterodimer with the T-cell factor (TCF) transcription factors.

Nuclear Receptors

Ligands for nuclear hormone receptors diffuse into the cell and bind their receptors either in the cytoplasm or the nucleus. The ligands include steroids, eicosanoids, retinoids, and thyroid hormone. The sex steroids, androgens such as testosterone and estrogen and progesterone, are ligands for the androgen receptor, estrogen receptor, and progesterone receptor, respectively. Inhibition of androgen receptor is central to treatment of prostate cancer, while inhibition of estrogen receptor is central to treatment of estrogen receptor–positive breast cancer. The receptors are transcription factors that have both DNA- and ligand-binding domains. The unliganded receptor is bound to heat shock proteins that are dissociated after ligand binding. Release from the chaperone complex and ligand association

lead to binding of the receptor to cofactors and DNA to regulate transcription.

Adhesion Receptors

Cell adherence, either to the extracellular matrix or to other cells, is mediated by receptors that function mechanically and stimulate intracellular signaling pathways, primarily through tyrosine kinases.[27] Integrins mediate adherence to extracellular matrix and are composed of heterodimers of α and β subunits. They bind to an arginine/glycine/aspartate or leucine/aspartate/valine motif found in matrix molecules. Binding to ligand leads to integrin clustering and activation. Structural studies show that inactive integrins adopt a conformation that inhibits ligand binding. In this conformation the intracellular regions are also hindered from binding effector molecules.[28] Binding of ligand opens the intracellular regions so that they bind to the molecules required to transmit integrin-dependent signals. Similarly, modification of the intercellular region, such as phosphorylation, affects the conformation of the extracellular region to favor ligand binding. This is an example of a receptor that signals both "outside-in" and "inside-out." Integrin signaling is necessary for cell movement, but, in contrast to other pathways, adherence in nonmotile cells provides a continuous signal. This signal is necessary for survival of most cells. The ability to circumvent the requirement for adherence-dependent survival plays a major role in the development of human cancers by allowing tumor survival in inappropriate locations.

Propagation of Signals to the Cell Interior

Although the structures and mechanisms of the various receptors and ligands that initiate cell signaling are very different, most receptors activate a set of common downstream molecules to transmit their signals. The molecules that transmit signals include protein and lipid kinases, GTPases, phospholipases, proteases, adaptors, and adenylate cyclases (Table 5.3). These pathways lead to a broad array of responses, including changes in transcription and translation, enzymatic activities, and cell motility.

REGULATION OF PROTEIN KINASES

The balance between protein kinase and phosphatase activity controls protein phosphorylation. Protein kinases themselves, transcription factors, and cytoskeletal components are a few examples of proteins regulated by phosphorylation (Fig. 5.3).

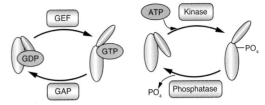

TABLE 5.3

ENZYME CLASSES STIMULATED BY ACTIVATED RECEPTORS

Enzyme Classes	Examples
PROTEIN KINASES	
Tyrosine	Jak
Serine, threonine	ERKs
PROTEIN PHOSPHATASES	
Tyrosine	SHP-2
Serine, threonine	Calcineurin
LIPID KINASES	
Phosphatidylinositol	PI3-kinase
LIPID PHOSPHATASES	
Phosphatidylinositol	SHIP, PTEN
PHOSPHOLIPASES	
A	CPLA2
C	PLCγ
D	
G PROTEINS	
Heterotrimeric	Gs, Gi
Ras-like	Ras, Rac
NUCLEOTIDE CYCLASES	
Adenylate	
Guanylate	

ERKs, Extracellular signaling-regulated kinases; PI3-kinase, phosphoinositide 3 kinase; PLC, phospholipase C.

FIGURE 5.3 Regulation of protein activity by phosphate. The exchange of guanosine triphosphate (GTP) for guanosine diphosphate (GDP) bound to G proteins induces an activating conformational change dependent on the additional γ phosphate of GTP. Guanine nucleotide exchange factors catalyze GDP/GTP exchange. GTPase-activating proteins (GAPs) accelerate the hydrolysis of GTP to GDP to remove the γ phosphate and attenuate G-protein signaling. Protein kinases add phosphate to proteins, resulting in conformational changes and changes in enzymatic activity. Protein phosphatases remove the phosphate to inhibit the signal. G proteins and protein kinase substrates undergo a similar cycle of phosphate addition and removal to regulate their activity. ATP, adenosine triphosphate; GEF, guanine nucleotide exchange factor.

Protein kinases are classified by the residues they phosphorylate. Eukaryotic cells have protein tyrosine kinases, protein serine-threonine kinases, and dual-specificity kinases that phosphorylate serine, threonine, and tyrosine residues. Important issues in understanding the role and regulation of protein phosphorylation are how specificities or kinases and phosphatases are determined and how phosphorylation alters the function of substrates. Work at the structural and functional levels has provided preliminary answers to these questions.

Most signal transduction pathways require protein tyrosine kinases. Receptors that are not themselves tyrosine kinases use several cytoplasmic tyrosine kinases, including the Src, Syk, and Jak families. Phosphorylation of proteins on tyrosine can either stimulate or inhibit enzymatic activity. In addition, phosphorylation of proteins on Tyr can lead to new protein-protein interaction. An example of how tyrosine phosphorylation regulates enzymatic activity is found in the Src family of protein tyrosine kinases, which are regulated positively and negatively by tyrosine phosphorylation.[29] Phosphorylation of a tyrosine residue in the C-phosphotyrosine and the Src homology 2 (SH2) domain blocks access of substrate to the catalytic domain. In contrast, phosphorylation of a tyrosine in the transactivation loop (T loop) of the catalytic domain stimulates the kinase activity by stabilizing the catalytic pocket in an active conformation.

The activity of many other tyrosine and serine-threonine protein kinases is regulated by phosphorylation of the activation, or T, loop. The T loop forms a lip of the catalytic pocket and may occlude the active site, preventing access of the substrate. In the case of the insulin receptor, the unphosphorylated T loop also appears to interfere with adenosine triphosphate (ATP) binding.[30] Crystallographic studies indicate that the T loop is mobile and thus is probably not always in an inhibitory confirmation, providing kinases with some constitutive activity. Low basal activity is sufficient to phosphorylate a nearby kinase (e.g., autotransphosphorylation of a partner in a dimeric receptor). After phosphorylation, the T loop undergoes a conformational change that provides much more efficient substrate access to the catalytic site.

Once a protein kinase is active, only specific substrates are phosphorylated. Specificity is determined on two properties: colocalization of the kinase with the substrate (discussed later in this chapter) and the presence of particular motifs in a substrate that can be phosphorylated by the kinase. A proline following the serine or threonine residue to be phosphorylated is absolutely required for MAP kinase substrates. In other cases, particular motifs are favored as phosphorylation sites. These motifs probably fit best into the catalytic cleft of the kinase. In some cases, sequences distant from the site of phosphorylation mediate low-affinity association of a kinase with its substrate and thereby enhance phosphorylation.

Most signaling pathways activate serine kinases, but there is also a high level of constitutive phosphorylation of proteins on serine and threonine residues. The relevance of this basal phosphorylation is still unclear. Myriad cellular functions are regulated by serine phosphorylation, ranging from the activity of transcription factors and enzymes to the polymerization of actin. Serine kinases themselves are regulated in a variety of ways. Mammalian serine-threonine kinases have been subdivided into 11 subfamilies based on primary sequence homology, which has also been predictive of related function.[31] Localization, phosphorylation, and ligand binding regulate serine kinases. Activation by ligand binding characterizes some classes of serine protein kinases. For example, cyclic nucleotides (e.g., cyclic adenosine monophosphate [cAMP]) activate the protein kinase A superfamily. Calcium and diacylglycerol (DAG) activate members of the protein kinase C (PKC) family. The protein kinase B or Akt family is activated by phosphatidylinositol (PtdIns) phosphate products of phosphoinositide-dependent kinase 1 (PDK1) to phosphorylate the activation, or T, loop. Association with cyclins activates the cyclin-dependent kinase family, and the calcium-calmodulin–dependent kinases are activated by calcium. Kinase cascades also are important in providing multiple levels of regulation and amplification of serine kinase activity. For example, MAP kinases are activated by phosphorylation of the T loop after activation of upstream kinases: Activation of Raf leads to phosphorylation and activation of MEK1, which phosphorylates and activates the extracellular signaling-regulated kinases (ERKs) (Fig. 5.4).

Protein kinase signals are generally attenuated by phosphatases, metabolism of activating second messengers, or both. Dephosphorylation of the T-loop site markedly reduces the activity of most kinases, and dephosphorylation of motifs required for protein-protein binding prevents kinases from interacting with their substrates. Phosphatases also counteract the phosphorylation of substrate molecules, reversing the effects of the kinases.

Regulation of Protein Phosphatases

Protein phosphatases remove the phosphate residues from proteins, which can either activate or inhibit signaling pathways. Protein phosphatases are divided into the same three groups as the kinases on the basis of their substrates: tyrosine phosphatases, serine-threonine phosphatases, and dual-specificity phosphatases, which use a cysteinylphosphate intermediate, whereas the serine-threonine phosphatases are metal-requiring enzymes that dephosphorylate in a single step.[32]

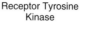

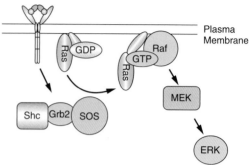

FIGURE 5.4 Activation of the extracellular signaling-regulated kinases (ERK) pathway. Many receptors activate the ERKs. Most receptor tyrosine kinases stimulate the activity of the Ras guanine nucleotide exchange factor son of sevenless (SOS), which associates with the linker proteins Shc and Grb2. The activation of Ras by SOS stimulates a protein serine kinase cascade initiated by Raf, which stimulates MEK. MEK then activates the ERKs. ERKs phosphorylate transcription factors to regulate gene expression. GDP, guanosine diphosphate; GPT, guanosine triphosphate.

Structural work has revealed how the activity of some nonreceptor tyrosine phosphatases is regulated.[33] The SHP2 phosphatase has, in addition to the catalytic domain, two SH2 domains. These domains (discussed later in this chapter) mediate binding to other proteins by direct association with phosphorylated tyrosine residues. In the inactive state, the catalytic cleft of SHP2 is blocked by the N-terminal SH2 domain. Binding of the N-terminal SH2 domain to a phosphotyrosine residue of a target protein induces a conformational change that allows substrate access to the catalytic domain. Tyrosine phosphatases act to attenuate signals that require tyrosine phosphorylation and to activate pathways inhibited by tyrosine phosphorylation. An example of the negative regulatory function of tyrosine phosphatases is the role of SHP1 (a homologue of SHP2) in inhibiting cytokine and B-cell receptor signaling. In contrast, SHP2 is necessary for cytokine stimulation of cells. On the basis of the ability of phosphatase inhibitors (e.g., vanadate) to activate tyrosine kinase-dependent signaling in the absence of ligands, acute inactivation of specific tyrosine phosphatases may play an important role in regulating the balance of tyrosine phosphorylation and dephosphorylation that controls signaling pathways. Reactive oxygen generated in response to many signals can inhibit tyrosine phosphatases by oxidizing the catalytic cysteine.

Protein phosphatase 1 (PP1), PP2, PP2B, and PP2C are the major serine-threonine phosphatases; PP1 and PP2A are composed of catalytic and regulatory subunits. PP1 affects many pathways from glycogen metabolism to the cell cycle. PP2B binds to calmodulin and is regulated by calcium.

Phosphorylation of either the regulatory or catalytic subunit affects the activity of serine phosphatases. More than 100 PP1 regulatory subunits function to target the catalytic domain to different cellular locations and mediate activation or inhibition. This illustrates how a single catalytic activity can perform multiple specific functions as a result of targeting by a regulatory subunit.

Guanosine Triphosphate-Binding Proteins

Protein-protein interaction is also an important mechanism of signal transduction. G proteins, which bind GTP, are the best-studied protein mediators that regulate other proteins by direct binding.[21] GTP-binding proteins function as digital switches. GTP binding results in a conformational change that allows G proteins to bind to effector molecules and transmit a signal (Fig. 5.3). GTP hydrolysis to GDP ultimately returns the protein to its inactive conformation. GTP-binding proteins regulate the same molecules activated by receptors: protein and lipid kinases, phosphatases, and phospholipases. GTP-binding proteins are categorized into two large classes: the heterotrimeric GTP-binding proteins and the Ras-like GTP-binding proteins. Activation of GTP-binding proteins is regulated by guanine nucleotide exchange factors that catalyze the release of GDP and allow GTP to bind. Since the concentration of GTP in the cell far exceeds that of GDP, proteins (GAPs) accelerate GTP hydrolysis, inactivating GTP-binding proteins. All GTP-binding proteins have lipid modifications that promote membrane association.

Heterotrimeric GTP-binding proteins have three subunits and are activated by GPCRs. In the inactive state, the α, β, and γ subunits form a heterotrimer. In mammalian cells, 20 α subunits, 6 β subunits, and 12 γ subunits are known. The heterotrimeric forms are divided into four classes on the basis of function. Gαs stimulates adenylate cyclase, Gαi inhibits adenylate cyclase, and Gαq activates PLC β. G12 and G13 form a related group. In general they activate the small GTPase RhoA. GPCRs have GDP/GTP exchange activity, and binding of ligand stimulates GTP binding to the subunit of heterotrimeric G proteins. In response to GTP loading, the α and β/γ subunits dissociate. The α subunits and the β/γ complex each send signals. Release of the β/γ dimmer from the α subunit exposes surfaces that allow β/γ to bind to effectors. The α and β/γ subunits regulate a wide range of downstream effectors, including ion channels, protein kinases, and phospholipases. Domains termed *regulators of G-protein signaling* act as GAPs toward the α subunit and attenuate the signal by catalyzing hydrolysis of GTP to GDP.

Ras-like GTP-binding proteins are monomeric and usually of lower molecular weight than are the heterotrimeric GTP-binding proteins. Ras-like GTP-binding proteins are classified into five families: the Ras, Rho, Rab, Arf, and Ran families. The Ras and Rho families regulate cell growth, transcription, and the actin cytoskeleton; the Arf family regulates PLD and vesicle trafficking; the Rab family regulates vesicle trafficking; and the Ran family regulates nuclear import. Ras-like GTP-binding proteins are activated in a manner similar to that of the α subunit of heterotrimeric G proteins. Exchange of GTP for GDP results in a conformational change that promotes binding to the effector molecules. In contrast to heterotrimeric G proteins, nucleotide exchange for Ras-like GTP-binding proteins is not catalyzed directly by receptor or in response to specific cellular events. Signals are attenuated by the action of GAPs, analogous to regulators of the G protein-signaling domain-containing proteins that catalyze GTP hydrolysis.

GTP-binding proteins affect the activity of their targets by causing conformational changes and perhaps by serving to localize the target. Crystal structures of the catalytic domain of adenylate cyclase bound to G proteins illustrate the conformational change.[34] Gαs binds to the C2a domain of adenylate cyclase, causing rotation of the C1a domain, which positions the catalytic residues more favorably for conversion of ATP to cAMP. Although crystal structures of small G proteins bound to portions of their targets also have been solved, the effect on the activity of target molecules as a result of binding has not yet been explained. Studies of the role in Ras in the interaction of Raf suggest that an important role of Ras is localization of Raf to the membrane, but Ras also may help to activate Raf directly.[35]

SMALL-MOLECULE SECOND MESSENGERS

Small molecules transmit signals by binding noncovalently to protein targets and affecting their function. These molecules are called *second messengers* because they are generated within the call in response to a first messenger, such as a growth factor, binding to a cell surface receptor.

cAMP was the first of the second messengers discovered. Adenylate cyclase, activated by heterotrimeric G proteins, catalyzed the synthesis of cAMP from ATP.[36] The primary target of cAMP is protein kinase A, and the activation of protein kinase A by cAMP demonstrates how second messengers function. The inactive form of protein kinase A is a tetramer of two catalytic and two regulatory subunits; the regulatory subunit contains two cAMP-binding sites. Binding of cAMP to the first site causes a conformational change that exposes the second site. Binding of cAMP to the second site results in dissociation of the regulatory and catalytic subunits. The free catalytic subunits are then active.

Phospholipase C proteins (PLCs) are common downstream effectors of signaling.[37] They cleave PtdIns-4,5-P_2 to generate two small molecule signals: inositol-1,4,5-trisphosphate (IP_3) and diaclyglycerol (DAG). All three families of PLC-β, -γ, and -δ are activated by calcium. PLC-β is also activated by the α and β/γ subunits of heterotrimeric G proteins, and PLC-γ is activated by tyrosine phosphorylation. DAG interacts with the C1 domain of PKCs to mediate their membrane localization and activation. IP_3 binds to a calcium channel in the endoplasmic reticulum (ER) and stimulates the release in cytoplasmic calcium from intracellular stores.[38] The initial increase in cytoplasmic calcium is followed by an influx of extracellular calcium via capacitive calcium channels at the plasma membrane. In unstimulated cells, cytosolic calcium is much lower than in the extracellular space of ER (100 nM vs. 1 mM), and, therefore, opening channels in the ER or plasma membrane allows calcium to flood into the cytoplasm, temporarily raising the cytoplasmic calcium to micromolar concentrations. Ultimately, calcium returns to basal levels as a result of the channels closing and removal of cytosolic calcium by both extracellular transport and pumping calcium into intracellular compartments. Calcium has a multitude of cellular effects, including directly regulating enzymatic activities, ion channels, and transcription. Several calcium-binding domains are known, including the C2 domain and EF hands. Calcium binds directly to enzymes and regulates their activity or to regulatory subunits, such as calmodulin.

Eicosanoids are ubiquitous signaling molecules that bind to GPCRs and transcription factors.[39] Eicosanoid synthesis occurs in response to a number of stimuli and is an example of rapid cell-to-cell signaling. Unlike most second messengers, eicosanoids produced in one cell escape that cell and diffuse to nearby cells and either bind to receptors or are metabolized further. Eicosanoid synthesis is regulated by the production of arachidonic acid, which is produced from DAG via diglyceride lipases or from phospholipids by PLA. PLA2s clear the sn-2 acyl group of phospholipids to produce a free fatty acid and a lysophospholipid. The calcium-regulated form of PL2 shows a preference for substrates containing arachidonic acid. The further metabolism of arachidonic acid results in the synthesis of prostaglandins and leukotrienes.

The Phosphatidyl Inositol 3′ Kinase Pathway

The phosphatidyl inositol 3 (PI3)-kinase pathway is central to intracellular signaling.[40,41] The intracellular messenger PIP3 is produced by PI3-kinase proteins, encoded by the *PIK3CA* and *PIK3R1* genes for the catalytic and regulatory subunits, respectively. PIP3 is cleaved by the lipid phosphatase protein, PTEN. PI3 signaling leads to activation of the Akt kinase and the related PDK1 kinase, and then signals through the tuberous sclerosis 1 and 2 (TSC1/TSC2) complex to the mammalian target of rapamycin (mTOR) protein (Fig. 5.5).

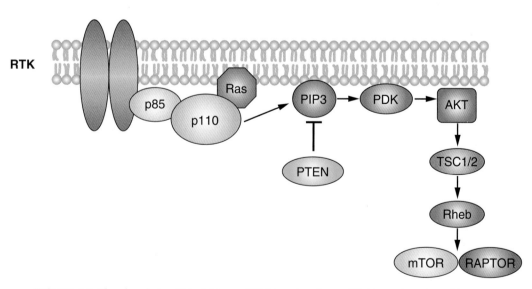

FIGURE 5.5 The phosphoinositide 3 kinase (PI3-kinase) pathway. PI3-kinase is activated by many growth factor receptors and leads to the formation of the intracellular messenger PI3. The lipid phosphatase tumor suppressor PTEN dephosphorylates PI3K. Downstream effectors include the mammalian target of rapamycin (mTOR) kinase.

EFFICIENCY AND SPECIFICITY: FORMATION OF MULTIPROTEIN SIGNALING COMPLEXES

Compartmentalization

The ability of a signal transduction pathway to transmit a signal is dependent on the probability that a protein finds its target. The likelihood of any two proteins coming into contact is proportional to their concentrations. Recruiting a protein to a specific compartment in a cell markedly increases the local concentration of that protein, thereby enhancing the probability that it will interact with other proteins or small molecules that are recruited to or generated in the same compartment. Colocalization of proteins in a signaling pathway is achieved by recruitment to the same membrane surface or organelle (e.g., plasma membrane vs. ER) and by protein-protein interactions. Conversely, separating proteins or second messengers (or both) into distinct compartments runs off signaling pathways.

Transport of signaling proteins into the nucleus is important in a number of signal transduction pathways, and it illustrates the concept of colocalization in the same organelle.[42] Nuclear transport proceeds through nuclear pores. Proteins of less than about 40 kD cross by simple diffusion, but transport of larger molecules requires a nuclear localization signal to which the importin proteins bind. The importins target the protein to the nuclear pore, and the complex is transported into the nucleus. The Ran G protein dissociates the importins from their cargo once they are in the nucleus. Regulated export of proteins from the nucleus is similar to import. A nuclear export signal is recognized by the protein exportin, which then transports the cargo out of the nucleus. A specific example is nuclear localization of the transcription factor nuclear factor of activated T cells (NFAT), which is required for its transcriptional activity.[43] In response to T-cell activation and a rise in intracellular calcium, NFAT is dephosphorylated by the calcium-responsive phosphatase calcineurin. Dephosphorylation allows the nuclear localization signal in NFAT to bind to the importins, and NFAT, along with calcineurin, is imported into the nucleus. NFAT also contains a nuclear export signal, and phosphorylation appears to allow the nuclear export signal to bind to exportin, resulting in transport to the cytoplasm.

Protein compartmentalization also occurs on a smaller scale in the form of protein-protein complexes, which serve either to target proteins to particular parts of the cell or to promote efficient signal transmission. Well-studied examples of the use of protein-protein interaction to determine the localization of enzymes include the A kinase anchoring proteins that bind to protein kinase A, a family of proteins that bind to PCK, and the subunits of PP2A.[44]

Lipid rafts are regions where sphingolipids and cholesterol are concentrated in the outer leaflet of the plasma membrane and are important sites for signaling.[45] The lipid composition provides structural cohesiveness. Rafts both concentrate and exclude proteins, promoting the formation of signaling complexes. Glycosylphosphatidylinositol-linked proteins on the extracellular surface of the plasma membrane concentrate in lipid rafts, as do acylated proteins on the intracellular surface. Transmembrane receptors can be recruited into rafts following their activation, along with their targets, leading to efficient signal generation.

Domains that Mediate Protein-Protein Binding

The regulated assembly of protein-protein complexes has several functions in signal transduction, including the formation of complexes allowing proteins to signal to each other, forming a "solid state" module that does not require diffusion to transmit a signal. Protein-protein interactions also localize an enzyme near its substrate: the binding of PLC $\gamma 1$ to the PDGF receptor brings the enzyme to the plasma membrane where its substrate, PtdIns-4, 5-P$_2$, is concentrated. These interactions are often mediated by conserved domains that recognize phosphorylated tyrosine or serine residues or proline-rich sequences (Table 5.4).

SH2 and phosphotyrosine-binding domain bind to motifs that contain phosphorylated tyrosine residues.[46] The crystal structures of several SH2 domains have been determined and reveal a pocket that binds the phosphotyrosine and a groove that determines binding specificity based on the fit of the residue's C-terminal (or, in a few cases, N-terminal) to the phosphotyrosine. Tyrosine kinases and phosphatases regulate the formation of complexes involving these domains. Tyrosine kinases themselves serve as docking sites for other proteins, which is most evident with tyrosine kinase receptors that recruit PI3-kinase, p120 Ras GAP, PLCγ, and SHP-2 through SH2 domain–dependent interactions. Tyrosine kinases phosphorylate adaptors such as the IRS and Gab families of proteins also recruit other signaling molecules through phosphotyrosine-based interactions. In addition to mediating protein-protein interactions, binding of SH2 domains also bind to intramolecular phosphotyrosines, as in the case of Src, to inhibit catalytic activity.

Phosphotyrosine-binding domains are functionally analogous to SH2 domains in that they bind phosphotyrosine sequence or structural similarity to SH2 domains. Thus, they represent an independent evolutionary solution to phosphotyphotyrosine-binding, and SH2 domains bind to a

TABLE 5.4

PROTEIN-PROTEIN INTERACTION DOMAINS AND MOTIFS

Motifs	Domains that Bind Motif	Examples of Proteins that Contain the Domain
Phosphotyrosine	SH2	Scr, PI3-kinase, SHP-2
	PTB	IRS Family, SHC
Phosphoserine	WD40	Telomerase, APAF-1, Coatamer
	14-3-3	
	WW	Pin1
	FHA	Rad53
Proline-rich	SH3	Src, PI3-kinase
	WW	YAP, Dystrophin
	EVH1	VASP, ENA, WASp
C-terminal sequences	PDZ	ZO-1, lim kinase

PI3-kinase, phosphoinositide 3 kinase; SH2, src homology 2; SH3, src homology 3.

tyrosine-containing motif in the absence of phosphorylation.

Recognition of phosphoserine motifs is also an important means of protein-protein interaction. Forkhead-associated domains, 14-3-3 proteins, and some WD40 and WW domains bind to regions of proteins containing phosphothreonine or phosphoserine.[47] WD40 domains in members of the F-box and ubiquitination and subsequent proteolysis of proteins. A prominent example of this pathway is degradation of the inhibitor of κB (IκB), which regulates the activity of the transcription factor nuclear factor κB (NF-κB). The 14-3-3 proteins are a family of small proteins whose primary function is binding to phosphoserine or phosphothreonine motifs. An example of the importance of this interaction is the role of 14-3-3 in regulating the nuclear location of the phosphatase Cdc25 that regulates the cell cycle. Binding of 14-3-3 to phosphorylated Cdc25 leads to its export from the nucleus and blocks the cell cycle.

Src homology 3 (SH3), WW, and ena-vasp homology domains are structurally distinct, but all bind to proline-rich sequences. Many proteins that contain SH3 domains also have proline-rich regions that could be involved in intramolecular binding, suggesting that a conformational change in the protein could disrupt intramolecular binding and allow the SH3 domain to interact with other proteins. Similarly, the accessibility of proline-rich regions to SH3 domains may be regulated by conformational changes that expose the proline-rich region or disrupt an intramolecular interaction.

PDZ domains recognize motifs in the C-termini of proteins and bind to each other and lipids.[48] These C-terminal motifs are found in cytoplasmic proteins, many of which also contain multiple PDZ domains. PDZ domain-containing proteins function to aggregate transmembrane proteins, such as the glutamate receptor. Group I PDZ domains bind to a consensus sequence, T/S-X-V/I, where V/I is the C-terminus of the protein. In some cases, phosphorylation of the S or T in this motif disrupts PDZ domain binding. For example, phosphorylation of this serine in the β_2-adrenergic receptor was shown to lead to a loss of PDZ domain–mediated binding to EBP50, which regulates endocytic sorting of receptor.

Domains that Mediate Protein Binding to Membrane Lipids

Localization of proteins to membranes greatly limits the space in which they can diffuse and increases the probability that enzymes and substrates will contact each other. A variety of domains have evolved to bind phospholipids as a means of membrane localization (Table 5.5). C1 domains present in PKCs and some other signaling molecules bind to DAG, thereby recruiting PKCs to the membrane.[49] Membrane recruitment of PKCs is also aided by the C2 domain, which binds to anionic phospholipids in the presence of calcium. This pathway is controlled by DAG production by PLC-dependent hydrolysis of PtdIns-4,5-P$_2$.

Several different domains bind to phosphoinositides, localizing the proteins that contain them to membranes.[50] These domains include pleckstrin homology (PH), Phox, FYVE, FERM, and ENTH domains. Particular PH domains bind specific phosphoinositides, including PtdIns-3-P, PtdIns-4,5-P$_2$, PtdIns-3,4-P$_2$, and PtdIns-3,4,5-P$_3$. Phox and FYVE domains typically bind to PtdIns-3-P.

TABLE 5.5

DOMAINS THAT BIND PHOSPHOLIPIDS

Phospholipid	Domains that Bind
Diacylglycerol	C1
Phosphatidic acid	PX
PtdIns-4-P	PH
PtdIns-3-P	PX, PH, FYVE
PtdIns-3,4-P_2	PH, PX
PtdIns-3,5-P_2	PH
PtdIns-4,5-P_2	PH, Tubby, FERM, Sprouty, ENTH, ANTH
PtdIns-3,4,5-P_3	PH

PH, pleckstrin homology.

FERM and ENTH domains bind to PtdIns-4,5-P_2. The accessibility of the domain and the availability of PtdIns phosphates regulate these interactions. Phosphoinositide kinases synthesize phosphoinositides. PtdIns4-kinases synthesize PtdIns-4-P from PtdIns. Type I PtdIns phosphate kinases phosphorylate PtdIns-4-P at the 5 position to make PtdIns-4,5-P_2. Phosphoinositide levels are also regulated by phosphatases. PTEN and related phosphatases remove the phosphate from the 3 position of the PtdIns-3,4,5-P_3. PtdIns-3,4-P_2, and PtdIns-3-P.[51] PTEN thus counteracts PI3-kinase signals, and cells lacking PTEN expression have increased signaling through PI3-kinase–dependent pathways. A family of phosphatases that removes the phosphate from the 5 position of PtdIns-3,4,5-P_3, the SH2 inositol phosphatases (SHIP1 and SHIP2), also regulates phosphoinositide signaling pathways.[52]

Acute production of specific phosphoinositides in a membrane compartment results in the recruitment of proteins containing PH domains that recognize that phosphoinositide. Colocalization of a subset of proteins allows them to interact more efficiently. An example of the role of PH domains in such a pathway is the activation of Akt by PDK1.[53] PDK1 and Akt are protein serine-threonine kinases that contain PH domains that bind PtdIns-3,4-P_2 or PtdIns-3,4,5-P_3. Activation of PI3-kinase leads to local synthesis of PtdIns-3,4-P_2 and PtdIns-3,4,5-P_3, which causes recruitment of Akt and PDK1 to the same membrane location. This localization facilitates phosphorylation and activation of Akt by PDK1.

Regulation of Protein Levels: Transcription, Translation, and Proteolysis

In addition to influencing the activity of proteins in the cell, signal transduction pathways also regulate the type and levels of proteins expressed in cells. This sort of regulation is necessary for development, differentiation, and the specific function of distinct cell types. Whether a protein is expressed at all in a cell is regulated at the transcriptional level, whereas transcription, translation, and proteolysis have a role in determining the concentration of a protein in a cell.

Ultimately, most signal transduction pathways regulate gene transcription and, thus, the level and type of proteins expressed in the cell. Analysis of the effects of stimuli on gene expression profiles using microarray analysis has shown that a single stimulus affects the transcription of hundreds of genes. The ability to transcribe a gene is regulated at multiple levels, including the structure of chromatin in the region of the gene, modifications of the promoter regions, and the activity of transcription factors and coactivators. Signal transduction pathways regulate histone acetylases and deacetylases that determine the accessibility of chromatin to the transcriptional apparatus. Recent work has shown that a number of signals lead to histone hyperacetylation that disrupts the nucleosome to allow transcription. These pathways cooperate with the activation of transcription factors.

Signal transduction pathways regulate transcription factors in numerous ways. The binding of ligands to the nuclear receptor family of transcription factors causes dissociation of the receptor from a complex with heat shock proteins and allows the receptor to bind to DNA. Tyrosine phosphorylation of the STAT family of transcription factors by Jak kinases in response to stimulation of cytokine receptors allows them to dimerize through their SH2 domains, enter the nucleus, and bind to DNA.[54] TGF-β receptors activate transcription by phosphorylating SMAD proteins on serine residues. Phosphorylation of SMAD proteins promotes heterodimerization with SMAD4 and exposes the DNA-binding domain. Activated SMADs translocate to the nucleus complex with a protein called Fast1 and bind to DNA to regulate transcription.

Activation of transcription factors also occurs much farther downstream from the receptor. Stimulation of the transcriptional activity of Elk-1 by EGF requires a Ras exchange factor, which leads to activation of Ras. Active Ras stimulates Raf. Raf in turn phosphorylates and activates MEK1, which phosphorylates and activates ERK. Active ERK translocates to the nucleus and phosphorylates Elk-1.

Translation is controlled at several levels.[55] The sequences of some RNAs result in stable tertiary structures that bind proteins to regulate location or translation. The ability of these types of RNAs to be translated is regulated by protein kinase cascades. A common mechanism is phosphorylation of initiation factor eIF-4E. p70[56] kinase regulates the translation of specific RNAs containing a 5′ terminal oligopyrimidine tract by phosphorylation of the ribosomal S6 protein. This increases the ability of the ribosome to process such messages.

The levels of some proteins are regulated by proteolysis, which occurs either via the proteosome or the lysosome. Ubiquitination targets proteins to the proteosome but can also regulate other aspects of protein function.[56] An example of the role of ubiquitination is the regulation of IκB levels (introduced previously). Phosphorylation of IκB is stimulated by a number of receptor-mediated signaling pathways and leads to its dissociation from NF-κB and allows NF-κB to enter the nucleus and bind DNA. After phosphorylation, the β-transducin repeat-containing protein binds to IκB, recruiting ubiquitin ligase that catalyzes the ubiquitination of IκB and leads to its recognition and degradation by the proteosome.

The second major pathway of protein degradation is the lysosomal pathway. An early response to the stimulation of receptors is their internalization into endosomes. Some receptors continue to signal following endocytosis.[57] In the case of receptor tyrosine kinases, ligand-dependent kinase activity is necessary for endocytosis, mediated by clathrin-coated pits. After endocytosis, receptors recycle to the plasma membrane of the endosomes and fuse with lysosomes, leading to degradation of the receptor.

SIGNALING NETWORKS

Although signaling pathways are usually depicted as linear cascades, nearly all signaling pathways are highly interconnected and form networks that allow dynamic regulation of the timing, strength, and duration of signaling. In addition, both feed forward and feed backward loops provide the means to self-regulate signaling or to integrate signaling from multiple signals simultaneously.

As a consequence, the same signal may induce different outcomes depending on the particular cell or cell state. For example, TGFβ can stimulate cell proliferation or arrest in different cells. With the development of small molecule and antibody inhibitors that show exquisite specificity for their targets, inhibition of one part of a signaling cascade may lead to cell death in some contexts and paradoxical proliferation in others. For example, a small molecule inhibitor of the serine-threonine kinase BRAF in some melanomas that harbor an activated mutant BRAF leads to cell death, while this same inhibitor can lead to increased proliferation in tumor cells that contain a normal BRAF gene but instead have an activating mutation in KRAS.[58–60] Thus, deciphering specific pathways as well as their interconnections is necessary to understand how cells and tissues respond to physiologic and pathologic stimuli as well as to predict the response to therapy.

Selected References

The full list of references for this chapter appears in the online version.

1. Kao J, Rosenstein BS, Peters S, Milano MT, Kron SJ. Cellular response to DNA damage. Ann N Y Acad Sci 2005;1066:243.
2. Ferrell JE Jr. Self-perpetuating states in signal transduction: positive feedback, double-negative feedback and bistability. Curr Opin Cell Biol 2002;14:140.
3. Schlessinger J. Cell signaling by receptor tyrosine kinases. Cell 2000;103:211.
4. Rothenberg SM, Engelman JA, Le S, et al. Modeling oncogene addiction using RNA interference. Proc Natl Acad Sci U S A 2008;105:12480.
5. Fretto LJ, Snape AJ, Tomlinson JE, et al. Mechanism of platelet-derived growth factor (PDGF) AA, AB, and BB binding to alpha and beta PDGF receptor. J Biol Chem 1993; 268:3625.
6. de Vos AM, Ultsch M, Kossiakoff AA. Human growth hormone and extracellular domain of its receptor: crystal structure of the complex. Science 1992;255:306.
7. Spivak-Kroizman T, Lemmon A, Dikic A, et al. Heparin-induced oligomerization of FGF molecules is responsible for FGF receptor dimerization, activation, and cell proliferation. Cell 1994;79:1015.
8. Schlessinger J. Ligand-induced, receptor-mediated dimerization and activation of EGF receptor. Cell 2002;110:669.
10. Harris RC, Chung E, Coffey RJ. EGF receptor ligands. Exp Cell 2003;284:2.
11. Zhang X, Pickin KA, Bose R, et al. Inhibition of the EGF receptor by binding of MIG6 to an activating kinase domain interface. Nature 2007;450:741.

12. Zhang X, Gureasko J, Shen K, Cole PA, Kuriyan J. An allosteric mechanism for activation of the kinase domain of epidermal growth factor receptor. Cell 2006;125:1137.
13. Kerr IM, Costa-Pereira AP, Lillemeier BF, Strobl B. Of JAKs, STATs, blind watchmakers, jeeps and trains. FEBS Lett 2003;546:1.
14. Mustelin T, Abraham RT, Rudd CE, Alonso A, Merlo JJ. Protein tyrosine phosphorylation in T cell signaling. Front Biosci 2002;7:d918.
15. Gauld SB, Dal Porto JM, Cambier JC. B cell antigen receptor signaling: roles in cell development and disease. Science 2002;296:1641.
16. Shi Y, Massague J. Mechanisms of TGF-beta signaling from cell membrane to the nucleus. Cell 2003;113:685.
17. Tonks NK. Protein tyrosine phosphatases: from genes, to function, to disease. Nat Rev Mol Cell Biol 2006;7: 833.
19. Pierce KL, Premont RT, Lefkowitz RJ. Seven-transmembrane receptors. Nat Rev Mol Cell Biol 2002;3:639.
21. Wettschureck N, Offermanns S. Mammalian G proteins and their cell type specific functions. Physiol Rev 2005;85: 1159.
24. Murad F. Shattuck lecture. Nitric oxide and cyclic GMP in cell signaling and drug development. N Engl J Med 2006; 355:2003.
26. van Amerongen R, Nusse R. Towards an integrated view of Wnt signaling in development. Development 2009;136: 3205.
27. Arnaout MA, Mahalingam B, Xiong JP. Integrin structure, allostery, and bidirectional signaling. Annu Rev Cell Dev Biol 2005;21:381.

29. Bjorge JD, Jakymiw A, Fujita DJ. Selected glimpses into the activation and function of Src kinase. *Oncogene* 2000;19:5620.

30. Hubbard SR. Protein tyrosine kinases: autoregulation and small-molecule inhibition. *Curr Opin Struct Biol* 2002;12:735.

31. Manning G, Whyte DB, Martinez R, Hunter T, Sudarsanam S. The protein kinase complement of the human genome. *Science* 2002;298:1912.

32. Barford D, Das AK, Egloff MP. The structure and mechanism of protein phosphatases: insights into catalysis and regulation. *Annu Rev Biophys Biomol Struct* 1998;27:133.

33. Barford D, Neel BG. Revealing mechanisms for SH2 domain mediated regulation of the protein tyrosine phosphatase SHP-2. *Structure* 1998;6:249.

34. Simonds WF. G protein regulation of adenylate cyclase. *Trends Pharmacol Sci* 1999;20:66.

35. Chong H, Vikis HG, Guan KL. Mechanisms of regulating the Raf kinase family. *Cell Signal* 2003;15:463.

37. Rhee SG. Regulation of phosphoinositide-specific phospholipase C. *Annu Rev Biochem* 2001;70:281.

39. Soberman RJ, Christmas P. The organization and consequences of eicosanoid signaling. *J Clin Invest* 2003;111:1107.

40. Bunney TD, Katan M. Phosphoinositide signalling in cancer: beyond PI3K and PTEN. *Nat Rev Cancer* 2010;10:342.

41. Grant S. Cotargeting survival signaling pathways in cancer. *J Clin Invest* 2008;118:3003.

42. Lei EP, Silver PA. Protein and RNA export from the nucleus. *Dev Cell* 2002;2:261.

43. Hogan PG, Chen L, Nardone J, Rao A. Transcriptional regulation by calcium, calcineurin, and NFAT. *Genes Dev* 2003;17:2205.

44. Virshup DM. Protein phosphatase 2A: a panoply of enzymes. *Curr Opin Cell Biol* 2000;12:180.

46. Schlessinger J, Lemmon MA. SH2 and PTB domains in tyrosine kinase signaling. *Sci STKE* 2003;2003(191):RE12.

47. Yaffe MB, Elia AE. Phosphoserine/threonine-binding domains. *Curr Opin Cell Biol* 2001;13:131.

48. Nourry C, Grant SG, Borg JP. PDZ domain proteins: plug and play! *Sci STKE* 2003;2003(179):RE7.

50. Hurley JH. Membrane binding domains. *Biochim Biophys Acta* 2006;1761:805.

51. Maehama T, Taylor GS, Dixon JE. PTEN and myotubularin: novel phosphoinositide phosphatases. *Annu Rev Biochem* 2001;70:247.

52. Rohrschneider LR, Fuller JF, Wolf I, Liu Y, Lucas DM. Structure, function, and biology of SHIP proteins. *Genes Dev* 2000;14:505.

53. Mora A, Komander D, van Aalten DM, Alessi DR. PDK1, the master regulator of AGC kinase signal transduction. *Semin Cell Dev Biol* 2004;15:161.

54. Levy DE, Darnell JE Jr. Stats: transcriptional control and biological impact. *Nat Rev Mol Cell Biol* 2002;3:651.

55. Dever TE. Gene-specific regulation by general translation factors. *Cell* 2002;108:545.

56. Kerscher O, Felberbaum R, Hochstrasser M. Modification of proteins by ubiquitin and ubiquitin-like proteins. *Annu Rev Cell Dev Biol* 2006;22:159.

57. Di Fiore PP, De Camilli P. Endocytosis and signaling. an inseparable partnership. *Cell* 2001;106:1.

58. Hatzivassiliou G, Song K, Yen I, et al. RAF inhibitors prime wild-type RAF to activate the MAPK pathway and enhance growth. *Nature* 2010;464:431.

59. Poulikakos PI, Zhang C, Bollag G, Shokat KM, Rosen N. RAF inhibitors transactivate RAF dimers and ERK signalling in cells with wild-type BRAF. *Nature* 2010;464:427.

60. Heidorn SJ, Milagre C, Whittaker S, et al. Kinase-dead BRAF and oncogenic RAS cooperate to drive tumor progression through CRAF. *Cell* 2010;140:209.

GENERAL PRINCIPLES

CHAPTER 6 CELL CYCLE

STEVEN I. REED

Cell division is a process that must be carried out with absolute fidelity. The program of generating an adult organism from a single zygote involves countless cell duplications, each requiring the precise partitioning of genetic material and most other cellular components to daughter cells. The division process then continues during adult life to replenish essential cells restricted to a limited lifespan. As a result, organisms have evolved cell-duplication strategies that include redundant safeguards to prevent errors or, if errors occur, to correct them. Nevertheless, errors do occur at a measurable frequency, and mutations accumulated over time can weaken protective mechanisms, rendering the genome increasingly vulnerable to challenges. The resulting loss of genetic and genomic stability has serious implications for survival in that it is a major contributing factor to the development of malignancy. Indeed, cancer is one of the leading causes of mortality in humans.

In this chapter, the basic principles of mammalian cell division and the mechanisms that have evolved to safeguard the integrity of the process are reviewed. Then there is a discussion of how the normal control mechanisms of cell division and protective safeguards become subverted in cancer cells. It is hoped that, ultimately, detailed knowledge of cell division in normal and cancer cells will lead to rational effective therapeutic approaches.

CELL-CYCLE ENGINE

Although the details of cell division vary considerably across phylogenetic lines and even in different cell types within the same organism, the underlying infrastructure that mediates and controls the cell division process is remarkably conserved. If one compares yeast cells and mammalian cells in culture, perhaps the two most aggressively studied model cell division systems are not only the respective cell division cycles organized along a similar scheme, but many of the proteins used in the cell division pathway are easily recognizable as being evolutionarily related. Indeed, some of these proteins are so highly conserved that they are functional in the heterologous organism despite a billion years of divergent evolution.

Phases of the Cell Cycle

As alluded to previously, the basic organization of the cell cycle is highly conserved in eukaryotic evolution. In 1951, Howard and Pelc,[1] studying the division of plant root cells, separated the process into four phases eventually referred to as *GAP1*, *synthetic phase*, *GAP2*, and *mitosis*. The shorthand that emerged from this descriptive work (G_1, S phase, G_2, and M phase or mitosis) has been the lens through which all subsequent dividing cells have been observed, and the four successive phases are referred to collectively as the *cell cycle*. The key observation made by these investigators was that the events that together make up the cell division process do not all occur continuously. Specifically, although growth and protein synthesis occur constantly for the most part, synthesis of DNA occurs only during a discrete interval. The preceding phase was designated *GAP1* or G_1, and the subsequent phase before cell division was referred to as *GAP2* or G_2. Although at the time little could be said concerning what a cell did during these silent "gap" phases, it is now known that these are not idle periods in a cell's life but the intervals in which most regulation of the cell cycle is specifically exerted. A large amount of information, originating from the external environment and the cell's internal milieu, is integrated during the G_1 and G_2 intervals and used to determine whether and when to proceed into S phase and M phase, respectively.

Mitosis, the most visibly dynamic interval of the cell cycle, has itself been traditionally subdivided into five phases: prophase, prometaphase, metaphase, anaphase, and telophase. In metazoans and plants (as opposed to fungi) mitosis entails a particularly dramatic change of state for the cell. During prophase most of the internal membranous compartments of the cell, including the nucleus, are disassembled and dispersed. Replicated chromosomes (chromatids) are condensed into paired compact rods, and a bipolar microtubule spindle is assembled. Biosynthesis of proteins (transcription and translation) largely ceases. During prometaphase, chromosomes form bivalent attachments to the spindle, driving them to the cellular equator. Proper alignment of paired chromatids on the spindle is indicative of metaphase. During anaphase, the paired sister chromatids lose cohesion and microtubule forces separate the chromatids and pull them to opposite poles of the cell. During telophase, the events of prophase are reversed: The nuclei and other membrane structures reassemble, the chromosomes decondense, and protein synthesis resumes. After mitosis, the two daughter cells pull apart and separate in a process known as *cytokinesis*.

Current knowledge of the cell cycle has accrued historically from a number of different experimental approaches and systems. In the early 1970s, experiments carried out by fusing mammalian cells in different cell-cycle phases revealed the existence of dominant inductive activities for the S phase and the M phase.[2,3] Shortly thereafter, similar inductive activities were isolated from mature frog eggs arrested at meiotic metaphase II and shown to be capable of inducing G_2 oocytes to enter into meiotic divisions,[4] equivalent in many respects to mitosis. At the same time, genetic analysis of cell division in yeast revealed that the products of individual genes controlled specific events in the cell cycle and that these events could be organized in pathways, much like metabolic pathways.[5] Eventually, all of these lines of investigation converged in the 1980s, leading to the discovery of cyclin-dependent kinases (CDKs).

Cyclin-Dependent Kinases

Arguably the most significant advance in understanding cell-cycle regulation was the discovery of CDKs.[6] These are binary, proline-directed, serine-threonine–specific protein kinases that consist of a catalytic subunit (the CDK) that has little if any intrinsic enzymatic activity and a requisite positive regulatory subunit known as a *cyclin*. In yeast, one CDK and numerous cyclins carry out cell-cycle regulatory functions, whereas in mammals, these same functions are carried out by a number of different CDKs and cyclins. In yeast, in which multiple cyclins activate the same CDK (CDK1, also known as Cdc28 or Cdc2, depending on the species) for distinct cell-cycle tasks, it is clear that most if not all substrate specificity beyond a rather degenerate primary structure target consensus lies in the cyclin subunit. In mammals, it is likely that substrate specificity is shared by CDK and cyclin subunits. Although not all pairwise combinations are permitted, there are enough combinatorial possibilities to create a significant level of substrate specificity.

CDKs have a structure similar to that of other protein kinases, consisting of two globular domains (the N-lobe and C-lobe) held together by a semi-flexible hinge region. Protein substrates bound by the active enzyme are thought to fit into a cleft between the two domains. The N-lobe contains the adenosine triphosphate (ATP)–binding site. Studies comparing CDKs and CDK-cyclin complexes based on x-ray diffraction crystallography indicate that the primary role of the cyclin, in addition to substrate docking functions, is to realign critical active site residues into a catalytically permissive configuration and to open the catalytic cleft to accommodate substrates.[7] Once bound to a cyclin, the CDK active site is configured similarly to other protein kinases that do not require cyclin binding.

The known CDKs and cyclins and their presumptive intervals of function in the mammalian cell cycle are summarized in Figure 6.1. For the

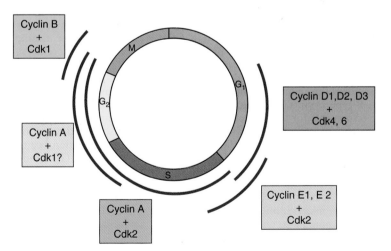

FIGURE 6.1 Windows of cyclin-dependent kinase (CDK) function in the cell cycle. D-type cyclins (cyclins D1, D2, and D3) activate CDK4 and CDK6 for functions extending from middle G_1 to the G_1/S-phase transition. E-type cyclins (cyclins E1 and E2) activate CDK2 for functions at the G_1/S-phase boundary, probably extending into early S phase. Cyclin A activates CDK2 for functions extending from the G_1/S-phase boundary and extending into G_2. Cyclin A is known to interact with CDK1 as well; however, no specific function for this complex has been identified. Finally, cyclin B activates CDK1 at the G_2/M-phase boundary with activity that lasts until cyclin B is degraded during anaphase.

most part, the functional intervals of CDKs are determined by the accumulation and disappearance of cyclins. Whereas CDKs tend to be expressed at a constant level through the cell cycle, cyclin accumulation is usually dynamic, regulated at the level of biosynthesis and degradation (discussed in greater detail in "Cell-Cycle Machinery"). To summarize, three partially redundant D-type cyclins (D1, D2, and D3) activate two partially redundant CDKs (CDK4 and CDK6). Although, unlike most other cyclins, D-type cyclins do not appear to be expressed with high periodicity in cycling cells, the interval at which their primary activating function is thought to occur is from mid-to-late G_1 to direct phosphorylation of the cell-cycle inhibitor pRb and related proteins p107 and p130. Phosphorylation of these proteins by cyclin D–CDK4/6 inactivates their negative regulatory functions, allowing progression into S phase.[8,9]

Unlike D-type cyclins, E-type cyclins (E1 and E2) are expressed with high cell-cycle periodicity, accumulating in late G_1 and declining during S phase. E-type cyclins activate CDK2, and the fact that premature expression of cyclin E1 leads to accelerated entry into S phase[10,11] has suggested that the target(s) must be proteins responsible for initiation of DNA replication. However, the essentiality of cyclin E–CDK2 in this context has been put into question by the demonstration that cells from cyclin E1/E2 nullizygous mouse embryos can cycle with reasonably normal kinetics and can certainly initiate DNA replication.[12] The most likely explanation for the dispensability of E-type cyclins for S phase functions is redundancy with cyclin A, which also activates CDK2.

Cyclin A accumulates initially at the G_1/S-phase boundary and persists until prometaphase of mitosis. It has been best characterized as an activator of CDK2; however, it has also been reported to form complexes with CDK1. It is presumed that CDK2, activated by E-type cyclins and cyclin A, promotes cell-cycle progression from the G_1/S boundary through the G_2 interval.

At this time, B-type cyclins, in conjunction with CDK1, are responsible for getting cells into and through mitosis. Although mammalian cells express a number of B-type cyclins, only cyclin B1 appears to be essential. Cyclin B1 accumulates through S phase and G_2 and then is degraded at the metaphase-anaphase transition. It should be pointed out that the CDK family is extensive and that eukaryotes possess many additional CDKs that ostensibly have nothing to do with cell-cycle regulation.

The blueprint for CDK function through the mammalian cell cycle presented here is based on a large body of experimental evidence and most likely accounts for primary activities at each cell-cycle stage. However, this model does not account for potential redundancy of CDK function. Recently, however, it has been demonstrated that

a *CDK2*-nullizygous mouse is viable, and furthermore, relatively normal.[13,14] Investigation of embryonic fibroblasts from these mice has suggested that in the absence of CDK2, CDK1 can carry out the functions normally attributed to CDK2.[15] However, the contribution of CDK1 to these functions in unperturbed cells remains to be determined.

Modes of Cyclin-Dependent Kinase Regulation

Because the activity of CDKs is central to cell survival, these enzymes are, of necessity, highly regulated.[6] As a result, a number of diverse regulatory mechanisms have evolved to allow for integration of environmental and internal signals (Fig. 6.2). A primary mode of CDK regulation is the availability of activating cyclins, as alluded to previously. For most cell-cycle regulatory CDKs, the relevant cyclins exhibit a distinct temporal program of accumulation and degradation, determining a precise window of CDK activation. Although D-type cyclins tend not to be highly regulated in cycling cells, they are strongly down-regulated as cells exit the cell cycle into a nonproliferative state and then resynthesized in response to mitogen stimulation and cell-cycle re-entry. The genes encoding cyclin E1 and E2 are transcribed periodically late in G_1 and up to the G_1-S phase transition. This, coupled with ubiquitin-mediated proteolysis of cyclin E in active cyclin E–CDK2 complexes, creates the observed window of cyclin E accumulation from late G_1 to mid-S phase.

Like cyclin E, the accumulation of cyclin A is determined by periodic transcription. However, unlike cyclin E, cyclin A remains stable in active CDK2 complexes. The timing of ubiquitin-mediated proteolysis of cyclin A is determined by activation of a protein-ubiquitin ligase known as the *anaphase-promoting complex/cyclosome* (APC/C) in prometaphase. Thus, the window of cyclin A accumulation is from the G_1-S transition until early in mitosis. Finally, B-type cyclin accumulation is also linked to periodic transcription. In this case, transcription begins in late S phase and persists through G_2. Similarly to cyclin A, B-type cyclins are targeted for ubiquitin-mediated proteolysis by the APC/C during mitosis, although their disappearance occurs slightly later in mitosis than that of cyclin A.

It is interesting to note that periodic transcription of cyclins E, A, and B mRNAs relies primarily on negative regulation. For cyclin E, an element known as *CERM* (cyclin E repressor module) binds a repressor complex containing the repressive member of the E2F family of transcription factors, E2F4, as well as the Rb-related protein p107 and a histone deacetylase.[16] Inactivation of the repressive complex in late G1 via phosphorylation of p107

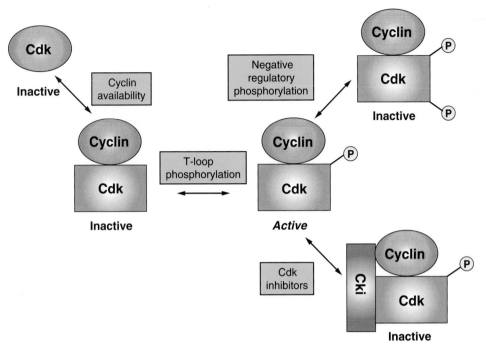

FIGURE 6.2 Principles of cyclin-dependent kinase (CDK) regulation. Because CDK catalytic subunits are inactive when unbound to cyclins, the first level of regulation is through the expression and availability of cyclins. The second level of regulation appears to constitute a housekeeping function in that cyclin binding stimulates an essential phosphorylation of a threonine within a structural feature known as the *T loop*. Binary complexes with phosphorylated T loops are active. Such active kinase complexes can be subjected to negative regulation in two ways. Additional phosphorylation events on threonine 14 and tyrosine 15 (or the equivalent residues) render the kinase inactive. In addition, the formation of ternary complexes with CDK inhibitory proteins (Ckis) promotes an inactive state. One class of Cki, INK4, specific for CDK4 and CDK6, can inhibit by forming binary complexes directly with the CDK.

by CDK4/6 allows the constitutive transcription factor, Sp1, to drive cyclin E transcription. Transcription of cyclin A and B mRNAs is similarly regulated. In this case, the repressor element is known as cell cycle genes homology region (CHR)[17] but the corresponding repressor complex has not yet been well characterized. However, once repression is relieved, transcription of both cyclin A and B mRNAs is driven the constitutive transcription factor, NF-Y.

A second important mode of CDK regulation is by phosphorylation. CDKs require an activating phosphorylation on a structural feature designated the *T loop*. Phosphorylation induces a movement of the T loop that has global effects on CDK structure, including an increase in CDK-cyclin contacts and changes in the substrate-binding site.[18] In most if not all instances, T-loop phosphorylation appears to constitute a housekeeping function that occurs concomitant with cyclin binding. However, negative regulatory phosphorylation of CDKs is a highly dynamic process. Proper cell-cycle regulation of CDK1, in particular, requires phosphorylation on two residues within the N-lobe, adjacent to the ATP-binding site: threonine 14 and tyrosine 15. During the normal course of the cell cycle, as

cyclin B–CDK1 complexes accumulate, they are immediately phosphorylated at these sites and thereby kept inactive. This allows stockpiling of the large numbers of cyclin B–CDK1 complexes required for efficient entry into mitosis and maintaining them in an inactive state during late S phase and G_2. At the G_2/M-phase boundary, there is concerted dephosphorylation of these residues, causing cells to advance rapidly into mitosis. Although CDK2 and CDK4 have also been reported to undergo negative regulatory phosphorylation at the homologous residues, the function(s) of this regulation are not as clear-cut (but see "DNA Damage Checkpoints").

A third mode of CDK regulation is through the action of inhibitory proteins that can form either binary complexes with CDKs or ternary complexes with cyclin-CDK dimers. These exist in three major families. The INK4 family consists of four members (p15, p16, p18, and p19). All are composed of a series of conserved structural motifs known as *ankyrin repeats* and they specifically target CDK4 and CDK6. The mechanism of action of these inhibitors is to bind the CDK subunit and, by causing a rotation of the N-lobe relative to the C-lobe, constraining the kinase in an inactive conformation and, in addition, precluding cyclin binding.[19] The Cip/Kip family consists of three members in mammals: p21[Cip1], p27[Kip1], and p57[Kip2]. All contain a conserved amino terminal cyclin–CDK–binding inhibitory domain and a divergent C-terminal domain possessing other less well-characterized functions. Although these have been characterized primarily as potent inhibitors of CDK2 and have more recently been shown to also be effective CDK1 inhibitors, the case for inhibition of CDK4 and CDK6 is less certain. Whereas Cip/Kip inhibitors are clearly capable of inhibiting CDK4 and CDK6 at high concentration, it is not clear that these conditions are met *in vivo*, and the situation is further complicated by the finding that Cip/Kip inhibitor binding is actually required to provide a chaperonin or assembly function for the efficient formation of active cyclin D–CDK4 complexes.[20] In the case of cyclin A–CDK2, where structural studies have been carried out, it appears that the Cip/Kip inhibitors first anchor via a high-affinity interaction with the cyclin.[21] This then allows the inhibitor polypeptide to invade and deform the N-lobe, thus interfering with ATP binding and catalysis.[16] The final class of inhibitors consists of two members of the pRb protein family, p107 and p130. Although these proteins have well-characterized functions as transcriptional inhibitors, they also are potent cyclin E/A–CDK2 inhibitors. p107 and p130 each contain cyclin-binding and CDK-binding sites that collaborate to confer inhibitory activity.

A final mode of CDK regulation is via control of nuclear import/export. This level of regulation is most obvious for cyclin B–CDK1 complexes, which are kept out of the nucleus via active nuclear export until late G_2, when phosphorylation inactivates *cis*-acting nuclear export signals allowing nuclear accumulation.[22] Sequestration of cyclin B–CDK1 in the cytoplasm is a redundant mechanism, along with negative regulatory phosphorylation of CDK1, for preventing premature phosphorylation of mitotic targets.

INDUCTION OF CELL-CYCLE PHASE TRANSITIONS

The cell cycle is composed of two action phases, S phase and M phase, in which the genetic material is duplicated and the components of a mother cell are divided into two daughter cells, respectively. The intervening phases, G_1 and G_2, are thought to exist primarily to allow time for cell growth and for regulatory inputs. Therefore, from the point of view of regulatory theory, cell proliferation is controlled operationally at two key transitions: that between G_1 and S phase and that between G_2 and M phase. The important characteristic of these two transitions is that, once initiated based on integration of regulatory signals, they must be executed decisively to maintain genetic and genomic integrity. This is accomplished by using a combination of positive and negative modulators to set up the equivalent of a molecular capacitor.

In cycling mammalian cells, the programmed accumulation of cyclins E and A via transcriptional induction provides the positive impetus for the G_1-S phase transition. However, these kinases are kept in check by the action of Cip/Kip family inhibitors. If the internal and external environments are permissive for proliferation, the continued accumulation of cyclins will eventually titrate the inhibitors, allowing the latter to be phosphorylated by free cyclin-CDK complexes. Phosphorylation then marks these inhibitors as targets of ubiquitin-mediated proteolysis. The concerted destruction of CDK inhibitors and concomitant activation of the entire pool of CDK complexes assure that the transition into S phase is rapid and irreversible.

Although the details of its regulation are somewhat different, the strategy underlying control of the G_2-M transition is similar. Cyclin B–CDK1 complexes accumulate starting near the end of S phase but are held in check not by CDK inhibitors but by negative regulatory phosphorylation of CDK1. This phosphorylation on threonine 14 and tyrosine 15 is carried out by kinases Wee1 and Myt1. Entry into M phase is signaled by the rapid dephosphorylation of T14 and Y15, resulting in activation of CDK1. This dephosphorylation is carried out by specialized protein phosphatases, CDC25B and CDC25C. The concerted dephosphorylation of CDK1 depends on activation of CDC25 isoforms by phosphorylation, as well as ubiquitin-mediated proteolysis of Wee1, also in response to phosphorylation. Although the initial activation of CDC25 isoforms is thought to be carried out by other protein kinases, such as Plk1, CDC25B and C are also activated by cyclin B–CDK1, establishing a positive feedback loop. These positive feedback dynamics leading to the simultaneous activation of a large accumulated pool of cyclin B–CDK1 assures that entry into mitosis is decisive. The turnover of Wee1 enforces irreversibility. Because entry into mitosis involves dismantling many of the cell's components and organelles, as well as construction and use of a complex apparatus for segregating the cell's genetic material, mitosis is a period of particular vulnerability, and therefore it is important that this transition and subsequent events be carried out rapidly and efficiently.

An important secondary transition that occurs within M phase is that between metaphase and anaphase (Fig. 6.3).[23] To preserve genomic integrity, all duplicated chromosomes must be aligned along the cell's equator and properly attached to microtubules of the mitotic spindle. The trigger for separation of sister chromatids and their movement to opposite poles of the cell is the activation of the protein-ubiquitin ligase APC/C. This

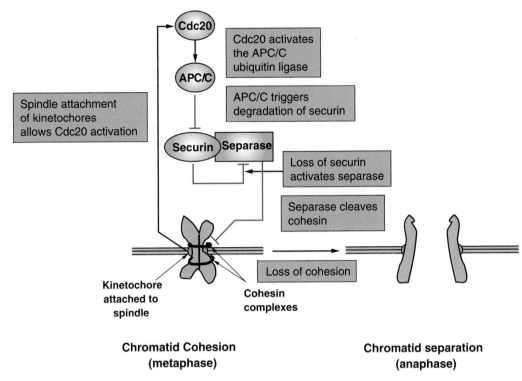

Chromatid Cohesion
(metaphase)

Chromatid separation
(anaphase)

FIGURE 6.3 Regulation of the metaphase-anaphase transition. After replication, paired sister chromatids are held together by a complex of proteins, known collectively as *cohesin*, thus preventing anaphase. However, once paired chromatids have formed bivalent attachments to a functional mitotic spindle, inhibition of CDC20 mediated by the chromosome kinetochores is relieved. CDC20 is an essential cofactor of the protein-ubiquitin ligase anaphase-promoting complex/cyclosome (APC/C), which now becomes active. The primary initial target of the APC/C is securin, an inhibitor of the protease separase. Ubiquitin-mediated proteolysis of securin releases separase to cleave the cohesin subunit Scc1. This event releases paired chromatids from cohesion, thereby allowing anaphase to proceed.

is achieved via CDK1 activation, but more importantly by the binding of a key cofactor, CDC20, whose availability is linked to the proper attachment of chromosomes and the integrity of the spindle. The targets of the APC/C are a protein known as *securin* as well as cyclin B, both of which inhibit a specialized protease, separase. The key target of separase is a complex that binds sister chromatids together: cohesin. Cleavage of the Scc1 subunit of cohesin leads to a rapid execution of anaphase. It is the ability to stockpile a large pool of inactive securin-separase complexes that can be rapidly mobilized by irreversible proteolysis of securin and cyclin B that allows for a rapid irreversible metaphase-anaphase transition.

UBIQUITIN-MEDIATED PROTEOLYSIS

It is becoming increasingly evident that much of the regulation of cell-cycle phase transitions depends on ubiquitin-mediated proteolysis.[24] Ubiquitin is a 76-amino acid polypeptide that can

be covalently linked to lysines of other proteins via the formation of an isopeptide bond with its C-terminal carboxylate. Additional ubiquitin molecules can then be attached to the lysines of already conjugated ubiquitin to form polyubiquitin chains. Polyubiquitylated proteins are usually targeted for rapid proteolysis by a large multisubunit protease known as the *proteasome*. The enzymes that transfer ubiquitin to target proteins are known as *protein-ubiquitin ligases*. From the perspective of cell-cycle control, two families of protein-ubiquitin ligases have predominant roles. The first family, SCF (Skp1-Cullin–F-box protein), specifically targets proteins that are marked for destruction by phosphorylation. This allows degradation of specific proteins to be regulated at a separate level from the protein-ubiquitin ligase itself, which can be expressed constitutively and used to target a large number of substrates independently. SCF ligases consist of three invariant core components and one of a number of specificity factors (F-box proteins) that recognize phosphorylated substrates. A few notable examples of SCF protein-ubiquitin ligases are SCF[Skp2] (containing the F-box protein Skp2), which targets p27[25] and p130,[26] and SCF^{CDC4} (containing the F-box protein CDC4, also known as FBXW7), which targets cyclin E.[27-29] The second family of protein-ubiquitin ligases that is critical for cell-cycle control is known collectively as the *APC/C*. The APC/C is a large complex consisting of 12 core subunits and 1 of 2 specificity factors, CDC20 and CDH1. Unlike SCF ubiquitin ligases, targeting of substrates by the APC/C is determined by ligase activation rather than substrate activation. APC^{CDC20} is active from metaphase until the end of mitosis as a result of periodic accumulation and degradation of CDC20 itself. APC^{CDH1}, on the other hand, which is negatively regulated by CDK-mediated phosphorylation, is activated on mitotic exit and during the subsequent G$_1$ interval when CDKs are inactive. In this manner, important mitotic targets, such as cyclin A, cyclin B, and securin (as well as many others), are degraded during mitosis and prevented from reaccumulating during the subsequent G$_1$ interval.

REGULATION OF THE CELL CYCLE

To preserve organismic function and integrity, the cell cycle must be regulated at a number of levels. These include entry into and exit from proliferation mode, coordination of cell-cycle events, and specialized responses that increase the probability of surviving a variety of environmental and internally generated insults.

Quiescence and Differentiation

The most fundamental aspect of cell-cycle control is the regulation of entry and exit. For mammalian cells, the decision to enter or exit the proliferative mode is based on environmental signals such as mitogens, growth factors, hormones, and cell-cell contact, as well as on internal differentiation programs. If the state of cell-cycle exit is reversible, it is referred to as *quiescence*. If it is in the context of terminal differentiation, cell-cycle exit may merely be one component of a differentiation program. Although cells entering quiescence and postmitotic differentiation vary from each other in many respects, from the perspective of cell-cycle control, they have much in common. First, cell-cycle exit is usually associated, at least initially, with an accumulation of G$_1$/S CDK inhibitors. Members of the INK4 family, targeting CDK4 and CDK6 and members of the Cip/Kip family, as well as the Rb-related protein p130, all targeting CDK2, are up-regulated. This causes accumulation of cells in G$_1$, from where cell-cycle exit can occur. Next, or simultaneously, the positive cell-cycle machinery is dismantled by downregulation of CDKs and cyclins, primarily at the transcriptional level. In the case of quiescence, cell-cycle exit is paralleled by a reduced rate of protein synthesis, indicative that cells have entered a resting state.

Entry into and exit from quiescence are mediated largely by growth factors and mitogens that interact with cell surface receptors. These in turn are linked to intracellular signaling cascades that up-regulate the rate of protein synthesis as well as the transcription of genes that promote proliferation, such as those encoding CDKs and cyclins. The two best-characterized signaling pathways in this context are the mitogen-activated protein kinase/extracellular signaling–regulated kinase pathway[30] and the phosphoinositide 3 (PI3) kinase/ AKT pathway,[31] shown in Figure 6.4. Whereas the mitogen-activated protein kinase/extracellular signaling–regulated kinase pathway tends to stimulate expression of genes required for proliferation, the PI3-kinase/AKT pathway primarily stimulates protein synthesis and growth but also affects key cell-cycle regulatory proteins. Just as the presence of growth factors and mitogens stimulates these pathways, promoting cell-cycle entry, their removal shuts down these pathways, promoting quiescence. This is the basis for the reversibility of the quiescent state.

Antimitogenic Signals

An important aspect of control of cell division in mammals is antimitogenic signaling. Just as mitogens and growth factors bind to transmembrane receptors and use signal transduction pathways and downstream transcriptional programs to stimulate proliferation, parallel systems antagonize proliferation. The classic example of an antimitogenic signal is the effect of transforming growth factor-β (TGF-β) on epithelial cells (Fig. 6.5).[32] TGF-β, a cytokine, binds to a specific heterodimeric transmembrane receptor that, when occupied by ligand, phosphorylates a class of transcription factors, known as *SMADs*. These phosphorylated SMADs heterodimerize with non–receptor-interactive SMADs and translocate to the nucleus, where they complex with DNA-binding transcription factors and coactivators to transactivate specific genes. Relevant to cell-cycle regulation, stimulation of the TGF-β signaling pathway promotes transcription of the gene encoding p15. p15 is an INK4 class CDK inhibitor that specifically inactivates CDK4 and CDK6. However, the effects of p15 accumulation on cell-cycle regulators are more global than inhibition of CDK4/6.[33] INK4 inhibitors such as p15 have a secondary effect of displacing a pool of the Cip/Kip inhibitor p27 from cyclin D–CDK4/6 complexes, allowing it to then target and inactivate cyclin E–CDK2 and cyclin A–CDK2 (Fig. 6.5). Thus, exposure of epithelial cells to TGF-β has the effect of inhibiting G$_1$ and S phase CDK activities, thereby causing G$_1$ arrest.

Interestingly, in many cancers of epithelial origin, the response to TGF-β has been abrogated,

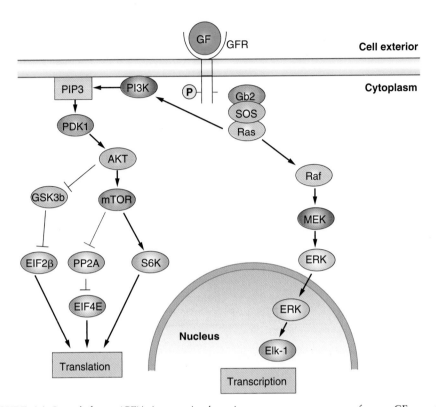

FIGURE 6.4 Growth factor (GF)/mitogen stimulator in response to occupancy of many GF receptors (GFRs) by ligand depends on the small guanosine triphosphatase transducer Ras. Receptor activation leads to phosphorylation of the receptor cytoplasmic domain. The phosphorylated receptor assembles a complex that includes Ras and its activated nucleotide exchange factor, son of sevenless (SOS), leading to activation of Ras. Activated Ras can then stimulate two important signal transduction pathways: the extracellular signaling–regulated kinase (ERK) pathway and the phosphoinositide 3 kinase (PI3K) pathway. Activated Ras stimulates the protein kinase activity of Raf, activating a protein kinase cascade consisting of Raf, MEK, and ERK. Activated ERK then translocates into the nucleus, where it phosphorylates and activates transcription factors, notably Elk-1. Genes important for growth and division are then transcribed. Activated Ras also stimulates PI3K activity, leading to the accumulation of phosphatidylinositol 3,4,5-triphosphate. This in turn stimulates the protein kinase activity of phosphoinositide-dependent kinase 1 (PDK1), activating a protein kinase cascade consisting of PDK1, AKT, and mTOR. Activation of this signal transduction pathway has the effect of stimulating translation and growth. AKT phosphorylates and inhibits the protein kinase glycogen synthase kinase 3 (GSK3β), thereby activating EIF2B required for translational initiation. mTOR phosphorylates and inhibits the protein phosphatase PP2A, thereby activating EIF4E, also required for translational initiation. Finally, mTOR phosphorylates and activates pp70S6 kinase, which in turn phosphorylates and activates ribosomal subunit S6.

suggesting that this and similar response pathways have an important role in maintaining control of proliferation. Interferons comprise another class of cytokines that have antiproliferative effects on many cell types. Although the receptors used and signaling pathways are distinct from those used by TGF-β, the ultimate effects on the cell-cycle machinery are similar: up-regulation of CDK inhibitors and down-regulation of cyclins.

Checkpoints

Cells are constantly faced with insults, resulting in damage that can threaten their survival. These insults can be generated internally as chemically active by-products of metabolism or can originate in the external environment; for example, chemical agents or radiation. As a result, mechanisms have evolved to remove damaged molecules and make necessary repairs. In instances in which cell-cycle progression would be harmful or catastrophic before repair of damage, further mechanisms have evolved to delay progression pending repair. These are called *cell-cycle checkpoints*.[34] The necessity of checkpoints can be easily envisioned for genotoxic agents. Cells are particularly susceptible to the harmful effects of DNA damage at two points in the cell cycle: S phase and M phase. Unrepaired DNA damage poses a number of problems for cells undergoing DNA replication. Chromosomal lesions present

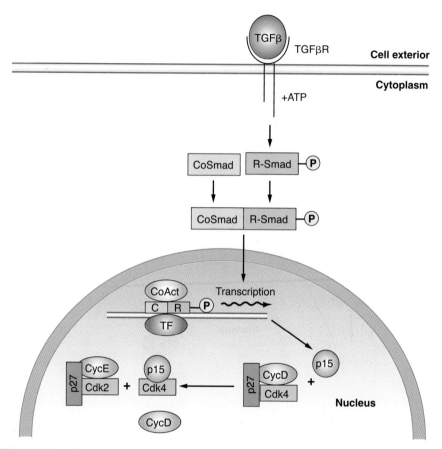

FIGURE 6.5 Transforming growth factor-β (TGF-β) antimitogenic pathway. Occupancy of the heterodimeric TGF-β receptor by ligand leads to phosphorylation of a class of transcription factor known collectively as *R-SMADs*. Phosphorylated R-SMADs then dimerize with nontargeted cofactors known as *CoSMADs* and translocate to the nucleus. There the R-SMAD/CoSMAD dimers complex with DNA-binding transcription factors and transcriptional coactivators to stimulate transcription of specific genes. One of the key targets of TGF-β signaling is the gene encoding p15/INK4b, a CDK4/6 inhibitor. p15, by binding to CDK4 and CDK6, inhibits these kinases and displaces a large pool of CDK4/6-bound p27, which is then free to inhibit CDK2 complexes. The result is G_1 arrest. ATP, adenosine triphosphate; TF, transcription factor; CoAct, coactivator.

physical barriers to replication forks. Replication that does traverse regions of unrepaired DNA damage is likely to be error-prone, resulting in accumulation of mutations. Likewise, segregation of severely damaged chromosomes at mitosis might lead to loss of genetic information, seriously threatening the survival or integrity of daughter cells. Therefore, cells possess mechanisms for preventing DNA replication and mitosis in response to genotoxic stress. Although the scope of this review does not permit a detailed description of all known checkpoints, those thought to be most basic to cell survival are characterized here.

DNA Damage Checkpoints

Although DNA damage exists in many forms, ranging from chemical adducts to double-strand breaks, they all pose similar problems for proliferating cells. As previously stated, impeded and error-prone DNA replication and loss of genetic material during mitosis are some of the likely consequences in the absence of DNA damage checkpoints. Therefore, cell-cycle progression is blocked at three points: before S phase entry (the G_1 DNA damage checkpoint), during S phase (the intra-S phase DNA damage checkpoint), and before M phase entry (the G_2 DNA damage checkpoint). Although the responses to different types of DNA damage are not identical, they are similar enough to generalize. DNA damage of various forms is first detected by DNA-bound protein complexes that serve as sensors. In mammalian cells, two related atypical protein kinases that share homology with lipid kinases, ATM and ATR,[35] are primary signal transducers that are activated by DNA damage at all points in the cell cycle. A key effector of the G_1 and G_2 checkpoint responses is a transcription factor known as *p53*.[36,37] In response to DNA damage, p53 is activated and stabilized leading to increased levels. The principal transcriptional target of p53 in the context of the G_1 checkpoint is the Cip/Kip inhibitor p21[Cip1]. The resulting high levels of p21 block CDK2 activity and possibly CDK4 and CDK6 activity, leading to G_1 arrest. An additional transcriptional target of p53, GADD45, inhibits CDK1, thereby contributing to the G_2 DNA damage checkpoint. Another p53-dependent mechanism contributing to checkpoint-mediated G_2 arrest is through transcriptional repression of the genes encoding cyclin B1 and CDK1. This occurs via direct interaction p53 and NF-Y, the positive transcriptional activator of these genes. However, although p53-dependent mechanisms are required for long-term maintenance of arrest, the primary mechanism underlying the immediate G_2 DNA damage checkpoint is p53-independent. It involves one of two effector protein kinases known as *chk1* and *chk2* that have the effect of inhibiting CDC25C,[38] which carries out the activating dephosphorylation of CDK1. Therefore, in response to DNA damage, G_2 cells accumulate inhibited cyclin B–CDK1 complexes and are incapable of entering into mitosis. The intra-S phase DNA damage checkpoint response appears to be p53-independent but requires the chk1 or chk2 kinases, or both. A key target is CDC25A, responsible for activating CDK2 by dephosphorylation. In response to DNA damage, phosphorylation of CDC25A by chk1 or chk2 leads to its destabilization via ubiquitin-mediated proteolysis and thus the accumulation of inactive CDK2 complexes[39] phosphorylated on threonine 14 and tyrosine 15. Because ongoing DNA replication requires the activity of CDK2, DNA synthesis ceases until damage is repaired.

Replication Checkpoint

Under normal circumstances, DNA replication is complete well before the time when the accumulation and activation of cyclin B–CDK1 would drive cells into mitosis. However, through the action of toxins or the rare but finite probability that the duration of S phase will be excessively long, situations can be encountered in which completion of replication extends beyond the normal time of mitotic induction or replication is blocked entirely. Under such circumstances, it is necessary to delay or block entrance into M phase accordingly, as segregation of incompletely replicated chromosomes would be catastrophic, leading to chromosome breaks and/or nondisjunction events. Although the signaling pathways are somewhat different, the replication checkpoint ultimately functions like the G_2 DNA damage checkpoint in that mitotic entry is blocked by inhibiting CDC25C via the action of chk1, thus preventing activation of CDK1.

Spindle Integrity Checkpoint

The actual act of division is a dangerous time for a cell. It requires aligning duplicated chromosomes by attaching them via bipolar attachments to the spindle and then separating the chromatids so that each daughter cell gets a full complement. Errors result in aneuploidy, an extremely undesirable outcome. As a result, assembling a mitotic spindle and attaching chromosomes to it are extensively monitored processes. The mechanism of delay at prometaphase or metaphase in response to spindle defects or improper chromosome attachment is referred to as the *spindle integrity checkpoint*.[40] The sensor for this checkpoint consists of a number of proteins that reside at the chromosome kinetochores, sites of spindle microtubule attachment. The target is the essential APC/C cofactor, CDC20. Unattached or improperly attached kinetochores not experiencing an appropriate level of tension indicative of bipolar attachment inhibit CDC20 function. This in turn prevents the ubiquitylation and degradation of the anaphase inhibitors, securin and cyclin B. As a result, cells are prevented from initiating anaphase until all kinetochores are properly attached to a bipolar spindle (Fig. 6.3).

Restriction Point

Cells deprived of an essential nutrient or growth factor are blocked from cell-cycle progression at a point in mid-G_1.[41] Cells that have already passed this point, termed the *restriction point* or *R*, enter into S phase and complete the current cell cycle before arresting in the subsequent G_1 interval. In contrast, G_1 cells that have not reached the restriction point arrest immediately. The molecular basis for the restriction point has remained elusive. Initially it was thought that passage through the restriction point was a manifestation of G_1 CDK activation and/or phosphorylation the pRb family of transcriptional inhibitors. However, more recent work has indicated that CDK activation and pRb phosphorylation occur after passage through the restriction point.[42,43] Significantly, most malignant cells do not have a functional restriction point, which presumably helps them evade normal growth control signals.

Senescence

All normal mammalian cells have a finite proliferative lifespan. As cells approach the end of their proliferative capacity, they enter a state referred to as *replicative senescence*.[44,45] Although the reasons for programmed senescence are not known, it has been speculated that restricting cells to a finite number of divisions may be a protective mechanism against malignant growth. Although the rationale for senescence is not known, the mechanism has been largely elucidated, particularly for human cells. It is based on the requirement for a specialized replicase, telomerase, in the replication of the ends of chromosomes known as *telomeres*. Whereas germ line cells express telomerase, most if not all somatic cells do not. As a result, because of the topology of telomeres and the requirements of conventional DNA replication, progressive telomere shortening or attrition occurs with each cell cycle. Although linear chromosome ends create a discontinuity, which topologically is indistinguishable from a chromosome break, telomere-specific DNA sequences are shielded from the DNA damage checkpoints. However, when sufficient telomere attrition has removed these protected sequences, cells enter into a chronic checkpoint response, which is the molecular basis for senescence. Senescence is characterized by the accumulation of high levels of CDK inhibitors and ultimately permanent G_1 arrest. It should be noted that one of the requirements of malignant transformation of cells is to overcome the senescence barrier so as to provide tumor cells with unlimited proliferative capacity.

Regulation of DNA Replication

Entry into S phase is one of the key regulatory points of the cell cycle. The actual triggering of replication is attributed to the activation of CDK2 by cyclins E and A. However, the transcription of a large number of genes whose products are required for DNA replication requires the activity of CDK4 or CDK6, or both, driven by D-type cyclins. Mechanistically, this is based on the function of pRb and related proteins p130 and p107 serving as transcriptional repressors when bound to E2F family transcription factors (Fig. 6.6).[8] Phosphorylation by cyclin D–CDK4/6 relieves this repression. Once cells have synthesized all the necessary enzymes and initiated DNA replication, another serious regulatory problem is encountered. To maintain genomic integrity, cells must replicate all genomic sequences only once per cell

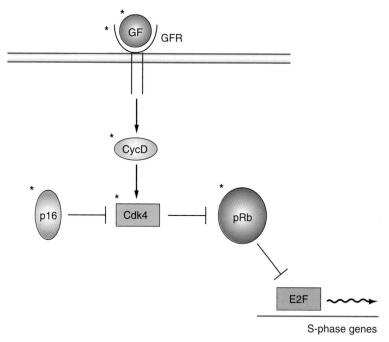

FIGURE 6.6 pRb pathway. pRb is a critical negative cell-cycle regulator that links growth factor (GF) signaling pathways to cell-cycle progression. One of the principal functions of pRb is to interact with E2F family transcription factors and, by recruitment of corepressors, to maintain many genes encoding proteins that are important for cell-cycle progression in a tightly repressed state. GF and mitogen-signaling pathways relieve this repression by stimulating accumulation of D-type cyclins on receptor occupancy. The resulting activation of CDK4 and CDK6 leads to phosphorylation of pRb and concomitant inactivation of its repressive functions. p16 is a CDK inhibitor of the INK4 family that down-regulates this pathway by inhibiting CDK4. It should be noted that all elements marked by an *asterisk* are found mutated or deregulated, or both, in human cancer. GFs, GF receptors (GFRs), and D-type cyclins are frequently overexpressed or deregulated. p16 is often not expressed or is underexpressed. Mutant versions of CDK4 that cannot bind p16 have been identified in human cancers. Finally, the gene encoding pRb is frequently mutated in cancer.

cycle, necessitating that origins of replication, sites where DNA synthesis begins, are used once during each S phase. This is accomplished by requiring that replication origin preparation and firing are mediated, respectively, by distinct CDK environments.[46] Pre-replication complex assembly is triggered by low or absent CDK activity and therefore normally occurs as cells exit mitosis. This process requires the successive loading of proteins, CDC6, ctd1, and six MCM proteins (MCM2–7) to another complex of proteins, known as the *origin recognition complex*, which marks the origin site. Because of the requirement for low CDK activity, the permissive window for this process extends from the end of mitosis (telophase) until the point in G_1 when CDK activity begins to rise. The activation of CDK2 in late G_1 has the dual effect of blocking further pre-replication complex assembly and causing DNA replication to initiate at primed origins. The maintenance of high levels of CDK activity (CDK2 followed by CDK1) for the remainder of the cell cycle assures that no new pre-replication complex assembly can occur until the end of mitosis, when CDK levels once again decline, and in doing so restricts origin function to once per cell cycle. Indeed, inhibiting CDK1 activity during G2 or early M phase is sufficient to promote a round of DNA replication without cell division.

CELL CYCLE AND CANCER

Cancer is partly a disease of uncontrolled proliferation. Because the proliferation of cells within an organism is normally tightly controlled by redundant regulatory pathways, it is not surprising that cell-cycle and checkpoint genes are often found misregulated or mutated in cancer. Genes in which mutations give rise to a gain of function or an enhanced level of function, leading to malignancy, are referred to as *protooncogenes*. Protooncogenes usually encode growth- or division-promoting proteins. Genes that give rise to loss of function mutations that lead to malignancy are referred to as *tumor suppressor genes*. Tumor suppressor genes usually encode negative regulators of growth and proliferation that protect cells from malignancy. Some cell-cycle genes commonly mutated or misregulated in cancer are listed in Table 6.1. Whereas mutations that create oncogenes tend to be dominant, mutations in tumor suppressor genes are usually recessive. This has led to the two-hit model of carcinogenesis (Fig. 6.7).[47] Briefly, recessive mutations occur in tumor suppressor genes but are latent because of the persistence of a wild type allele. The tumor suppressor phenotype, therefore, requires mutation or loss of the second allele, a process known as *loss of*

TABLE 6.1

CELL-CYCLE GENES COMMONLY MUTATED OR ALTERED IN EXPRESSION IN HUMAN CANCER

Gene	Protein	Function	Alteration in Cancer
CCND1,2,3	D cyclins	Positive regulator of CDK4/6	Overexpressed
CCNE1	Cyclin E1	Positive regulator of CDK2	Overexpressed, deregulated
CDKN2A	p16, INK4a[a]	CDK4/6 inhibitor	Mutated, deleted, methylated
CDKN1B	p27[Kip1]	CDK2 inhibitor	Underexpressed
CDKN1C	p57[Kip2]	CDK2 inhibitor	Underexpressed, methylated
SKP2	Skp2	Turnover of p27	Overexpressed
CDK4	CDK4	Inactivates pRb	p16-resistant mutations
hCDC4	hCdc4	Turnover of cyclin E	Mutated, deleted
RB1	pRb	Represses E2F transcription	Mutated, deleted
RB2	p130	Inhibits CDKs, represses E2F	Mutated, deleted
CKS1,2	cks1, cks2	CDK-binding proteins	Overexpressed
AURKA	Aurora A	Mitotic kinase	Overexpressed
PLK	Plk1	Mitotic kinase	Overexpressed
PTTG1	Securin	Anaphase inhibitor	Overexpressed
TP53	p53	Checkpoints, apoptosis	Mutated, deleted
MTBP	MDM-2	Inhibitor of p53	Overexpressed
CDKN2A	p14[Arf, a]	Activator of p53	Mutated, deleted
ATM	ATM	Checkpoints, repair	Mutated, deleted
CHK2	chk2	Checkpoints	Mutated
NBS1	Nbs1	Checkpoints, repair	Mutated

[a]Interestingly, the p16[INK4A] and p14[Arf] are encoded by the same gene via alternative reading frames and different promoters.

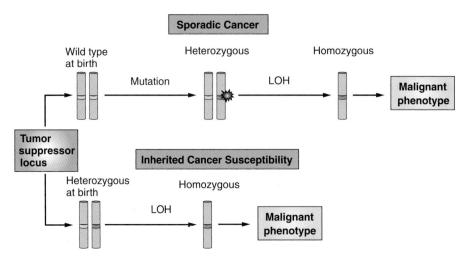

FIGURE 6.7 The two-hit model of tumor suppression. Tumor suppressors are proteins that are thought to provide protection from malignancy. Depicted is a chromosome carrying a tumor suppressor–encoding locus shown in white. At birth, normal individuals carry two wild type alleles (*yellow bands*) at tumor suppressor loci. Over time, however, spontaneous mutations occur at these loci (*red flash*) that render one allele nonfunctional (*orange band*). However, because such mutations are expected to be recessive to the wild type allele that is still present, there is no phenotypic consequence. Over time, additional events can lead to loss of the wild type allele, a phenomenon referred to as *loss of heterozygosity* (LOH). LOH then provides a tangible contribution to the malignant phenotype. However, because spontaneous mutations at specific loci and specific secondary allelic losses are rare events, malignancy usually develops only after a very long latency period. On the other hand, some individuals are born with inherited tumor suppressor mutations. Because only LOH is then required for expression of the tumor suppressor–null phenotype, cancer with decreased latency and higher penetrance develops in such individuals.

heterozygosity. Alternatively, the second allele of a tumor suppressor gene can be silenced epigenetically without a direct genetic alteration. A number of genes encoding negative regulators of the cell cycle conform to this two-hit paradigm.

In theory, to achieve uncontrolled cell division, two basic requirements must be met. First, cells need a strong constitutive proliferation signal capable of overriding the environmental and internal restraints on division that normal cells experience. Second, the barrier of senescence needs to be dismantled to render tumor cells immortal. Mutations in a large variety of cell-cycle control and related genes are associated with malignancy, and most of these can be accommodated within this framework. This model of tumorigenesis has been confirmed in rodent tissue culture–based *in vitro* models. Transfection of primary rodent fibroblasts with individual plasmids programmed to express proteins that promote either growth or immortalization does not result in malignant transformation. However, cotransfection of two plasmids, one in each category, does promote transformation (Fig. 6.8). However, these results need to be interpreted cautiously in the context of human cancer because immortalization of rodent cells in culture most likely does not involve telomeres, which are much longer in rodents than in humans.[48] One idea that has emerged is that strong growth signals and other environmental pressures exerted on premalignant cells produce potent stress responses, leading to cell-cycle block-

ade or cell death.[49] Phenotypically, such stress-induced effects on fibroblasts closely resemble those associated with replicative senescence; therefore, this phenomenon has been termed *stress-induced senescence* (see following discussion). Therefore, genetic alterations are likely required to neutralize these stress responses to immortalize rodent cells. Transformation of human cells requires these same genetic alterations, but also telomere attrition must be reckoned with, requiring additional mutations.

Alterations in Pathways Affecting Growth and Proliferation

Mutations that regulate cell growth and proliferation can occur at many levels, ranging from cell surface receptor–mediated signaling pathways that control proliferation to elements of the core cell-cycle machinery itself.

Growth and Proliferation Signaling Pathways

Because a large number of receptors and pathways can influence cell proliferation, many mutations in elements of these pathways have been recovered in human malignancies. Only a few examples are cited here. One way to provide a strong constitutive proliferation signal is to overexpress or deregulate

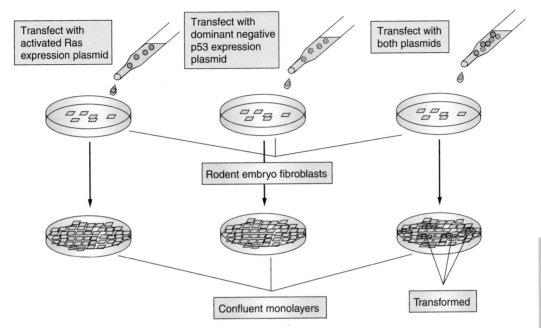

FIGURE 6.8 Malignant transformation requires multiple genetic alterations. Depicted is an *in vitro* experiment using primary rodent embryonic fibroblasts. Cells transfected with a plasmid programmed to express an activated Ras allele eventually grow to form a confluent monolayer, at which time proliferation ceases because of inhibition mediated by cell-cell contact. Similarly, cells transfected with a plasmid programmed to express a dominant-negative allele of p53 (encoding a protein that can complex with and inactivate endogenous wild type p53) from a confluent monolayer. However, cells transfected simultaneously with both plasmids from a confluent monolayer, out of which grow transformed foci. These piles of cells are no longer subject to the controls that restrict fibroblast proliferation and, as such, resemble cancer cells. The requirement for two perturbations in this system supports a mechanism whereby activated Ras stimulates growth and proliferation, and dominant negative p53 inactivates stress pathways that would cause these cells to have a limited proliferative lifespan.

growth factor receptors. HER2/neu, a transmembrane tyrosine kinase receptor found on many epithelial cell types, is often overexpressed because of gene amplification in breast and other cancers.[50] Presumably the amplitude of proliferation signaling is abnormally high or completely deregulated in such tumors. Similarly, signaling elements downstream of mitogen receptors can be mutated to produce constitutive signaling. Perhaps the best-known example is the case of the Ras family guanosine triphosphatases, which serve as signal transducers for a number of key proliferation pathways. Dominant mutations in Ras isoforms that stabilize the activated state confer strong constitutive proliferation signaling. One of the pathways stimulated by Ras is the PI3-kinase pathway. A PI3 phosphatase, PTEN, normally reverses this phosphorylation, keeping the signal in check. Consistent with this, mutational loss of PTEN similarly to oncogenic mutations in Ras can lead to constitutive signaling contributing to carcinogenesis.

Cell-Cycle Machinery

Signaling pathways that stimulate proliferation impinge on the cell-cycle machinery by stimulating the biosynthesis of D-type cyclins and promoting the degradation of CDK inhibitors. Accumulation of D-type cyclins and concomitant activation of CDK4 and CDK6 have been shown to activate the cell-cycle program primarily by phosphorylation and inactivation of the retinoblastoma protein, pRb, and related proteins p107 and p130. These proteins form potent repression complexes with transcription factors that are critical for S-phase entry and progression, notably the E2F family, effectively blocking cell-cycle progression. In addition, INK4 family inhibitors specifically downregulate CDK4 and CDK6, buffering their capacity to phosphorylate pRb and related proteins. Virtually all components of this pathway have been found to be misregulated or mutated in cancer to provide a constitutive proliferation signal (proteins with asterisks in Fig. 6.6).[51] The genes encoding D-type cyclins are found amplified in a broad spectrum of tumors. On the other hand, the gene encoding the INK4 inhibitor, p16, is mutated and lost in some types of cancer, whereas CDK4 has been found to be mutated so as not to bind p16. In many instances p16, although not genetically altered, is downregulated at the epigenetic level. The p16 promoter contains a CpG island that is subject to repression via methylation. Finally, pRb is the tumor suppressor on which the so-called two-hit hypothesis was originally formulated. Inherited mutations in the *RB* gene and subsequent loss of heterozygosity invariably lead to childhood retinoblastoma and eventually other malignancies. However, somatic mutation of *RB1* and loss of heterozygosity are found in many sporadic noninherited cancers, underscoring the critical nature of negative cell-cycle regulation by pRb.

Like D-type cyclins, cyclin E is frequently found up-regulated in cancer. The fact that deregulated expression of cyclin E can drive cells prematurely into S phase suggests that cyclin E provides a growth/division stimulus during carcinogenesis. Furthermore, cells from cyclin E nullizygous mice are resistant to malignant transformation in tissue culture models.[12] However, other evidence suggests that deregulation of cyclin E may promote carcinogenesis principally by inducing genomic instability rather than by promoting growth (see "Mutations Causing Genetic and Genomic Instability"). Likewise, the CDK2 inhibitor p27^{Kip1} is often found down-regulated in cancer, although never behaving as a classic tumor suppressor inactivated through mutation and allelic loss. However, as with cyclin E deregulation, it is not clear whether low p27 levels have an impact on carcinogenesis by promoting growth or genomic instability. While the CDK-inhibitory functions of p27 are restricted to the nucleus, hyperphosphorylation leads to cytoplasmic translocation, where non–CDK-bound p27 promotes cell migration. This may explain why p27 is rarely deleted in cancer, as cytoplasmic functions may be important for invasion and metastasis.[52]

Alterations in Pathways Affecting Senescence

In addition to a constitutive growth stimulus that overrides natural restraints, tumors need to have the capacity for unlimited proliferation. Normally, the limited lifespan of somatic cells imposed by the process of replicative senescence constitutes a natural barrier to tumorigenesis. Therefore, genes that mediate senescence are commonly mutated in cancer. However, the issue of senescence is complicated by functional overlap between senescence pathway genes and oncogenic stress pathway genes that also require inactivation.[48,49] Because senescence is a result of checkpoint responses to acute telomere attrition, genes that encode DNA checkpoint signaling elements and transducers are targeted. One of the most commonly mutated genes in human cancer encodes the checkpoint effector p53.[36] Inherited mutations in *TP53*, the gene encoding p53, confer a syndrome known as *Li-Fraumeni* characterized by early-onset cancer.[53] However, the majority of sporadic cancers are also mutated at the p53 locus. The role of p53 mutation in cancer as a promoter of immortalization is supported by the finding that cells from p53 nullizygous mice are immortal.[54] However, this conclusion is complicated by the fact that p53 is central to cellular stress responses that also require inactivation during malignant transformation, and as previously stated, telomere attrition is not likely to be a significant issue for immortalization in mice. Nevertheless, an observation supporting the idea that checkpoint genes likely to be triggered by telomere attrition are targeted to immortalize premalignant cells is that chk2, a signaling element of the DNA damage checkpoint response, is mutated in a subset of patients with Li-Fraumeni syndrome[53] rather than p53.

Mutation of the gene encoding Nbs1, required for activation of chk1 and chk2 kinases, is also associated with a hereditary cancer syndrome,[55] Nijmegen disease, as well as sporadic cancers, although the interpretation of this result is complicated by the fact that Nbs1 is also involved in DNA damage repair (see "Mutations Causing Genetic and Genomic Instability"). However, the most direct strategy to bypass senescence is to induce directly the expression of telomerase in somatic cells. c-Myc, a transcription factor linked to stimulation of proliferation, has also been shown to be a positive regulator of the gene encoding telomerase reverse transcriptase (hTERT), the catalytic subunit of telomerase.[56] This may explain the high frequency of human tumors exhibiting c-Myc amplification or overexpression, or both. However, there appear to be a number of different mutational targets that can lead to derepression of the *hTERT* gene.[57]

Mutations Neutralizing Stress Responses

Abnormally strong growth and proliferation signals provoke antagonistic stress responses leading to cell-cycle arrest or cell death. For example, it has been observed that expression of mutationally activated Ras alleles in nontransformed human fibroblasts leads to a cell-cycle arrest phenotype that closely resembles replicative senescence. As stated in "Alterations in Pathways Affecting Senescence," cellular stress responses are intimately related to checkpoint responses. Therefore, it is difficult to clearly categorize mutations that affect both. An example is p53, which is required for DNA damage checkpoint responses but also is a key effector of cellular stress responses.[37,48,49] In the case of activated Ras previously cited, the stress-activated MAP kinase pathway promotes phosphorylation and activation of p53 leading to cell-cycle arrest. Therefore, mutations that directly or indirectly inactivate p53 can promote oncogenesis by bypassing stress-dependent cell-cycle arrest or cell death. Murine double-minute gene-2, which is frequently amplified and overexpressed in human cancer, promotes turnover of p53, consistent with a role in neutralizing stress responses.[58] Conversely, p14[Arf], a protein that stabilizes p53 by antagonizing murine double-minute gene-2, is frequently found mutated or underexpressed in cancer.[58] Indeed, the p53 pathway is so frequently inactivated in human cancer most likely because loss of p53 function simultaneously antagonizes stress pathways and helps override cellular responses to telomere attrition. pRb may have a parallel function in maintenance of senescence, as loss of pRb has recently been shown to cause fibroblasts rendered senescent by expression of activated Ras to undergo DNA replication[59]. Thus, mutation of *RB* in cancer may contribute to escape from oncogene-induced senescence.

Mutations Causing Genetic and Genomic Instability

The pathway to malignancy minimally requires several mutations. In the case of tumor suppressor mutations, secondary genetic events mediating allelic loss are necessary. Therefore, any mutation that itself can confer genetic or genomic instability, or both, is likely to promote carcinogenesis.[60,61] Mutations in genes required for DNA repair result in a mutator phenotype linked to hyperaccumulation of secondary mutations. In this context, strong association between mutation of the gene encoding Nbs1, which is required for efficient DNA repair as well as checkpoint signaling, and carcinogenesis is easily understood.[55] Similarly, the association between mutation of components of the spindle integrity checkpoint, such as Bub1, and carcinogenesis can be rationalized.[62] Cells defective in this checkpoint experience deregulated mitosis, leading to chromosome instability and ultimately aneuploidy. In principle, aneuploidy potentiates amplification at oncogenic loci and allelic losses at tumor suppressor loci.

An interesting link between the core cell-cycle machinery and genomic instability is the case of cyclin E. Cyclin E is found overexpressed and deregulated in a broad spectrum of malignancies.[63] Although this correlation might be interpreted in the context of simply promoting proliferation, experiments on cells in culture have revealed that deregulation of cyclin E expression causes chromosome instability leading to aneuploidy and polyploidy.[64] This occurs because expression of cyclin E at inappropriate times in the cell cycle leads to impairment of DNA replication as well as of mitosis. Therefore, one possible role that cyclin E might play in promoting oncogenesis is to accelerate loss of heterozygosity at tumor suppressor loci. This was tested in a transgenic mouse mammary carcinogenesis model and, consistent with this idea, cyclin E deregulation led to accelerated loss of heterozygosity at the *TP53* locus (encoding p53),

which correlated with higher tumor incidence.[65] Interestingly, an essential component of the ubiquitin ligase responsible for cell cycle–dependent targeting of cyclin E for proteolysis, hCDC4 (also known as FBXW7), is often found mutated in cancer,[27,29,66] and its deletion has been shown to also cause genomic instability in cultured cells.[67] Thus, genetic alterations that interfere with proper regulation of cell-cycle machinery have the potential of affecting not only the cell cycle itself, but also the genetic and genomic integrity of the cell.

MICRORNAs, THE CELL CYCLE, AND CANCER

Although discovered in the nematode *Caenorhabditis elegans* many years ago, the importance of microRNAs (miRs) in mammalian cells and human cancer has only recently begun to be appreciated.[68,69] These small RNAs target specific mRNAs via degradation or inhibition of translation. They confer unique regulatory possibilities in that they usually target several different mRNAs simultaneously, allowing for coordination of multiple pathways. At least five groups or clusters of miRs have been shown to target mRNAs encoding cell-cycle regulatory proteins. The miR-15a/16 cluster targets cyclin E1, cyclin D1, and cyclin D3, as well as CDK6. Not surprisingly, this miR cluster has been shown to have tumor suppressive functions in several different types of cancer. The miR-17/20 cluster, which targets cyclin D1 and E2F transcription factors, and let-7, which targets cyclin D1, cyclin D3 cyclin A, CDK4, and CDK6, have been also been shown to be tumor suppressive. Conversely, the miR-221-222 cluster and mir-21, which target a number of CDK inhibitors, has oncogenic properties. Understanding of the regulation and roles of miRs in normal cell function and cancer etiology is largely incomplete, and filling in the gaps poses a significant research challenge for the coming years.

THE CELL CYCLE AND CANCER THERAPY

Because cancer cells must proliferate, essential cell-cycle proteins have been suggested as targets for therapeutic exploitation. Notably, CDKs have been extensively screened for small-molecule inhibitors, some of which are in clinical trials. It is too early, however, to judge the efficacy of this approach beyond its success using *in vitro* models. An alternative approach being explored is to develop agents that undermine checkpoint responses. The presumption is that cancer cells, because of their highly proliferative state, might be more susceptible to loss of essential controls. This idea remains to be confirmed. However, it is noteworthy that many therapeutic approaches currently use compounds that normally trigger checkpoint responses, such as genotoxic agents or spindle poisons. It is assumed that these treatments are effective because tumor cells are actually impaired in their defensive checkpoint responses. An interesting approach that initially showed promise in model systems but has proven disappointing in clinical trials, uses the fact that a large percentage of malignancies are defective for p53 function in order to evade checkpoint and stress responses. A common human lytic virus known as *adenovirus,* expresses an essential gene, E1B p55K, specifically to down-regulate p53 in order to allow a productive infection. Oncolytic adenoviruses have therefore been engineered to not express E1B p55K.[70] These adenoviruses are harmless to normal cells but can productively infect and lyse p53-defective tumor cells in tissue culture and mouse xenograft models. However, technical issues such as low tumor infectivity, rapid viral clearance, and neutralizing immune responses in clinical trials

have limited the efficacy of this approach.[70] On the other hand, if new generations of oncolytic viruses that circumvent these problems can be developed, this may constitute one of the more promising new therapeutic approaches.

Circadian rhythms may present another interesting link between cancer therapeutics and the cell cycle. Although circadian rhythms regulate virtually every aspect of human physiology, it is clear that cell-cycle regulatory gene expression and the cell cycle itself are entrained to the day-night cycle.[71] It has also been shown that tumor cells have largely lost this regulation. This difference, therefore, may be exploitable therapeutically. Indeed, the tolerance and efficacy of a variety of genotoxic chemotherapeutic agents varies with time of day, suggesting a possible link between the time of administration and the cell-cycle position of cells in healthy tissues. More detailed understanding of circadian regulation of the cell cycle may provide an avenue for optimization of current therapeutics.

Selected References

The full list of references for this chapter appears in the online version.

2. Johnson RT, Rao PN. Mammalian cell fusion: induction of premature chromosome condensation in interphase nuclei. *Nature* 1970;226:717.
3. Rao PN, Johnson RT. Mammalian cell fusion: studies on the regulation of DNA synthesis and mitosis. *Nature* 1970; 225:159.
4. Masui Y, Markert CL. Cytoplasmic control of nuclear behavior during meiotic maturation of frog oocytes. *J Exp Zool* 1971;177:129.
5. Hartwell LH, Culotti J, Pringle JR, et al. Genetic control of the cell division cycle in yeast. *Science* 1974;183:46.
6. Harper JW, Adams PD. Cyclin-dependent kinases. *Chem Rev* 2001;101:2511.
7. Jeffrey PD, Russo AA, Polyak K, et al. Mechanism of CDK activation revealed by the structure of a cyclinA-CDK2 complex. *Nature* 1995; 376:313.
8. Stevens C, La Thangue NB. E2F and cell cycle control: a double-edged sword. *Arch Biochem Biophys* 2003;412: 157.
9. Stiegler P, Giordano A. The family of retinoblastoma proteins. *Crit Rev Eukaryot Gene Expr* 2001;11:59.
10. Ohtsubo M, Roberts JM. Cyclin-dependent regulation of G1 in mammalian fibroblasts. *Science* 1993;259:1908.
11. Resnitzky D, Gossen M, Bujard H, et al. Acceleration of the G1/S phase transition by expression of cyclins D1 and E with an inducible system. *Mol Cell Biol* 1994;14:1669.
12. Geng Y, Yu Q, Sicinska E, et al. Cyclin E ablation in the mouse. *Cell* 2003;114:431.
13. Berthet C, Aleem E, Coppola V, et al. CDK2 knockout mice are viable. *Curr Biol* 2003;13:1775.
14. Ortega S, Prieto I, Odajima J, et al. Cyclin-dependent kinase 2 is essential for meiosis but not for mitotic cell division in mice. *Nat Genet* 2003;35:25.
18. Russo AA, Jeffrey PD, Pavletich NP. Structural basis of cyclin-dependent kinase activation by phosphorylation. *Nat Struct Biol* 1996;3:696.
19. Russo AA, Tong L, Lee JO, et al. Structural basis for inhibition of the cyclin-dependent kinase CDK6 by the tumour suppressor p16INK4a. *Nature* 1998;395:237.
20. Cheng M, Olivier P, Diehl JA, et al. The p21(Cip1) and p27(Kip1) CDK inhibitors are essential activators of cyclin

D-dependent kinases in murine fibroblasts. *EMBO J* 1999; 18:1571.
24. Reed SI. Ratchets and clocks: the cell cycle, ubiquitylation and protein turnover. *Nat Rev Mol Cell Biol* 2003;4:855.
25. Carrano AC, Eytan E, Hershko A, et al. SKP2 is required for ubiquitin-mediated degradation of the CDK inhibitor p27. *Nat Cell Biol* 1999;1:193.
26. Tedesco D, Lukas J, Reed SI. The pRb-related protein p130 is regulated by phosphorylation-dependent proteolysis via the protein-ubiquitin ligase SCF(Skp2). *Genes Dev* 2002;16: 2946.
27. Strohmaier H, Spruck CH, Kaiser P, et al. Human F-box protein hCdc4 targets cyclin E for proteolysis and is mutated in a breast cancer cell line. *Nature* 2001;413:316.
28. Koepp DM, Schaefer LK, Ye X, et al. Phosphorylation-dependent ubiquitination of cyclin E by the SCFFbw7 ubiquitin ligase. *Science* 2001;294:173.
30. Davis RJ. Transcriptional regulation by MAP kinases. *Mol Reprod Dev* 1995;42:459.
31. Chang F, Lee JT, Navolanic PM, et al. Involvement of PI3K/Akt pathway in cell cycle progression, apoptosis, and neoplastic transformation: a target for cancer chemotherapy. *Leukemia* 2003;17:590.
32. Shi Y, Massague J. Mechanisms of TGF-beta signaling from cell membrane to the nucleus. *Cell* 2003;113:685.
34. Elledge SJ. Cell cycle checkpoints: preventing an identity crisis. *Science* 1996;274:1664.
35. Yang J, Yu Y, Hamrick HE. ATM, ATR, and DNA-PK: initiators of the cellular genotoxic stress responses. *Carcinogenesis* 2003;24:1571.
36. Vousden KH. Activation of the p53 tumor suppressor protein. *Biochim Biophys Acta* 2002;1602:47.
37. Taylor WR, Stark GR. Regulation of the G2/M transition by p53. *Oncogene* 2001;20:1803.
38. Bartek J, Lukas J. Chk1 and Chk2 kinases in checkpoint control and cancer. *Cancer Cell* 2003;3:421.
39. Sorensen CS, Syljuasen RG, Falck J, et al. Chk1 regulates the S phase checkpoint by coupling the physiological turnover and ionizing radiation-induced accelerated proteolysis of Cdc25A. *Cancer Cell* 2003;3:247.
40. Allshire RC. Centromeres, checkpoints and chromatid cohesion. *Curr Opin Genet Dev* 1997;7:264.
41. Blagosklonny MV, Pardee AB. The restriction point of the cell cycle. *Cell Cycle* 2002;1:103.

42. Ekholm SV, Zickert P, Reed SI, et al. Accumulation of cyclin E is not a prerequisite for passage through the restriction point. *Mol Cell Biol* 2001;21:3256.

43. Martinsson HS, Starborg M, Erlandsson F, et al. Single cell analysis of G1 check points—the relationship between the restriction point and phosphorylation of pRb. *Exp Cell Res* 2005;305:383.

44. Smith JR, Pereira-Smith OM. Replicative senescence: implications for in vivo aging and tumor suppression. *Science* 1996;273:63.

45. Harley CB, Sherwood SW. Telomerase, checkpoints and cancer. *Cancer Surv* 1997;29:263.

46. Woo RA, Poon RY. Cyclin-dependent kinases and S phase control in mammalian cells. *Cell Cycle* 2003;2:316.

47. Knudson AG Jr. Hereditary cancer. *JAMA* 1979;241:279.

49. Schmitt CA. Cellular senescence and cancer treatment. *Biochim Biophys Acta* 2007;1775:5.

51. Ortega S, Malumbres M, Barbacid M. Cyclin D-dependent kinases, INK4 inhibitors and cancer. *Biochim Biophys Acta* 2002;1602:73.

52. Lee J, Kim SS, The function of p27^{KIP1} during tumor development. *Ex. Mol Med* 2009;41:765.

53. Varley J. TP53, hChk2, and the Li-Fraumeni syndrome. *Methods Mol Biol* 2003;222:117.

58. Zhang Y, Xiong Y. Control of p53 ubiquitination and nuclear export by MDM2 and ARF. *Cell Growth Differ* 2001;12:175.

60. Loeb KR, Loeb LA. Significance of multiple mutations in cancer. *Carcinogenesis* 2000;21:379.

61. Vessey CJ, Norbury CJ, Hickson ID. Genetic disorders associated with cancer predisposition and genomic instability. *Prog Nucleic Acid Res Mol Biol* 1999;63:189.

63. Donnellan R, Chetty R. Cyclin E in human cancers. *FASEB J* 1999;13:773.

64. Spruck CH, Won KA, Reed SI. Deregulated cyclin E induces chromosome instability. *Nature* 1999;401:297.

68. Migliore C, Giordano S. MiRNAs as new master players. *Cell Cycle* 2009;8:2185.

69. Yu Z, Baserga R, Chen L, et al. microRNA, cell cycle and human breast cancer. *Am J Pathol* 2010;176:1058.

71. Levi F, Alper O, Dulong S, et al. Circadian timing in cancer treatments. *Annu Rev Pharmacol. Toxicol* 2010;50:377.

GENERAL PRINCIPLES

CHAPTER 7 MECHANISMS OF CELL DEATH

VASSILIKI KARANTZA AND EILEEN WHITE

Cell death has historically been subdivided into genetically controlled (or programmed) and unregulated mechanisms. Apoptosis has been recognized as a fundamental type of programmed cell death that is activated and repressed by specific genes and pathways. In contrast, necrosis has traditionally been considered an unregulated process and the result of cell death by acute physical trauma or overwhelming stress that is incompatible with cell survival. More recently, however, this strict classification of cell death mechanisms has been revisited, as mechanisms considered "programmed" were in certain instances shown to modulate necrosis and result in a regulated nonapoptotic cell death displaying necrotic morphology (necroptosis). It is also becoming apparent that disabling programmed cell death reveals novel survival mechanisms such as the catabolic autophagy pathway used by cancer cells to tolerate stress and starvation. Thus, cancer cells that acquire defects in programmed cell death are not merely "undead" but rather mobilize a novel physiologic state that actively enables survival. We review here the key aspects of the different cell death mechanisms and their regulation, and how they impact cancer development, progression, and treatment response.

APOPTOSIS

Apoptosis (or type I programmed cell death) is a genetic pathway for rapid and efficient killing of unnecessary or damaged cells that was initially described by Vogt (1842), and then Kerr et al.[1] and Wyllie et al.[2] They detailed a novel morphologic process for cell death that included swiftly executed cell shrinkage, blebbing of the plasma membrane, chromatin condensation, and intranucleosomal DNA fragmentation, after which cell corpses are engulfed by neighboring cells and professional phagocytes and degraded. Apoptosis (commonly pronounced ap-a-tow'-sis), a term coined from the Greek *apo* or from, and *ptosis* or falling, to make the analogy of leaves falling off a tree. Although underappreciated at the time, once the genes that controlled apoptosis were identified in model organisms and humans, and it was shown that perturba-

tion of this program disturbed development and provoked disease, the importance of apoptosis was generally realized.

Cell death by apoptosis is involved in sculpting tissues in normal development. These developmental cell deaths span the removal of the interdigital webs and tadpole tails, to selection for and against specific B- and T-cell populations essential for controlling the immune response. Proper regulation of apoptosis is critical in that excessive apoptosis is associated with degenerative conditions, while deficient apoptosis promotes autoimmunity and cancer. Furthermore, apoptosis is required for eliminating damaged or pathogen-infected cells as a mechanism for limiting disease, especially cancer. In turn, tumors and pathogens have also evolved elegant mechanisms for disabling apoptosis to facilitate their persistence, often promoting disease progression. In human cancers, multiple mechanisms to disable apoptosis include loss of function of the apoptosis-promoting *p53* tumor suppressor and gain of function of the apoptosis-inhibitory and oncogenic B-cell chronic lymphocytic leukemia/lymphoma 2 (*BCL2*). It became apparent then that cancer progression was aided not only by increasing the rate of cell multiplication through activation of the *c-myc* oncogene, for example, but also by decreasing the rate of cell elimination through apoptosis, exemplified by gain of *BCL2* expression (Fig. 7.1). Indeed, activation of oncogenes such as *c-myc* or *E1A*,[3–5] or loss of tumor suppressor genes such as *Rb*,[6] can promote apoptosis, providing an explanation for the necessity for inactivation of the apoptotic pathway in many tumors. This may create a physiological state of cancer cells being "primed for death" where the necessity to up-regulate antiapoptotic mechanisms such as BCL2 to oppose oncogene activation poises cancer cells to reactivation of apoptosis providing a therapeutic window for cancer therapy.[7]

The effectiveness of many existing anticancer drugs involves or is facilitated by triggering the apoptotic response. Thus, a detailed understanding of the components, molecular signaling events, and control points in the apoptotic pathway has enabled rational approaches to chemotherapy aimed at restoring the capacity for apoptosis to

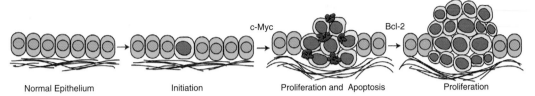

FIGURE 7.1 Tumor progression through cooperation of proliferative and antiapoptotic functions. In normal cells in epithelial tissues (*green cells*) initiating mutational events such as deregulation of *c-myc* expression deregulate cell growth control and promote abnormal cell proliferation (*yellow cells*) while triggering a proapoptotic tumor suppression (*red apoptotic cells*) mechanism that can restrict tumor expansion. Subsequent acquisition of mutations that disables the apoptotic response, exemplified by *Bcl-2* overexpression, prevents this effective means of culling emerging tumor cells, thereby favoring tumor expansion. Similar oncogenic events occur in lymphoid tissues.

tumor cells. Identification of the molecular means by which tumors inactivate apoptosis has led to cancer therapies directly targeting the apoptotic pathway. These drugs are now being used in the clinic to specifically reactivate apoptosis in tumor cells in which it is disabled to achieve tumor regression.

Model Organisms Provide Mechanistic Insight into Apoptosis Regulation

Key to elevating the field of programmed cell death from a descriptive to a mechanism-based process

was the discovery of genes in the nematode *Ceanorhabditis elegans* that control cell death, the cell death defective or *ced* genes.[8] Genetic analysis revealed that *ced-4* and *ced-3* promote cell death, as worms with defective mutations in these genes possessed extra cells. In contrast, the *ced-9* gene inhibited the death-promoting function of *ced-4* and *ced-3*, thereby maintaining cell viability.[9] *ced-9* in turn was inhibited by *egl-1*, thereby promoting cell death. This creates a linear genetic pathway controlled upstream by cell-specific death specification regulators, and downstream by cell corpse engulfment and degradation mechanisms (Fig. 7.2).[10] These findings helped propel work in mammalian systems when it became apparent that Ced-9 was homologous to BCL2,[11] Ced-3 was

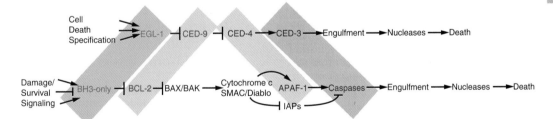

FIGURE 7.2 Analogous pathways regulate programmed cell death/apoptosis in metazoans. Regulation of programmed cell death in the nematode *Ceanorhabditis elegans* (**top**) and regulation of apoptosis in mammals (**bottom**). Shaded regions highlight corresponding homologous genes and protein families. In *C. elegans*, numerous cell death specification genes can up-regulate the transcription of the BH3-only protein Egl-1, which interacts with the antiapoptotic Bcl-2 homologue Ced-9 inhibiting is interaction with Ced-4. Ced-4, the Apaf-1 homologue, in turn, activates the caspase Ced-3, leading to cell death. A variety of engulfment gene products are then responsible for apoptotic corpse elimination and nucleases degrade the genome. In mammals, many survival, damage, and stress events impinge on the numerous members of the BH3-only class of proapoptotic proteins to either activate them to promote apoptosis or suppress their activation to enable cell survival. BH3-only proteins interact with and antagonize the numerous Bcl-2-related multidomain antiapoptotic proteins that serve to sequester proapoptotic Bax and Bak and may also contribute directly to Bax/Bak activation. Bax or Bak is essential for signaling apoptosis by permeabilizing the outer mitochondrial membrane to allow the release of cytochrome *c* and second mitochondrial-derived activator of caspase (SMAC). Cytochrome *c* acts as a cofactor for Apaf-1-mediated caspase activation in the apoptosome, and the SMAC amino-terminal four amino acids bind and antagonize the inhibitors of apoptosis proteins that interact with and suppress caspases, leading to their activation, widespread substrate cleavage, and cell death. Many engulfment gene products are responsible for corpse elimination and caspase-activated nucleases in the apoptotic cell itself, and additional nucleases within the engulfing cell are responsible for degradation of the genome.

homologous to interleukin1-β–converting enzyme, a cysteine protease that would later be classified as a member of the caspase family of aspartic acid proteases,[12] Egl-1 was a BH3-only protein homologue,[10] and that the proapoptotic factor apoptotic protease-activating factor (APAF-1)-1 identified in mammals was homologous to Ced-4.[13]

A similar cell death pathway in the fruit fly *Drosophila melanogaster* identified Reaper, Hid and Grim as inhibitors of the inhibitors of apoptosis proteins (IAPs) that negatively regulate caspase activation. This eventually led to the identification of their mammalian counterpart second mitochondrial-derived activator of caspase (SMAC), also known as direct IAP-binding protein with low pI (DIABLO).[14] These and other studies established the paradigm whereby proapoptotic BH3-only proteins inhibit antiapoptotic Bcl-2 proteins that prevent APAF-1-mediated caspase activation suppressed by IAPs, and the caspase-mediated proteolytic cellular destruction leads rapidly to cell death. It would later be realized that in mammals BH3-only proteins could also act as direct activators of the proapoptotic machinery (see later discussion).

Discovery of Bcl-2 and its Role as an Apoptosis Inhibitor in B-cell Lymphoma

To identify mechanisms of oncogenesis, the *bcl-2* gene was cloned from the site of frequent chromosome translocation t(14;18):(q32;q21) in human follicular lymphoma.[15–17] This chromosome rearrangement places *bcl-2* under the transcriptional control of the immunoglobulin heavy chain locus causing abnormally high levels of *bcl-2* expression. Distinct from other oncogenes at the time, instead of promoting cell proliferation, *bcl-2* promoted B-cell tumorigenesis by the novel concept of providing a survival advantage to cells stimulated to proliferate by *c-myc*.[18] Indeed, engineering high Bcl-2 expression in the lymphoid compartment in mutant mice promotes follicular hyperplasia that progresses to lymphoma upon *c-myc* translocation, and *bcl-2* synergizes with *c-myc* to produce lymphoid tumors, paralleling events in human follicular lymphoma.[19,20] Bcl-2 localizes to mitochondria where it has broad activity in promoting cell survival through suppression of apoptosis,[21] provoked by numerous events, including oncogene activation (*c-myc*, *E1A*), tumor suppressor activation (*p53*), growth factor and cytokine limitation, and cellular damage. It also became clear that inactivation of the retinoblastoma tumor suppressor (*Rb*) pathway promotes a *p53*-mediated apoptotic response, suggesting that apoptosis was part of a tumor suppression mechanism that responded to deregulation of cell growth.[6,22,23] Indeed, apoptotic defects acquired by a variety of means are a common event in human tumorigenesis.

Control of Apoptosis by Bcl-2 Family Members

Bcl-2 is the first member of what is now a large family of related proteins that regulate apoptosis and are conserved among metazoans including worms, flies, and mammals, and also viruses.[24–28] Multidomain Bcl-2 family members containing Bcl-2 homology regions 1-4 (BH1-4) are either antiapoptotic (Bcl-2, Bcl-x_L, Bcl-w, Mcl-1, and Bfl-1/A1, and virally encoded Bcl-2 homologues such as E1B 19K), or proapoptotic (Bax and Bak). Antiapoptotic proteins can block apoptosis by binding and sequestering Bax and Bak or by indirectly preventing Bax and Bak activation (Fig. 7.3).[25,29,30]

Bax and Bak are functionally redundant and required for signaling apoptosis through mitochondria, and deficiency in Bax and Bak produces a profound defect in apoptosis. Bax and Bak are considered the core apoptosis machinery controlled directly or indirectly by antiapoptotic Bcl-2-like proteins and proapoptotic BH3-only proteins. Remarkably, mice deficient in both Bax and Bak develop relatively normally, suggesting that other death mechanisms can compensate for loss of apoptosis in development.[31] In healthy cells, Bak is bound and sequestered by Mcl-1 and Bcl-x_L at cellular membranes, whereas Bax resides in the cytosol in a latent form and requires activation and translocation to membranes, where it is either sequestered by antiapoptotic Bcl-2-like proteins or otherwise induces apoptosis (Fig. 7.3).

Control of Multidomain Bcl-2 Family Proteins by the BH3-only Proteins

Bax and Bak deficiency abrogates the ability of BH3-only proteins to induce apoptosis, placing them upstream and dependent on the core apoptosis machinery.[32] BH3-only protein Bcl-2 family members (Bim, Bid, Nbk/Bik, Puma, Bmf, Bad, and Noxa) are proapoptotic and antagonize the survival activity of antiapoptotic Bcl-2-like proteins by binding and displacing Bax and Bak to allow apoptosis (BH3-only proteins as neutralizers of Bcl-2) (Fig. 7.4).[30] The different BH3-only proteins respond to specific stimuli to activate apoptosis (Fig. 7.3). For example, Bim induces apoptosis in response to taxanes, Puma and Noxa are transcriptional targets of and mediate apoptosis in response to *p53* activation, Bad signals apoptosis on growth factor withdrawal, Nbk/Bik promotes apoptosis in response to inhibition of protein synthesis, and Bid is required for apoptosis signaled by death receptors. All of these signals are transduced from the BH3-only proteins to other members of the Bcl-2 family by protein-protein interactions.

The BH3 region of BH3-only proteins binds to a hydrophobic cleft in the multidomain Bcl-2-like antiapoptotic proteins that also supports Bax and Bak binding,[33,34] causing their displacement (neutralization mode; Fig. 7.4).[30] Differential binding specificities among the BH3 regions of the different BH3-only proteins determine whether they bind one or more Bcl-2-like proteins and displace Bax or Bak or both.[35] Noxa binds and antagonizes Mcl-1, whereas Bad binds and antagonizes Bcl-2 and Bcl-x_L, necessitating cooperation between Noxa and Bad function for efficient apoptosis. In contrast, Bim, Bid, and Puma have broader binding specificity and antagonize Mcl-1, Bcl-2, and Bcl-x_L to release both Bax and Bak to induce apoptosis. Bim, the active form of Bid (truncated Bid or tBid) and possibly Puma can

also be direct activators of Bax and Bak. For example, tBid can bind to latent, inactive Bax and promote its conformational change and translocation to the mitochondrial membrane that is required for apoptosis.[36] BH3-only proteins can inhibit Bcl-2-like proteins, releasing these direct activators of Bax and Bak to promote apoptosis in the de-repression mode (Fig. 7.4). BH3-only proteins that only interact with Bcl-2-like proteins can release activator BH3-only proteins to promote apoptosis in the sensitizer mode (Fig. 7.4). Thus, apoptosis induction by BH3-only proteins can occur through neutralization, de-repression and sensitizer functions.[28]

Importantly, it is this BH3 interaction with Bcl-2 that is the molecular basis for the BH3-mimetic class of proapoptotic, Bcl-2–antagonizing

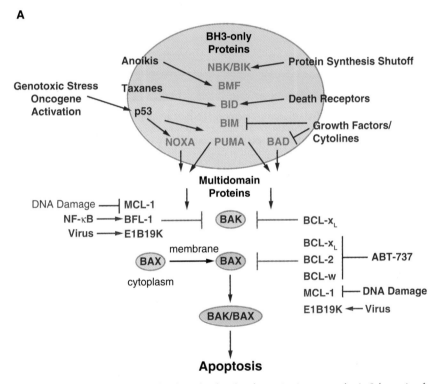

A

Apoptosis

FIGURE 7.3 Regulation of apoptosis by the Bcl-2 family of proteins in mammals. **A:** Schematic of apoptosis regulation by the Bcl-2 family. Cytotoxic events activate, while survival signaling events suppress the activity of the BH3-only class of Bcl-2 family members (*orange*). BH3-only proteins are controlled at the transcription level and also by numerous posttranscriptional events that modulate phosphorylation, proteolysis, localization, sequestration, and protein stability. Once activated, BH3-only proteins disrupt functional sequestration of Bak and Bax by the multidomain antiapoptotic Bcl-2-like proteins (*blue*) and may also directly facilitate Bax/Bak activation. Although Bak is commonly membrane-associated in a complex with Mcl-1 and Bcl-x_L in healthy cells, Bax resides in the cytoplasm as an inactive monomer with its carboxy-terminus occluding the BH3-binding hydrophobic cleft.[138] Bax activation thereby additionally requires a change in protein conformation and membrane translocation by an unknown mechanism that may be facilitated by tBid binding. Binding specificity among BH3-only proteins for antiapoptotic Bcl-2-like proteins determines which complexes are disrupted, with some BH3-only proteins having broad specificity and others do not. Survival and death signaling events can also modulate apoptosis by targeting the multidomain antiapoptotic proteins either by antagonizing their function to promote apoptosis or induction their function to promote survival. ABT-737 is a rationally designed BAD BH3 mimetic that can bind Bcl-2, Bcl-x_L, and Bcl-w but not Mcl-1 that can promote apoptosis where survival does not depend on Mcl-1. Once activated, Bax or Bak oligomerization promotes apoptosis. (*continued*)

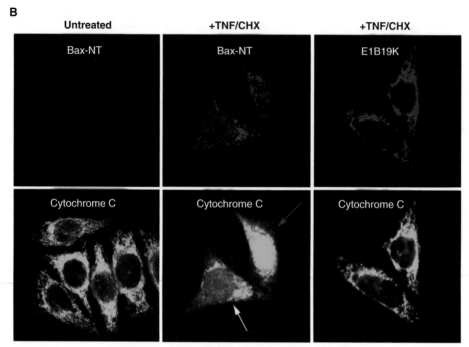

FIGURE 7.3 (*Continued*) **B:** Tumor necrosis factor-α (TNF-α) apoptotic signaling induces mitochondrial membrane translocation and a conformational change exposing the amino-terminus of Bax (visualized here by the Bax-NT antibody) and apoptosis, which is blocked by sequestration of Bax by the antiapoptotic viral Bcl-2 homologue E1B 19K. The human cancer cell line (HeLa cells) with or without E1B 19K expression, were then left untreated or treated with TNF/CHX. The localization of conformationally altered Bax (Bax-NT) and cytochrome *c* (left and middle panels), or E1B 19K and cytochrome *c* (right panel), are shown. The proapoptotic stimulus (TNF/CHX) induces Bax activation, mitochondrial translocation, and cytochrome *c* release from mitochondria that leads to caspase activation and apoptotic cell death, whereas expression of E1B 19K sequesters Bax thereby blocking cytochrome *c* release from mitochondria, caspase activation, and apoptotic cell death. The *yellow* and *red* arrows, respectively, mark cells with partial or complete cytochrome *c* release from mitochondria upon TNF/CHX treatment.

anticancer drugs (Fig. 7.5).[33,37–39] This detailed understanding of the Bcl-2 family member protein interactions and function is allowing rational, apoptosis-targeted therapy (see later discussion).

Role of Mitochondrial Membrane Permeabilization in Apoptosis

Once activated, Bax and Bak oligomerize in the mitochondrial outer membrane, rendering it permeable to proapoptotic mitochondrial proteins cytochrome *c* and SMAC.[40–44] How Bcl-2 family members permeabilize membranes is not entirely clear but it is likely related to a change in topology of the proteins in the membrane and formation of a channel or pore. Once released into the cytoplasm, cytochrome *c* interacts with the WD40 domains of APAF-1 in the apoptosome, a wheel-like particle with sevenfold symmetry that serves as a scaffold for caspase-9 activation.[45] SMAC functions to antagonize the caspase inhibitors, the IAP proteins, to facilitate caspase activation. The amino-terminus of SMAC binds to IAPs, neutralizing their caspase-inhibitor function. Subsequent effector caspase activation (e.g., caspase-3), leads to the rapid, orderly dismantling of the cell and cell death without activating the innate immune response.[46]

Control of Apoptosis by Death Receptors

One of the apoptotic pathways being modulated in cancer therapies is that belonging to the death receptors. Ligands related to tumor necrosis factor-α (TNF-α), including Fas/Apo1 (Fas) and tumor necrosis factor-related ligand (TRAIL) and their cognate receptors were identified as potent activators of apoptosis, and this pathway is critical for regulating the immune response.[47] Engagement of the receptor by soluble or membrane-localized ligand activates the death-inducing signaling complex composed of adaptor proteins such as FADD, which promotes activation of

Neutralization Mode

BH3-only ——|Bcl-2-like ——|Bax——▶Apoptosis

De-repression Mode

Bcl-2-like ——|BH3-only——▶Bax——▶Apoptosis

Sensitizer Mode

BH3-only ——|Bcl-2-like ——|BH3-only ——▶Bax——▶Apoptosis

FIGURE 7.4 Modes of apoptosis activation by BH3-only proteins. The neutralization mode (**top**), de-repression mode (**middle**), and sensitizer mode (**bottom**). See text for explanation.

caspase-8 (Fig. 7.5). Caspase-8, in turn, cleaves the BH3-only protein Bid to its truncated or activated form tBid, which then antagonizes the antiapoptotic function of Bcl-2-like proteins, promoting Bax and Bak activation.[36] This process signals cytochrome c and SMAC release from mitochondria and caspase-9 and -3 activation and cell death. In some cell types that do not require this Bcl-2 family protein-regulated, mitochondrial amplification step, active caspase-8 can directly cleave and activate caspase-3 to cause cell death by apoptosis. Execution of apoptotic cell death is extremely rapid and efficient, resulting in cell death in less than 1 hour in mammalian cells.

pathway to therapeutically induce apoptosis preferentially in tumor cells. Although TNF-α and Fas proved highly toxic to both normal and tumor cells, tumor cells display preferential sensitivity to TRAIL, which has now entered clinical trials (Fig. 7.6).[48–52] Moreover, in cases in which apoptosis is blocked at the mitochondrial level in tumors, SMAC-mimetics have proved useful in stimulating the activity of TRAIL by antagonizing the caspase-inhibitory function of IAPs to facilitate direct caspase-3 activation by caspase-8 (Fig. 7.6).[53–56] Thus, defining this pathway to apoptosis regulation has revealed novel opportunities to rational therapy designed to activate apoptosis preferentially in tumor cells.

Modulation of the Death Receptor Pathway in Cancer Therapy

The ability of soluble ligands to activate the apoptotic response has stimulated interest in using this

Drugs Targeting the Bcl-2 Family for Chemotherapy

In addition to Bcl-2 up-regulation in B-cell lymphoma as previously described, there are other

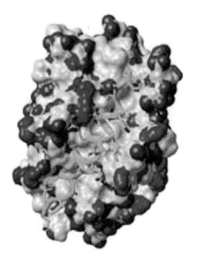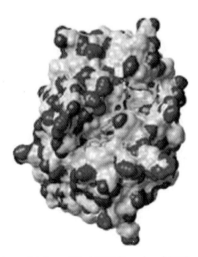

FIGURE 7.5 Three-dimensional structure of Bcl-x$_L$ with bound Bad BH3 ligand and ABT-737. Space-filling model of Bcl-x$_L$ illustrating the hydrophobic cleft binding the 25-mer peptide (*green helix*) of the Bad BH3 (**left**) or the rationally designed BH3-mimetic ABT-737 (**right**). (Reprinted from ref. 33, with permission.)

GENERAL PRINCIPLES

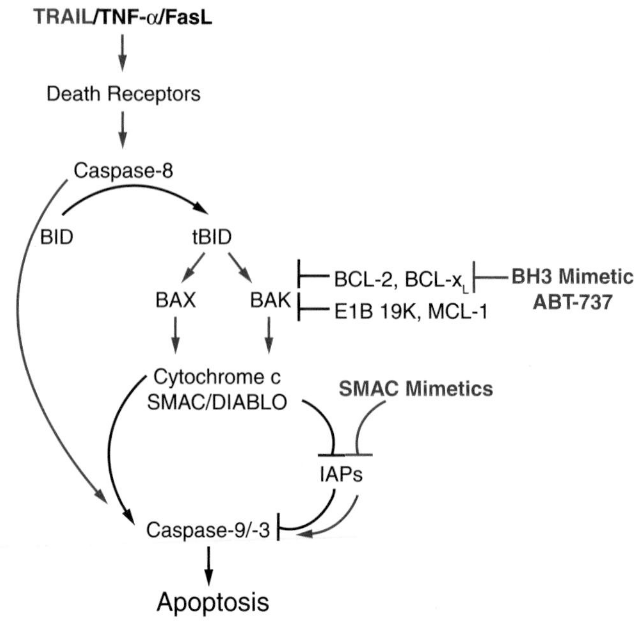

FIGURE 7.6 Therapeutic modulation of the apoptotic pathway downstream of death receptors. Tumor necrosis factor-related ligand (TRAIL) and related death-promoting ligands engage their cognate death receptors and activate caspase-8, which then cleaves Bid to active tBid. tBid can bind Bcl-2 and related antiapoptotic proteins to release Bax and Bak and may also directly promote their activation to permeabilize the mitochondrial outer membrane to release the APAF-1 cofactor cytochrome c, and the inhibitors of apoptosis protein antagonist second mitochondrial-derived activator of caspase (SMAC) for promote caspase-9 and -3 activation and cell death. BH3-mimetics such as ABT-737 can promote apoptosis-induction by TRAIL by relieving the protective capacity of the antiapoptotic Bcl-2-like proteins. In cells that do not depend on the mitochondrial apoptotic signal, TRAIL-mediated caspase-8 activation can directly promote downstream caspase activation and can synergize with SMAC mimetics in this case.

mechanisms for directly or indirectly inactivating apoptosis in tumors that facilitate tumor progression and treatment resistance. Inactivation of the *p53* tumor suppressor, or the *p53* pathway through the gain of function of the *p53* inhibitor MDM-2, is a common occurrence in tumors that results in the loss of the proapoptotic and growth arrest functions of *p53*.[57,58] The BH3-only proteins Puma and Noxa are transcriptional targets of *p53*, the loss of which prevents induction of the *p53*-mediated response to genotoxic stress in tumors as a mechanism of tumor suppression. Various means for restoration of *p53* function in tumors are, therefore, an attractive therapeutic approach.[59–61]

Activation of the MAP kinase pathway is also common in tumors and results in stimulation of tumor cell proliferation, but also the phosphory-

lation and proteasome mediated degradation of the BH3-only protein Bim. This Bim inactivation promotes tumor growth, while also producing resistance to the taxane class of chemotherapeutic drugs. This loss of Bim function is rectified by blocking Bim degradation with a proteasome inhibitor (bortezomib) (Fig. 7.7).[62] Similarly, direct inhibition of MAP kinase pathway signaling with inhibitors (sorafenib, UO126) can also restore apoptotic function in addition to suppressing the proliferative response (Fig. 7.7). Receptor tyrosine kinase pathway activation in tumors also promotes tumor cell proliferation in part through MAP kinase pathway activation downstream and in part through Bim and thereby apoptosis inactivation. In chronic myelogenous leukemia in which chromosomal translocation and activation of the Bcr/Abl tyrosine kinase also leads

FIGURE 7.7 Therapeutic regulation of Bim and the MAP kinase pathway in cancer chemotherapy. Bim protein stability is regulated by Erk phosphorylation and proteasome-mediated degradation. Therapeutic modulation of the MAP kinase pathway (imatinib, sorafenib, and UO126) or proteasome function (bortezomib) can restore Bim protein levels and apoptosis function. Taxanes also stimulate Bim expression and promote Bim-mediated apoptosis, synergizing with the aforementioned inhibitors.

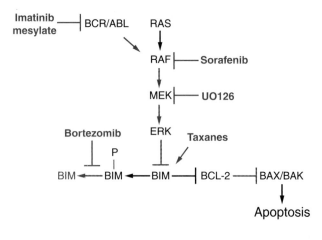

to BIM inhibition, blocking kinase signaling with imatinib mesylate restores Bim and also Bad apoptotic function as a therapeutic strategy (Fig. 7.7).[63] Activation of the PI-3 kinase pathway commonly through loss of *PTEN* tumor suppressor function and AKT activation results in phosphorylation and inactivation of the BH3-only protein Bad and reduction of Bim transcription through inhibition of forkhead factors, resulting in down-regulation of apoptosis.[64] Thus, inhibitors of the PI-3 kinase pathway can restore apoptosis and facilitate tumor regression.[65] NF-κB, a cytokine-responsive transcription factor, also promotes tumor growth while turning on the expression of antiapoptotic regulators Bcl-x$_L$, Bfl-1 and IAPs (Fig. 7.3).[66] Strategies to inhibit NF-κB are likely to promote tumor regression in part through restoration of apoptotic function.[67]

Direct Modulation of Bcl-2 with BH3-mimetics

The observation that antiapoptotic Bcl-2 family members bound and sequestered BH3-regions in a hydrophobic cleft as a means to suppress apoptosis activation (Fig. 7.5) revealed the opportunity for the rational design of small molecules that occlude the cleft and disrupt this Bcl-2-like protein/proapoptotic protein interaction, thereby promoting apoptosis.[33] This was accomplished and resulted in ABT-737, which binds the BH3 binding pocket of Bcl-2, Bcl-x$_L$, and Bcl-w, but not Mcl-1, similarly to the Bcl-2 family protein binding by Bad (Fig. 7.5). ABT-737 exhibited activity as a single agent against human lymphoma and small cell lung cancer cell lines *in vitro* and in mouse xenographs *in vivo*,[37] and in combination with various cytotoxic agents against acute myeloid leukemia,[68] multiple myeloma,[69] chronic lymphocytic leukemia,[70] and small cell lung cancer.[71] ABT-263, an orally bioavailable form of ABT-737, exhibited similar preclinical activity,[72] and has now entered clinical trials as a single agent or in combination with other anticancer drugs. Not surprisingly, given that ABT-737 does not bind to Mcl-1, resistance to ABT-737 has been associated with Mcl-1, as well as Bfl-1, up-regulation,[73] indicating that combinatorial treatment with anticancer agents that target Mcl-1[74] or Bfl-1 could be therapeutically beneficial. Alternate chemical approaches to generating BH3-mimetics to promote apoptosis in cancer cells are also producing encouraging results in the preclinical setting.[39] Thus, deciphering the mechanisms of apoptosis regulation in tumor cells is yielding novel opportunities for rational drug design and therapeutic intervention. These analyses can help predict which tumors have the potential to respond to apoptosis modulation and the types of drug combinations they may respond to.

Killing the Unkillable Cells: Alternate Approaches to Achieving Tumor Cell Death

An apoptotic response to therapy in tumors may not always be possible to achieve; therefore, it is important to determine alternate cell death processes and how to access them specifically in tumor cells. One intrinsic difference between normal and tumor cells is their altered metabolism and prevalence of aerobic glycolysis, which is an inefficient means for generation of adenosine triphosphate (ATP) required for sustaining homeostasis but an efficient means to generate synthetic precursors to support cell proliferation.[75,76] This tumor cell-specific altered metabolism can provide novel approaches to therapeutically target cancer but not normal cells.[75] Altered tumor cell metabolism is frequently coupled with high energy demand due to a rapid cell growth, with the potential to render tumor cells susceptible to cell death because of metabolic catastrophe where cellular energy consumption exceeds production.[77]

The means to specifically drive tumor cells toward metabolic catastrophe is through therapeutic nutrient deprivation that may be an additional consequence of the use of angiogenesis, growth factor, nutrient transporter, and metabolic pathway inhibitors. In addition, inhibition of the catabolic process of autophagy may similarly create metabolic deprivation and promote tumor cell death. Importantly, induction of cell death by interfering with metabolism can occur independently of an intact apoptotic response, suggesting that modulation of tumor cell metabolism may be therapeutically advantageous.

AUTOPHAGY

Role of Autophagy in Promoting Cell Survival to Metabolic Stress

Autophagy is an evolutionarily conserved, stress-activated catabolic lysosomal pathway that results in degradation of long-lived proteins and organelles. This process involves formation of the "autophagosome," a double-membrane vesicle in the cytosol that engulfs organelles and cytoplasm and then fuses with the lysosome to form the "autolysosome," where the sequestered contents are degraded and recycled to generate building blocks for macromolecular synthesis and maintenance of energy homeostasis.[78,79] Hence the name autophagy (commonly pronounced aw-tof´ə-je), a term coined from the Greek *auto* or oneself, and *phagy* or eating, accurately depicts the process. Although autophagy can potentially induce cell death through progressive cellular consumption (autophagy is sometime referred to as type II programmed cell death), physiologic conditions in mammals where this occurs have not yet been identified. In most settings, autophagy is a survival pathway that can delay apoptosis, support metabolism in nutrient stress, and mitigate cellular damage by preventing the accumulation of damaged proteins and organelles. In tumor cells with defects in apoptosis, it has recently become apparent that autophagy supports long-term survival of tumor cells,[80,81] newly revealing opportunities to target not only apoptosis, but also the mechanism by which cells survive once apoptosis is disabled.[82]

Autophagy is regulated by mTOR in the PI3-kinase/AKT pathway that functions to link nutrient availability to cellular metabolism.[83] Under conditions of nutrient limitation, normal cells use this pathway to turn down growth and protein synthesis while activating the catabolic process of autophagy to maintain energy and biosynthetic homeostasis.[79] Thus, autophagy is a temporary survival mechanism during starvation, as self-digestion provides an alternative energy source.[80,84–86]

On growth factor deprivation, hematopoietic cells activate autophagy, which is essential for maintenance of ATP production and cellular survival.[81] In normal mouse development, amino acid production by autophagic degradation of "self" proteins allows maintenance of energy homeostasis and survival during neonatal starvation.[87] Chronically ischemic myocardium induces autophagy, which inhibits apoptosis and may function as a cardioprotective mechanism.[88] These and other examples indicate that autophagy is essential for the maintenance of cellular energy homeostasis that enables survival particularly during stress and starvation.

Autophagy is not only involved in recycling of normal cellular constituents to support cellular metabolism, but is also essential for the removal of toxic-damaged proteins and organelles. The importance of this toxic garbage disposal mechanism is exemplified by the observation that defects in autophagy result in the accumulation of ubiquitin-positive and p62-positive protein aggregates, abnormal mitochondria, and deformed cellular structures associated with production of reactive oxygen species and cellular degeneration.[89–93] This protein and organelle quality control function of autophagy is important in preserving cellular health and viability in conjunction with metabolic support via catabolism.

Autophagy also contributes to innate immunity by protecting cells against infection with intracellular pathogens[94–97] and to acquired immunity by promoting T-lymphocyte survival and proliferation[98] and by affecting antigen presentation in dendritic cells and bacterial handling.[99] Moreover, autophagy is involved in cellular development and differentiation,[100,101] and may have a protective role against aging and age-related pathologies.[102,103]

Progressive autophagy can potentially lead to cell death in limited circumstances when allowed to proceed to completion, and when cells unable to undergo apoptosis are triggered to die. Unfortunately, it is often unclear whether autophagy is directly involved in initiation and/or execution of cell death or if it merely represents a failed or exhausted attempt to preserve cell viability.[104] Recent studies indicate that autophagy may play an active role in programmed cell death, but the conditions under which autophagy promotes cell death versus cell survival remain to be resolved.[105–108]

Role of Autophagy in Tumorigenesis

Defective autophagy has been implicated in tumorigenesis, as the essential autophagy regulator *becn1* is monoallelically deleted in human breast, ovarian, and prostate cancers[109] and some human breast cancers have decreased Beclin1 levels.[110] *Becn1* is the mammalian orthologue of the yeast *atg6/vps30* gene, which is required for autophagosome formation.[111] *Becn1* complements the autophagy defect present in *atg6/vps30*-disrupted yeast and in human MCF7 breast cancer cells, the latter in association with inhibition of MCF7-induced tumorigenesis in nude mice.[110] *Becn1*[−/−] mice die early in embryogenesis, whereas aging *Becn1*[+/−] mice have increased incidence of lymphoma and carcinomas of the lung and liver[112,113] In addition, mammary tissue from *Becn1*[+/−] mice shows hyperproliferative, preneoplastic changes.[113] Tumors forming in *Becn1*[+/−] mice express wild type Beclin1 mRNA and protein, indicating that *Becn1* is a haploinsufficient tumor suppressor.[112]

Recent studies revealed that autophagy enables tumor cell survival *in vitro* and *in vivo* that is particularly obvious in tumor cells when apoptosis is inactivated.[80,85,86] When angiogenesis is insufficient, autophagy localizes to the resulting hypoxic tumor regions where it supports tumor cell viability (Fig. 7.8).[80,85,86] This process of autophagy during nutrient deprivation allows recovery of growth and proliferative capacity with remarkably high fidelity when nutrients, oxygen, and growth factors are restored. Thus, autophagy may be a fundamental obstacle to tumor eradication.[80]

How inactivation of a survival pathway promotes tumorigenesis has been an intriguing question. The apparently conflicting pro-survival and pro-death functions of autophagy can, however, be reconciled if one considers autophagy a prolonged but interruptible pathway to cell death on stress and starvation, where nutrient restoration prior to its culmination can provide cellular salvation. This contrasts the death processes of apoptosis and necrosis, which are executed rapidly and are irreversible. As such, the identification of the precise mechanism by which autophagy supports survival is critical.

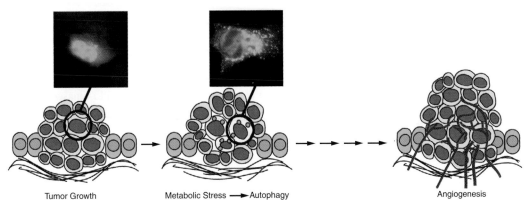

Tumor Growth   Metabolic Stress ⟶ Autophagy   Angiogenesis

FIGURE 7.8 Role of autophagy in enabling survival of tumor cells to metabolic stress. As epithelial tumor cells proliferate and multiple cell layers accumulate, the initial absence of a blood supply produces metabolic stress in regions most distal to the supply of nutrients and oxygen often in the center of the tumor mass. In tumor cells with apoptosis defects, this allows tumor cells in these metabolically stressed tumor regions to survive through autophagy. Subsequent angiogenesis relieves metabolic stress, obviating the need for autophagy, fueling tumor growth.

Autophagy not only provides an alternate means for energy generation during periods of starvation, but also has a role in cellular damage mitigation through promotion of protein and organelle quality control, especially under conditions of stress in which proteins and organelles become damaged. By degrading damaged proteins and organelles, autophagy prevents their accumulation, which can be toxic. This function of autophagy is particularly critical in stressed tissues and tumors, which are regularly subjected to metabolic stress by their dependence on the inefficient process of aerobic glycolysis and by their intermittently limited blood supply during rapid tumor growth or metastasis. Thus, autophagy defects in tissues and tumors reduce cellular fitness and render cells prone to DNA damage, mutation, and genomic instability,[85,86,92] which in turn contribute to tumor initiation and progression.[82,114,115]

In addition to these cell-autonomous mechanisms, defective autophagy can promote tumorigenesis in a non–cell-autonomous way by reducing tumor cell survival that causes chronic cell death and inflammation in tumors.[80,92,115] Autophagy can thereby be thought of as a double-edged sword. On the one hand, autophagy promotes tumor cell survival through maintaining energy homeostasis and mitigating oxidative damage by preventing the accumulation of aggregated proteins and abnormal organelles. On the other hand, defects in autophagy elevate oxidative stress, DNA damage, and mutation, and promote chronic cell death and inflammation, all of which are linked to promotion of cancer initiation and progression.[115] These observations have led to the notions that autophagy stimulation can prevent cancer, whereas inhibiting autophagy-mediated survival is an approach to treating established, aggressive cancers.[82,114]

Autophagy Modulation for Cancer Treatment

As autophagy can enable tumor cell survival to stress,[80,81] the means to block autophagy has the potential to promote cell death that may be therapeutically advantageous.[82,114] Moreover, both targeted and cytotoxic antineoplastic agents have been observed to induce autophagy in human cancer cell lines,[116,117] possibly as a survival mechanism in response to treatment-induced stress. Thus, autophagy inhibitors are expected to deprive cancer cells of an essential survival mechanism and consequently render them more susceptible to cell death. This novel paradigm in cancer therapy has been validated in several preclinical studies.[118–126] This approach is now under investigation in phase 1/2 clinical trials involving autophagy inhibition by the antimalarial drug hydroxychloroquine, which blocks lysosome degradation of the products of autophagy, in combination with standard chemotherapy.

NECROSIS

Recent evidence suggests that tumor cells in which apoptosis has been disabled can be diverted to necrosis, which has traditionally been considered an unregulated (and thus, not programmed) form of cell death implicated in pathologic states, such as ischemia, trauma, and infection.[127] Recent evidence is calling the unregulated nature of necrosis into question.

Necrosis is derived from the Greek word *nekros* for corpse, and it involves rapid swelling of the cell, loss of plasma membrane integrity, and release of the cellular contents into the extracellular environment, resulting in an acute inflammatory response. Necrosis is largely viewed as an accidental and unregulated cellular event triggered by cellular trauma (direct physical injury), acute energy depletion, or extreme stress.[128] Recently, a type of programmed necrotic cell death, called *necroptosis*,[129] has been identified as induced by interaction of death domain receptors with their respective ligands under conditions of defective or inhibited downstream apoptotic machinery.[130] Necroptosis depends on the serine/threonine kinase activity of the death domain receptor-associated adaptor Rip1 and its relative Rip3.[131–136] Necroptosis is potently inhibited by the Rip1 kinase inhibitors, the necrostatins.[133] In a genome-wide siRNA screen for necroptosis regulators, a set of 432 genes with enriched expression in the immune and nervous systems was identified and cellular sensitivity to necroptosis was found to depend on the same signaling network that mediates innate immunity.[131] Harnessing necroptosis to induce cell death in cancer is an exciting new prospect, the exploitation of which will require a deeper mechanistic insight into the process and its regulation.

Regarding necrosis as a therapeutic end point, tumor cell fate in response to treatment with DNA-damaging agents depends on the effect of the DNA repair protein poly(ADP-ribose) polymerase (PARP) on cellular metabolism. PARP activation by DNA-damaging alkylating agents causes PARP-mediated β-nicotinamide adenine dinucleotide (NAD) consumption, ATP depletion, and metabolic stress. The glycolytic state (Warburg effect) and inefficient mode of energy production in most cancer cells renders them sensitive to this ATP depletion in response to PARP activation, resulting in induction of necrotic cell death of apoptosis-defective tumor cells.[137] Tumor cells with defects in both apoptosis and autophagy may be particularly susceptible to death by necrosis as loss of autophagy potential deprives cells of an alternate energy source for maintenance of metabolism and viability in metabolic stress that is compounded by the Warburg effect.[80]

Manipulation of tumor cell metabolism is an appealing therapeutic approach, as it can be used to induce cancer cell death by metabolic catastrophe.[77] This is particularly relevant for tumors with increased proliferative capacity and high bioenergetic requirements, such as tumors with constitutive activation of the PI3-kinase/Akt pathway, which are unable to down-regulate metabolism and to activate autophagy in response to starvation. Thus, the very properties that confer cancer cells with the capacity for rapid growth may also render them susceptible to metabolic stress pharmacologically induced by a wide variety of means, including nutrient deprivation, angiogenesis inhibition, glycolysis inhibition, accelerated ATP consumption, or autophagy inhibition. Furthermore, necrotic cell death can be genetically determined indirectly through manipulation of cellular bioenergetics (decreased energy production through autophagy and catabolism inhibition, increased metabolic demand through elevated consumption, or decreased nutrient availability) or directly by activating Rip kinases or PARP. It will be of great interest to see if necrosis, like apoptosis, can be exploited for cancer therapy.

It is becoming clear that cells possess multiple death mechanism, and establishing how these are altered in tumors and can be activated with therapy is essential. Defining at the molecular level how apoptosis is regulated has led to the development of novel cancer therapies aimed at triggering or restoring apoptotic function in tumor cells, and this progress is likely to continue. Moreover, defining the mechanisms by which common mutations in human tumors inactivate apoptosis has yielded novel opportunities for tumor-genotype–specific rational chemotherapy targeting the apoptotic pathway. In tumor cells where apoptosis is disabled, it is apparent that alternate forms of cell death can be activated, including necrosis, the process by which remains poorly characterized. Finally, the catabolic process of autophagy can promote tumor cell survival to metabolic stress, providing new opportunities for therapeutic intervention, in part capitalizing on the altered metabolic state intrinsic to tumor cells.

Selected References

The full list of references for this chapter appears in the online version.

3. Rao L, Debbas M, Sabbatini P, Hockenbery D, Korsmeyer S, White E. The adenovirus E1A proteins induce apoptosis, which is inhibited by the E1B 19-kDa and Bcl-2 proteins. *Proc Natl Acad Sci U S A* 1992;89:7742.
4. Fanidi A, Harrington EA, Evan GI. Cooperative interaction between c-myc and bcl-2 proto-oncogenes. *Nature* 1992;359:554.
5. Evan GI, Wyllie AH, Gilbert CS, et al. Induction of apoptosis in fibroblasts by c-myc protein. *Cell* 1992;69:119.

6. Morgenbesser SD, Williams BO, Jacks T, DePinho RA. p53-dependent apoptosis produced by Rb-deficiency in the developing mouse lens. *Nature* 1994;371:72.
7. Certo M, Del Gaizo Moore V, Nishino M, et al. Mitochondria primed by death signals determine cellular addiction to antiapoptotic BCL-2 family members. *Cancer Cell* 2006;9:351.
9. Hengartner MO, Ellis RE, Horvitz HR. *Caenorhabditis elegans* gene ced-9 protects cells from programmed cell death. *Nature* 1992;356:494.
12. Yuan J, Shaham S, Ledoux S, Ellis HM, Horvitz HR. The *C. elegans* cell death gene ced-3 encodes a protein similar

to mammalian interleukin-1 beta-converting enzyme. *Cell* 1993;75:641.

13. Zou H, Henzel WJ, Liu X, Lutschg A, Wang X. Apaf-1, a human protein homologous to C. elegans CED-4, participates in cytochrome c-dependent activation of caspase-3. *Cell* 1997;90:405.

15. Bakhshi A, Jensen JP, Goldman P, et al. Cloning the chromosomal breakpoint of t(14;18) human lymphomas: clustering around JH on chromosome 14 and near a transcriptional unit on 18. *Cell* 1985;41:899.

16. Cleary ML, Smith SD, Sklar J. Cloning and structural analysis of cDNAs for bcl-2 and a hybrid bcl-2/immunoglobulin transcript resulting from the t(14;18) translocation. *Cell* 1986;47:19.

17. Tsujimoto Y, Gorham J, Cossman J, Jaffe E, Croce CM. The t(14;18) chromosome translocations involved in B-cell neoplasms result from mistakes in VDJ joining. *Science* 1985;229:1390.

18. Vaux DL, Cory S, Adams JM. Bcl-2 gene promotes haemopoietic cell survival and cooperates with c-myc to immortalize pre-B cells. *Nature* 1988;335:440.

19. McDonnell TJ, Korsmeyer SJ. Progression from lymphoid hyperplasia to high-grade malignant lymphoma in mice transgenic for the t(14; 18). *Nature* 1991;349:254.

20. Strasser A, Harris AW, Bath ML, Cory S. Novel primitive lymphoid tumours induced in transgenic mice by cooperation between myc and bcl-2. *Nature* 1990;348:331.

22. Debbas M, White E. Wild-type p53 mediates apoptosis by E1A, which is inhibited by E1B. *Genes Dev* 1993;7:546.

23. Lowe SW, Ruley HE. Stabilization of the p53 tumor suppressor is induced by adenovirus 5 E1A and accompanies apoptosis. *Genes Dev* 1993;7: 535.

31. Wei MC, Zong WX, Cheng EH, et al. Proapoptotic BAX and BAK: a requisite gateway to mitochondrial dysfunction and death. *Science* 2001;292:727.

32. Zong WX, Lindsten T, Ross AJ, MacGregor GR, Thompson CB. BH3-only proteins that bind pro-survival Bcl-2 family members fail to induce apoptosis in the absence of Bax and Bak. *Genes Dev* 2001;15:1481.

34. Muchmore SW, Sattler M, Liang H, et al. X-ray and NMR structure of human Bcl-xL, an inhibitor of programmed cell death. *Nature* 1996;381:335.

37. Oltersdorf T, Elmore SW, Shoemaker AR, et al. An inhibitor of Bcl-2 family proteins induces regression of solid tumours. *Nature* 2005;435:677.

40. Du C, Fang M, Li Y, Li L, Wang X. Smac, a mitochondrial protein that promotes cytochrome c-dependent caspase activation by eliminating IAP inhibition. *Cell* 2000;102:33.

42. Kluck RM, Bossy-Wetzel E, Green DR, Newmeyer DD. The release of cytochrome c from mitochondria: a primary site for Bcl-2 regulation of apoptosis. *Science* 1997;275:1132.

43. Verhagen AM, Ekert PG, Pakusch M, et al. Identification of DIABLO, a mammalian protein that promotes apoptosis by binding to and antagonizing IAP proteins. *Cell* 2000;102:43.

44. Yang J, Liu X, Bhalla K, et al. Prevention of apoptosis by Bcl-2: release of cytochrome c from mitochondria blocked. *Science* 1997;275:1129.

56. Fulda S, Wick W, Weller M, Debatin KM. Smac agonists sensitize for Apo2L/TRAIL- or anticancer drug-induced apoptosis and induce regression of malignant glioma in vivo. *Nat Med* 2002;8:808.

59. Xue W, Zender L, Miething C, et al. Senescence and tumour clearance is triggered by p53 restoration in murine liver carcinomas. *Nature* 2007;445:656.

60. Ventura A, Kirsch DG, McLaughlin ME, et al. Restoration of p53 function leads to tumour regression in vivo. *Nature* 2007;445:661.

62. Tan TT, Degenhardt K, Nelson DA, et al. Key roles of BIM-driven apoptosis in epithelial tumors and rational chemotherapy. *Cancer Cell* 2005;7:227.

68. Konopleva M, Contractor R, Tsao T, et al. Mechanisms of apoptosis sensitivity and resistance to the BH3 mimetic ABT-737 in acute myeloid leukemia. *Cancer Cell* 2006; 10:375.

80. Degenhardt K, Mathew R, Beaudoin B, et al. Autophagy promotes tumor cell survival and restricts necrosis, inflammation, and tumorigenesis. *Cancer Cell* 2006;10:51.

81. Lum JJ, Bauer DE, Kong M, et al. Growth factor regulation of autophagy and cell survival in the absence of apoptosis. *Cell* 2005;120:237.

86. Mathew R, Kongara S, Beaudoin B, et al. Autophagy suppresses tumor progression by limiting chromosomal instability. *Genes Dev* 2007;21:1367.

87. Kuma A, Hatano M, Matsui M, et al. The role of autophagy during the early neonatal starvation period. *Nature* 2004; 432:1032.

90. Komatsu M, Waguri S, Chiba T, et al. Loss of autophagy in the central nervous system causes neurodegeneration in mice. *Nature* 2006;441: 880.

91. Hara T, Nakamura K, Matsui M, et al. Suppression of basal autophagy in neural cells causes neurodegenerative disease in mice. *Nature* 2006;441:885.

92. Mathew R, Karp CM, Beaudoin B, et al. Autophagy suppresses tumorigenesis through elimination of p62. *Cell* 2009; 137:1062.

93. Komatsu M, Waguri S, Koike M, et al. Homeostatic levels of p62 control cytoplasmic inclusion body formation in autophagy-deficient mice. *Cell* 2007;131:1149.

102. Lee JH, Budanov AV, Park EJ, et al. Sestrin as a feedback inhibitor of TOR that prevents age-related pathologies. *Science* 2010;327:1223.

112. Yue Z, Jin S, Yang C, Levine AJ, Heintz N. Beclin 1, an autophagy gene essential for early embryonic development, is a haploinsufficient tumor suppressor. *Proc Natl Acad Sci U S A* 2003;100:15077.

113. Qu X, Yu J, Bhagat G, et al. Promotion of tumorigenesis by heterozygous disruption of the beclin 1 autophagy gene. *J Clin Invest* 2003;112:1809.

114. White E, DiPaola RS. The double-edged sword of autophagy modulation in cancer. *Clin Cancer Res* 2009; 15:5308.

122. Degtyarev M, De Maziere A, Orr C, et al. Akt inhibition promotes autophagy and sensitizes PTEN-null tumors to lysosomotropic agents. *J Cell Biol* 2008;183:101.

123. Maclean KH, Dorsey FC, Cleveland JL, Kastan MB. Targeting lysosomal degradation induces p53-dependent cell death and prevents cancer in mouse models of lymphomagenesis. *J Clin Invest* 2008;118:79.

124. Carew JS, Nawrocki ST, Kahue CN, et al. Targeting autophagy augments the anticancer activity of the histone deacetylase inhibitor SAHA to overcome Bcr-Abl-mediated drug resistance. *Blood* 2007;110:313.

125. Amaravadi RK, Yu D, Lum JJ, et al. Autophagy inhibition enhances therapy-induced apoptosis in a Myc-induced model of lymphoma. *J Clin Invest* 2007;117:326.

130. Degterev A, Huang Z, Boyce M, et al. Chemical inhibitor of nonapoptotic cell death with therapeutic potential for ischemic brain injury. *Nat Chem Biol* 2005;1:112.

133. Degterev A, Hitomi J, Germscheid M, et al. Identification of RIP1 kinase as a specific cellular target of necrostatins. *Nat Chem Biol* 2008;4:313.

135. Cho YS, Challa S, Moquin D, et al. Phosphorylation-driven assembly of the RIP1-RIP3 complex regulates programmed necrosis and virus-induced inflammation. *Cell* 2009; 137:1112.

136. He S, Wang L, Miao L, et al. Receptor interacting protein kinase-3 determines cellular necrotic response to TNF-alpha. *Cell* 2009;137:1100.

138. Suzuki M, Youle RJ, Tjandra N. Structure of Bax: coregulation of dimer formation and intracellular localization. *Cell* 2000;103:645.

GENERAL PRINCIPLES

CHAPTER 8 CANCER METABOLISM

MATTHEW G. VANDER HEIDEN

One of the first distinctions noted between cancer tissues and normal tissues was a difference in metabolism. In the 1920s, the biochemist Otto Warburg observed that when provided with glucose, cancer tissues generate large amounts of lactate regardless of whether oxygen is present. This finding is in contrast to most normal tissues that only ferment glucose to lactate in the absence of oxygen. This metabolic difference between cancer cells and normal cells is referred to as the Warburg effect, and along with other metabolic alterations that characterize cancer cells, it remains an incompletely understood aspect of cancer biology. The metabolic phenotype of cancer cells has been exploited for cancer diagnostics and led to the development of some of the first successful chemotherapies. However, despite the fact that altered metabolism is shared across many different cancer types, few therapies exist that exploit differences in cellular metabolism. Efforts to understand cancer metabolism are currently an active area of investigation and hold great promise as a source of novel targets for cancer treatment.

ALTERED METABOLISM IN CANCER CELLS

The regulation of metabolic pathways in tumor tissues is different from that observed in most adult tissues.[1] Rapidly dividing cells must balance energy production with macromolecular synthesis, while most nonproliferating adult tissues utilize a greater fraction of nutrients for energy production and require less nutrient uptake. Cancer cells rely primarily on glycolysis for their metabolism, while the majority of normal cells in adult tissues utilize aerobic respiration to completely catabolize glucose and generate cellular energy.[2–5] Most differentiated cells primarily metabolize glucose to carbon dioxide in the presence of oxygen and only produce large amounts of lactate under anaerobic conditions. Warburg observed that cancer cells produce large amounts of lactate regardless of oxygen availability (Fig. 8.1).[6,7] Because cancer cells use glycolysis to make lactate from glucose in the presence of oxygen, this form of metabolism observed in cancer cells is also called aerobic glycolysis.

The primary energy source for cells in most tissues is glucose. The concentration of glucose in the blood remains relatively constant at around 4–6 mM (72–110 mg/dL). Glucose uptake into cells is controlled most proximally by the expression of glucose transport proteins on the cell surface (Fig. 8.2).[8] Insulin-responsive tissues rely on the regulated delivery of Glut4 transporters to the cell surface to increase glucose uptake. Noninsulin responsive tissues, including most cancers, do not use Glut4, but instead use the homologous Glut1, Glut2, or Glut3 proteins to transport glucose into cells. All of these glucose transporters allow the diffusion of glucose across the plasma membrane. The transporters differ in their affinity for glucose and capacity for transport. Glut1 is responsible for the basal level of glucose uptake in most normal cells and is thought to be the transporter responsible for glucose uptake in most tumor cells. Expression of Glut3 and other less well characterized glucose transporters have also been described in some cancers.[9,10] How these transporters differ from Glut1 and whether these differences are important for tumor biology and metabolism remain active areas of investigation.

Glucose is trapped in the cytoplasm of cells by the addition of a phosphate group to form glucose-6-phosphate (Fig. 8.2).[11] This reaction is catalyzed by the enzyme hexokinase, which also has several isoforms with different normal tissue distributions and enzymatic properties. The various isoforms of hexokinase can associate with the outer surface of mitochondria, and this proximity to a source of adenosine triphosphate (ATP) has been suggested to be important for the high rate of glucose uptake observed in many cancer cells.[12] The association of hexokinase with mitochondria has also been implicated in the regulation of apoptosis such that hexokinase may constitute a molecular link between glycolysis and the cell death machinery.[13]

Once trapped in cells, glucose can be metabolized via glycolysis to generate pyruvate in the cytosol.[11] The rate of glycolysis is controlled by glucose flux into cells, cofactor availability, and the activity of glycolytic enzymes (Fig. 8.3). Both the phosphofructokinase and pyruvate kinase steps of glycolysis are highly regulated and have been implicated in the control of tumor cell metabolism

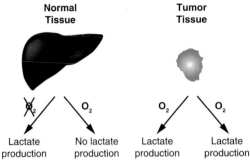

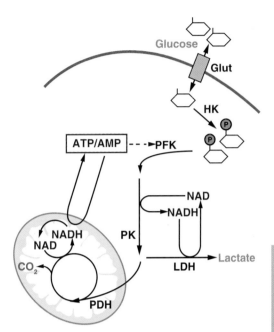

FIGURE 8.1 A graphic representation of Warburg's experiment is shown. Most normal tissues produce lactate in large quantities only when oxygen (O_2) is absent. In contrast, cancer cells tend to make lactate regardless of O_2 availability. This tendency of cancer cells to metabolize glucose to lactate (aerobic glycolysis) is often referred to as the Warburg effect.

(Figs. 8.3 and 8.4).[14-16] Another major determinant of glucose metabolism by glycolysis is the availability of oxidized nicotinamide adenine dinucleotide (NAD) to serve as the electron acceptor for the conversion of glyceraldehyde-3-phosphate to 1,3-bisphosphoglycerate. This reaction, catalyzed by glyceraldehyde-3-phosphate dehydrogenase reduces NAD to NADH (reduced nicotinamide adenine dinucleotide). Because the size of the NAD/NADH cofactor pool in cells is small relative to the flux of glucose through glycolysis, continued cycling of NADH back to NAD is critical

FIGURE 8.3 Cellular glucose metabolism is regulated at several steps. Uptake of glucose is regulated by glucose transporter expression (Glut). Glucose metabolism by glycolysis classically is considered to be regulated at three enzymatic steps: these include the reactions catalyzed by hexokinase (HK), phosphofructokinase (PFK) and pyruvate kinase (PK). The PFK step in glycolysis is a major point of regulation. One major allosteric input to PFK activity is the adenosine triphosphate: adenosine monophosphate (ATP:AMP) ratio. PFK activity and glycolysis are activated when the ATP:AMP ratio is low and inhibited when the ATP:AMP ratio is high. Glycolysis is also controlled by the availability of the cofactor nicotinamide adenine dinucleotide (NAD). NAD is reduced to NADH at the glyceraldehyde-3-phosphate dehydrogenase step of the pathway, and NADH must be recycled back to NAD to allow continued glycolysis. NADH can be converted to NAD by lactate dehydrogenase (LDH)-mediated conversion of pyruvate to lactate. NAD regeneration can also be coupled to the tricarboxylic acid (TCA) cycle and mitochondrial oxidative phosphorylation. Entry of pyruvate into the TCA cycle is controlled by pyruvate dehydrogenase (PDH) and allows the complete catabolism of glucose to carbon dioxide (CO_2) and maximum ATP production.

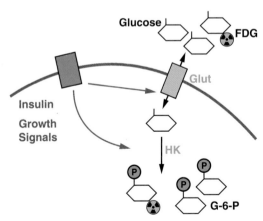

FIGURE 8.2 Glucose uptake is controlled in mammalian cells by the presence of glucose transporters on the cell surface (Glut). These transport proteins allow the diffusion of glucose across the plasma membrane where it is phosphorylated by the enzyme hexokinase (HK) and trapped in the cell. Glucose transporter expression is controlled by insulin signaling in insulin responsive tissues. Glucose uptake is also regulated by cell growth signals. A positron emission tomography (PET) scan can be used to monitor glucose uptake in the clinic. This assay uses the positron-emitting fluorine-18 (^{18}F)-conjugated glucose analogue fluoro-2-deoxyglucose (FDG), which can be phosphorylated by hexokinase and trapped in the cell but cannot be metabolized further.

to permit continued glycolysis (Fig. 8.3). NADH can be reoxidized to NAD through a series of reactions that shuttle reducing equivalents into mitochondria for use in oxidative phosphorylation. This process is coupled to the further metabolism of pyruvate in the mitochondrial tricarboxylic acid (TCA) cycle and can result in the generation of large amounts of ATP. ATP is used as a source of free energy for cells to enable otherwise unfavorable biochemical processes. Mitochondrial oxidative phosphorylation requires the presence of oxygen (O_2) as the final acceptor of electrons from NADH and therefore is also referred to as

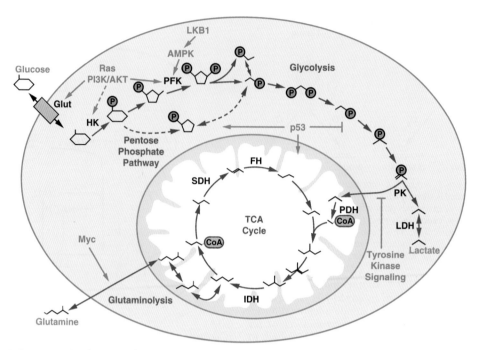

FIGURE 8.4 A schematic of central carbon metabolism is presented to show how glycolysis, the tricarboxylic acid (TCA) cycle, the pentose phosphate pathway, and glutamine metabolism are interconnected in cells. The major points of enzymatic regulation, along with the enzymes discussed in the text that have been demonstrated to be important in cancer, are shown for orientation within the pathways, Glut, glucose transporter; HK, hexokinase; PFK, phosphofructokinase; PK, pyruvate kinase; LDH, lactate dehydrogenase; PDH, pyruvate dehydrogenase; IDH, isocitrate dehydrogenase; SDH, succinate dehydrogenase; FH, fumarate hydratase. The site of regulation within these pathways by some of the major oncogenes and tumor suppressor genes is also shown.

aerobic respiration. Aerobic glycolysis also generates ATP; however, the ATP yield per molecule of glucose is much less than for aerobic respiration. The metabolism of glucose to pyruvate without mitochondrial respiration requires the enzyme lactate dehydrogenase (LDH) to produce lactate and regenerate NAD from NADH.

Several hypotheses for why aerobic glycolysis appears to be selected for in cancer cells have been proposed. Warburg hypothesized that cancer cells develop a defect in mitochondria that leads to impaired aerobic respiration and a subsequent reliance on glycolytic metabolism.[2] Although mutations in mitochondrial enzymes have been implicated in a subset of cancers (discussed in detail later in the chapter), subsequent studies demonstrated that mitochondrial function is not impaired in the majority of cancer cells.[17] Nevertheless, despite his hypothesis being incorrect, Warburg's original observation has held true with numerous reports describing that despite normally functioning mitochondria many cancer cells preferentially metabolize glucose via aerobic glycolysis.[4,18]

The growth of solid tumors is limited by the presence of an adequate blood supply to deliver oxygen and nutrients to support cell metabolism. Therefore, angiogenesis is an important process

for tumor growth, and targeting this process has been successful for cancer therapy.[19] Because many tumors are characterized by inefficient angiogenesis, cells must survive periods of relative hypoxia and nutrient deprivation during tumorigenesis.[5] Therefore, it has been proposed that the relative hypoxia of tumors selects for glycolytic metabolism.[3] However, aerobic glycolysis is observed at the earliest stages of tumorigenesis. It is a characteristic feature of leukemia and lung cancers that arises under conditions of normal to high oxygen tensions and is found in normal rapidly proliferating tissues during embryogenesis and immune responses.[1] Therefore, it is likely that aerobic glycolysis provides another benefit to cancer cells that is selected for during tumorigenesis.[1] Aerobic glycolysis may still facilitate tumor survival during periods of hypoxia. The same pathways that regulate angiogenesis also promote aerobic glycolysis, suggesting that important connections between these two processes exist.[20,21]

The selective pressure for aerobic glycolysis in cancer cells may be related to the reprogramming of metabolism to accommodate rapid cell division. Cells metabolize glucose for purposes other than generating ATP.[1] Intermediates derived from the metabolism of glucose are used in other metabolic pathways in cells and ultimately provide much of the carbon necessary to produce biomass. The production of nucleic acids, amino acids, lipids, and carbohydrates needed to duplicate all the components of the dividing cell is the major metabolic requirement that distinguishes rapidly proliferating cancer cells from most normal cells. If glucose is completely catabolized to carbon dioxide (CO_2), as occurs during oxidative metabolism, there are no metabolic intermediates available for biosynthetic reactions. Thus, aerobic glycolysis may reflect how metabolism is altered to permit anabolic metabolism.[1] Indeed, many microorganisms grow by fermentation when nutrients are abundant and display a metabolic phenotype analogous to aerobic glycolysis.[22]

ENERGETICS OF CELL PROLIFERATION

There is evidence that the rate of aerobic glycolysis, including the accompanying increased rate of glucose utilization, is not elevated in cancer cells solely to satisfy ATP demand. It has been suggested that glycolysis in tumors cells is limited by the rate of ATP consumption.[23,24] Cancer cells must balance the catabolism of nutrients to generate ATP with other metabolic needs to allow net biosynthesis and cell proliferation.[1] To produce a daughter cell, a proliferating cell must replicate the genome, duplicate the ribosomes and protein synthesis machinery, generate new organelles, and synthesize *de novo* enough lipids to duplicate cellular membranes. This imposes a large requirement of new nucleic acids, amino acids, and lipids for cell proliferation. While ATP hydrolysis provides free energy for many biosynthetic pathways, there are additional requirements to carry out these anabolic reactions. Synthesis of lipids and nucleic acids both require specific metabolite precursors and reducing equivalents provided by nicotinamide adenine dinucleotide phosphate (NADPH) (Fig. 8.5). In fact the need for NADPH and carbon skeletons on a molar basis exceeds the requirement for ATP in many biosynthetic reactions.[1] Aerobic glycolysis may allow cancer cells to balance the various metabolic requirements of proliferation.

Cancer Cells Can Metabolize Nutrients Other Than Glucose

Although tumor cell metabolism is adapted to facilitate anabolic metabolism for rapid proliferation, it is not clear why many cancer cells excrete lactate. Each lactate excreted wastes three carbons that might otherwise be recycled to fulfill some need in building a new cancer cell. It has been hypothesized that the excretion of lactate, which accompanies aerobic glycolysis, may enable faster

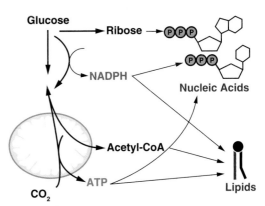

FIGURE 8.5 The generation of macromolecules requires several products of central carbon metabolism. In addition to adenosine triphosphate (ATP), the synthesis of nucleic acids and lipids both require reducing equivalents provided by nicotinamide adenine dinucleotide phosphate (NADPH) and carbon precursors that branch from different points of core metabolic pathways. Cancer cells must balance the production of specific macromolecular precursors such as ribose and acetyl-coa with the generation of enough NADPH and ATP to support proliferation.

proliferative metabolism.[1] In the early stages of tumorigenesis, cancer cells are not limited for nutrients. Cells that incorporate nutrients into biomass most efficiently will proliferate faster. Lactate production may provide other advantages to a tumor as well. Acidification of the tumor microenvironment has been shown to promote invasion and metastasis.[3] Lactate can also act as a nutrient for some cells in the tumor.[25] As tumors grow, cells in the less-well vascularized regions of a tumor can utilize lactate from neighboring cells as a carbon source to survive periods of cell stress.[26]

Despite an increased reliance on aerobic glycolysis, most tumor cells continue to metabolize at least some nutrients by oxidative phosphorylation. In fact, it is likely that in some cancer cells oxidative phosphorylation continues to generate much of the ATP required for biosynthetic reactions and cellular housekeeping functions.[4] Attempts to quantitate ATP production experimentally in cancer cells have estimated that 80% of the ATP generated is derived from oxidative pathways, while 20% comes from glycolysis,[27] and others report that up to 50% of the ATP in cancer cells can be derived from oxidative phosphorylation.[28]

Glucose is not the only substrate used by cancer cells for oxidative phosphorylation.[27,29] In fact, some human cancers do not demonstrate elevated glucose uptake. It has been proposed that at least some of these cancers may be dependent on the amino acid glutamine as a primary source of carbon. Glutamine can be metabolized via two transamination reactions to the TCA cycle intermediate α-ketoglutarate (Fig. 8.4), and glutamine is required for proliferation of many cancer cells.[30]

In addition to glucose and glutamine, other nutrients have been shown to be important in some tumors. Several clinical studies have demonstrated that some human cancers show increased uptake of acetate by positron emission tomography (PET) scan using carbon-11 (^{11}C)-acetate as a tracer (see below).[31] Acetate can be converted to acetyl-coA and serve as a precursor for lipid synthesis.[32] When production of lipids from glucose is blocked by inhibiting ATP citrate lyase, an enzyme required to convert glucose to cytosolic acetyl-coA, acetate can completely rescue lipid synthesis and cell growth. Acetate is not thought to be a major nutrient available to cancer cells in patients, but may reflect an increased dependence of some cancer cells on lipid metabolism. Other enzymes involved in lipid metabolism have been linked with cancer progression,[33,34] however, the exact mechanisms by which lipid metabolism promotes malignancy are not clear.

Nutrients such as amino acids and iron are also important for some tumors.[35,36] Cachexia, or the loss of body mass that cannot be reversed by increased nutrition, is associated with the late stages of some cancers. Cachexia is poorly understood, but in cancer patients it is characterized by the loss of adipose tissue and muscle mass.[37] This may reflect a derangement in whole body metabolism to supply specific nutrients to the cancer. Understanding how nutrients other than glucose contribute to cancer biology remains an active area of investigation.

IMAGING CANCER METABOLISM IN PATIENTS

The characteristic increased glucose uptake of cancer cells has been exploited to image cancer in the clinic. The glucose analogue 2-deoxyglucose is permeable to glucose transporters and trapped in cells when phosphorylated by hexokinase (Fig. 8.2). The 2-deoxyglucose-6-phosphate is unable to be further metabolized,[38,38] and thus 2-deoxyglucose-6-phosphate accumulation can be used to assess the rate of glucose uptake into cells. By conjugating the positron emitting isotope fluorine-18 (^{18}F) to 2-deoxyglucose, the uptake of glucose can be measured in patients using PET.[40] ^{18}F-fluoro-2-deoxyglucose (FDG)-PET is used widely in the clinic to visualize tumors. The current use of FDG-PET is primarily as a staging tool for cancers, however, it is also sometimes used to characterize lesions observed by other imaging modalities. FDG-PET is also increasingly being used as a marker of response to therapy (Fig. 8.6). At least for some treatments, there is mounting evidence that decreased uptake of FDG by PET scan following therapy is a predictor of clinical efficacy.[41,42]

In the clinic, FDG-PET scan can be used to classify tumors. Although many tumors are visible by FDG-PET scan, some tumors do not display elevated FDG uptake. This illustrates that different tumors can display distinct metabolic phenotypes related to their genetic background or site of origin. As discussed above, some tumors rely on nutrients other than glucose. For instance increased ^{11}C-acetate uptake has been observed by PET in prostate tumors that do not demonstrate elevated signal on FDG-PET scan.[43] However, increased uptake of ^{11}C-acetate is also seen in some benign prostate conditions, so whether ^{11}C-acetate uptake defines a characteristic of some prostate cancers or reflects the underlying biology of the prostate gland remains to be determined.[44] New methods to image tumor metabolism by PET or magnetic resonance imaging (MRI) are being developed. If successful, such efforts will better define distinct metabolic phenotypes in patient tumors.

GENETIC EVENTS IMPORTANT FOR CANCER INFLUENCE METABOLISM

Human cancer occurs as a consequence of genetic events that promote the inappropriate proliferation of cells.[45] These events lead to the expression of oncogenes or the loss of tumor suppressor genes that contribute to tumor formation and progression. Although alterations involving specific oncogenes or tumor suppressor genes are hallmarks of specific malignant phenotypes, many of these genetic events are found in numerous types of cancer. These genetic changes occur in diverse cellular signaling and transcriptional pathways, and it is unclear how the various mutations converge to allow inappropriate cell growth and proliferation. One common downstream consequence of these genetic changes is altered cellular metabolism.

Efforts to understand the predisposition to malignancy displayed by von Hippel-Lindau (VHL) syndrome patients identified a link between cancer genetics and the regulation of cell metabolism.[46] VHL syndrome results when patients inherit one mutated copy of the *VHL* gene, leading to a spectrum of benign and malignant tumors including clear cell carcinoma of the kidney. In these patient's tumors, the normal *VHL* allele is lost, consistent with *VHL* acting as a tumor suppressor gene. Subsequent work demonstrated that the *VHL* gene product is also commonly lost in sporadic renal clear cell carcinomas. Although the exact mechanism by which *VHL* loss leads to renal cell carcinoma and other tumors is not known, loss of *VHL* has a profound impact on metabolic gene regulation, and these effects are thought to be important in the pathogenesis of these cancers.

The *VHL* gene encodes the substrate recognition component of a ubiquitin E3 ligase.[46] As an E3 ligase, the VHL protein-containing complex

A
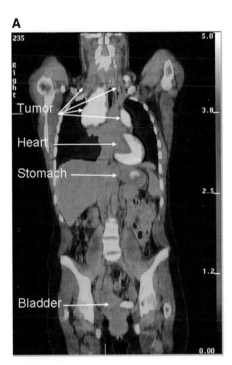

B
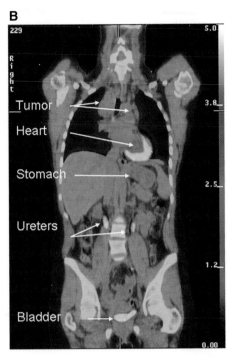

FIGURE 8.6 Early metabolic changes on ^{18}F-fluro-2-deoxyglucose position emission tomography/ computed tomography (FDG-PET/CT) are highly predictive of final treatment response. Fused coronal FDG-PET/CT images in a 44-year-old woman with stage IIA Hodgkin's lymphoma at presentation (**A**) and after two cycles of ABVD (doxorubicin, bleomycin, vinblastine, dacarbazine) chemotherapy (**B**). The tumor seen in the mediastinum and bilateral neck shows intense avidity for the glucose analogue FDG prior to therapy consistent with increased glucose uptake in (**A**). Although a residual tumor mass is still seen on CT after two cycles of ABVD chemotherapy (**B**), it is no longer FDG-avid, and the patient has been in remission for over 2 years since completion of therapy. Normal FDG uptake and excretion is seen in the stomach, heart, and urinary tract, respectively. (Image courtesy of Tricia Locascio, Katherine Zukotynski, and Annick D. Van den Abbeele, Department of Imaging, Dana-Farber Cancer Institute.)

facilitates the transfer of ubiquitin to specific target proteins to effect their degradation. Among the targets of the VHL protein is the hypoxia-inducible transcription factor-1α (HIF-1α) (Fig. 8.7). HIF-1α levels are regulated by oxygen tension.[21,47] In the presence of oxygen HIF-1α is hydroxylated. The hydroxylated form of HIF-1α is recognized by VHL, leading to ubiquitination and degradation of the protein. When oxygen is absent, or when VHL is lost, HIF-1α protein accumulates, dimerizes with HIF-1α, and promotes the transcription of a number of hypoxia inducible genes. These genes include factors that promote angiogenesis to improve tissue blood supply as well as glucose transporters and most of the enzymes in glycolysis. Thus, inappropriate HIF-1α activation leads to the characteristic increased glucose uptake and glycolysis that is observed in cancer. HIF-1α accumulation is a direct consequence of VHL loss, providing a link between the loss of a tumor suppressor gene and the altered metabolic phenotype of malignant cells.

Increased expression of HIF-1α-regulated genes is found in many different types of cancer and correlates with poor patient prognosis.[48] Expression profiling of transformed cells demonstrates that metabolic genes are among the most strongly up-regulated groups of genes.[49] Loss of expression of the HIF-1α target genes correlates with response to therapy in at least some models of cancer, suggesting that these genes are important for malignant cell proliferation and survival. Importantly, increased expression of glucose transporters and glycolytic enzymes under the control of HIF-1α are seen even in non-hypoxic tumors expressing VHL.[49,50] HIF-1α also drives expression of pyruvate dehydrogenase kinase, a negative regulator of the pyruvate dehydrogenase complex that catalyzes pyruvate entry into mitochondria.[51,52] Thus HIF-1α expression can promote aerobic glycolysis in cancer cells.

Transcription factors other than HIF-1α can promote the expression of metabolic enzymes. Expression of ChREBP-1, mondoA, and SREBP-1 has also been shown to be important in some cancers. ChREBP-1 is a key regulator of glycolytic enzyme expression and can promote anabolic

GENERAL PRINCIPLES

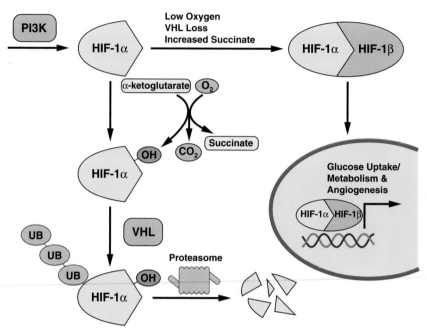

FIGURE 8.7 Transcription of many genes related to metabolism and angiogenesis is controlled by hypoxia-inducible transcription factor-1α (HIF-1α). HIF-1α levels are regulated by translational control downstream of phosphatidylinositol-3-kinase (PI3K) signaling and by the rate of proteosomal degradation. HIF-1α is marked for degradation by hydroxylation. This hydroxylation is sensitive to O_2, α-ketoglutarate, and succinate levels. The von Hippel-Lindau (VHL) protein facilitates ubiquitination and degradation of hydroxylated HIF-1α. Thus, PI3K signaling, hypoxia, succinate levels, and the presence of VHL all influence transcription of HIF-1a target genes. (Figure courtesy of Brooke J. Bevis, Whitehead Institute.)

metabolism.[53] MondoA is a key regulator of metabolic gene expression and coordinates glucose and glutamine metabolism.[54] Enzymes involved in cholesterol and lipid metabolism are controlled by the SREBP transcription factor,[55] and SREBP is induced as a result of oncogenic signaling.[56] Finally, increased HIF-1α–mediated gene transcription is observed in many cancers in the absence of hypoxia or VHL loss.[48] This has been attributed to increased production of HIF-1α that results from aberrant signaling downstream of phosphatidylinositol-3-kinase (PI3K), as discussed below.

Many Genetic Drivers of Cancer Increase Nutrient Uptake

Highlighting the central role that altered cellular metabolism plays in tumor biology, one shared consequence of many genetic events that promote cancer is increased glucose uptake and metabolism. Transformation is associated with elevated glucose uptake.[57,58] Activation of the PI3K signaling pathway is a common event in human cancer, and PI3K has a well-described role in glucose

metabolism through its action as a proximal mediator of insulin signaling that leads to glucose uptake.[59] However, even in noninsulin dependent tissues, PI3K signaling can regulate glucose uptake and utilization and appears to drive this process in many cancers.

PI3K is activated downstream of receptor tyrosine kinases and transfers a phosphate to the membrane lipid phosphatidylinositol.[59,60] When phosphorylated on the 3-position (to generate phosphatidylinositol-3,4,5-triphosphate), the phosphorylated inositol species can recruit other kinases to the membrane, including the protein kinase AKT (also known as protein kinase B). Activation of AKT leads to increased expression of glucose transporters such as Glut1 and enhances the proximal steps in glycolysis by increasing hexokinase and phosphofructokinase activity (Fig. 8.4). Point mutations that result in growth-factor independent activation of PI3K are found in many human cancers, including a significant percentage of breast, ovarian, and colon cancers.[60] Loss of phosphatases that degrade the phosphatidylinositol species, leading to activation of signaling downstream of PI3K, are also common events in human cancer. Loss of the phosphatidylinositol-3,4,5-triphosphate-3-phosphatase PTEN is frequently observed in human cancer, including a sizable fraction of prostate cancer, breast cancer, glioblastoma, and melanoma.[60] Similarly, loss of INPP4B, a phosphatidylinsolitol-3,4-bisphosphate-4-phosphatase, is seen in breast and ovarian cancers.[61]

In addition to regulating glucose uptake and capture through activation of AKT, PI3K activation also leads to increased expression of enzymes in glucose metabolism via increased production of HIF-1α.[62] Activation of the mTOR kinase, an event downstream of PI3K signaling, induces expression of HIF-1α target genes at least in part through increased translation.[63–65] This activation of glucose metabolism results in the propensity for tumors with PI3K activation to be FDG-avid on PET scan. Small molecules that disrupt PI3K signaling lead to decreased glucose uptake by the tumors as measured by FDG-PET, and the ability to inhibit tumor FDG uptake correlates with tumor regression in PI3K-driven animal models of cancer.[66]

Increased glucose uptake and metabolism are also characteristic features of tumors with activated RAS signaling. RAS activation is frequently observed across human cancers. Glucose deprivation has been shown to drive the emergence of cells harboring an activating mutation in the KRAS gene.[67] This has led to the hypothesis that increased glucose uptake via Glut1 expression is a major downstream mediator of RAS signaling that contributes to tumorigenesis. In addition to increasing glucose transporter expression, RAS activation leads to increased phosphofructokinase activity and stimulates the proximal metabolism of glucose (Fig. 8.4).[14] Though less well studied, activating mutations in B-Raf, a kinase downstream of RAS, also result in increased nutrient uptake.[67] Mutations in receptor tyrosine kinases cause increased signaling through both the RAS and PI3K signaling pathways and also cause increased nutrient uptake.

Increased MYC expression is another frequent event in human cancer. MYC is a transcription factor, and many of the transcriptional targets of MYC include metabolic genes.[50] MYC regulates the transcription of enzymes involved in glucose uptake and metabolism, including LDH, the enzyme responsible for production of lactate. MYC-dependent tumors are sensitive to LDH inhibition.[68] MYC also directly and indirectly regulates the uptake of glutamine,[30,69] and MYC-dependent cancer cells are particularly sensitive to glutamine withdrawal.[70] Genetic alterations that lead to activation of MYC, PI3K, RAS, Raf, and receptor tyrosine kinases are among the best-understood driver events in human cancers. These seemingly disparate genetic alterations that promote cancer and occur across cancer types all lead to a converging metabolic phenotype characterized by enhanced cell autonomous nutrient uptake (Fig. 8.8).

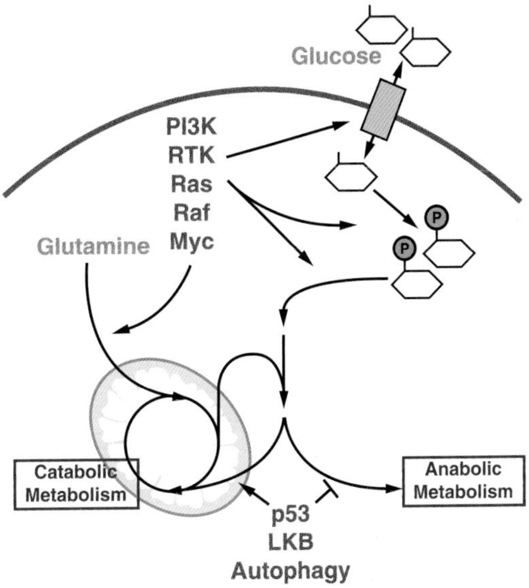

FIGURE 8.8 Many of the oncogenic events thought to drive cancer development influence metabolism by increasing glucose or glutamine uptake. Other genetic events and processes associated with cancer also influence metabolism but do not necessarily cause elevated nutrient uptake. Rather, these events appear to be involved in reprogramming of metabolism away from catabolic metabolism and promote the anabolic pathways necessary for cell growth and proliferation. Both the increase in nutrient uptake and the reprogramming of metabolism to support anabolism are required for cancer cells to proliferate. RTK, receptor tyrosine kinase.

Tumor Suppressor Gene Products Also Influence Cellular Metabolism

Many tumor suppressor gene products also regulate metabolism (Fig. 8.8). Loss of p53 function is among the most frequent genetic events in human cancer, and p53 expression influences metabolism (Fig. 8.4).[71] TIGAR, a gene induced by p53 expression, redirects glucose flux from glycolysis to the pentose phosphate pathway and promotes apoptosis.[72] Phosphoglycerate mutase, a glycolytic enzyme negatively regulated by p53, inhibits cell senescence.[73] Excess production of reactive oxygen species also promotes cellular senescence and apoptosis, and many of the genes induced by p53 are involved in adaptation to oxidative stress and regulation of mitochondrial metabolism.[74,75]

The tumor suppressor LKB1 is also involved in the adaptive response to cell stress. LKB1 is a kinase that is required for activation of adenosine monophosphate (AMP)-activated protein kinase (AMPK).[76–78] AMPK responds to cellular energy stress (by sensing a low ATP/AMP ratio) and initiates a signaling cascade that promotes increased ATP production and decreased ATP consumption.[79] AMPK also inactivates the mTOR protein kinase that acts as an important integrator of cell growth signals with nutrient availability to regulate cell growth.[80,81] In addition to AMPK, mTOR is regulated by PI3K signaling through the TSC1/TSC2 complex.[82,83] TSC1 and TSC2 are tumor suppressor genes that indirectly influence metabolism via effects on mTOR signaling.[84] mTOR is also regulated by amino acids such that the mTOR growth promoting activity is turned off under conditions of poor nutrient availability.[85] The response to cell stress also includes the induction of autophagy to catabolize existing cellular material for energy production and removal of damaged organelles.[86,87] Both mTOR signaling and nutrient stress regulate autophagy induction,[88] but the role of autophagy in cancer remains unclear. The use of mTOR inhibitors is gaining increasing use in the clinic to treat various cancers, yet the relationship between mTOR, autophagy, metabolic stress, and cancer is incompletely understood.

Other genetic changes may be important to promote anabolic metabolism in cancer cells. For instance, all cancer cells appear to express the M2 isoform of the glycolytic enzyme pyruvate kinase (PK-M2).[16,89] PK-M2 is normally expressed during embryonic development and is unique among the human pyruvate kinase isoforms in that it is regulated by tyrosine kinase signaling.[15] This regulation of PK-M2 by growth factor signaling promotes aerobic glycolysis in cells[89] and may constitute a molecular switch that allows cancer cells to metabolize glucose in a manner conducive to proliferation only when growth signals are present.

Mutations in Metabolic Enzymes Can Lead to Cancer

Altered cell metabolism can directly contribute to transformation as mutations in metabolic enzymes can promote cancer. Inherited loss of function mutations in genes that encode proteins involved in the proper assembly or function of the mitochondrial succinate dehydrogenase complex account for the subtypes of hereditary paraganglioma.[90–94] Succinate dehydrogenase

(SDH) is an enzyme complex in the TCA cycle that catalyzes the oxidation of succinate to fumarate and supplies electrons to the mitochondrial electron transport chain.[11] These mutations lead to decreased activity of SDH and succinate accumulation. The enzymes that carry out the oxygen-dependent hydroxylation of HIF-1α also convert α-ketoglutarate to succinate as part of their catalytic mechanism.[95] Thus, accumulation of succinate leads to a decrease in HIF-1α hydroxylation, less HIF-1α degradation, and increased expression of HIF-1α target genes (Fig. 8.7). Loss-of-function SDH mutations that cause this "pseudohypoxia" account for some cases of renal cell carcinoma expressing normal amounts of VHL, supporting the notion that HIF-1α expression is an important event in some cancers.[93,95] Mutations in the TCA cycle enzyme fumarate hydratase (FH), which further metabolizes the fumarate produced by the succinate dehydrogenase complex, have also been described in renal cell carcinoma, leiomyomas, and other rare cancers.[95–97]

Isocitrate dehydrogenase (IDH) is another metabolic enzyme that is mutated in cancer.[98–100] All reported cases of IDH mutation occur in only one allele, with preservation of wild-type enzyme expression from the other allele (Fig. 8.9).[101] These mutations are frequent events in low-grade gliomas and secondary glioblastomas.[98,99,102] Interestingly, IDH-mutant gliomas appear to have a better prognosis,[98] suggesting that gliomas harboring these mutations represent a distinct subset of glioma with a different response to therapy or natural history. IDH mutations are also found in patients with acute myelogenous leukemia (AML) and myelodysplastic syndrome (MDS) and define a distinct clinical subset of these patients without other cytogenetic abnormalities.[100,103–105] IDH mutations have been proposed to be an early event in the pathogenesis of both AML and glioma.[101,105,106] Sporadic mutations in other cancers have also been reported. A summary of IDH mutations in human cancer is shown in Table 8.1, and the frequency of IDH1 or IDH2 mutations in specific cancer subsets is shown in Table 8.2.

FIGURE 8.9 Mutations in isocitrate dehydrogenase-1 or -2 (IDH1 or IDH2) reported in human cancer are all monoallelic and involve a single residue in IDH1 or one of two residues in IDH2. (Figure adapted from Lenny Dang and Shengfang Jin, Agios Pharmaceuticals.)

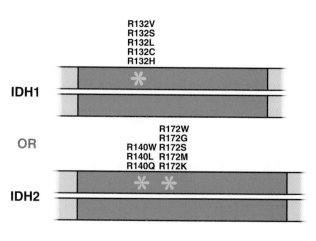

TABLE 8.1

MUTATIONS IN IDH1 AND IDH2 REPORTED IN HUMAN CANCERS

Cancer Type	IDH1 (Ref.)	IDH2 (Ref.)
Glioma	R132H (98,102,150–153) R132C (98,154,155) R132S (98,99) R132G (99) R132L R132V (102)	R172K R172M (99) R172G R172S (155)
Acute myeloid leukemia (AML)	R132H (103) R132G (105) R132C (107)	R140Q (103,105) R140W (105) R140L R172K (107)
Myelodysplastic syndrome (MDS)	R132H (156) R132C R132L (104) R132G	R140Q R140L (104) R172K
Acute lymphoblastic leukemia (ALL)	R132C (153)	
Prostate cancer	R132H (153) R132C	
Colorectal cancer	R132C (98)	
Paragangliomas	R132C (157)	
Thyroid cancer	R132H (109)	

Table provided by Lenny Dang and Shengfang Jin, Agios Pharmaceuticals. IDH, isocitrate dehydrogenase.

The IDH mutations associated with cancer involve point mutations in the active site of either IDH1 or IDH2.[98–100,105] Other less frequent mutations involving residues in IDH1 have been reported in rare cases,[105,107–109] however, whether these represent driver mutations or polymorphisms remains unclear. IDH1 mutations involve R132, and mutations in the analogous active site residue (R172) are found in IDH2. This arginine (R132 in IDH1, R172 in IDH2) coordinates the CO_2 group that is lost during oxidative decarboxylation of isocitrate to α-ketoglutarate.[110] The other mutated residue in IDH2 (R140) makes contacts with the same CO_2 group in the IDH2 active site.[105] All three mutations result in an alteration of enzyme activity that decreases the enzyme's ability to oxidatively decarboxylate isocitrate to α-ketoglutarate, but increases enzyme activity to reduce α-ketoglutarate. In the mutant enzymes, this reduction does not lead to incorporation of CO_2 to make isocitrate, but instead produces 2-hydroxyglutarate (2HG).[105,107,110] Because IDH mutations are monoallelic and the neomorphic activity acquired by the mutant enzyme is slow relative to the normal wild-type enzyme in these cells, the normal interconversion of isocitrate and α-ketoglutarate is not dramatically altered, and the main consequence of these mutations is 2HG production (Fig. 8.10).[105,107,110] The

2HG is produced in low levels in normal cells as an error product of various TCA cycle enzymes; however, in IDH mutant tumors 2HG accumulates to very high levels and has been linked with the pathogenesis of the disease.[110] Accumulation of 2HG has been demonstrated in rare patients with hereditary loss of the enzyme that degrades 2HG,[111] and gliomas have been described in a subset of these patients.[112] Mutations in IDH1 have been reported to result in HIF-1α accumulation,[113] however, the relationship among IDH mutation, 2HG accumulation, and HIF-1α accumulation remains unclear.

Recurrent mutations in yet another metabolic enzyme have recently been reported in colon cancer.[114] These are inactivating mutations of an enzyme involved in glucosamine metabolism, and signaling involving glucosamine-based protein modifications has been suggested to be important in cancer.[115] The exact mechanism by which the shunt from glucose to glucosamine impacts cellular metabolism and cancer remains to be determined.

TARGETING METABOLISM TO TREAT CANCER

The mechanisms by which cancer metabolism is regulated and how this regulation is impacted by

TABLE 8.2

FREQUENCY OF IDH1 AND IDH2 REPORTED IN HUMAN CANCERS

Tumor Classification	IDH1 Mutated (%)	IDH2 Mutated (%)
GLIOMA		
Secondary glioblastoma (grade IV)	73–88	—
Diffuse astrocytoma (grade II)	59–88	0.9
Oligodendroglioma (grade II)	68–82	2.3
Oligoastrocytoma (grade II)	50–94	1.3
Anaplastic astrocytoma (grade III)	52–78	0.9
Anaplastic oligodendroglioma (grade III)	60–86	3.4
Anaplastic oligoastrocytoma (grade III)	43–78	3.4
Primary glioblastoma (grade IV)	3–16	—
Primitive neuroectodermal tumor (grade IV)	6–33	—
Giant cell glioblastoma (grade IV)	*	—
Pediatric glioblastoma (grade IV)	*	—
Pilocytic astrocytoma (grade I)	*	—
Pleomorphic xanthoastrocytoma (grade II)	—	*
Compiled from references: (98, 99, 102, 106, 150, 153, 155, 158–161)		
HEMATOLOGIC MALIGNANCIES		
Acute myeloid leukemia (AML), all	4.4–9.1	15.4
AML, normal cytogenetics	7.1–16.2	19.3–19.4
AML, abnormal cytogenetics	0–5.4	—
Myelodysplastic syndrome/myeloproliferative neoplasm	1.1	5.8
B-acute lymphoblastic leukemia	2.0	—
Compiled from references: (100, 104, 105, 107, 108, 162–164)		

*Less than 50 cases reported, too few to determine percentage mutated.
IDH, isocitrate dehydrogenase; — indicates no reported cases.
Table provided by Patrick S. Ward and Craig B. Thompson, University of Pennsylvania.

genetic alterations known to be critical for cancer survival suggest cellular metabolic dependencies that could be exploited for cancer treatment. In fact, one of the first successful chemotherapies targeted folate metabolism. The observation that folate could enhance blood cell proliferation ultimately lead to the development of antifolates as chemotherapeutics.[116] Other active chemotherapeutics target purine metabolism. Although these agents are now thought of as "cytotoxic," they target metabolic dependencies of tumor cells and continue to play an important role in modern cancer therapy.

New therapies are being explored that directly or indirectly target cancer metabolism. A large fraction of human cancer is dependent on aberrant signaling through the PI3K/AKT pathway, and agents that target this pathway are being actively tested in the clinic.[117] The growing evidence that cancer cells depend on elevated glucose metabolism suggests that targeting key metabolic control points important for aerobic glycolysis might also be effective cancer therapies. Recent evidence suggests that drugs developed to treat metabolic diseases such as diabetes may provide a

benefit to patients with cancer. A number of retrospective clinical studies have found a benefit to the widely used diabetic drug metformin (Glucophage) both in the primary prevention of cancer as well as improved outcomes when used with other cancer therapies.[118–120] The exact mechanism by which metformin lowers blood glucose levels is not completely understood; however, metformin decreases gluconeogenesis in the liver. Recently, metformin was discovered to be an activator of AMPK, and this effect was shown to be critical for inhibiting gluconeogenesis in the liver.[121] In addition, metformin has been shown to inhibit mitochondrial complex I and impair oxidative phosphorylation in cells.[122,123] Inhibition of oxidative phosphorylation and the subsequent decrease in energy charge (ATP:AMP ratio) is likely how metformin activates AMP kinase.

Recently, two separate clinical studies have shown a reduction in cancer-related mortality with metformin use.[118,119] This effect appears to be independent of blood glucose level as patients with similar glucose levels treated with insulin do not derive the same benefit as patients taking metformin. Another study reported that diabetic

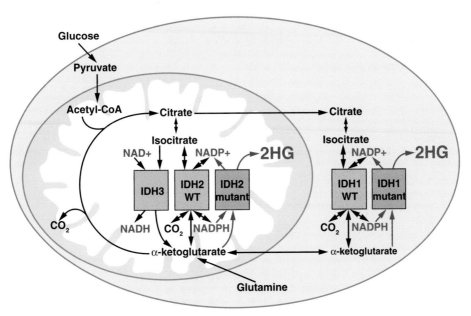

FIGURE 8.10 Human cancer associated mutations in isocitrate dehydrogenase-1 or -2 (IDH1 or IDH2) results in the neomorphic production of the metabolite 2-hydroxyglutarate (2HG). Because a wild-type version of both IDH1 and IDH2 remain even in IDH mutant cells, the normal activities of these enzymes persist despite the activity of the mutant enzyme to produce 2HG. The subcellular localization and enzymatic activities for all of the IDH isoforms is shown. (Figure courtesy of Patrick S. Ward and Craig B. Thompson, University of Pennsylvania.)

patients on metformin had a higher pathological complete response to neoadjuvant therapy for breast cancer than diabetic patients receiving other glucose lowering therapies.[120] Studies exploring metformin use for cancer therapy in numerous preclinical cancer models have suggested that these compounds may be selectively toxic to cancer cells with specific genetic backgrounds,[123–125] however, these compounds may also influence cancer therapy via their systemic effects on glucose metabolism. Increased insulin-like growth factor-1 (IGF1) levels, which accompany poor glucose control, may promote cancer growth.[126,127] Particularly in tumors with mutations that lead to activation of the PI3K pathway,[128] at least one effect of metformin may be to decrease the effect of IGF1 on cell growth.[129]

The success of FDG-PET scans as a diagnostic and predictive tool for treatment response in many cancers has lead some to suggest that targeting enzymes involved in metabolism may be an effective therapy.[130] Specific therapies may be possible for patients with mutations in metabolic enzymes that contribute directly to tumorigenesis.[130,131] In addition, metabolism may be sufficiently different in some cancers to target pathways such as glycolysis. 2-deoxyglucose is a competitive inhibitor of proximal glucose metabolism.[38,39] Cells exposed to sufficient amounts of 2-deoxyglucose undergo growth arrest or apoptosis,[132–134] and preclinical models show 2-deoxyglucose may

potentiate standard cytotoxic chemotherapy.[135] 2-deoxyglucose can be administered to patients,[136] but when given in combination with radiation therapy to glioblastoma patients at doses sufficient to limit glucose metabolism in cancer cells significant toxicity is observed.[137–139] However, other agents to block glucose metabolism are being investigated.[67,130,140–146] Whether a sufficient therapeutic window exists to target glycolysis directly remains to be determined.

It is possible to alter cellular metabolism in a tumor without causing unacceptable toxicity in patients. Dichloroacetate has been used to treat lactic acidosis in non-cancer patients with rare inborn errors of mitochondrial metabolism.[147,148] Dichloroacetate reduces lactate production by inhibiting pyruvate dehydrogenase kinase (PDK),[149] a negative regulator of the mitochondrial pyruvate dehydrogenase complex (PDH). PDH catalyzes the first step in mitochondrial metabolism of pyruvate (Fig. 8.4).[11] Thus, PDK inhibition that leads to activation of PDH diverts pyruvate away from lactate production. Because lactate production is the hallmark of aerobic glycolysis, it has been proposed that dichloroacetate might be a useful agent to target cancer metabolism.[148,149] Dichloroacetate is tolerated by cancer patients at dosages that can alter mitochondria in patient tumor samples. Studies are ongoing to understand the impact of these metabolic alterations on tumor biology and clinical outcome.

Selected References

The full list of references for this chapter appears in the online version.

1. Vander Heiden MG, Cantley LC, Thompson CB. Understanding the Warburg effect: the metabolic requirements of cell proliferation. *Science* 2009;324:1029.
2. Warburg O. On the origin of cancer cells. *Science* 1956;123:309.
3. Gatenby RA, Gillies RJ. Why do cancers have high aerobic glycolysis? *Nat Rev Cancer* 2004;4:891.
4. Deberardinis RJ, Lum JJ, Hatzivassiliou G, et al. The biology of cancer: metabolic reprogramming fuels cell growth and proliferation. *Cell Metab* 2008;7:11.
5. Hsu PP, Sabatini DM. Cancer cell metabolism: Warburg and beyond. *Cell* 2008;134:703.
7. Warburg O, Posener K, Negelein E. Ueber den Stoffwechsel der Tumoren. *Biochemische Zeitschrift* 1924;152:319.
12. Mathupala SP, Ko YH, Pedersen PL. The pivotal roles of mitochondria in cancer: Warburg and beyond and encouraging prospects for effective therapies. *Biochim Biophys Acta* 2010;1797:1225.
17. Weinhouse S. The Warburg hypothesis fifty years later. *Z Krebsforsch Klin Onkol Cancer Res Clin Oncol* 1976; 87:115.
19. Folkman J. Angiogenesis. *Annu Rev Med* 2006;57:1.
20. Bertout JA, Patel SA, Simon MC. The impact of O_2 availability on human cancer. *Nat Rev Cancer* 2008;8:967.
21. Semenza GL. Regulation of cancer cell metabolism by hypoxia-inducible factor 1. *Semin Cancer Biol* 2009;19:12.
24. Racker E. Why do tumor cells have a high aerobic glycolysis? *J Cell Physiol* 1976;89:697.
25. Sonveaux P, Vegran F, Schroeder T, et al. Targeting lactate-fueled respiration selectively kills hypoxic tumor cells in mice. *J Clin Invest* 2008;118:3930.
27. Guppy M, Leedman P, Zu X, et al. Contribution by different fuels and metabolic pathways to the total ATP turnover of proliferating MCF-7 breast cancer cells. *Biochem J* 2002;364:309.
29. DeBerardinis RJ, Mancuso A, Daikhin E, et al. Beyond aerobic glycolysis: transformed cells can engage in glutamine metabolism that exceeds the requirement for protein and nucleotide synthesis. *Proc Natl Acad Sci U S A* 2007;104:19345.
32. Hatzivassiliou G, Zhao F, Bauer DE, et al. ATP citrate lyase inhibition can suppress tumor cell growth. *Cancer Cell* 2005;8:311.
35. Lockart RZ Jr, Eagle H. Requirements for growth of single human cells. *Science* 1959;129:252.
37. Tisdale MJ. Mechanisms of cancer cachexia. *Physiol Rev* 2009;89:381.
40. Hawkins RA, Phelps ME. PET in clinical oncology. *Cancer Metastasis Rev* 1988;7:119.
41. Ben-Haim S, Ell P. 18F-FDG PET and PET/CT in the evaluation of cancer treatment response. *J Nucl Med* 2009; 50:88.
46. Kaelin WG Jr. The von Hippel-Lindau tumour suppressor protein: O_2 sensing and cancer. *Nat Rev Cancer* 2008;8:865.
47. Kaelin WG Jr, Ratcliffe PJ. Oxygen sensing by metazoans: the central role of the HIF hydroxylase pathway. *Mol Cell* 2008;30:393.
48. Rankin EB, Giaccia AJ. The role of hypoxia-inducible factors in tumorigenesis. *Cell Death Differ* 2008;15:678.
49. Majumder PK, Febbo PG, Bikoff R, et al. mTOR inhibition reverses Akt-dependent prostate intraepithelial neoplasia through regulation of apoptotic and HIF-1-dependent pathways. *Nat Med* 2004;10:594.

50. Dang CV, Kim JW, Gao P, et al. The interplay between MYC and HIF in cancer. *Nat Rev Cancer* 2008;8:51.
57. Flier JS, Mueckler MM, Usher P, et al. Elevated levels of glucose transport and transporter messenger RNA are induced by ras or src oncogenes. *Science* 1987;235:1492.
58. Birnbaum MJ, Haspel HC, Rosen OM. Transformation of rat fibroblasts by FSV rapidly increases glucose transporter gene transcription. *Science* 1987;235:1495.
60. Engelman JA, Luo J, Cantley LC. The evolution of phosphatidylinositol 3-kinases as regulators of growth and metabolism. *Nat Rev Genet* 2006;7:606.
71. Cheung EC, Vousden KH. The role of p53 in glucose metabolism. *Curr Opin Cell Biol* 2010;22:186.
75. Matoba S, Kang JG, Patino WD, et al. p53 regulates mitochondrial respiration. *Science* 2006;312:1650.
79. Hardie DG. AMP-activated/SNF1 protein kinases: conserved guardians of cellular energy. *Nat Rev Mol Cell Biol* 2007;8:774.
82. Tee AR, Blenis J. mTOR, translational control and human disease. *Semin Cell Dev Biol* 2005;16:29.
83. Dann SG, Thomas G. The amino acid sensitive TOR pathway from yeast to mammals. *FEBS Lett* 2006;580:2821.
85. Shaw RJ, Cantley LC. Ras, PI(3)K and mTOR signalling controls tumour cell growth. *Nature* 2006;441:424.
86. Kundu M, Thompson CB. Autophagy: basic principles and relevance to disease. *Annu Rev Pathol* 2008;3:427.
87. Jin S, White E. Tumor suppression by autophagy through the management of metabolic stress. *Autophagy* 2008;4:563.
88. Wang RC, Levine B. Autophagy in cellular growth control. *FEBS Lett* 2010;584:1417.
90. Baysal BE, Ferrell RE, Willett-Brozick JE, et al. Mutations in SDHD, a mitochondrial complex II gene, in hereditary paraganglioma. *Science* 2000;287:848.
95. King A, Selak MA, Gottlieb E. Succinate dehydrogenase and fumarate hydratase: linking mitochondrial dysfunction and cancer. *Oncogene* 2006;25:4675.
98. Parsons DW, Jones S, Zhang X, et al. An integrated genomic analysis of human glioblastoma multiforme. *Science* 2008;321:1807.
100. Mardis ER, Ding L, Dooling DJ, et al. Recurring mutations found by sequencing an acute myeloid leukemia genome. *N Engl J Med* 2009;361:1058.
101. Thompson CB. Metabolic enzymes as oncogenes or tumor suppressors. *N Engl J Med* 2009;360:813.
110. Dang L, White DW, Gross S, et al. Cancer-associated IDH1 mutations produce 2-hydroxyglutarate. *Nature* 2009; 462:739.
116. Farber S, Diamond LK. Temporary remissions in acute leukemia in children produced by folic acid antagonist, 4-aminopteroyl-glutamic acid. *N Engl J Med* 1948;238: 787.
118. Evans JM, Donnelly LA, Emslie-Smith AM, et al. Metformin and reduced risk of cancer in diabetic patients. *BMJ* 2005;330:1304.
127. Pollak M. Insulin and insulin-like growth factor signalling in neoplasia. *Nat Rev Cancer* 2008;8:915.
128. Kalaany NY, Sabatini DM. Tumours with PI3K activation are resistant to dietary restriction. *Nature* 2009;458:725.
132. Laszlo J, Humphreys SR, Goldin A. Effects of glucose analogues (2-deoxy-D-glucose, 2-deoxy-D-galactose) on experimental tumors. *J Natl Cancer Inst* 1960;24:267.
141. Kroemer G, Pouyssegur J. Tumor cell metabolism: cancer's Achilles' heel. *Cancer Cell* 2008;13:472.
148. Michelakis ED, Sutendra G, Dromparis P, et al. Metabolic modulation of glioblastoma with dichloroacetate. *Sci Transl Med* 2010;2:31.

ROBERT S. KERBEL AND LEE M. ELLIS

INTRODUCTION: ORIGINS OF THE CONCEPT OF ANTIANGIOGENIC THERAPY FOR CANCER

Among the most significant advances in medical oncology over the last 6 years is the U.S. Food and Drug Administration (FDA) approval of several antiangiogenic drugs for the systemic treatment of a variety of metastatic malignancies. Prior to the first successful randomized phase 3 clinical trial involving an antiangiogenic agent[1] (bevacizumab, the humanized monoclonal antibody to vascular endothelial growth factor [VEGF]), enthusiasm in the field had waned by a combination of high expectations but little success in several pivotal phase 3 clinical trials. However, the initial success of bevacizumab, in combination with chemotherapy in the first-line treatment of metastatic colorectal cancer, initiated a resurgence in the field, in both the laboratory and the clinic, that has led to variable degrees of improvement in the therapy for advanced breast cancer, renal cell carcinoma (RCC), colorectal cancer, non–small cell lung cancer, glioblastoma, hepatocellular carcinoma, and ovarian cancer. However, despite these successes, clinical trials evaluating the use of these agents in some other malignancies has not yet led to similar success, and even where there is success, the clinical benefits are modest, as most notably in the case for breast cancer. Thus, it is essential to continue investigating basic mechanisms and mediators of angiogenesis with the aim of advancing the care of patients with malignant disease.

The era of antiangiogenic drug development began with the publication in 1971 of a landmark hypothesis article in the *New England Journal of Medicine* by M. Judah Folkman.[2] He hypothesized that inhibition of blood vessel growth within a tumor could prolong tumor dormancy and improve survival of patients with minimal toxicity. Following publication of his hypothesis, Folkman and colleagues reported a significant number of discoveries that were instrumental in advancing the field, including defining the nature of the angiogenic "switch" in tumors, raising awareness of the presence of both pro- and anti-angiogenic factors that mediate both pathologic and physiologic processes.[3]

Although the hypothesis of the essential role of angiogenesis in tumor growth, and the proposed therapeutic benefit of antiangiogenic drugs for cancer treatment, have been partially validated, there have been many surprising twists and turns in the field over the ensuing decades necessitating some interesting modifications of the basic therapeutic concept.[4] These will be discussed in more detail later and include the following: (1) certain antiangiogenic drugs such as bevacizumab seem to have little or no clinical benefit when used as monotherapies to treat advanced disease of certain malignancies such as colorectal cancer, whereas they show clinical benefit only when used in combination treatments with other agents, particularly (thus far) chemotherapy[4–6]; (2) in addition to stimulators of angiogenesis, there are also a number of endogenous angiogenesis inhibitors, the expression of which may be down-regulated during tumor development, permitting a more robust angiogenic response[3]; (3) angiogenesis can also contribute to the growth of "liquid" hematologic malignancies, not just solid tumors[3,5,7]; (4) endothelial cells in developing blood vessels may be derived by incorporation and differentiation of systemically mobilized cells from the bone marrow, that is, circulating endothelial progenitor or precursor cells (CEPs) (Fig. 9.1.), not just by local division of pre-existing endothelial cells in resident vessels ("sprouting angiogenesis")[8,9]; and (5) there is not a single "TAF" but a large and diverse array of molecular mediators of angiogenesis.

SEQUENTIAL STEPS INVOLVED IN THE FORMATION OF BLOOD VESSEL CAPILLARIES IN TUMORS

There are a number of sequential and fairly well-defined steps involved in the development for new capillary blood vessels, and their subsequent formation into a functional network. The first step in the formation of a capillary sprout ("sprouting angiogenesis") from a pre-existing mature blood

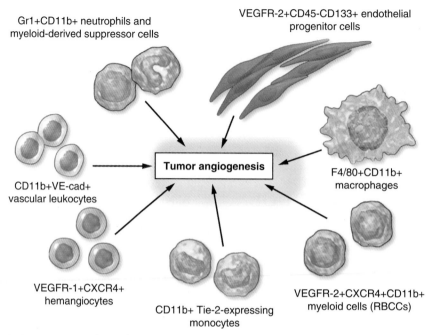

FIGURE 9.1 Circulating bone marrow–derived cell populations that stimulate or amplify tumor angiogenesis. The various hematopoietic (CD45-positive) cell types appear to have a perivascular location with respect to the tumor neovasculature, whereas the CD45-negative endothelial progenitor cells can become incorporated into the lumen of a growing blood vessel and differentiate into mature endothelial cells. In recent preclinical studies, neutrophils have also been shown to contribute to the induction of tumor angiogenesis. F4/80 is a pan macrophage cell-surface marker. CXCR4, CXC chemokine receptor 4; RBCCs, recruited bone marrow–derived circulating cells; VE-cad, vascular endothelial-cell cadherin (an adhesion molecule); VEGFR, vascular endothelial growth factor receptor. (From ref. 4, with permission.)

vessel is the localized degradation of the surrounding basement membrane of the parental postcapillary venule. This creates a break to allow the movement of differentiated endothelial cells toward the adjacent tumor cells and the stimuli produced by such cells. Localized degradation is likely the consequence of the ability of various proangiogenic growth factors secreted by the tumor cell population or reactive stromal cells to induce synthesis and export of a number of proteolytic enzymes such as matrix metalloproteinases, cathepsins, and urokinase plasminogen activator.

The next step involves the directed locomotion/migration of endothelial cells from the parental venule toward the angiogenic stimulus emanating from the tumor mass. This is followed by division of endothelial cells that, in concert with migration, lengthen the "stalk" of the endothelial cell sprout. Subsequently, lumen formation takes place with completion of capillary sprouts and loops, and the envelopment of nascent capillaries with new basement membrane structures along with recruitment of perivascular support cells, especially pericytes. Critical in this process are specialized endothelial cells at the ends of growing capillaries called *tip* cells, which fuse with other tip cells to create a fused (linked) network of new capillaries.[10] This sequence of events is thought to be quite similar to the formation of new blood vessel capillaries that occurs in developing embryos; however, the structure/morphology and function of many tumor-associated blood vessels can be highly irregular, heterogeneous, and functionally abnormal.[6]

Although this abbreviated description of sprouting angiogenesis is the most common view of angiogenesis, over the past 5 to 10 years, modifications or alternative views of angiogenesis have emerged. The mechanisms of angiogenesis may be organ- and/or tumor-specific. For example, in vascular-rich organs such as the brain, co-option may play an important role in providing a nutrient blood supply to the growing tumor.[11] It has been hypothesized that parts of the vessel wall in tumors such as ocular melanoma or glioblastoma may be composed or melanoma cells, either in part (mosaic vessels)[12] or full[13] ("vascular mimicry"). Also noteworthy are the large number and diversity of molecular changes detected in endothelial cells in tumor blood vessels during angiogenesis, many of which suggest possible new targets for development of antiangiogenic drugs.[14,15] Some of these molecular changes might be related to the recently reported genetic and cytogenetic abnormalities detected in endothelial cells isolated from the tumor vasculature[16] or by endothelial cell uptake of tumor cell–derived membrane vesicles.[17]

PERICYTES

Pericytes (our definition of pericytes is a single layer of periendothelial smooth muscle cells) modulate endothelial cell function, and are critical for the development of a mature vascular network. Pericytes regulate vascular function, including vessel diameter (and thus blood flow) and vascular permeability.[18] Pericytes also provide mechanical support and stability to the vessel wall and maintain endothelial cell survival through direct cell-cell contact and paracrine circuits.[18,19]

The role of pericytes within the tumor vasculature is currently an intense area of study. The degree of pericyte coverage of endothelial cells in human tumors is controversial and discrepancies among studies may be because a single marker is not sufficient to examine pericyte presence and morphology. Markers such as alpha-smooth muscle actin, desmin, NG2, and RGS5 are commonly used, and confocal imaging is necessary to observe the true relationship of pericytes to endothelial cells.

Because of the role of pericytes in mediating endothelial cell survival,[19] these cells have emerged as an important therapeutic target for antiangiogenic therapy. Studies of antiangiogenic agents targeting endothelial cell survival have demonstrated that such drugs result in increased apoptosis in endothelial cells that are *not* associated with pericytes, leading to a relative increase in the proportion of vessels with pericyte coverage.[20] These data have led to the hypothesis that pericytes mediate resistance to antiangiogenic therapy. If this hypothesis is correct, targeting both endothelial cells and pericytes will increase the efficacy of antiangiogenic therapy, and there is some evidence in support of this hypothesis in preclinical studies.[21,22] However, there is currently some growing doubt about the clinical impact of targeting pericytes using drugs such as multitargeting tyrosine kinase inhibitors (TKIs), for example, sunitinib, sorafenib, and pazopanib, which target platelet-derived growth factor (PDGF) receptors (which are expressed by pericytes) in addition to vascular endothelial growth factor receptors (VEGFRs). Thus, the therapeutic impact of such drugs does not appear to be significantly greater compared with specific anti-VEGF antibodies with the exception, currently, of hepatocellular carcinoma. Moreover, there is some limited preclinical evidence that inhibition of pericyte function and attachment to endothelial cells may actually facilitate metastasis by allowing tumor cell intravasation and extravasation.[23] Still others have shown that inhibition of pericyte stimulatory factors may actually increase tumor growth, as pericytes may induce endothelial cell quiescence. Pericyte biology remains an important area of research that needs to be investigated more thoroughly.

DYSFUNCTIONAL NATURE OF THE TUMOR VASCULATURE

Although tumors possess the means to recruit and develop a new vascular network, this is not to suggest, as already mentioned, that such blood vessels are normal in either structure or function. Indeed, the characteristics of the vasculature in solid tumors are associated with a number of prominent abnormalities, the consequences of which have been hypothesized to have a significant impact on tumor growth, progression, and response to various anticancer therapies. For example, the structural and morphologic abnormalities include excessively dilated blood vessels, other vessels with areas containing absent or abnormal basement membranes, or having extreme corkscrewlike tortuosities, a relative lack of supporting perivascular cellular elements such as pericytes, or abnormalities in the pericyte population, and excessive vascular leakiness.[24,25] These abnormalities can be quite variable within a solid tumor mass, and such heterogeneity can also extend to the relative density of blood vessels, which can be quite high in certain areas, and low in others.

As a result of all of these features, blood flow and perfusion within tumors can be highly heterogeneous and often sluggish, with some areas therefore being deprived of oxygen and nutrients leading to adjacent areas of elevated hypoxia. This may account for slow growth of tumors in some regions and more rapid growth in others. In addition, the marked leakiness/hyperpermeability of the tumor vasculature can lead to a marked extravasation of high-molecular-weight plasma proteins and fluid into the extracellular microenvironment within tumors, which can lead to elevated interstitial fluid pressures.[24] It has been hypothesized that this can limit or retard the diffusion of anticancer drugs, especially antibodies or gene therapy vectors, and immune effector cells from the blood through the interstitium of the tumors.[24] Thus, given their nature, tumor blood vessels, while necessary for progressive tumor growth and hematogenous metastasis, may also actually limit the efficacy of a broad and diverse array of anticancer drugs and treatments, including

GENERAL PRINCIPLES

chemotherapy, and oxygen required for optimal efficacy of radiation therapy.[24]

MOLECULAR MEDIATORS OF TUMOR ANGIOGENESIS: ANGIOGENIC STIMULATORS AND THEIR RECEPTORS

Several diverse families of growth factors (angiogenic factors) are now known to stimulate/mediate tumor angiogenesis. Some, like VEGF,[26] are primary, direct-acting factors that bind to cognate receptors that are primarily expressed on endothelial cells, especially when they are "activated." Other factors are likely secondary in nature, that is, indirect acting. In other words, they stimulate expression of one or more of the primary proangiogenic growth factors or recruit cells to sites of angiogenesis that amplify the angiogenic process. Included in this group are such molecules as transforming growth factor beta (TGF-β), TGF-α, hepatocyte growth factor, inflammatory cytokines such as interleukin-6 and interleukin-8, cytokines such as granulocyte-colony stimulating factor, chemokines such as stromal-derived factor-1, and sex hormones such as estrogens and androgens.[4] PDGFs have also been implicated as mediators of angiogenesis, for the most part through their effects on PDGF receptor-expressing pericytes, as previously mentioned. However, it is the primary, direct-acting factors, foremost among them VEGF,[26] that are considered to be the principal driving forces in stimulating both physiologic and pathologic angiogenesis, including tumor angiogenesis, in most cases.

Direct-acting, primary proangiogenic growth factors include the VEGF family and their cognate receptor tyrosine kinases,[26] the angiopoietins, especially angiopoietin-1 and -2 (ang-1/ang-2), and their cognate tyrosine kinase receptors, in particular tie-2 (see later discussion), and the Notch signaling receptor (specifically Notch 4) and its family of ligands, such as Deltalike ligand 4 (DLL4) and Jaggeds (see later discussion). All three systems have in common a high (but not absolute) degree of specificity for endothelial cells, and in particular activated endothelial cells associated with neovascularization. Another receptor tyrosine kinase-ligand system involved in angiogenesis is Eph receptor ephrin-B2.[27] Ephrin-B2 is a transmembrane ligand that is involved in "bidirectional signaling" whereby Eph receptors help regulate endothelial tip cell guidance in the sprouting and branching of new blood vessel capillaries. Ephrin-B2 mediates its effects, at least in part, by regulating VEGFR-2 function.[27]

Discovery of the VEGF family and their receptors (Fig. 9.2) represented a profound turning point in the field of tumor angiogenesis research and the development of antiangiogenic drugs.[26] Prior to the first published reports of VEGF, which was initially called vascular permeability factor,[28] basic fibroblast growth factor (bFG)F was considered to be the central mediator of angiogenesis, and was the first molecular mediator of angiogenesis to be identified.[3] However, bFGF lacks a signal sequence for cellular secretion, and therapeutic blockade of bFGF using antibodies did not cause consistent antitumor results, observations that raised doubts about a predominant role for bFGF in tumor angiogenesis.

VEGF was discovered in 1989 and reported to be a highly specific and potent mitogen for vascular endothelial cells.[26,29] When the genes for vascular permeability factor and VEGF were sequenced, it was realized they were the same molecule.[26] The vascular permeability function of VEGF is extremely potent (50,000-fold that of histamine) and probably accounts for much of the leakiness of the tumor vasculature. It is possible that enhanced permeability may be due to intercellular gaps between endothelial cells, decreased pericyte coverage (as a second barrier to permeability), and/or specialized endothelial cell organelles called *vesiculovacuolar organelles*,[30] transmembrane vacuoles that can form channels leading to extravasation of fluid and proteins. VEGF (VEGF-A) is the prototypical member of a family of ligands with ~40–80% homology: VEGF-A (also called simply VEGF), VEGF-B, VEGF-C, VEGF-D, and placental growth factor (PlGF) (Fig. 9.2). VEGF-A (hereafter called VEGF) actually exists in a number of variant isoforms based on RNA splicing. In humans, the most common splice variants are $VEGF_{121}$, $VEGF_{165}$, $VEGF_{189}$, and $VEGF_{206}$ (whereby the number denotes the number of amino acids in the mature protein). $VEGF_{121}$, the shortest isoform, is freely circulating, whereas $VEGF_{189}$ and $VEGF_{206}$ are strongly bound to heparin sulphate containing glycoproteins and thus remain cell-bound or sequestered in the extracellular matrix where they remain biologically inactive until mobilized by specific proteases. $VEGF_{165}$ has a heparin-binding sequence but can also freely circulate. Thus, $VEGF_{121}$ and $VEGF_{165}$ are generally considered to be the main VEGF family members that drive tumor angiogenesis. $VEGF_{121}$ and $VEGF_{165}$ bind to two tyrosine kinase receptors expressed by endothelial cells. These are known as VEGFR-1 (flt-1) and VEGFR-2 or KDR in humans (kinase insert domain receptor; with flk-1 being the KDR homolog in mice).[26] The major signaling receptor is VEGFR-2. In contrast, VEGFR-1 signals only weakly, after VEGF binding, despite the fact that it can bind VEGF with tenfold greater affinity compared with VEGFR-2. A naturally occurring soluble form of VEGFR-1 is thought to serve as a negative regulator in physiologic angiogenesis. In addition, neuropilins (e.g., neuropilin-1 and

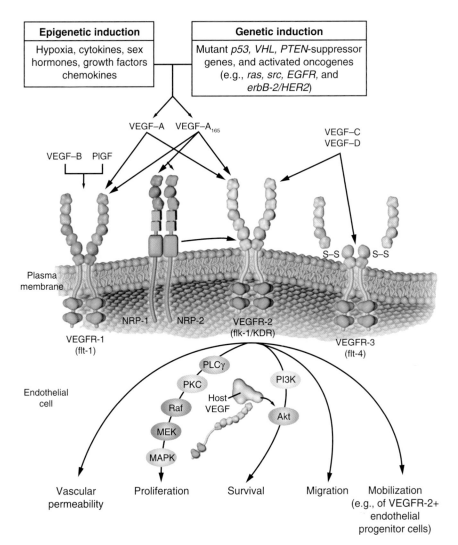

FIGURE 9.2 The family of vascular endothelial growth factor (VEGF) molecules and receptors. The major mediator of tumor angiogenesis is vascular endothelial growth factor A (VEGF-A, also called VEGF), specifically the circulating isoforms of VEGF, $VEGF_{121}$ and $VEGF_{165}$. These isoforms signal through VEGF receptor 2 (VEGFR-2), the major VEGF signaling receptor that mediates sprouting angiogenesis (called kinase-insert domain–containing receptor [KDR] in humans and fetal liver kinase 1 [flk-1] in mice). The role of VEGFR-1 in sprouting angiogenesis is much less clear. VEGF is expressed in most types of human cancer, and increased expression in tumors is often associated with a less favorable prognosis. Induction of or an increase in VEGF expression in tumors can be caused by numerous environmental (epigenetic) factors such as hypoxia, low pH, inflammatory cytokines (e.g., interleukin-6), growth factors (e.g., basic fibroblast growth factor), sex hormones (both androgens and estrogens), and chemokines (e.g., stromal cell–derived factor 1). Other causes include genetic inductive changes such as activation of numerous different oncogenes or loss or mutational inactivation of a variety of tumor suppressor genes. The binding of VEGF to VEGFR-2 leads to a cascade of different signaling pathways, two examples of which are shown, resulting in the upregulation of genes involved in mediating the proliferation and migration of endothelial cells and promoting their survival and vascular permeability. For example, the binding of VEGF to VEGFR-2 leads to dimerization of the receptor, followed by intracellular activation of the phospholipase C gamma–protein kinase C–Raf kinase–MEK–mitogen-activated protein kinase (MAPK) pathway and subsequent initiation of DNA synthesis and cell growth, whereas activation of the phosphatidylinositol 3′–kinase (PI3K)–Akt pathway leads to increased endothelial cell survival. Activation of *src* can lead to actin cytoskeleton changes and induction of cell migration. VEGF receptors are located on the endothelial cell surface; however, intracellular ("intracrine")-signaling VEGF receptors (VEGFR-2) may be present as well, and they are involved in promoting the survival of endothelial cells. The detailed structure of the intracellular VEGFR-2 in endothelial cells is not yet known, but it is shown as the full-length receptor that is normally bound to the cell surface. Binding of VEGF-C to VEGFR-3 mediates lymphangiogenesis. $VEGF_{165}$ can bind to neuropilin (NRP) receptors, which can act as coreceptors with VEGFR-2 (*horizontal arrow*) to regulate angiogenesis. EGFR, epidermal growth factor receptor; flt-1, fms-like tyrosine kinase 1; PlGF, placental growth factor; PTEN, phosphatase and tensin homologue; S–S disulfide bond; VHL, von Hippel–Lindau. (From ref. 4, with permission.)

neuropilin-2), which can bind class 3 semaphorins involved in axon guidance, can also bind the larger VEGF isoforms, as $VEGF_{121}$ lacks the domain that binds to neuropilin.[31] Neuropilin likely contributes to angiogenesis by serving as a coreceptor to VEGF and enhancing binding of VEGF-A to VEGFR-2.[32] Antibodies that target both VEGF and neuropilin-1 yield better antiangiogenic responses than targeting a single protein.[33]

Binding of VEGF to up-regulated endothelial cell VEGFR-2 sets in motion a unique intracellular signaling cascade.[34] Various investigators have identified autophosphorylation on tyrosine residues in VEGFR-2, including residues 951, 1054, 1059, 1175, and 1214. Phosphorylation of Y1175 leads to activation of phospholipase C gamma, that in turn stimulates the protein kinase C (PKC) pathway leading to inositol trisphosphate generation and calcium mobilization. In addition, this pathway, via $PKC\beta$, stimulates the c-Raf-MEK-MAP-kinase cascade.

Another member of the VEGF family, PlGF, binds to VEGFR-1, but not VEGFR-2, and there may be circumstances where it contributes to tumor angiogenesis. Interestingly, heterodimers of VEGF-A/PlGF may prevent angiogenesis by limiting VEGF-A signaling.[35] VEGF appears to be a key mediator of embryonic angiogenesis, as well as both physiologic and pathologic forms of angiogenesis in the adult. A landmark discovery in this regard was the finding that disruption and inactivation of only one of the two VEGF alleles leads to embryonic lethality associated with marked developmental abnormalities of the vasculature ("haploinsufficiency").[36,37] Homozygous disruption of flk-1/VEGFR-2 or VEGFR-1 also leads to embryonic lethality accompanied by prominent vascular defects.[26]

There are at least four proposed roles by which VEGF is thought to promote tumor angiogenesis[26]: it can stimulate endothelial division, induce locomotion/migration, enhance endothelial cell survival[38] by up-regulating various inhibitors of apoptosis,[39] and mobilize endothelial progenitor cells from the bone marrow to sites of angiogenesis.[4] In addition, the permeability enhancing effects of VEGF might also stimulate tumor angiogenesis by causing extravasation of large molecular proteins such as fibrinogen, that can be crosslinked to form a fibrin gel in the extracellular milieu of tumors serving as a matrix for endothelial cell migration and blood vessel formation.[40] VEGF also has secondary effects including up-regulation of second messengers such as nitric oxide.

VEGF is expressed by most, if not all, human (and animal) cancers, often (but not always) at much higher levels than in corresponding normal tissues. Moreover, there are many reports showing elevated VEGF is an unfavorable prognostic marker.[26] The ubiquitous and elevated expression of VEGF in both human and animal tumors is likely the consequence of many factors that are commonly associated with tumors, as shown in Figure 9.2. Among the most important is hypoxia, a prominent feature associated with the Gompertzian growth of solid tumors. Hypoxia can stabilize and hence up-regulate the levels of the hypoxia-inducible transcription factor called $HIF1\alpha$, which in turn regulates hundreds of genes, among the most important of which is VEGF.[41] In addition, a broad spectrum of oncogenes (e.g., ras, src, Her family members), and tumor suppressor genes, when they become mutated/inactivated or deleted, including p53, PTEN, and VHL, result in elevated VEGF expression.[4]

A second major growth factor signaling system that is known to be a major regulator of angiogenesis, especially for the later vessel maturation and stabilization stages, is the angiopoietin/tie-2 signaling pathway.[42] There are a number of members in the family including angiopoietins-1-4 (Ang) with Ang-1 and -2 being the best characterized.[43] Both of the latter bind to a highly specific endothelial cell-associated receptor tyrosine kinase, tie-2. Binding of Ang-1 to tie-2 causes an agonist effect whereas binding of Ang-2 is antagonistic. However, "pharmacologic levels" of Ang-2 may also serve as an agonist, which makes this system somewhat more complex and difficult to study.

Basic studies of this system suggest that Ang-1 is a stabilizing factor for endothelial cells; that is, it enhances endothelial cell survival and pericyte coverage. It is not truly a "proangiogenic" factor in the classic sense in that it does not promote endothelial cell proliferation. In fact, forced expression of Ang-1 in tumor cells leads to inhibited tumor growth from this "stabilizing" effect.[44] In contrast, Ang-2 is a destabilizing factor that, if present with VEGF, can promote angiogenesis. Hence, Ang-2 is a rationale for inhibiting tumor angiogenesis.[45] The tie-1 receptor remains an orphan receptor, with an undefined function. The Ang-1/tie-2 signaling pathway appears to be involved mainly in later stages of blood vessel formation, especially in the maturation and stabilization of vessels.[46]

Like VEGF and VEGF receptors, genetic disruption ("knockout") of either Ang-1 or tie-2 leads to embryonic lethality, although both alleles of Ang-1 (or tie-2) have to be silenced (homozygous disruption), unlike VEGF.[46] Studies of the role of Ang-1/tie-2 in tumor angiogenesis were hampered for many years by the inability to generate highly specific blocking antibodies or peptides. However, there are now a number of reports of the development not only of specific blocking peptides[47] ("peptibodies"), which have proceeded to clinical trial assessment,[45] but also monoclonal antibodies to Ang-2,[48] which cause robust antitumor activity; such reagents should help considerably in clarifying the role of this system in tumor angiogenesis.

There are a number of other factors implicated in the process of angiogenesis including interleukin-8, epidermal growth factor receptor ligands, basic and acidic FGF, PDGF, among many others. However, because of the need for brevity in this chapter, we have focused on a number of factors most relevant to clinical medicine, and perhaps the future of oncology. Some of the aforementioned factors may take on increasing importance as mediators of resistance to drugs that target the VEGF pathway of angiogenesis.[49,50]

ENDOGENOUS INHIBITORS OF TUMOR ANGIOGENESIS

In addition to the existence of multiple molecular stimulators of angiogenesis, there are a large number of endogenous and intrinsic inhibitors of angiogenesis. The existence of such inhibitors was first surmised by Folkman[3] on the basis of the observation that there are a number of tissues or organs that lack blood vessels and that also are rare sites of metastasis, such as cartilage or vitreous. It is also important to recognize the endogenous inhibitors are important in physiologic angiogenesis (wound healing, menstruation, luteal cycle) where a "stop" signal is necessary to prevent a pathologic condition.

A breakthrough in the field of endogenous inhibitors came with a series of reports by Dameron et al.[51] and Bouck et al.[52] beginning in 1989/1990. They reported a large glycoprotein that is a prominent member of the extracellular matrix, namely, thrombospondin-1 (TSP-1), which binds to CD36 receptors, and is a potent endogenous angiogenesis inhibitor. Moreover, the *p53* suppressor gene was found to up-regulate levels of TSP-1 in various cell types, and inactivation or loss of *p53* is associated with down-regulation of TSP-1 expression,[51] an observation that served to link the fields of cancer genetics—specifically the role of tumor suppressor genes and oncogenes in tumor development progression—with tumor angiogenesis.[3,4] Subsequently, a number of other proteins were identified as endogenous inhibitors of angiogenesis.[53–58] Many, if not most, are actually proteolytically cleaved fragments of larger proteins that are members of either the clotting/coagulation cascade family (e.g., angiostatin, which is a fragment of plasminogen[53]) or members of the extracellular matrix family of glycoproteins. Some examples of the latter category include endostatin,[54] tumstatin, and canstatin, fragments of type IV collagen.[55,56] Another endogenous inhibitor is known as vasostatin, which is a fragment of calreticulin.[57] Vasohibin is a secreted protein that is produced by endothelial cells on stimulation with an angiogenic stimulator such as VEGF. Vasohibin was the first example of an endogenous inhibitor that operates on the principles of a negative feedback mechanism.[58] A theory that has emerged from this body of work is that tumor angiogenesis likely requires two broad functional events: the induction or elevated expression of one or more proangiogenic growth factors, such as VEGF, coinciding with the downregulation with one or more endogenous inhibitors, such as TSP-1.[3,52,59]

A COOPERATIVE REGULATOR OF TUMOR ANGIOGENESIS: THE NOTCH RECEPTOR-DLL4 SIGNALING PATHWAY IN ENDOTHELIAL CELLS

During the last 5 years, the Notch/Notch ligand system has been shown to mediate embryonic and tumor angiogenesis.[60–65] Notch cell surface receptors (i.e., Notch 1, 2, 3, and 4) are expressed by a number of cell types and are involved in cell fate, differentiation, and proliferation. They interact with transmembrane-bound ligands (Jagged 1, Jagged 2, DLL 1, 3, and 4) on adjacent cells. The signaling aspects are unique: on ligand binding, the intracellular domain of Notch is cleaved by gamma secretase, where the Notch intracellular domain then translocates to the nuclear and acts as a transcription cofactor. It turns out that vascular endothelial cells express Notch 1 and Notch 4 receptors and Jagged 1, DLL1, and DLL4 ligands. Of these ligands, DLL4 is the only one that is selectively expressed by endothelial cells. It is expressed in small arteries and capillaries. Gene disruption experiments have shown that Notch/DLL4 signaling is absolutely essential for vascular development and arteriogenesis in embryos. Indeed, knockout of only one DLL4 allele (haploinsufficiency) is embryonic-lethal, similar to VEGF haploinsufficiency.[63] This would suggest that this system, like VEGF, would be a major stimulator of adult angiogenesis, including tumor angiogenesis. However, in some respects, Notch/DLL4 signaling is a *negative* regulator of tumor angiogenesis.[64] Thus, it turns out that DLL4 can be significantly up-regulated in the tumor vasculature in tumors, as a consequence of VEGF function. By using a combination of neutralizing antibodies to DLL4 or other types of approaches to block DLL4 function, blood vessel formation in tumors was found to be paradoxically increased, but these vessels are largely abnormal and functionally compromised such that blood flow and perfusion are impeded and tumor hypoxia increased.[60,64] This results in tumor growth inhibition. The impact of DLL4 signaling through Notch (Notch 1) is primarily restricted to tip cells at the leading edge of a growing vessel sprout or stalk, at least in the mouse retina.[61]

As a consequence of these biologic effects it appears that the Notch/DLL4 signaling pathway, though a "stimulator" of vasculogenesis and angiogenesis during early development, functions as an inhibitor of "productive" tumor angiogenesis in the adult. As such, it would seem that there is a sound therapeutic rationale for targeting the pathway to inhibit the growth of tumors, especially tumors that have become resistant to anti-VEGF therapies, by "converting" tumor blood vessels to a nonproductive or nonfunctional state.[60–64] It would appear that angiogenesis induced by VEGF can up-regulate DLL4 in endothelial cells of newly forming blood vessels and, in so doing, act as a negative feedback mechanism to prevent excessive functional angiogenesis.[62] Thus, vasohibin and DLL4 represent two negative feedback mechanisms to control/regulate tumor angiogenesis. However, the prospects of specifically targeting DLL4 received a setback recently when it was reported that chronic DLL4 blockade in mice using monoclonal antibodies caused the formation of subcutaneous vascular neoplasms and pathologic effects in organs such as the liver, thus raising critical safety concerns.[65] Hence, as always, one must carefully weigh the risk-benefit ratio of agents that may exhibit toxicities due to inhibition of pathways essential to homeostatic mechanisms.

STRATEGIES FOR DEVELOPMENT OF ANTIANGIOGENIC DRUGS

Given the aforementioned information, it can be appreciated that there are a number of possible strategies that have been developed to target tumor angiogenesis. These strategies have resulted in the discovery of an unusually large and diverse number of antiangiogenics.[25] The most obvious strategies would include developing drugs that neutralize proangiogenic growth factors such as VEGF, or block signaling from VEGFRs. In 1993, Kim et al.[66] reported that a highly specific neutralizing monoclonal antibody to human VEGF was capable of delaying the growth of VEGF expressing transplanted human tumor xenografts in immune-deficient mice, whereas it had no antiproliferative effect on the same tumor cells in cell culture, an observation consistent with an antiangiogenic mechanism of action. This was a seminal finding that opened the field of molecularly targeted anti-angiogenic drugs for the treatment of cancer.

All of the currently approved antiangiogenic drugs either target VEGF or VEGFR tyrosine kinase receptors. For example, bevacizumab, as previously discussed, is a humanized derivative of a mouse monoclonal antibody that was developed to neutralize human VEGF.[26] There are also antibodies to VEGFR-2, which are in advanced clinical development,[67] a murine precursors of which has been studied extensively in preclinical studies.[68] Another antiangiogenic approach is the fusion of the extracellular binding domains of VEGFR-1 and -2 to an Fc backbone to create a "VEGF trap" molecule that primarily binds VEGF-A, but potentially binds other VEGFR-1 ligands as well such as PlGF.[69]

In addition to antibody/protein therapeutics a large number of small-molecule oral receptor tyrosine kinase inhibitors have been developed that block VEGF receptor phosphorylation. Such drugs, currently approved by the FDA, include sorafenib, sunitinib, and pazopanib.[70–72] These latter drugs are also known to affect other structurally similar receptor tyrosine kinases, including PDGF-α/β, c-kit, flt-3, CSF-1R, and the serine threonine (in the case of sorafenib), raf kinase. The antibody-based drugs, which clearly target a single pathway, rarely cause tumor regressions in preclinical models, whereas in contrast, there are instances where the small-molecule multikinase inhibitors can cause regressions of even large established tumors.[73] However, in such situations, the tumor responses induced may be a consequence of not only inhibition of angiogenesis, but also as a result of direct inhibition of tumor cell receptor tyrosine kinases involved in cell growth and survival. Furthermore, because they target PDGF receptors, the function of pericytes in stabilizing blood vessels may be compromised and this could conceivably also increase the initial efficacy of such drugs.[74]

It is important to note that at the present time it is not possible to determine which type of drug (antibody versus TKI) is optimal. With TKIs, multiple kinases may be affected, thus this class of drugs typically lead to many types of off-target toxicity and generally are more toxic than antibodies. In addition, it is more likely that there will be more patient-to-patient variation in drug exposure to small-molecule TKIs than antibodies (antibodies are dosed based on patient mass, whereas TKIs are dosed with a standard dose such as milligram per day and so forth).

A second broad approach to antiangiogenesis involves the administration of an endogenous angiogenesis inhibitor using recombinant genetically engineered protein. In this regard, there have been phase 1 clinical trials evaluating such drugs as endostatin, angiostatin, and TSP-1 peptide mimetics.[75] In general, this approach has not yet shown obvious clinical benefit in clinical trials.

Another important point about antiangiogenic drugs for the treatment of cancer is the concept of "accidental" angiogenesis inhibitors.[76] This refers to the idea that many anticancer drugs, both old and new, that were not developed with the intention of inhibiting angiogenesis, may in fact do so, which contributes to their overall antitumor effects. By way of example, chemotherapy drugs have been shown to have antiangiogenic effects.[77]

There are at least two ways this can happen: either by directly targeting dividing endothelial cells present in growing tumor blood vessels,[78] or circulating bone marrow-derived endothelial progenitor cells and possibly other types of pro-angiogenic bone marrow derived circulating cells.[79] The nature of these different targets is important with respect to maximizing the antiangiogenic effects of chemotherapy. For example, there is limited preclinical evidence which shows that maximum tolerated doses of a chemotherapy drug can cause apoptosis of endothelial cells in the growing tumor vasculature of transplantable mouse tumors.[78] However, such a potential antiangiogenic effect is reversed during the subsequent drug-free break periods. This "repair" process may be mediated by a rapid mobilization and homing of endothelial progenitor cells to the drug-treated tumors.[5,80] By shortening the break periods or even eliminating them altogether, this process can be minimized or prevented. However, this requires giving relatively low doses of chemotherapy, that is, "metronomic chemotherapy," the antitumor effects of which can be markedly enhanced by combination with a targeted antiangiogenic drug.[81,82]

Metronomic chemotherapy has now been evaluated in phase 2 both randomized and non-randomized clinical trials in a number of indications, with encouraging results, which will have to be validated in larger randomized phase 3 trials,[83–85] although there are examples of successful adjuvant metronomic chemotherapylike phase 3 trials, such as the daily oral administration of UFT, a 5-fluorouracil prodrug (comprising tegafur plus uracil) for 2 years with no breaks for non–small cell lung cancer[86] or breast cancer.[87]

ENHANCEMENT OF CHEMOTHERAPY EFFICACY AND OTHER THERAPEUTIC MODALITIES BY ANTIANGIOGENIC DRUGS

A concern in the early days of antiangiogenic drug development was that such drugs would not be useful for combination treatments involving chemotherapy or radiation therapy. By compromising blood flow/perfusion antiangiogenic drugs would "starve" tumors of oxygen, thus increasing levels of tumor hypoxia, a resistance factor to radiation and chemotherapy. However, in 1992 Teicher et al.[88] reported the first of a series of studies showing that the antitumor effects of chemotherapy on transplantable mouse tumors were actually enhanced by combination with a drug known to have antiangiogenic properties. The preclinical efficacy results were subsequently confirmed in many other studies, and foreshadowed the clinical benefit successes of bevacizumab in randomized phase 3 clinical trials in which the drug was combined with various chemotherapy regimens for the treatment of metastatic colorectal,[1] non–small cell lung[89] and breast cancers.[90] Consequently there has been considerable interest in unraveling the basis by which an antiangiogenic drug such as bevacizumab enhances the efficacy of chemotherapy. In addition, preclinical studies have shown that inclusion of an antiangiogenic drug with other therapeutic modalities— such as radiation,[91] signal transduction inhibitors,[92] oncolytic virus therapy,[93] and vascular disrupting agents[80]—can enhance the antitumor activity of all these aforementioned therapies as well as others.

With respect to the mechanistic basis by which antiangiogenic drugs enhance the efficacy of other types of anticancer therapy, most studies thus far have dealt with chemotherapy or dealing with radiation therapy, and a number of hypotheses have been proposed. One proposes that a proportion of the chaotic dysfunctional tumor-associated vasculature, which is responsible for heterogeneous and often sluggish blood flow within regions of tumors, and hence regional areas of hypoxia, can be transiently "normalized" by an antiangiogenic drug, in this case, a VEGF-targeted agent.[24] This can result in a paradoxical transient increase in regional blood flow, decreased hypoxia, and increased tumor cell proliferation.[24] If tumors are exposed to chemotherapy or radiation during the period of "vascular normalization," their efficacy will be increased. In addition, VEGF inhibition may decrease permeability, leading to a reduction in the high tumor interstitial fluid pressures, allowing better perfusion of tumor vessels.

The overall combined effect of all these changes would be transient episodes of increased tumor oxygenation and cell proliferation coinciding with an increased ability of the tumors to take up certain chemotherapy drugs during the "window" of vascular normalization, thus increasing the ability to affect a greater proportion of the tumor cell population than otherwise would be the case in the absence of the VEGF inhibition.[24,91] However aspects of this hypothesis have yet to be confirmed clinically. Thus, paradoxical increases in blood flow may not occur in all tumors, as single-agent anti-VEGF therapy for RCC is not associated with an increase in size prior to regression. Furthermore, clinical studies involving imaging (magnetic resonance imaging, computed tomographic scan) have not demonstrated an increase in blood flow with single-agent anti-VEGF therapy.

In addition, consistent evidence that the intratumoral delivery and distribution of conventional chemotherapy drugs is improved by normalization induced by antiangiogenic drugs is still lacking, especially with respect to clinical studies. A second theory is that the presence of an antiangiogenic drug during the extended drug-free break

periods following each cycle of maximum tolerated dose chemotherapy will slow down the rate
of tumor cell repopulation that inevitably follows
tumor shrinkage, as repopulating tumor cells
would require oxygen and nutrients normally
supplied by the tumor vasculature.[94] In addition,
there is some limited evidence that bolus injec-
tions of some cytotoxic chemotherapeutic drugs
such as cyclophosphamide can cause a rapid
mobilization of some of the bone marrow-derived
cell populations shown in Figure 9.1 including
CEPs.[79] Should some of these cells then home to
sites of tumor angiogenesis in the drug-treated
tumors, tumor cell repopulation would be accelerated.[5] There is some limited preclinical evidence
that suggests this occurs after administration of a
cytotoxiclike vascular disrupting agent or various
chemotherapy drugs: tumor vascular disrupting
agent (VDA)-induced CEPs home to the viable
tumor rim that typically remains after VDA treatment and contributes to rapid tumor repopulation, a process that can be blocked by treatment
with an antiangiogenic drug just before administration of the VDA.[80] Such systemic CEP responses
constitute a form of "rebound vasculogenesis"
and can occur after maximum tolerated dose chemotherapy as well.[95,96]

A third theory is that tumor stem or stemlike
cells (self-renewing "tumor-initiating" cells) may
reside in a vascular niche within tumors and
depend on the vasculature for normal function
and survival, as appears to be the case for glioma
stem cells.[97] Disruption of the vascular niche can
occur as a result of treatment with an antiangiogenic drug; the "compromised" tumor stem cell
population might then be more sensitive to the
chemotherapy than would otherwise be the case,
provided chemotherapy retained access to the
tumor.[98] This possibility also highlights an emerging area of research in tumor angiogenesis, namely
the link between tumor stem cells and tumor
angiogenesis, given the potent tumorigenic
(tumor-initiating) property of the tumor stem cell
subpopulation. There is growing interest in their
proangiogenic phenotype in comparison to the
bulk non tumor stem cell population.[97,99] On the
contrary, there is also evidence in some systems
that cancer stem cells may have an angiogenic-in-
dependent phenotype by adapting to hypoxic
environments and using metabolic pathways that
involve increased conversion of glycose to pyruvate and lactate.[100] This is an area of research that
merits further analysis.

A fourth theory is that chemotherapy itself
might be capable of causing direct damage to the
dividing, activated endothelial cells of the tumor's
growing vasculature, where the extent of such a
vascular targeting effect is amplified by concurrent therapy with an antiangiogenic drug, such as
an anti-VEGF antibody that would neutralize the
prosurvival function of VEGF for endothelial
cells, making endothelial cells more susceptible to

the toxicity of chemotherapy.[81,101] However, even
with single-agent anti-VEGF therapy, responses
are noted in patients with metastatic RCC, providing indirect evidence that single-agent anti-
VEGF therapy can lead to vascular regression.[102]

Finally, a fifth possibility is related to the fact
that VEGF may act as a direct autocrine survival
factor for certain tumor cell population by virtue
of their expression of receptors that can bind
VEGF, for example, VEGFR-1, VEGFR-2, or neu-
ropilin-1.[103] Hence, blockade of VEGF signaling
on tumor cells could conceivably directly render
the cells more sensitive to chemotherapy in such
cases.[103,104]

When considered together, these different theories serve to illustrate how difficult it is to dissect
the mechanism of action of VEGF-targeted agents,
despite its successes in the clinic. In addition, there
are also clinical failures, and the successes
observed in the clinic remain relatively modest as
will be described later; thus there is a clear need
to better understand mechanism(s) of action to
improve efficacy and limit toxicity.

RESISTANCE TO ANTIANGIOGENIC DRUGS OR TREATMENTS

One of the theoretical advantages for antiangiogenic therapy of cancer hypothesized over 15
years ago was the possibility that this type of
treatment strategy would be less susceptible to
being rendered ineffective over time as a result of
the development of acquired drug resistance.[105]
However, preclinical experiments as well as clinical outcomes with angiogenesis inhibitors have
shown that acquired resistance represents a significant problem, similar in nature to virtually
every other anticancer drug or treatment modal-
ity. Intrinsic resistance is also a problem. In this
regard, several investigators have shown that
tumor endothelial cells from tumor neovasculature may not always be genetically stable, as was
initially proposed. Klagsbrun and colleagues have
shown that tumor endothelial cells are aneuploid,
whereas others have actually reported similar
genetic mutations in tumor cells and tumor associated endothelial cells.[106,107]

With respect to the clinical results, with rare
exception, tumors of patients that initially show
good responses to VEGF-targeted agents eventually stop responding. Preclinical investigations
have revealed a number of mechanisms by which
resistance to a drug such as bevacizumab or
VEGF-targeted TKIs can develop when such
drugs are administered as monotherapies, some of
which are summarized in Figure 9.3.[108] Some of
these resistance factors are discussed here.

(1) *Proangiogenic growth factor redundancy.*
There are, as summarized earlier, many different

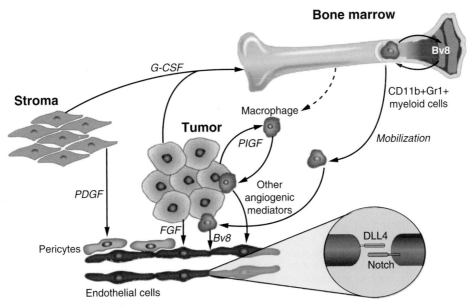

FIGURE 9.3 Some possible resistance pathways to vascular endothelial growth factor (VEGF)-targeted therapy. VEGF signaling plays a central role in tumor angiogenesis, but numerous compensatory angiogenic factors and cell types contribute to resistance to VEGF-targeted therapy. Mediators of resistance to VEGF-targeted therapy include soluble angiogenic factors such as fibroblast growth factor, placental growth factor, and Bv8; cell-bound Delta-like ligand 4 that can activate Notch on adjacent endothelial cells; pericytes that directly support endothelial cell survival; macrophages that secrete numerous angiogenic factors; and bone marrow–derived myeloid cells that also secrete soluble angiogenic factors. (From ref. 108, with permission.)

growth factors that can stimulate angiogenesis, and moreover, the number and diversity of such growth factors expressed by tumors can increase with disease progression.[109] Thus, targeting a single proangiogenic pathway, especially in the context of advanced disease, by using a drug such as a monospecific antibody to VEGF or to VEGFR-2 can lead to the selection, and eventual overgrowth, of variants that can sustain angiogenesis despite persistence of VEGF/VEGFR-2 blockade.[50,110] By way of example, an alternative proangiogenic growth factor, such as bFGF, can assume control and begin to induce tumor angiogenesis during anti-VEGFR-2 antibody therapy, even though decreases in phosphorylated VEGFR-2 are detected in tumors that initially responded to the drug.[50,110] The bFGF was induced in the tumor cell population, probably as a consequence of elevated levels of hypoxia induced by drug treatment, and thus up-regulation of various growth factors known to be regulated by hypoxia.[50] Such findings would appear to support a theoretical advantage of using multitargeting TKI antiangiogenic drugs that block several proangiogenic pathways simultaneously as a means of significantly delaying or circumventing this type of acquired resistance. However, as previously mentioned, resistance to such drugs (e.g., sunitinib or sorafenib, as in RCC) eventually occurs in all patients who initially respond to treatment. One recent report

implicated up-regulation of interleukin-8 as a mechanism for resistance to sunitinib in a model of RCC.[111] In some cases the source of a compensatory growth factor may be the tumor stroma, such as fibroblast-derived PDGF-C.[110] In addition, drugs such as sunitinib can induce elevated levels of multiple cytokines, chemokines, and growth factors such as granulocyte-colony stimulating factor, stromal-derived factor-1-1, PlGF, and VEGF in a tumor-independent fashion, and it is conceivable, but not yet proven, that these drug-induced changes could contribute to acquired resistance.[112]

(2) *Selection for hypoxia-resistant cells.* Cancer cells, as a result of certain genetic mutations (e.g., *p53* mutation/inactivation), can acquire an enhanced ability to survive under relatively hypoxic conditions, as would be expected to occur during an effective and long-term antiangiogenic therapy.[113] Thus, over time there could be a selection for mutant/variant subpopulations that depend less on tumor angiogenesis for survival, and possibly even cell growth.[113]

(3) *Co-option of normal organ vasculature.* It has been proposed that the ability of tumors to grow in certain vascular-rich organs such as the lung, brain, or liver might not be affected significantly by antiangiogenic drugs by virtue of the tumor cells exploiting ("co-opting") the existing mature normal vasculature to obtain the necessary

oxygen and nutrients for robust growth[11]; this might also contribute to "mixed" responses in patients in whom tumors in one organ location respond to antiangiogenic treatment, but do not do so in a different organ.

(4) *Vascular remodeling.* Antiangiogenic drugs tend to preferentially target relatively immature growing neovasculature and have much reduced or even no efficacy on established/more mature vessels.[114] It has been reported that antiangiogenic therapy in preclinical tumor models can accelerate the maturation and remodeling of blood vessels, which become progressively less sensitive to the therapy.[114] The remodeled vasculature may be driven by increased expression of various factors that contribute to vessel stabilization and maturation (e.g., PDGF-BB and angiopoietin-1).[114]

With respect to development of new strategies that could have promise in dealing with tumors that are either intrinsically resistant to VEGF-targeted therapies, several strategies are being evaluated, such as sequential or salvage therapy with different antiangiogenic drugs (e.g., patients whose RCC stops responding to sunitinib may respond to sorafenib, or vice versa).[70] Combining VEGFR-2 pathway targeting drugs with other antiangiogenic drugs that block a different, complementary pathway (e.g., the tie-2/Ang2 pathway),[115] may be a promising strategy. Similarly, one might use drugs that target HIF-1α and the hypoxic tumor microenvironment, a consequence of VEGF-targeted therapies.

BIOMARKERS FOR TUMOR ANGIOGENESIS AND ANTIANGIOGENIC THERAPY

A challenge associated with the development and clinical use of antiangiogenic drugs, which is similar in nature to many other types of anticancer therapeutic modalities, especially "targeted" therapies, is the need for predictive and surrogate biomarkers to improve overall therapeutic benefit, including increasing efficacy, reducing toxicity, and improving cost-effectiveness.[116] It is important to make the distinction between predictive and surrogate markers. Predictive markers are identified prior to treatment to identify patients who may or may not benefit from therapy (predictive markers may also be used to identify patients who may develop toxicity). A surrogate marker is one that changes after initiation of therapy whereby the change may indicate target modulation and, hopefully, clinical benefit.[116]

Although there are a number of *in vivo* assays to monitor angiogenesis and hence inhibition of angiogenesis that are commonly used in mice, none of these are of practical use for use in humans.

Potential biomarkers for antiangiogenic therapies markers under investigation include circulating proteins, for example, VEGF or other proangiogenic growth factors, and soluble VEGF receptors.[116–118] In addition, circulating cells thought to be relevant to angiogenesis have been studied, including circulating endothelial cells and circulating endothelial progenitor cells.[4,9] Finally, another intensively studied approach is based on noninvasive imaging of blood flow or vascular permeability using such methods as dynamic contrast enhanced magnetic resonance imaging, computed tomographic scans incorporating flow parameters, or high-frequency microultrasound, among others.[103,116] Thus far, none of these approaches has yet been validated in prospective randomized clinical trials. However, recent studies have implicated the possibility that certain single nucleotide polymorphisms in angiogenesis-related genes (e.g., the *vegf* gene) may have promise as predictive markers for VEGF pathway targeting drugs such as bevacizumab, both for predicting clinical benefit as well as certain toxicities such as hypertension, a common side effect of VEGF inhibition.[119,120] Indeed, elevated hypertension is also currently being evaluated as a relatively simple and inexpensive surrogate biomarker, although this remains a point of controversy.[121]

To illustrate the nature of the considerable challenges involved in developing biomarkers for antiangiogenic drugs, attempts to exploit VEGF as a predictive marker for possible clinical benefit in patients receiving anti-VEGF monoclonal antibody (bevacizumab) therapy provides a compelling example. There is abundant literature reporting elevated levels of tumor VEGF are associated with a poor prognosis, so it might be anticipated that examining VEGF levels in tumors or in the circulation would be a relatively single predictive assay: the higher the levels of VEGF, the target of bevacizumab, the more likely a patient would benefit from bevacizumab therapy. However, neither VEGF expression in tumor tissue or circulating VEGF levels is predictive of clinical benefit for patients receiving either bevacizumab or other drugs that target the VEGF pathway.[122,123]

ANTIANGIOGENIC/ ANTI-VEGF DRUG-BASED CLINICAL TRIALS

Research over the last two decades has shed a tremendous amount of light on the process of angiogenesis, which in turn has led the successful application of this knowledge to the care of patients with advanced-stage malignancies. All of the FDA-approved drugs considered to be antiangiogenic interfere with VEGF signaling, whereas the effectiveness of other agents remains to be determined. Because VEGF plays such diverse roles in regulating vascular development, function, and morphology, it is important at this stage in time to differentiate anti-VEGF therapy from other agents considered to be antiangiogenic. Anti-VEGF therapy can theoretically be of benefit to patients by numerous mechanisms,[124] as discussed earlier in this chapter. Thus, it is appropriate to refer to agents that inhibit VEGF signaling as "anti-VEGF agents" or "VEGF-targeted therapies," providing a distinction from "generic" antiangiogenic agents that primarily target tumor endothelial cell proliferation.

Anti-VEGF therapy, despite all its high profile, does not always lead to patient benefit. A few prin-ciples derived from phase 3 clinical trial results deserve mention (Tables 9.1 and 9.2), with details of clinical trials being presented in other chapters in this text. First, for tumors other than RCC, anti-VEGF therapy is of benefit only to patients when combined with chemotherapy. The benefit to patients with RCC may be because there is a well-defined, dominant molecular alteration (loss of von Hippel–Lindau function) leading to tumors highly dependent on VEGF signaling. Second, despite the fact that anti-VEGF therapy appears to augment the effects of chemotherapy, this is not always the case. Tyrosine kinase inhibitors for

TABLE 9.1

PHASE 3 TRIALS: CHEMOTHERAPY WITH OR WITHOUT VASCULAR ENDOTHELIAL GROWTH FACTOR (VEGF) TARGETED THERAPIES

Trial	Disease Site	Line of Rx	Total Patients on Trial	Primary End Point Met	ΔPFS
5-FU/LCV ± SU5416	mCRC	First	NA	No	NP
IFL ± BV	mCRC	First	923	Yes	4.4
FOLFOX ± PTK/ZK	mCRC	First	1168	No	0.2
XELOX/FOLFOX ± BV	mCRC	First	1400	Yes	1.4
FOLFOX ± BV	mCRC	Refractory	829	Yes	2.6
Capecitabine ± BV	mCRC	First	313	Yes	1.8
FOLFOX ± PTK/ZK	mCRC	Refractory	855	No	1.5
FOLFIRI ± sunitinib	mCRC	First	768	No	0.4–0.6
Chemo +/ cediranib vs chemo + BV[a]	mCRC	First	1,422	No	?
Chemo ± BV/BV	Stage II/III	Adjuvant	3,451	No	NA
FOLFOX ± BV/BV	Stage II/III CRC	Adjuvant	2,710	No	NA
5-FU/cisplatin ± BV	Gastric	First	774	No	1.4
Paclitaxel ± BV	mBreast Ca	First	715	Yes	5.9
Docetaxel ± BV	mBreast Ca	First	736	Yes	0.7–0.8
Capecitabine ± BV	mBreast Ca	Refractory	462	No	0.7
Chemo ± BV	mBreast Ca	First	1237	Yes	1.2–2.9
Chemo ± BV	M Breast Ca	First	684	Yes	1.3–2.2
Docetaxel ± sunitinib	mBreast Ca	First	?	No	?
Capecitabine ± sunitinib	mBreast Ca	Refractory	?	No	?
Carbo/Paclitaxel ± BV/ BV	Ovarian	First	1,873	No/yes	0.9/3.8
Carbo/Paclitaxel ± BV/BV	Ovarian	First	1,528	Yes	?
Carbo/Paclitaxel ± BV	Melanoma	First	?	No	1.4
Gem ± BV	Pancreatic Ca	First	602	No	0
Gem ± axitinib	Pancreatic Ca	First	597	No	2.3
Gem ± VEGF-Trap	Pancreatic Ca	First	?	No	?
Gemcitabine/erlotinib ± BV	Pancreatic Ca	First	301	No	1.0
Docetaxel ± BV	Prostate CA	Hormone-refractory	1050	No	2.4
Carbo/paclitaxel ± BV	NSCLC	First	878	Yes	1.9
Gem/Cis ± BV	NSCLC	First	1043	Yes	0.4–0.6
Carbo/paclitaxel ± sorafenib	NSCLC	First	926	No	−0.8

PFS, progression-free survival; 5-FU, 5-fluorouracil; LCV, mCRC, metastatic colorectal cancer; NP, not published at the time of writing; IFL, irinotecan, fluorouracil, leucovorin; FOLFOX, fluorouracil, leucovorin, oxaliplatin; BV, bevaci-zumab; PTK/ZK, PTK787/ZK222584; FOLFIRI, folinic acid, 5-FU, irinotecan, recently reported in press release but not yet presented at major meeting; NA, not available; Chemo, chemotherapy; Ca, cancer; Carbo, carboplatin; NSCLC, non–small cell lung cancer; Gem, gemcitabine; Cis, cisplatin.
[a]Head-to-head comparison.

TABLE 9.2

PHASE 3 TRIALS: VASCULAR ENDOTHELIAL GROWTH FACTOR-TARGETED THERAPIES (SINGLE AGENT OR WITH A BIOLOGIC)

Trial	Disease Site	Line of Rx	Total Patients on Trial	Primary End Point Met	ΔPFS
Sunitinib vs IFN-α	RCC	First	750	Yes	5.9
Sorafenib vs placebo	RCC	Refractory	903	Yes	2.7
IFN ± BV	RCC	First	641	Yes	4.8
Pazopanib vs placebo	RCC	Both	435	Yes	5.0
Sorafenib vs placebo	HCC	First	602	Yes	2.7
Sorafenib vs placebo	HCC	First	226	Yes	1.4
Sunitinib vs sorafenib	HCC	First	?	No	?
Sunitinib vs placebo	Pancreatic NET	First	170	Yes	5.9
Prednison ± Sunitinib	Prostate cancer	Hormone refractory	?	No	?

TPFS, progression-free survival; RCC, renal cell carcinoma; IFN, interferon; BV, bevacizumab; HCC, hepatocellular cancer; ?, recently reported in press release but not yet presented at major meeting; NET, neuroendocrine tumors.

patients with various types of metastatic cancer have so far failed to demonstrate improved efficacy over chemotherapy alone in multiple randomized phase 3 clinical trials, many of which have not yet been reported or published.[125,126] In addition, in trials in patients with metastatic breast cancer, bevacizumab augments the effects of paclitaxel in patients in the front-line setting, but in later lines of therapy the addition of bevacizumab provided no benefit when added to capecitabine. Lastly, anti-VEGF therapy leads to specific and sometimes unexpected toxicities, such as hypertension, proteinuria, bowel perforations, hemorrhage, arteriothrombotic events, and others. Some of these adverse effects may be due to our understanding of basic biology. For example, many investigators believe that hypertension associated with anti-VEGF therapy is due to inhibition of endothelial cell-derived nitric oxide, known pathway mediated by VEGFR-2 activation. However, the basis of other toxicities, such as bowel perforation, remain a mystery.[127]

It is important to point out that the benefits obtained with anti-VEGF/angiogenic therapy are incremental; cures are rare and tumor dormancy, if it occurs, is short-lived and rarely lasts beyond a year. The use of anti-VEGF therapy as "maintenance therapy" (after maximal tumor response with chemotherapy) has only recently been tested in a clinical trial.[128] Furthermore, the use of anti-VEGF/angiogenic therapy in the adjuvant setting is under study, but with one exception (Table 9.1), results from most such trials will not be available for several years. The exception comes from the results of the first randomized phase 3 trial involving an antiangiogenic drug, which was recently announced.[129] The trial evaluated bevacizumab in combination with chemotherapy for 6 months followed by bevacizumab maintenance therapy

for 6 additional months. The trial did not meet its primary end point of a progression-free survival benefit at 3 years despite prior interim analyses showing a transient benefit in the bevacizumab arm.[129] This benefit gradually disappeared over time, suggesting that there may be a change in the biological aggressiveness of tumor growth after the bevacizumab therapy has been completed.

Similarly, many recent phase 3 trials of bevacizumab plus chemotherapy have shown a benefit in progression-free survival but not overall survival. This has been reported for a number of trials in metastatic breast cancer, for example,[90] and also for trials in colorectal cancer,[130] gastric cancer,[131] and ovarian cancer.[128] The lack of overall survival benefit may be because of subsequent lines of therapy diluting the effect of front-line therapy. However, others have hypothesized that these findings suggest a possible change in the biology of tumor growth after an initial tumor response that reduces some of the initial clinical benefit. In this regard several recent preclinical studies have shown that there may be circumstances in which treatment with an antiangiogenic drug may accelerate tumor growth once treatment is stopped, and may also cause an increase in tumor cell invasion and/or metastasis.[112,132] With the possible exception of glioblastoma,[133,134] evidence for such increased malignant aggressiveness in the clinic has not yet been reported when drugs such as bevacizumab (plus chemotherapy) or single-agent antiangiogenic TKIs are used to treat various types of cancer. Moreover, if and when such increases in malignant aggressiveness occur, this does not mean that survival is decreased, but rather that the overall clinical benefits attained may be less than would otherwise be the case.[132] One theory to explain increases in malignant aggressiveness is that the elevated tumor hypoxia induced by antiangiogenic drug treatments will result in up-regulation of HIF-1α, which regulates numerous genes that contribute to tumor cell motility, invasion, and metastasis.[132,135,136]

LOOKING AHEAD: NEW TARGETS, NEW DRUGS, AND NEW STRATEGIES FOR ANTIANGIOGENIC THERAPY

We have stressed that, thus far, all approved antiangiogenic drugs involve the VEGF pathway as the only or primary target. Despite their successes, the limitations of such drugs highlight the need to develop alternative or complementary approaches to blocking tumor angiogenesis and improving the effects of existing drugs. With respect to new targets, there is currently considerable effort being put into defining molecular signatures of activated endothelial cells that may reveal new drivers of angiogenesis and/or promising molecular targets, especially those that are independent of the VEGF pathway. Some promising developments in this regard include the discovery and functional characterization of microRNAs—small noncoding RNA molecules that regulate gene expression at the post-transcriptional level—in vascular endothelial cells or tumor cells, and which thus can either stimulate or suppress angiogenesis.[137–139] For example, members of the microRNA-17-92 cluster have an antiangiogenic effect in endothelial cells[140] whereas *mir*-126, an endothelial-specific microRNA, can contribute to activation of VEGF signaling.[141]

Likewise, genomic and proteomic profiling of endothelial cells,[142] especially those isolated from the tumor vasculature, represents another approach being undertaken to uncover new molecular mediators of tumor angiogenesis.[15] With respect to new strategies, numerous possibilities exist, among them is the combining of antiangiogenic drugs with therapeutic modalities other than chemotherapy. For example, VEGF may have an impact on regulating components of the immune system, acting mainly as an immunosuppressive-regulating element.[143] Hence, VEGF inhibition may stimulate the immune system, making VEGF pathway targeting drugs ideal to combine with tumor vaccines or other immunotherapeutic methodologies. Many other types of combination treatment involving antiangiogenic drugs are currently under preclinical and clinical investigation.[93] Lastly, identifying patients likely to respond (or not respond) to current antiangiogenic therapies will lead to improvements in outcomes in those patients deemed likely to benefit from such therapies, while allowing other patients to be eligible for alternative antineoplastic approaches.

GENERAL PRINCIPLES

Selected References

The full list of references for this chapter appears in the online version.

1. Hurwitz H, Fehrenbacher L, Novotny W, et al. Bevacizumab plus irinotecan, fluorouracil, and leucovorin for metastatic colorectal cancer. *N Engl J Med* 2004;350: 2335.
2. Folkman J. Tumor angiogenesis: therapeutic implications. *N Engl J Med* 1971;285:1182.
3. Folkman J. Angiogenesis: an organizing principle for drug discovery? *Nat Rev Drug Discov* 2007;6:273.
4. Kerbel RS. Tumor angiogenesis. *New Engl J Med* 2008; 358:2039.
5. Kerbel RS. Antiangiogenic therapy: a universal chemosensitization strategy for cancer? *Science* 2006;312:1171.
6. Jain RK, Duda DG, Clark JW, Loeffler JS. Lessons from phase III clinical trials on anti-VEGF therapy for cancer. *Nat Clin Pract Oncol* 2006;3:24.
14. St. Croix B, Rago C, Velculescu V, et al. Genes expressed in human tumor endothelium. *Science* 2000;289:1197.
22. Bergers G, Song S, Meyer-Morse N, Bergsland E, Hanahan D. Benefits of targeting both pericytes and endothelial cells in the tumor vasculature with kinase inhibitors. *J Clin Invest* 2003;111:1287.
23. Xian X, Hakansson J, Stahlberg A, et al. Pericytes limit tumor cell metastasis. *J Clin Invest* 2006;116:642.
24. Jain RK. Normalization of tumor vasculature: an emerging concept in antiangiogenic therapy. *Science* 2005;307:58.
25. Kerbel RS, Folkman J. Clinical translation of angiogenesis inhibitors. *Nat Rev Cancer* 2002;2:727.
26. Ferrara N. Timeline: VEGF and the quest for tumour angiogenesis factors. *Nat Rev Cancer* 2002;2:795.
27. Sawamiphak S, Seidel S, Essmann CL, et al. Ephrin-B2 regulates VEGFR2 function in developmental and tumour angiogenesis. *Nature* 2010;465:487.
28. Senger DR, Galli S, Dvorak AM, Perruzzi CA, Harvey VS, Dvorak HF. Tumor cells secrete a vascular permeability factor that promotes accumulation of ascites fluid. *Science* 1983;219:983.
29. Leung DW, Cachianes G, Kuang W-J, Goeddel DV, Ferrara N. Vascular Endothelial Growth Factor is a secreted angiogenic molecule. *Science* 1989;246:1306.
32. Ellis LM. The role of neuropilins in cancer. *Mol Cancer Ther* 2006;5:1099.
34. Shibuya M, Claesson-Welsh L. Signal transduction by VEGF receptors in regulation of angiogenesis and lymphangiogenesis. *Exp Cell Res* 2006;312:549.
36. Ferrara N, Carver-Moore K, Chen H, et al. Heterozygous embryonic lethality induced by targeted inactivation of the VEGF gene. *Nature* 1996;380:439.
37. Carmeliet P, Ferreira V, Breier G, et al. Abnormal blood vessel development and lethality in embryos lacking a single VEGF allele. *Nature* 1996;380:435.
38. Alon T, Hemo I, Itin A, Pe'er J, Stone J, Keshet E. Vascular endothelial growth factor acts as a survival factor for newly formed retinal vessels and has implications for retinopathy of prematurity. *Nat Med* 1995;1(10): 1024.
41. Semenza GL. Targeting HIF-1 for cancer therapy. *Nat Rev Cancer* 2003;3:721.

46. Hanahan D. Signaling vascular morphogenesis and maintenance. *Science* 1997;277:48.

47. Oliner J, Min H, Leal J, et al. Suppression of angiogenesis and tumor growth by selective inhibition of angiopoietin-2. *Cancer Cell* 2004;6:507.

48. Brown JL, Cao ZA, Pinzon-Ortiz M, et al. A human monoclonal anti-ANG2 antibody leads to broad antitumor activity in combination with VEGF inhibitors and chemotherapy agents in preclinical models. *Mol Cancer Ther* 2010;9:145.

49. Bergers G, Hanahan D. Modes of resistance to anti-angiogenic therapy. *Nat Rev Cancer* 2008;8:592.

50. Casanovas O, Hicklin D, Bergers G, Hanahan D. Drug resistance by evasion of antiangiogenic targeting of VEGF signaling in late stage pancreatic islet tumors. *Cancer Cell* 2005;8:299.

52. Bouck N, Stellmach V, Hsu SC. How tumors become angiogenic. *Adv Cancer Res* 1996;69:135.

60. Noguera-Troise I, Daly C, Papadopoulos NJ, et al. Blockade of Dll4 inhibits tumour growth by promoting non-productive angiogenesis. *Nature* 2006;444:1032.

61. Hellstrom M, Phng LK, Hofmann JJ, et al. Dll4 signalling through Notch1 regulates formation of tip cells during angiogenesis. *Nature* 2007;445:776.

66. Kim KJ, Li B, Winer J, et al. Inhibition of vascular endothelial growth factor-induced angiogenesis suppresses tumour growth *in vivo*. *Nature* 1993;362:841.

68. Prewett M, Huber J, Li Y, et al. Antivascular endothelial growth factor receptor (fetal liver kinase 1) monoclonal antibody inhibits tumor angiogenesis and growth of several mouse and human tumors. *Cancer Res* 1999;59:5209.

69. Lockhart AC, Rothenberg ML, Dupont J, et al. Phase I study of intravenous vascular endothelial growth factor trap, aflibercept, in patients with advanced solid tumors. *J Clin Oncol* 2010;28:207.

70. Rini BI, Atkins MB. Resistance to targeted therapy in renal-cell carcinoma. *Lancet Oncol* 2009;10:992.

78. Browder T, Butterfield CE, Kraling BM, Marshall B, O'Reilly MS, Folkman J. Antiangiogenic scheduling of chemotherapy improves efficacy against experimental drug-resistant cancer. *Cancer Res* 2000;60:1878.

80. Shaked Y, Ciarrocchi A, Franco M, et al. Therapy-induced acute recruitment of circulating endothelial progenitor cells to tumors. *Science* 2006;313:1785.

81. Klement G, Baruchel S, Rak J, et al. Continuous low-dose therapy with vinblastine and VEGF receptor-2 antibody induces sustained tumor regression without overt toxicity. *J Clin Invest* 2000;105:R15.

89. Sandler A, Gray R, Perry MC, et al. Paclitaxel-carboplatin alone or with bevacizumab for non-small-cell lung cancer. *N Engl J Med* 2006;355:2542.

90. Miller K, Wang M, Gralow J, et al. Paclitaxel plus bevacizumab versus paclitaxel alone for metastatic breast cancer. *N Engl J Med* 2007;357:2666.

97. Calabrese C, Poppleton H, Kocak M, et al. A perivascular niche for brain tumor stem cells. *Cancer Cell* 2007;11:69.

103. Hicklin DJ, Ellis LM. Role of the vascular endothelial growth factor pathway in tumor growth and angiogenesis. *J Clin Oncol* 2005;23:1011.

109. Relf M, LeJeune S, Scott PA, et al. Expression of the angiogenic factors vascular endothelial cell growth factor, acidic and basic fibroblast growth factor, tumor growth factor beta-1, platelet-derived endothelial cell growth factor, placenta growth factor, and pleiotrophin in human primary breast cancer and its relation to angiogenesis. *Cancer Res* 1997;57:963.

110. Ferrara N. Pathways mediating VEGF-independent tumor angiogenesis. *Cytokine Growth Factor Rev* 2010;21:21.

112. Ebos JML, Lee CR, Cruz-Munoz W, Bjarnason GA, Christensen JG, Kerbel RS. Accelerated metastasis after short-term treatment with a potent inhibitor of tumor angiogenesis. *Cancer Cell* 2009;15:232.

116. Murukesh N, Dive C, Jayson GC. Biomarkers of angiogenesis and their role in the development of VEGF inhibitors. *Br J Cancer* 2010;102:8.

120. Chen HX, Cleck JN. Adverse effects of anticancer agents that target the VEGF pathway. *Nat Rev Clin Oncol* 2009;6:465.

132. Paez-Ribes M, Allen E, Hudock J, et al. Antiangiogenic therapy elicits malignant progression of tumors to increased local invasion and distant metastasis. *Cancer Cell* 2009;15:220.

134. Norden AD, Young GS, Setayesh K, et al. Bevacizumab for recurrent malignant gliomas: efficacy, toxicity, and patterns of recurrence. *Neurology* 2008;70:779.

136. Pennacchietti S, Michieli P, Galluzzo M, Mazzone M, Giordano S, Comoglio PM. Hypoxia promotes invasive growth by transcriptional activation of the met protooncogene. *Cancer Cell* 2003;3:347.

137. Heusschen R, van GM, Griffioen AW, Thijssen VL. MicroRNAs in the tumor endothelium: novel controls on the angioregulatory switchboard. *Biochim Biophys Acta* 2010;1805:87.

139. Bonauer A, Boon RA, Dimmeler S. Vascular microRNAs. *Curr Drug Targets* 2010;11:943.

CHAPTER 10 INVASION AND METASTASIS

ANDY J. MINN AND JOAN MASSAGUÉ

Many of the gains in our understanding of the genetics and molecular mechanisms of cancer have been driven by the quest to understand characteristic anatomic and cellular traits of the disease. Pathologists have long observed that cancer seemingly can evolve from hyperplasia through a series of increasingly disorganized and invasive-appearing tumors that can then colonize distant organs in a nonrandom fashion. This spread of cancer from the organ of origin (primary site) to distant tissues is called *metastasis*. Much of the complex knowledge that has been acquired about cancer biology has been from a reductionistic approach that has focused on the inner workings of cancer cells with limited regard to interactions with the microenvironment and host biology. Although our understanding about cell proliferation, cell death, genomic instability, and signal transduction pathways has rapidly progressed, detailed understanding about the molecular mechanisms of metastasis has lagged considerably behind.

Inherent difficulties in studying metastasis have been due to technological limitations in analyzing a complex *in vivo* process rich with heterotypic interactions. Invasion, survival in the circulation, and growth in distant organs are not amenable to methods that primarily use *in vitro* models. Despite technical challenges, elegant experiments that started in the 1950s were done with mouse xenograft models and resulted in an important descriptive understanding of the biology of metastasis. With the accumulation of knowledge from studying cancer cells in isolation, subsequent advances in metastasis built on the classic studies. Unfortunately, metastasis remains responsible for the vast majority of cancer-related morbidity and mortality. Therefore, advancing our scientific and clinical understanding of metastasis is a high priority. In this chapter, we will first review the classic paradigm of cancer metastasis and then describe recent advances that are starting to better characterize metastasis on the molecular, cellular, and organismal level.

THE EVOLUTION AND PATHOGENESIS OF METASTASIS

Somatic Evolution of Cancer

Hyperplastic and dysplastic lesions need not always progress to cancer, but when they do, it can take years if not decades for this to occur. This protracted course to malignancy is consistent with epidemiologic studies that show an age-dependent increase in the incidence of cancer.[1] Mathematically, this precipitous rise can be explained by the accumulation of many stochastic events. These ideas have contributed to the widely accepted view that cancer requires several genetic alterations during a course of somatic evolution. However, the mutation frequency of human cells is thought to be too low to explain the high prevalence of the disease if so many stochastic genetic alterations are needed. To account for this disparity, cancer cells are widely believed to have a "mutator phenotype," a concept with much experimental support.[2]

Driven by increased mutability of the genome, the dynamics of tumor progression depend on mutation, selection, and tissue organization.[3] Mutations can result in activation of oncogenes or loss of tumor suppressor genes that increase fitness and cell autonomy. To oppose the accumulation of cells with tumorigenic mutations, tissue architecture often limits the spread of mutant cells that have reached fixation. For example, large compartments containing many cells accumulate advantageous mutations more rapidly than smaller compartments. Similarly, if there are only a limited number of precursor cells that have self-renewal capabilities (stem cells), this also has the effect of reducing the risk of enriching for tumorigenic mutations. However, despite the sequential mutations and steps predicted by the somatic evolution of cancer, the nature and/or sequence of genes that are altered during this evolution are mostly unknown.

143

Clinical, Pathologic, and Anatomic Correlations

Metastasis is often associated with several clinical and pathologic characteristics. Among these, tumor size and regional lymph node involvement are consistently associated with distant relapse. For tumor size, no clear threshold exists but trends are clear. For example, metastatic risk for breast cancer rises sharply after 2 cm,[4] while distant metastasis in sarcoma is more common for tumor sizes larger than 5 cm.[5] The involvement of regional lymph nodes is often, but not always, a harbinger for increased risk of distant metastasis. For head and neck cancer, the association between lymph node involvement and metastasis is predictable. Metastasis rarely occurs without prior involvement of cervical neck lymph nodes, and the lower down in the neck nodal involvement occurs, the more likely distant metastasis becomes.[6] For breast cancer, the presence of positive lymph nodes is the strongest clinicopathologic prognostic marker for distant relapse. Like head and neck cancer, the extent of nodal involvement is telling, as a precipitous rise in metastatic risk is observed for patients with more than four axillary lymph nodes.[4] However, lymph node metastasis does not always precede distant relapse. In sarcomas, for example, metastasis is often seen in the absence of nodal disease.[5]

When tumor cells appear to have aggressive traits on microscopic analysis, this often translates into increased risk for distant disease. Although many histopathologic traits for different cancer types have been reported to associate with poor prognosis, there are several that consistently appear to track with metastatic risk across various tumor types. These traits include: (1) *Tumor grade.* Tumors that are poorly differentiated, or retain few features of their normal tissue counterparts, are generally considered to be high grade. High-grade tumors often exhibit infiltrative rather than pushing borders and show signs of rapid cell division. Breast cancer and sarcomas are well recognized for displaying a markedly elevated risk of metastasis with higher tumor grade. (2) *Depth of invasion beyond normal tissue compartmental boundaries.* Some cancers like melanoma and gastrointestinal malignancies are staged by how deeply they extend beyond the basement membrane. Violation of deeper layers of the dermis, or invasion through the lamina propria, muscularis mucosa, and serosa, represent progressively more extensive invasion and higher risk of metastasis. (3) *Lymphovascular invasion.* Tumor emboli seen in the blood or lymphatic vessels generally carry a poorer prognosis than cancer without these features. Breast cancer and squamous cell cancers of the head and neck or female cervix are examples.

Tissue Tropism and the Seed and Soil Hypothesis

Despite apparent similarities in clinical and/or histologic features, different cancer types do not exhibit the same proclivity to metastasize to the same organs, and the same cancer type can preferentially metastasize to different organs (Table 10.1). This tissue tropism has long been recognized and has intrigued clinicians and pathologists to seek an explanation. In 1889, Stephen Paget proposed his "seed and soil" hypothesis (reviewed in ref. 7). This stated that the propensity of different cancers to form metastases in specific organs was due to the dependence of the seed (the cancer) on the soil (the distant organ). In contrast, James Ewing and others argued that tissue tropism could be accounted for based on mechanical factors and circulatory patterns of the primary tumor. For example, colorectal cancer can enter the hepatic-portal system, explaining its propensity for liver metastasis, and prostate cancer can traverse a presacral plexus that connects the periprostatic and vertebral veins, explaining its propensity for metastases to the lower spine and pelvis. Supporting the arguments for both views, current understanding would suggest that both seed and soil factors and anatomic ("plumbing") considerations contribute to metastatic tropism. A modern interpretation of the seed and soil hypothesis is an active area of investigation, with molecular definitions accumulating for both the cancer and the microenvironment.

Basic Steps in the Metastatic Cascade

From clinical, anatomic, and pathologic observations of metastasis, a picture of the steps involved in a metastatic cascade emerges. Numerous prerequisites and steps can be envisioned.

1. *Invasion and motility.* Normal tissue requires proper adhesions with basement membrane and/or neighboring cells to signal to each other that proper tissue compartment size and homeostasis is being maintained. Tumor cells display diminished cellular adhesion, allowing them to become motile, a fundamental property of metastatic cells. Tumor cells use their migratory and invasive properties in order to burrow through surrounding extracellular stroma and to gain entry into blood vessels and lymphatics.
2. *Intravasation and survival in the circulation.* Once tumor cells enter the circulation, or intravasate, they must be able to withstand the physical shear forces and the hostility of sentinel immune cells. Solid tumors are not accustomed to surviving as single cells without attachments

TABLE 10.1

STEREOTYPIC PATTERNS OF METASTASIS TO DISTANT ORGANS BY CANCER TYPE

Cancer Type	Site of Metastasis
Breast carcinomas	Primarily bone, lung, pleura and liver; less frequently brain and adrenal. ER-positive tumors preferentially spread to bone; ER-negative tumors metastasize more aggressively to visceral organs.
Lung cancers	The two most common types of lung cancer have different etiologies. SCLC disseminates rapidly to many organs including the liver, brain, adrenals, pancreas, contralateral lung, and bone. NSCLC often spreads to the contralateral lung and the brain, and also to adrenal glands, liver, and bones.
Prostate carcinoma	Almost exclusively to bone; forms osteoblastic lesions filling the marrow cavity with mineralized osseous matrix, unlike the osteolytic metastasis caused by breast cancer.
Pancreatic cancer	Aggressive spread to the liver, lungs, and surrounding viscera.
Colon cancer	The portal circulation pattern favors dissemination to the liver and peritoneal cavity, but metastasis also occurs in the lungs.
Ovarian carcinoma	Local spread in the peritoneal cavity.
Sarcomas	Various types of sarcoma; mesenchymal origin; mainly metastasize to the lungs.
Myeloma	Hematologic malignancy of the bone marrow that causes osteolytic bone lesions, sometimes spreading to other organs.
Glioma	These brain tumors display little propensity for distance organ metastasis, despite aggressively invading the central nervous system.
Neuroblastoma	Pediatric tumors arising from nervous tissue of the adrenal gland. Forms bone, liver, and lung metastases, which spontaneously regress in some cases.

ER, estrogen receptor; SCLC, small cell lung cancer; NSCLC, non–small cell lung carcinoma.

and often interact with each other or blood elements to form intravascular tumor emboli.

3. *Arrest and extravasation.* Once arrested in the capillary system of distant organs, tumor cells must extravasate, or exit the circulation, into foreign parenchyma.

4. *Growth in distant organs.* Successful adaptation to the new microenvironment results in sustained growth. Of all the steps in the metastatic cascade, the ability to grow in distant organs has the greatest clinical impact and lies at the core of the seed and soil hypothesis. Accomplishing this step may be rate-limiting and may determine whether distant relapse occurs rapidly or dormancy ensues.

Heterogeneity in Cancer Metastasis and Rarity of Metastatic Cells

Because numerous sequential steps are needed for metastasis, multiple genetic changes are envisioned. A failure in any step would prevent metastasis altogether. Accordingly, tumor cells that can accumulate a full complement of needed alterations to endow them with metastatic ability should be rare. These ideas are supported by early experiments. Work by Fidler and colleagues[7] showed that subpopulations of tumor cells exist that display significant variation in their metastatic ability and metastatic

lesions likely arose from single progenitor cells. Early cell fate studies revealed that less than 0.01% of tumor cells gave rise to metastases. More recent studies using *in vivo* video microscopy to visualize and quantitate cell fate confirmed that metastasis is an inefficient process (reviewed in ref. 8). Thus, important early studies helped to establish the idea that primary tumors are heterogeneous in their metastatic ability and that tumor cells that can successfully metastasize are exceedingly rare.

The Traditional Progression Model for Metastasis and Its Implications

A synthesis of clinical observation, deduced steps in the metastatic cascade, and early studies of experimental metastasis in mice led to a traditional model for metastatic progression.[7] In this view, primary tumor cells undergo somatic evolution and accumulate genetic changes. Because numerous steps are required for metastasis, the number of genetic changes that are needed for full metastatic competency is large; hence, tumor cells that have acquired these changes are rare. Many clinicopathologic traits such as lymphovascular invasion and regional lymph node involvement represent successful completion of some of the steps in the metastatic cascade but not necessarily all. The clinical observation that metastatic risk increases with tumor size is explained by mathematical considerations predicting that genetic changes accumulate faster with increased population size. Larger tumors are more likely to contain rare cells that are metastatically competent, making metastasis a late event in tumorigenesis.

One of the primary objectives in the clinical management of cancer is to prevent or decrease the risk of metastasis. How this objective is approached is shaped by empiricism and perceptions about how metastasis proceeds. The idea that metastasis occurs as a late event in tumorigenesis argues that early detection and early eradication of the primary tumor will prevent metastasis and be sufficient for cure. Screening programs, radical versus more limited surgical excisions, and the use of adjuvant radiation to the surgical bed can be justified based on the idea that cancers caught early have not likely spread. Metastatic heterogeneity within the primary tumor and the rarity of tumor cells that can complete all the sequential steps in the metastatic cascade suggest that the detection of tumor cells caught in the act of undergoing an early step in the cascade may still represent an opportunity to stop metastasis in its tracks. This is a rationale for oncologic surgeries that include regional lymph node dissections and the use of regional radiation therapy. The likely emergence of rare metastatic cells late during tumorigenesis provides reason to add adjuvant systemic chemotherapy after local treatment of larger and more advanced primary tumors rather than smaller tumors with less aggressive features.

Alternative Models

Although the traditional model for metastasis has enjoyed favor, alternative models have been proposed. The clinical data for breast cancer has inspired a long-standing debate on whether metastasis follows a traditional progression model or a predetermination paradigm—also known as the Halsted model versus the Fisher model (discussed in ref. 9) for metastasis.[9] Both models seek to justify and explain clinical data looking at the benefit of aggressive local treatment of the primary tumor and draining lymph nodes versus the early use of adjuvant systemic chemotherapy. Although more anatomic than cellular in nature, the Halsted model looked at breast cancer from a traditional vantage point and imposed on it an orderly anatomic spread pattern from primary site, to regional lymph nodes, to distant organs. This orderly progression would make complete eradication of the primary and regional tumor burden sufficient to stop metastasis. In contrast, Fisher hypothesized that whether distant relapse occurs in breast cancer is predetermined from the onset of tumorigenesis (discussed in ref. 9). This view emphasizes breast cancer as a systemic disease for those tumors so fated and the importance of adjuvant systemic chemotherapy. The data from randomized trials for adjuvant treatment and from breast cancer screening programs do not clearly rule-out one model or the other.[10] To reconcile the clinical data, Hellman[9] proposed that breast cancer is best considered a spectrum of diseases bound by predetermination models and traditional progression models. Other models that conceptually differ from the traditional progression model include the clonal dominance model[11] and the dynamic heterogeneity model.[12]

Compatibility of Metastasis Models with Somatic Evolution

Both alternative and traditional progression models alike need to be compatible with the paradigm of somatic evolution, which presents a potential problem. Because it is not obvious why metastasis genes that promote growth at a distant site should have a fitness advantage for a primary tumor, the likelihood that multiple metastasis-specific genes will become fixed in a primary tumor would seem unlikely. To reconcile this, it has been suggested that the genes selected to drive primary tumor formation and progression are also the genes that mediate metastasis.[13] This notion would imply that metastasis is a predetermined property of primary tumors that principally depends on the history of oncogenes and tumor suppressor genes that the primary tumor acquires. Such early onset of metastatic ability could explain phenomenon like cancers of unknown primary and support earlier predetermination metastasis models for breast cancer. However, as previously mentioned, predetermination models are not always consistent with clinical data, in particular the ability of screening and early detection to decrease cancer mortality. Furthermore, the phenomenon of metastatic dormancy, whereby metastasis remains inactive and undetectable for years if not decades after treatment of the primary tumor, is difficult to explain unless further metastasis-promoting changes occur after the primary tumor has been removed.

AN INTEGRATED MODEL FOR METASTASIS

Different concepts on how metastasis progresses have individual merits and limitations. A clearer understanding of metastasis requires sophisticated insight on a molecular level. Recent advances in the field of metastasis research are beginning to bring together an integrated and more complex paradigm (Fig. 10.1) whereby elements from different models may be interconnected.[14] At the heart of this integrated paradigm are the principles of somatic evolution. Somatic evolution selects for functions and not directly for specific genes. Therefore, during primary tumor growth, the principal functions that are selected are *tumorigenic*

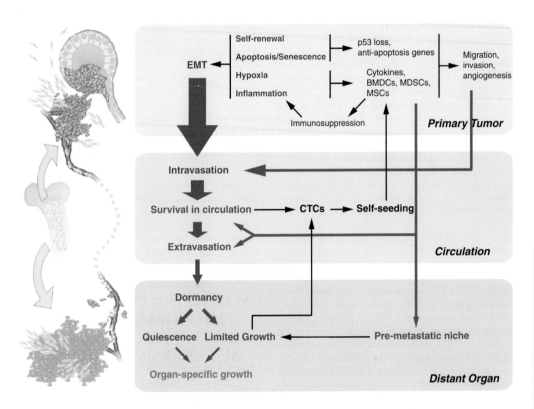

Metastasis Initiation Genes: **TWIST1, SNAI1, ZEB1, ZEB2, miR-10b, miR-200, miR-126**

Metastasis Progression Genes: **PTGS2, EREG, MMP1, LOX, ANGPTL4, CXCR4, CCL5/CCR5, VEGF, FSCN1, IL-6, IL-8, SRC, HBEGF**

Metastasis Virulence Genes: **IL11, SPARC, PTHRP, IL13RA2, IL-6, TNFα**

FIGURE 10.1 Selective pressures and steps from primary tumor growth to metastasis. Selective pressures at the primary tumor (labeled in *magenta*) can determine metastatic potential. Cancer is initiated by oncogenic changes. Of particular relevance to metastatic potential may be self-renewal pathways and the need to overcome apoptosis and senescence. Hypoxia and inflammation have important roles and lead to tumor cells co-opting bone marrow-derived cells (BMDCs), myeloid-derived suppressor cells (MDSCs), and mesenchymal stem cells (MSCs), to name a few. These cells and the cytokines that they produce enhance the ability of the tumor to migrate, invade, overcome hypoxia, and maintain an immunosuppressed environment. The ability of primary tumor cells to undergo an epithelial-to-mesenchymal transition (EMT) is also influenced by the selective pressures faced during primary tumor growth. EMT results in migration, invasion, and intravasation. Such functions (labeled in *red*) are examples of metastasis initiation functions. Although non–EMT-related migration and invasion can also lead to intravasation, EMT is likely a principle means by which circulating tumor cells (CTCs) are promoted. Further steps in the metastatic cascade are shown by *green arrows*, with the size of the arrow representing the likelihood that the step is successfully completed for many cancer types (e.g., breast cancer). Selective pressures encountered from the local microenvironment shape metastatic proclivity by selecting for tumorigenic functions that secondarily help cells navigate the metastatic cascade (metastasis-progression functions). Hypoxia and inflammation-related events contribute to metastasis-progression functions (labeled in *purple*) by enhancing the ability of CTCs to survive in the circulation, extravasate, and form a premetastatic niche. CTCs can either self-seed the primary tumor, which results in augmentation of tumor mass and further selection of metastatic traits, or extravasate into distant organs. Although a premetastatic niche facilitates adaptation to the foreign microenvironment of distant organs, further selection is needed for full colonization. This results in a period of dormancy whereby micrometastases remain quiescent or growth is counterbalanced by apoptosis and the lack of angiogenesis. Further somatic evolution within the distant organ can eventually result in selection of macrometastatic-colonization functions (labeled in *blue*) and organ-specific growth. On the bottom of the figure are examples of specific genes that play a role in metastasis initiation, metastasis progression, and macrometastatic colonization.

GENERAL PRINCIPLES

functions that can be met by a large repertoire of oncogenic mutations. Examples of these tumorigenic functions include proliferative and metabolic autonomy, self-renewal ability, resistance to cell death, resistance to inhibitory signals, immune evasion, motility, invasion, and angiogenesis. Most of these traits were enumerated by Hanahan and Weinberg[15] as being hallmarks of cancer. Many of these tumorigenic functions allow transformed cells to attract supporting stroma and migrate and invade surrounding tissue, regardless of whether or not cells reside in the primary tumor. This subset of tumorigenic functions is a prerequisite for metastasis because such functions are needed for cells to invade, penetrate blood vessels, and give rise to circulating tumor cells. These functions are shared by primary tumors and metastasis and are defined as *metastasis initiation functions*. A prominent example includes epithelial-to-mesenchymal transition (EMT).

It is evident how genes with tumorigenic functions and genes with metastasis initiation functions can be selected for during primary tumor growth. However, how are metastasis-specific functions (i.e. functions that are not characteristic of general tumorigenesis) selected during growth at the primary site? Metastasis-specific functions include survival in the circulation, extravasation, survival in the microenvironment of distant organs, and organ-specific colonization. Recent experimental evidence reveals that some genes can mediate tumorigenic functions and secondarily serve metastasis-specific functions either in a general way or with particular organ selectivity.[16,17] These types of functions are called *metastasis-progression functions* and genes with this duality are defined as *metastasis-progression genes*. Metastasis-progression genes form the basis for predetermination models for metastasis. When metastasis-progression genes are selected for, their expression by the primary tumor will track with increased risk of metastasis. These genes will also mechanistically couple certain traits of primary tumor progression (e.g., rapid growth, invasiveness, resistance to hypoxia) with distant spread.

Cancer cells that have acquired metastasis-progression genes can undergo additional selective pressure during life away from the primary tumor. Functionally, genes selected by the pressures of a distant site are similar to metastasis-progression genes but they are not coupled to tumorigenic genes and so confer no advantage to a primary tumor. Therefore, altered expression of these genes would be rare or absent in the primary tumor and discernible only in the metastatic lesion. These genes are called *macrometastatic-colonization genes* and provide *macrometastatic-colonization functions*. Macrometastatic-colonization genes form the basis of traditional progression models for metastasis.

In this integrated view that stratifies genes into tumorigenic, metastasis initiation, metastasis progression, and macrometastatic colonization, the selection for tumorigenic functions during primary tumor growth provides essential prerequisites for future metastasis. Certain biases in the genes that are selected to fulfill particular tumorigenic functions may result in genes that can also fulfill specific metastatic functions, leading to an early proclivity toward distant spread. The further selection of metastasis-specific functions after infiltration of distant organs can continue to modify metastatic behavior through the acquisition of macrometastatic-colonization genes. Although the emerging evidence does not always allow clear delineation between genes that serve tumorigenic versus metastasis initiation versus metastasis-progression functions, recent molecular understanding and insight offer the underpinnings of this integrated view.

SELECTIVE PRESSURES AT THE PRIMARY TUMOR DRIVING ACQUISITION OF METASTASIS FUNCTIONS

Of all the tumorigenic functions required by aggressive primary cancers, several may additionally select for metastasis initiation or metastasis-progression genes (Fig. 10.1). Experimental and clinical evidence point toward the following factors.

Hypoxia

In order to disrupt tissue homeostasis during primary tumorigenesis, many barriers that can limit growth must be overcome. A near-universal need is for tumors to respond to hypoxia (reviewed in refs. 18 through 20). Normal tissue such as epithelium is separated from blood vessels by a basement membrane. When preinvasive tumor growth occurs, hypoxia can ensue because oxygen and glucose typically can only diffuse 100 to 150 microns, resulting in portions of the expanding mass becoming hypoxic. This can be seen in comedo-type ductal carcinoma *in situ* (DCIS) of the breast, whereby a necrotic center characterizes these preinvasive breast tumors. The fact that DCIS can take years to progress to invasive cancer, or never progresses to cancer, suggests that hypoxia can be a significant barrier.

Although there are multiple paths that cancer cells can take to adapt to hypoxia, the hypoxia-inducible factor (HIF) transcription factors have a central role. Under hypoxic conditions, HIF-1α and HIF-2α become stabilized, resulting in the transcription of over 100 HIF-α regulated genes. These target genes are involved in angiogenesis, glycolysis, and invasion, which together help hypoxic cells adapt. Up-regulated angiogenesis genes include vascular endothelial growth factor (VEGF) and platelet-derived growth factor (PDGF). These factors cause quiescent blood vessels to undergo remodeling, including the laying down of a matrix that activated endothelial cells use to form newly vascularized areas. Various glycolysis genes are expressed and their metabolic by-products lead to acidification of the extracellular space. This is normally toxic to cells and requires further adaptation either by up-regulation of H^+ transporters or acquired resistance to apoptosis. To assist in invasion toward newly vascularized areas, HIF-α up-regulates matrix metalloproteinase 1 and 2 (MMP1, MMP2), lysyl oxidase (LOX), and the chemokine receptor CXCR4. Degradation of the basement membrane by MMP2 and alteration of the extracellular matrix (ECM) by MMP1 and LOX clears away a barrier to migration. The activation of CXCR4 then stimulates cancer cells to migrate to regions of angiogenesis. Thus, if these series of events can be successfully completed, not only will preinvasive tumors successfully deal with hypoxia, but they will also likely invade through the basement membrane in the process. Invasion through the basement membrane defines invasive carcinomas.

Inflammation

When normal tissue homeostasis and architecture are disrupted, this can lead to vessel injury, hypoxic zones, extravasation of blood proteins, and the entry of foreign pathogens (reviewed in refs. 21 and 22). A rapid response is mounted by a front line composed of immune and bone marrow-derived cells (BMDCs) such as lymphocytes, neutrophils, macrophages, dendritic cells, eosinophils, and natural killer (NK) cells. The purpose is to restore homeostasis through several phases: inflammation, tissue formation, and tissue remodeling. In the initial phase, tissue breakdown attracts neutrophils to infiltrate the wounded area and release various proinflammatory cytokines such as interleukin (IL)-8, IL-1β, and tumor necrosis factor-α (TNF-α). In addition, reactive oxygen species and proteases such as urokinase-type plasminogen activator (uPA) are produced by neutrophils to fight pathogens and debride devitalized tissue. After a few days, neutrophils begin to undergo cell death and are replaced by macrophages that are either resident or recruited from circulating monocytes in response to proinflammatory cytokines and chemotactic gradients. Activated macrophages are thought to play an integral part in coordinating the wound response by providing matrix remodeling capabilities (uPA, MMP9), synthesis of growth factors (fibroblast growth factor [FGF], PDGF, transforming growth factor beta [TGF-β]), and production of angiogenesis factors (VEGF). These factors activate

fibroblasts to synthesize new ECM and promote neovascularization in the formation of granulation tissue. Other cells that are important in wound healing include mesenchymal stem cells.[23] These fibroblastoidlike cells can be mobilized from the bone marrow or from niches within various tissues in order to aid wound healing by differentiating into different connective tissue cell types.

Cancer cells are often surrounded by activated fibroblasts and BMDCs. Because of the resemblances between primary tumors and normal tissue wound response, cancer has been described as a "wound that does not heal." Although Virchow hypothesized in the 1850s that inflammation was the cause of cancer, the presence of an inflammatory response has generally been interpreted as evidence that the immune system actively fights the cancer as it does with invading bacterial or viral pathogens. Under this scenario, the inflammatory response would apply significant selective pressure on the tumor to evade immune-mediated attack, and the nonhealing nature of the response suggests a back-and-forth struggle. Tumors that progress do so by orchestrating an immunosuppressive environment, a process known as *immunoediting*.[24]

To facilitate an immunosuppressive environment, the tumor microenvironment selects for cells that favor production of immunomodulatory factors like TGF-β, cyclooxygenase-2 (COX2), CSF-1 (macrophage growth factor, colony-stimulating factor-1), IL-10, and IL-6. These cytokines inhibit maturation of dendritic cells and promote tumor-associated macrophages (TAMs) that are immunosupressed.[25] Tumors also recruit BMDCs that have immunosuppressive properties such as myeloid-derived suppressor cells (MDSCs).[26] These cells are recruited through signaling events that involve stromal cell-derived factor-1 (SDF-1, also known as CXCL12) and its ligand CXCR4 and CXCL5/CXCR2, another chemokine/receptor pair. On arrival, the MDSCs increase local production of TGF-β, block T-lymphocyte function, and inhibit the activation of NK cells.[27] Thus, although the inflammatory response undoubtedly can help to limit cancer growth, cancers seem to select for cells that create immunosuppressive surroundings.

Rather than simply suppress the inflammatory response, cancer cells actually develop mechanisms to both co-opt and perpetuate it. For example, at the same time MDSCs are contributing to immunosuppression, these cells also facilitate tumor invasion by residing at the invasive front and secreting MMPs. The comingling of various stromal cells and other BMDCs with the cancer also actively contributes to tumor growth in a similar fashion. For example, TAMs are often found at points of basement membrane breakdown and, like MDSCs, end up at the invasive front to help tumors degrade extracellular proteins using uPA and MMPs or stimulate tumor growth and motility through EGF receptor ligands and PDGF. As in normal wound healing, growth factors secreted by the TAMs

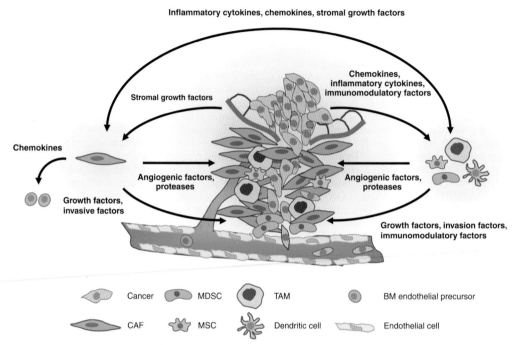

FIGURE 10.2 Interactions between cancer and stroma that promote invasion and metastasis. Cancerized stroma consists of fibroblasts, inflammatory cells, and other bone marrow-derived cells that have been conscripted to aid the tumor in overcoming hypoxia and in invasion and migration. Tissue breakdown, hypoxia, and inflammatory cytokines and chemokines secreted by the tumor cells result in recruitment of tumor-associated macrophages (TAMs), carcinoma-associated fibroblasts (CAFs), mesenchymal stem cells (MSCs), and myeloid-derived suppressor cells (MDSCs). TAMs and MDSCs can be found at points of basement membrane breakdown and at the invasive front of the tumor. These cells produce angiogenic factors to promote vascularization, proteases to degrade the extracellular matrix, and growth factors that stimulate tumor invasion and motility. CAFs also produce similar angiogenic factors, protease, and tumor growth factors. In addition, CAFs recruit bone marrow-derived endothelial precursors for angiogenesis. The cytokines and growth factors that TAMs and CAFs secrete are mutually beneficial to each other as part of an inflammatory/woundlike response. Cancers have been described as "wounds that do not heal." This chronic state is maintained by immunomodulatory cytokines that suppress immune functions to ensure a protumorigenic environment.

activate fibroblasts. These activated fibroblasts become carcinoma-associated fibroblasts (CAFs) and promote primary tumor growth by secreting CXCL12 to stimulate CXCR4 on tumor cells. Angiogenesis is also aided by the action of CAFs through recruitment of endothelial progenitor cells by CXCL12 and by the action of TAMs that are recruited to areas of hypoxia to produce VEGF. Figure 10.2 presents a summary of this interaction. Thus, although the question of whether the immune system is a friend or foe of malignancies is not a new one, it would seem that recent answers suggest that cancers actually find ways to turn an enemy into an accomplice.

Escaping Apoptosis and Senescence

A major mechanism to safeguard against a breakdown in tissue homeostasis due to cells that stray, become damaged, or spent, is to have these cells commit programmed cell death, or apoptosis.[28] This form of cell suicide is genetically regulated and can be triggered by a variety of signal transduction pathways linked to proteins that monitor environmental cues or act as damage sensors. Common cell intrinsic triggers for apoptosis include oncogene activation or tumor suppressor gene loss. For example, the inappropriate activation of c-MYC or the loss of Rb results in programmed cell death that must be countered by overexpression of antiapoptosis genes such as *Bcl-2* or loss of proapoptotic regulators like *p53*.[29] Extrinsic triggers for apoptosis include hypoxia, low pH, reactive oxygen species, loss of cell contact, and immune-mediated killing. Members of the TNF-receptor family can act as death receptors that mediate activation of proapoptotic proteases called *caspases* in response to loss of ECM adhesion[30] or after being engaged by immune cells for elimination. Cancer cells invariably ignore these cues, and their ability to resist cell death likely contributes to successful establishment of tumors.

In addition to apoptosis, senescence is another important barrier to cancer. This exit from the pool of proliferating cells results from telomere erosion, oncogene induction, and DNA damage. Similar to some forms of apoptosis, senescence is *p53*-dependent. Thus, pressure to escape senescence can result in the loss of *p53* or mutations in *p53*.

Self-Renewal Ability

Normal tissues result from the differentiation of precursor cells called *stem cells*, which are multipotent cells with self-renewal ability. In the adult, mature differentiated cells serve specialized tasks and have limited proliferative potential. However, adult tissue still undergoes turnover and is maintained through the self-renewal and multilineage differentiation of adult stem cells. Examples of this include skin, mucosa, and hematopoietic cells whereby a limited and spatially restricted pool of adult stem cells asymmetrically divides. One daughter cell maintains the stem cell pool by self-renewal, and the other daughter cell starts the process of terminal differentiation for tissue maintenance. The majority of cancers maintain some resemblance to their tissue of origin by virtue of persistent differentiation, albeit in an abnormal way. Thus, many cells in a tumor population may have limited proliferative potential and be incapable of sustained self-renewal, similar to their normal counterparts. The idea that only a limited subset of cells in a cancer is capable of self-renewal is called the *cancer stem cell hypothesis*.

The existence of cancer stem cells was first demonstrated in acute myeloid leukemia and recently shown in breast cancer, glioblastoma, and other cancer types.[31] These studies use cell surface markers to enrich for putative stem cell populations. In the case of breast cancer, CD44[high]/CD24[low] cells were found to form tumors when injected into immunocompromised mice in low numbers and give rise to a diverse population that contained additional CD44[high]/CD24[low] cells. In contrast, the injection of thousands of cells from other populations was nontumorigenic. Thus, the need for cancer cells to acquire self-renewal ability is paramount to the productive growth of the tumor. In principal, however, there is no advantage for cancer to keep this subpopulation of tumor-initiating cells small or fixed. Thus, tumors may contain a large proportion of cells with a tumor-perpetuating stem phenotype,[32] and this phenotype may be subject to back-and-forth reprogramming.

COUPLING TUMORIGENESIS WITH METASTASIS INITIATION

The selective pressures previously described that are encountered during primary tumor growth—hypoxia, inflammation, apoptosis, senescence, and need for proliferative, metabolic, and self-renewal sufficiency—drive primary tumors to acquire tumorigenic alterations that support aggressive growth. These same pressures collaterally support the initial stems of metastasis, and remain important throughout the subsequent malignant steps. One of the most striking types of metastasis initiation functions is EMT.

Selecting for Epithelial-to-Mesenchymal Transition

During development, the generation of many adult tissues and organs results from a series of EMT events and the reverse process, a mesenchymal-to-epithelial transition (MET).[33] For example, gastrulation and delamination of the neural crest are early developmental processes that layout the three germ layers (ectoderm, mesoderm, and endoderm) and give rise to diverse cell lineages (craniofacial cartilage and bone, smooth muscles, neurons, melanocytes), respectively. Both of these developmental events are characterized by epithelial cells loosening their cell-cell adhesion, losing cell polarity, and gaining the ability to invade and migrate under controlled cues. Important regulators include Notch and Wnt/β-catenin pathways, TGF-β family members, and FGF proteins that serve to set up regulatory networks involving EMT transcription factors such as Snail and Twist. These networks do not necessarily regulate cell fate, but rather drive morphogenetic movements by repression of the cell-cell adhesion protein E-cadherin, promoting cytoskeletal rearrangement, and increasing MMP activity. After cells complete EMT-mediated morphogenetic migration, they can then transiently differentiate into epithelial structures by repressing Snail and undergoing a MET. An example of cells that undergo a primary EMT that is followed by a MET includes neural crest cells giving rise to somites. These epithelial somites that have already experienced a primary EMT that is followed by a MET can then initiate a secondary EMT, which eventually results in development of muscle cells.

Growing evidence points toward EMT as an important characteristic of metastasis-prone cancers. EMT in cancer is not a concrete and tidy single process but rather a collection of cell reprogramming phenomena that share the property of down-regulating epithelial cell markers and, for convenience, the collective denomination of EMT. Hypoxia can induce Snail and Twist, a direct target of HIF-1α.[34] Low oxygen enhances β-catenin activity by inhibiting the activity of glycogen synthase kinase-3β, which normally induces the destruction of β-catenin. Accordingly, the presence of enhanced β-catenin signaling promotes Snail expression and subsequent EMT. Interestingly, the ability of hypoxia to liberate active β-catenin may set in place a feed-forward loop to help maintain EMT. Activation of Snail represses E-cadherin, which can then further enhance β-catenin and reinforce Snail expression.

Similar to hypoxia, the inflammatory microenvironment can also promote EMT. It has recently been demonstrated that TNF-α, which is an inflammatory mediator secreted by TAMs, sets into motion a signaling cascade that funnels through NF-κB and glycogen synthase kinase-3β to stabilize Snail and β-catenin, and thus, enhances cancer cell migration.[35] This ability of cancer cells to awaken an EMT program by co-opting an inflammatory microenvironment may be further reinforced by EMT itself. Snail-induced EMT is able to generate an environment of immunosuppressive T-regulatory cells and impaired dendritic cells partly through TGF-β and thrombospondin-1, helping to further perpetuate the inflammatory surroundings.[36]

Besides hypoxia and inflammation, the need for primary cancers to resist apoptosis and overcome senescence may be additional reasons to flip an EMT switch. Cells that have undergone EMT are associated with increased resistance to apoptosis, possibly through prosurvival activity conferred by Snail and Twist.[37,38] EMT can also help cancer overcome oncogene-induced senescence. Both Twist transcription factors and ZEB1 have been shown to suppress p21^{cip1} and/or p16^{ink4a}, two p53-regulated cell cycle proteins that are critical in restraining oncogene-transformed cells via senescence.[39] These findings suggest that the pressure to resist apoptosis and bypass senescence can result in activation of EMT transcriptional regulators.

Acquiring the ability to sustain long-term self-renewal would provide an enormous advantage to cells in a growing tumor mass. Recent data suggest that selection for cells that are capable of undergoing EMT may provide a pool of cells with stemlike features.[40] Stem cell-enriched subpopulations with a CD44^{high}/CD24^{low} cell surface marker profile have significantly higher levels of many EMT-related transcription factors, such as Snail and Twist, when compared with their CD44^{low}/CD24^{high} counterparts. Furthermore, these EMT transcription factors are able to directly increase the number of cells with stemlike characteristics. Although it remains to be determined whether EMT is occurring in cancer stem cells or whether EMT occurs in non–self-renewing cells that then give them stemlike properties, these data argue

for a another compelling reason for cancer cells to acquire EMT properties.

Epithelial-to-Mesenchymal Transition in Metastasis Initiation

Although the ability to awaken an EMT program would seem to offer numerous advantages for cells trying to expand within a primary tumor, it is not clear that primary tumor growth and invasion requires EMT. In fact, EMT-independent mechanisms have been shown to operate and allow carcinomas to invade and migrate at invasive fronts.[41] Despite this, mounting evidence suggests that for cancer cells that do satisfy tumorigenic functions with expression of EMT genes, these cells are also endowed with metastasis initiation functions. Early evidence that EMT genes can be dispensable for primary tumor growth but essential for metastasis has come from analyses of Twist.[42] In a breast cancer model, inhibition of Twist was shown to have no effect on primary tumor growth but potently reduced the number of metastatic lesions in the lung. Consistent with these findings, inhibiting Twist in either hypoxic cells or in cells overexpressing HIF-1α reversed both EMT and metastasis,[34] and inhibiting Snail decreased metastasis induced by inflammatory signals.[35] In total, these observations suggest that when imposing forces like hypoxia and inflammation select for cells capable of EMT, EMT genes become important in metastasis.

What makes EMT cells particularly adept at initiating early metastatic events? A careful analysis of the effect of Twist on metastasis revealed a role for Twist in establishing high levels of circulating tumor cells through enhancing intravasation and/or survival in the circulation.[42] The ability of cells undergoing EMT to intravasate is consistent with observations that EMT occurs at the invasive front of tumors whereby cells lose E-cadherin, detach, invade, and break down the basement membrane. Accordingly, experiments that directly analyzed EMT and non-EMT cells showed that only the EMT cells were able to penetrate surrounding stroma and intravasate.[43]

Another reason that EMT can make cells susceptible to distant spread may be related to the ability of EMT to confer stemlike properties. For the same reasons that primary tumors may rely on cancer stemlike cells for continued self-renewal, metastasis formation may also rely on cancer stemlike cells. Using pancreatic cancer models, it has been shown that a distinct subpopulation of CD133$^+$/CXCR4$^+$ cells localizes to the invasive edge of tumors and is more migratory than CD133$^+$/CXCR4$^-$ cells.[44] Interestingly, although both populations were equally capable of instigating primary tumor growth, only the CD133$^+$/CXCR4$^+$ cells could metastasize to the liver.

Targeting CXCR4 either through depletion or pharmacologic targeting interfered with spontaneous metastasis formation. In breast cancer patients, CD44^{high}/CD24^{low} cells, which are increased by EMT and express EMT markers, display stemlike properties and can be enriched both in the circulation and in the bone marrow.[45] Thus, EMT may play a role in metastasis initiation by ensuring that distant outgrowths are maintained with a pool of stemlike cells.

Prevalence of Primary Tumors with Metastasis-Initiation Functions and Early Dissemination

Considering that EMT can be selected by hypoxia and inflammation, resulting in invasive cancer cells that can intravasate and self-renew, one expectation might be that primary tumors can acquire metastasis-initiation functions early during tumorigenesis because EMT is acquired early. Indeed, recent evidence suggests that initial steps in metastasis can frequently occur far earlier than previously thought. By using transgenic mouse models of breast cancer, it has been shown that disseminated tumor cells (DTCs) can be found in bone marrow and lung tissue even before morphologic evidence of primary tumor invasion.[46,47] Closer inspection with electron microscopy reveals individual tumor cells from preinvasive atypical hyperplastic lesions breaching the basement membrane. Furthermore, preinvasive lesions also displayed high levels of Twist and MMP expression. These early DTCs progressed in parallel with the primary tumor and could give rise to metastatic lesions. Such experimental observations are consistent with clinical findings that patients with preinvasive DCIS also have cytokeratin-positive tumor cells in the bone marrow, as do a significant fraction of patients with early-stage breast cancers. However, despite these findings, patients with DCIS rarely develop metastasis, which highlights that metastasis-initiation functions are not sufficient to complete the metastatic cascade and indicates the need for metastasis-progression and macrometastatic-colonization genes.

COUPLING TUMORIGENESIS WITH METASTASIS PROGRESSION

The selection of genes that primarily fulfill tumorigenic functions may also result in genes that secondarily aid cancer cells after they have found their way into the circulation. In other words, when genes are selected to help the primary tumor grow, some of these genes have a collateral effect of benefiting the cancer after it disseminates by providing metastasis-specific tools. Such genes can be classified as metastasis-progression genes; however, a clear distinction with metastasis-initiation genes may not always be evident. In this section, we describe functions that can be classified as metastasis-progression functions.

Premetastatic Niche

Even before tumor cells colonize distant organs, they can help prepare foreign soil for the subsequent arrival of DTCs by remotely coordinating a "premetastatic niche" from the primary tumor.[48] These niches are often located within distant organs around terminal veins and are characterized by newly recruited hematopoietic progenitor cells of the myeloid lineage and by stromal cells. This niche provides an array of cytokines, growth factors, and adhesion molecules to help support metastatic cells on their arrival.

The remote coordination of the premetastatic niche by the primary tumor appears to be through cytokines and growth factors associated with the inflammatory and hypoxic microenvironment of the primary cancer. Through the secretion of cytokine profiles that include VEGF and placental growth factor, primary tumor cells can direct VEGFR1$^+$ myeloid cells to mobilize from the bone marrow and preferentially localize to areas in target organs with increased fibronectin.[49] If the primary tumor secretes VEGF, this promotes fibronectin deposition in the lung and directs the construction of the premetastatic niche there, while the combination of VEGF and placental growth factor leads to a more widespread pattern of niche assembly. Similarly, VEGF, TGF-β, and TNF-α produced at the primary tumor site can signal production of inflammatory proteins like S100A8 and S100A9 specifically within the lung parenchyma.[50,51] This results in the infiltration of myeloid cells into the lung and subsequent formation of the niche. Besides inflammatory signals from the primary tumor, LOX produced by a hypoxic primary tumor environment can also direct formation of a premetastatic niche.[52]

Once myeloid and activated stromal cells form the premetastatic niche, the local environment in the distant organ is altered by the production of inflammatory cytokines and MMPs, which begins bearing an evolving resemblance to the primary site. Consequently, when primary tumor cells start wandering in the circulation, the target organs with an established premetastatic niche become a better soil in which to attach, survive, and grow. Indeed, if the formation of the niche is disrupted, metastasis is inhibited. In this way, the shower of cytokines and growth factors that accompany inflammatory and hypoxic responses at the primary tumor not only selects for cancer cells that can flourish in the primary site but has the secondary effect of creating a more welcoming environment in distant organs after dissemination. Such a scenario would argue that the mechanism of premetastatic niche formation has properties consistent with metastasis-progression functions.

Survival in the Circulation

From experimental model systems, it has been estimated that approximately one million cancer cells per gram of tumor tissue can be introduced daily into the circulation.[53] Direct inoculation of tumor cells into mice demonstrates that metastasis can be an inefficient process because despite large numbers of circulating tumor cells (CTCs), relatively few metastases form.[8] In humans, the inefficiency of CTCs to give rise to detectable metastases was inadvertently demonstrated in ovarian cancer patients who received peritoneal-venous shunts for palliation of malignant ascites.[54] Despite the re-routing of millions of cancer cells from the peritoneum to the venous circulation, for years in some cases, the majority of the patients did not develop widespread metastases. Thus, even if cancer cells acquire metastasis-initiation functions like EMT, the ability to merely enter into the circulation often is not a rate-limiting step in metastasis. Other obstacles must be overcome.

After intravasation into the circulation from the primary tumor, tumor cells encounter significant physical stress due to shear forces or mechanical arrest in small-diameter vessels. The hepatic sinusoids can be activated by the mechanical restriction of tumor cells to secrete nitric oxide. Nitric oxide can cause apoptosis of arrested tumor cells and has been shown to be required for the massive cell death of experimentally injected melanoma cells.[55] Endothelial cells can also guard against wandering tumor cells through expression of DARC, a Duffy blood group glycoprotein.[56] DARC interacts with *KAI1* expressed on circulating tumor cells causing them to undergo senescence. *KAI1* was originally identified as a metastasis suppressor gene. The immune system can also actively attack circulating tumor cells.[57] For example, NK cells can engage and kill cancer cells via TNF-related molecules such as TRAIL or CD95L. In total, these mechanical and cell-mediated stresses can result in a short half-life for CTCs. Estimations derived from the enumeration of CTCs before and after removal of the primary tumor in patients with localized breast cancer demonstrate that the half-life can be as short as a few hours.[58]

How can CTCs evade cell death to enhance their metastatic potential? Growth at the primary tumor site will involve a selection for increased resistance to apoptosis. Antiapoptosis genes such as *BCL2* or *BCL-X_L*, or the loss of proapoptotic genes and genes downstream of the TNF-related receptor family, can result in increased metastasis.[59,60] Part of this may be the result of

survival both in the circulation and shortly after extravasation. Both CTCs and platelets can also express the $\alpha v\beta 3$ integrin to promote aggregation of these cells to form tumor emoboli.[61] This aggregation not only facilitates arrest but can protect against shear forces and NK cell-mediated killing. Activation of $\alpha v\beta 3$ can result from CXCL12/CXCR4 signaling and has been shown to be required for formation of tumor emboli and metastasis.[62,63] Thus, the ability of a primary tumor to respond to apoptosis, senescence, and inflammatory signals can secondarily make cancer cells better able to survive in the circulation once metastasis has been initiated.

Extravasation and Colonization

After arresting in capillaries, tumor cells that are able to survive can grow intravascularly. This can lead to a physical disruption of the vessels.[64] However, more selective processes of extravasation exist. Cancer cells can mimic leukocytes and bind to endothelial E- and P-selectins.[65] Molecular mediators of extravasation include the cytoskeletal anchoring protein Ezrin, which links the cell membrane to the actin cytoskeleton and engages the cell with its microenvironment. Ezrin was discovered to promote metastasis in osteosarcoma by preventing cell death during migration into the lung.[66] VEGF expression by the tumor can also lead to disruptions in endothelial cell junctions and facilitate extravasation of cancer cells through enhanced vascular permeability. This is likely mediated by the activation of SRC family kinases in the endothelial cells, which is consistent with decreased lung metastasis in SRC nullizygous mice.[67] Expression of hypoxia-induced CXCR4 on CTCs allows for the selective extravasation into certain organs. This selectivity is due to the expression of its ligand CXCL12 by certain organs that include the lung, liver, bone, and lymph nodes.[68] Thus, the selection to successfully deal with hypoxia during primary tumor growth may bias the pattern of distant spread through the CXCR4-CXCL12 pathway.

The steps of extravasation and establishment of micrometastases help to illustrate a more concrete example of the concept of metastasis-progression genes. Using a mouse model system for breast cancer metastasis, a gene expression signature for aggressive lung metastasis was discovered that not only mediated experimental lung metastasis but was also expressed by primary human breast cancers with increased risk of metastasis selectively to the lung.[17] Four members of this lung metastasis gene expression signature (LMS), namely *EREG* (an EGF receptor ligand), *MMP1*, *MMP2*, and *COX2*, were selected during primary tumor growth and conferred a growth advantage by facilitating the assembly of new blood vessels.[16] The vascular remodeling program coordinated by these four genes was also critical to the extravasation of circulating breast cancer cells into the lung parenchyma, as its inhibition resulted in the intravascular entrapment of single cells. Another LMS gene that is a mediator of lung extravasation is the cytokine angiopoietin-like 4 (*ANGPTL4*).[69] *ANGPTL4* promotes the dissociation of endothelial cell-cell junctions and, consistent with it being a metastasis-progression gene, *ANGPTL4* is induced by TFG-β produced in the primary tumor microenvironment. The combined examples of VEGF, CXCR4, and several LMS genes illustrate how metastasis-progression genes can arise during primary tumor growth through the acquisition of genes that can cope with or respond to selective pressures at the primary site.

Cancer cells that have initiated the metastatic cascade can also epigenetically acquire metastasis-progression functions through paracrine factors secreted by the microenvironment of primary tumors. Mesenchymal stem cells recruited to the inflammatory stroma of a primary tumor have been shown in a xenograft model to produce CCL5 as a result of heterotypic interaction with neighboring breast cancer.[70] CCL5 can then act in a paracrine fashion to enhance motility, invasion, and extravasation into the lung. Accordingly, the prometastatic effects mediated by CCL5 were reversible when interactions with MSCs were removed. Thus, metastasis-progression functions acquired through events that occur in the primary tumor need not be accompanied by somatic changes in metastasis-progression genes.

Tumor Self-Seeding

As cancer cells selected by the inflammatory and hypoxic surroundings of the primary tumor wander through the circulation, might the most hospitable and likely destination for extravasation be the primary tumor from which they came? At least in theory, it would seem that compared with uncharted foreign environments or even premetastatic niches, the primary tumor would impose the least resistance to colonization.[71] Support for this concept of tumor self-seeding has recently been provided using mouse model systems and a variety of different cancer types by demonstrating that CTCs can seed the primary tumor and contribute to its mass.[72] The ability to self-seed is promoted by IL-6 and IL-8, common prometastatic cytokines found in the tumor microenvironment. The cancer cell expression of *MMP1* and Fascin-1, two previously identified lung metastasis genes, facilitates transendothelial migration and tumor self-seeding. In fact, metastatic cells in general are more efficient seeders, which may result from a direct cause and effect. Subpopulations of cancer cells selected to be efficient seeders can express an array of multiorgan metastasis genes. These observations suggest that disseminated cells capable of

successfully navigating a round-trip rather than a one-way excursion help the primary tumor select for cells with metastatic functions.

FROM METASTASIS PROGRESSION TO MACROMETASTATIC COLONIZATION

Because metastasis-initiation functions and metastasis-progression functions are coupled to tumorigenic functions, the accumulating evidence that primary tumors can exhibit metastatic traits early on during primary tumorigenesis and with such high prevalence may not be surprising. However, despite the ability of EMT to drive invasion, intravasation, and self-renewal, and despite the remote influence the primary tumor has on survival in the circulation, extravasation, and premetastatic niche formation, the completion of the metastatic cascade is still relatively infrequent for many cancer types. This suggests an important requirement for macrometastatic colonization functions, or functions selected at distant sites for organ-specific colonization.

Dormancy

A major limiting step in metastasis is acquiring the ability to sustain growth within a distant site after extravasation. Many cancers such as breast and prostate will not give rise to metastasis until years or even decades after eradication of the primary tumor. Clinically, there is also a clear discrepancy between the proportion of patients with preinvasive or early-stage cancers that have cytokeratin-positive cells in the bone marrow and the proportion that develop overt metastasis. Experimentally, it has been shown that the vast majority of extravasated cancer cells do not form macrometastasis.[8] In aggregate, these observations of latency are referred to as *metastatic dormancy* and point toward the bottleneck that forms prior to outgrowth of macrometastasis.

A distinction has been made between tumor mass dormancy, which describes the process that inhibits expansion of a dividing tumor population, and cellular dormancy, which describes when cancer cells enter a state of growth arrest.[73] Tumor mass dormancy has been attributed to the existence of preangiogenic micrometastasis in which cell division is balanced by apoptosis.[74] Clinical evidence for this comes from one study whereby breast cancer patients with no evidence of disease years after mastectomy and considered candidates for having metastatic dormancy were shown to have detectable CTCs.[58] Later acquisition of angiogenic properties may allow such micrometastases to become vascularized and emerge from their occult state. Work with experimental models suggests that indolent metastasis may also be activated by coexisting with more aggressive metastasis secrete systemic factors like osteopontin (OPN).[75] Mechanisms that contribute to cellular dormancy may relate to the balance between the RAF-MEK-ERK pathway and the p38 MAPK pathway. Inhibition of the former and activation of the latter is associated with cellular quiescence in a G0-G1 state, and the exact balance between the two may depend on cross-talk between the tumor and the new microenvironment. Genes that may be important in blocking productive cross-talk between dormant metastasis and its microenvironment include metastasis suppressor genes such as *NME23, MKK4,* and *RKIP,* to name a few.[73,76] This functional class of genes specifically prevents growth of metastasis without influencing primary tumor growth.

Regardless of the nature of the dormancy, dormant cells must acquire genetic or epigenetic changes during residency at foreign sites in order to evolve into gross metastases. Tumor cells that are detected in the bone marrow and likely disseminated from the primary tumor at an early stage during tumorigenesis have been shown to undergo a separate evolution under separate selective pressures. Comparative genomic hybridizations of single breast cancer cells isolated from bone marrow were shown to be genetically heterogeneous in patients without overt metastasis.[77,78] These cells also showed few genetic features in common with matched primary tumors. In contrast, bone marrow-derived breast cancer cells from patients with overt metastatic disease displayed a marked reduction in genetic heterogeneity compared with patients with occult disease. These results are consistent with disseminated tumor cells departing from the primary tumor early on and being driven by different selective pressures found in the distant organ. Different metastatic sites that host dormant cells likely contribute unique selective pressures. This paves the way for the acquisition of macrometastatic colonization functions.

Organ Selective Growth

Bone

Homeostasis of the bone is maintained by a constant state of remodeling such that no net gain or loss of bone occurs. The mineralized bone matrix is reabsorbed by osteoclasts and filled in by osteoblasts. The differentiation of osteoclasts from bone marrow mononuclear cells is controlled by CSF-1 and the RANK receptor (reviewed in refs. 79 and 80). RANK interacts with its ligand RANKL produced by osteoblasts, leading to a tight coupling of these two cells with opposing actions. The activity of RANKL can also be controlled by osteoprotegerin (OPG). OPG is a secreted antagonist of RANKL and prevents interaction with RANK and resulting osteoclastogenesis. The differentiation of osteoblasts results from bone marrow mesenchymal stem cells under the control of a variety of regulators including insulin-like growth factor (IGF), endothelin-1, bone morphogenetic proteins, and WNT proteins.

The bone is one of the most common sites of distant spread. However, the latency period that precedes the development of gross osseous metastasis can be years, as illustrated by the high proportion of breast cancer patients with dormant cancer cells in the bone marrow. One factor that provides the ability to sustain this latency period is the SRC kinase, which is required for CXCL12- and IGF-mediated survival signals that protect indolent breast cancer cells in the bone marrow from TRAIL-mediated apoptosis.[81] Presumably, the sustained survival and dormancy afforded by SRC would allow time for the acquisition of bone-specific macrometastatic colonization genes.

When the dormancy period expires, gross osseous metastases are characterized by two basic types: osteoblastic and osteolytic. Many tumors such as lung, kidney, and breast carcinomas typically produce osteolytic lesions. Breast cancer cells achieve osteolytic metastasis competency by secreting factors including parathyroid hormone-related protein (PTHrP), TNF-α, IL-1, IL-6, IL-8, and IL-11 in order to orchestrate a vicious cycle of enhanced osteoclast activation, degradation of bone matrix, and the release of matrix-associated cytokines that stimulate the cancer cells[79,80] (Fig. 10.3). The secretion of PTHrP leads to the production of the membrane-bound RANKL on osteoblasts, resulting in RANK-mediated osteoclast activation. Other proinflammatory cytokines such as TNF-α, IL-1, IL-6, and IL-11 that are secreted by the tumor cell can lead to a synergistic effect on RANK-mediated signaling and may also inhibit production of OPG. Interestingly, RANK is also expressed on cancer cells and stimulates migratory activity.[82] On degradation of the bone matrix, embedded growth factors are released, including TGF-β and IGF. These liberated growth factors can further stimulate the tumor cells and enhance the entire vicious cycle.

A genomewide screen for genes involved in breast cancer bone metastasis uncovered IL-11, MMP1, ADAMTS1, CXCR4, connective tissue growth factor (CTGF), and OPN as mediators of osteolytic bone metastasis.[83] CXCR4 may enhance colonization of breast cancer cells to bone, MMP1 and ADAMTS1 proteolytically activate EGF receptor ligands,[84] and OPN and IL-11 may promote osteoclast differentiation. The expression of IL-11, CTGF, and PTHrP in breast cancer cells are targets for TGF-β, which is released by the bone matrix.[85] In total, these experimental data illustrate how tumor cells can survive and grow in the foreign environment of the bone by coercing resident cells to release secreted factors that are

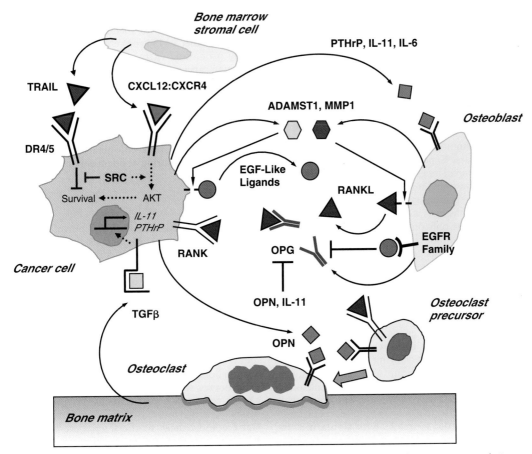

FIGURE 10.3 Interactions between cancer and the bone microenvironment lead to a "vicious cycle." Cancer cells can migrate to the bone microenvironment under the influence of CXCL12 (*blue triangle*), which also leads to cell activation and migration via its receptor CXCR4. The CXCL12:CXCR4 interaction promotes survival of metastatic cancer cells through AKT and SRC by counteracting proapoptotic stimuli directed by TRAIL (*red triangles*) and its receptor DR4/5. Survival can lead to dormancy, utilization of acquired metastasis-progression functions, and opportunities to accumulate additional macrometastatic-colonization genes. Surviving metastatic cells secretes factors such as PTHrP, IL-11, and IL-6 (*green squares*) that lead to production of membrane-bound RANKL (*brown triangles*) on osteoblasts. Tumor cell secretion of MMP1 (*red hexagon*) and ADAMST1 (*yellow hexagon*) can mobilize RANKL from osteoblasts and EGF-like ligands (*magenta circles*) from tumor cells. RANKL:RANK interaction stimulates tumor cells and promotes osteoclast differentiation and activation. RANKL can be antagonized by the decoy receptor osteoprotegerin, or OPG (*red-colored receptor*), that is normally produced by osteoblasts. Engagement of EGF receptor family members can inhibit OPG expression and thereby promote osteoclast activation and metastatic growth. Other tumor-derived factors like osteopontin, or OPN (*orange squares*), also promote osteoclast activation. Activation of osteoclasts leads to degradation of the bone matrix and release of TGF-β (*yellow square*). This further stimulates the tumor cells to transcriptionally activate genes such as *IL-11* and *PTHrP*, which contributes to the vicious cycle.

advantageous to the tumor. This cooperative situation between tumor cells and bone marrow cells is similar to that in the primary tumor whereby BMDCs and stromal cells act as accomplices.

Unlike osteolytic bone metastasis, osteoblastic metastasis is less common and typified by prostate cancer. Osteoblastic lesions result from the preferential stimulation of osteoblasts and/or the inhibition of osteoclasts. Like breast and other cancers that cause osteolytic lesions, prostate cancer also hijacks homeostatic regulation of bone remodeling to its advantage (reviewed in ref. 86). Various paracrine factors secreted by prostate cancer cells can regulate osteoblast proliferation or differentiation, including bone morphogenetic proteins, WNT, TGF-β, IGF, PDGF, FGF, and VEGF. Many of these signals converge on activation of RUNX2, a transcription factor that is essential for bone formation. In turn, the osteoblasts produce factors that stimulate the proliferation of prostate cancer as demonstrated by coculture experiments with either osteoblasts or their conditioned media. The exact factors that drive progression of prostate cancer metastasis have not been firmly established. Nonetheless, these results support the paradigm that a reciprocal relationship exists between the cancer cell and the cells of the microenvironment that contribute to bone-selective metastasis.

Lung

Lung is a common site of metastasis for many different cancers. Experimentally, colonization and growth in animal lungs has been used extensively to study metastasis and invasion by the direct inoculation of tumor cells into the venous circulation. With this method, the lung is the first organ encountered and may be the only organ encountered because of entrapment of tumor cells by the lung capillary bed. Although the list of genes that can contribute to enhanced experimental lung metastasis studied in this way is extensive, it can be difficult to know whether the genes are regulating a generic invasion pathway or contributing to organ-specific growth.

In a study seeking to gain insight into organ-selective metastasis genes, single cell-derived clones from a human breast cancer cell line were discovered to exhibit varying degrees of metastatic ability to the bone and to the lung.[87] Although there was no correlation between clones that metastasized well to the lung and those that metastasized effectively to the bone, metastatic tissue tropism did correlate with similarities in global gene expression patterns among the clones. These observations lead to the discovery of an LMS.[17] Several of these genes (some have already been discussed) were shown to cooperatively mediate experimental lung metastasis and consisted of secreted factors (*EREG, CXCL1, ANGPTL4,* and *SPARC*), cell surface receptors (*VCAM1* and *IL13Rα2*), extracellular matrix protein (*TNC*) and proteases (*MMP1* and *MMP2*), and intracellular effectors (*ID1, Fascin-1,* and *COX2*). Although these genes mediated lung metastasis, they did not enhance bone metastasis and were largely distinct from a previously defined bone metastasis gene expression signature from the same cell line.

Many of the LMS genes are also expressed in a subset of primary human breast cancers. These patients with LMS-expressing tumors are at a higher risk for lung metastasis but not metastasis to bone or various other visceral sites.[17,88] In addition, LMS-expressing tumors are larger at the time of diagnosis compared with LMS-negative tumors, which is consistent with experimental data showing that LMS genes were selected for during growth in the mouse mammary gland. Mechanistically, the coupling of tumorigenic function and metastatic function is provided by the LMS genes *EREG, COX2, MMP1,* and *MMP2*. As described already, these genes are prototypical metastasis-progression genes in that they assist the primary tumor by promoting the assembly of new blood vessels.[16] However, as part of the metastatic cascade, these genes and other LMS genes enhance lung metastasis by promoting extravasation and by priming departing cancer cells for the lung parenchyma.[69,89] Some of the LMS genes such as *IL13Rα2* and *SPARC* do not enhance primary tumor growth and are not among the LMS genes expressed by primary tumors that track with lung metastasis; however, these genes do promote lung metastasis, making them macrometastatic-colonization genes that may be selected during residence away from the primary site.

Liver

The liver is supplied by both the portal and the systemic circulations. Metastasis to the liver is commonly seen with colorectal cancer and this bias is likely favored by the portal circulation for this organ. Metastasis from other cancers such as melanoma and breast and lung carcinomas generally occurs via the systemic circulation. Besides the bias for liver metastasis from the portal circulation, there is evidence that the microenvironment of the liver may be particularly favorable for metastasis from gastrointestinal tumors. Extracellular matrix extracted from primary rat hepatocytes was found to stimulate colorectal cancer cell lines better than ECM from fibroblasts.[90] Furthermore, CAFs isolated from metastatic colon cancer to the liver were found to secrete factors that enhance proliferation of colon cancer to a greater extent than the conditioned media from fibroblasts isolated from uninvolved liver or skin.[91] DNA microarray analysis demonstrated that the CAFs were more genetically similar than uninvolved fibroblasts and preferentially expressed genes associated in ECM remodeling (proteoglycan 1), proteases/protease inhibitors (tissue plasminogen activator, tissue plasminogen activator inhibitor type 1), growth factors (PDGF, FGF, CTGF, VEGF, TGF-β2), cytokines (IL-6, MCP-1), and intracellular mediators like COX2. This alteration in the microenvironment as a potential contributor to liver metastasis was also demonstrated for hepatocellular carcinoma, which tends to recur with intrahepatic metastasis. By comparing noninvolved hepatic tissue from patients with and without metastasis, genes associated with inflammation and/or immune responses were found to be associated with a "metastasis-inclined microenvironment." A major difference was noted in the cytokine profile of the metastasis-inclined tissue, which was strongly biases to a T_H2 rather than a T_H1 cytokine profile.[92] The latter is associated with cytotoxic T-cell activity and the former is associated with a humoral immune response. These different cytokine milieus may be driven in part by high levels of CSF-1.

Besides local microenvironmental influences on liver metastasis, contributing signaling molecules

expressed by cancer cells have also been implicated. In a screen for genes associated with colon cancer metastasis to the liver, the *PRL-3* tyrosine phosphatase was identified.[93] Experimentally, *PRL-3* can trigger angiogenesis and enhance invasion. Clinically, its expression is found in primary colorectal tumors and correlates with metastasis. It is unclear whether *PRL-3* selectively mediates metastasis to the liver, as its expression is also found in other distant organs to which colorectal cancer relapses.[94]

Brain

The principal sources of brain metastasis are lung and breast carcinomas. Melanoma, colorectal, and renal cell carcinomas also can relapse in the brain, whereas some cancer types like prostate cancer rarely do. The microenvironment of the brain is unique in the sense that vascular access is more restricted because of the blood–brain barrier. This barrier is composed of tightly adjoined endothelial cells that are lined by basal lamina and astrocyte foot processes. The blood–brain barrier is a special consideration for pharmacologic intervention, but to what extent it uniquely deters circulating tumor cells from colonizing the brain is unclear. Once in the parenchyma, microenvironmental interactions occur with glial cells. Coculture experiments demonstrate enhanced adhesion and growth when astrocytes are partnered with cell lines from brain metastasis compared with lung metastasis.[95] This may involve IL-6, TGF-β, and IGF-1. Melanoma cells that metastasize to the brain have high STAT3 transcriptional activity compared with cutaneous metastases or primary melanoma specimens.[96] Manipulation of STAT3 activity was able to alter brain metastasis in animal models. Altered STAT3 affects expression of basic FGF, VEGF, and MMP2, and influences melanoma angiogenesis and invasion. Because of the dearth of cross-comparison studies with other organs, the selectivity of these effects for brain metastasis is unclear. Indeed, STAT3 has also been associated with metastasis to other visceral organs.[97]

In order to identify specific mediators of brain metastasis, a mouse model for breast cancer was used that incorporated both established cell lines and patient-derived samples.[98] Several genes were found to mediate metastasis to the brain, including *COX2*, the EGFR ligand *HBEGF*, and the α2,6-sialyltransferase, *ST6GALNAC5*. Notably, some of the newly identified brain metastasis genes overlapped with previously identified lung metastasis genes, a finding that is consistent with the known propensity for patients to develop synchronous or metachronous metastases to both organs. Accordingly, passage through the nonfenestrated capillaries of the brain and lungs could be promoted by *COX2* and *HBEGF*. In contrast, the specificity of the gene signature for the brain could be attributed to *ST6GALNAC5* and other associated genes that normally have a brain-restricted expression pattern. *ST6GALNAC5* enhances the ability of breast cancer cells to pass through the blood–brain barrier, although the exact mechanism remains unknown. Patients who express the genes in the brain metastasis signature also have a higher risk of succumbing to brain metastasis.

Lymphatics

The physiological function of the lymphatic system is to collect extravasated fluid, proteins, and immune cells from draining organs in order to return them for transport by the circulation. Lymphatics are low shear force vessels composed of a single layer of endothelial cells with little or no basement membrane and sparsely coated with pericytes. Lymphangiogenesis involves VEGF-C, VEGF-D, and their receptor VEGFR-3 (reviewed in ref. 99). In contrast to angiogenesis mediators like VEGF-A that responds to both inflammation and hypoxia, VEGF-C/D expression is induced by inflammation but not hypoxia. For example, macrophages that respond to inflammatory signals are a rich source of VEGF-C/D. Thus, angiogenesis can occur without lymphangiogenesis but under most circumstances lymphatic vessels grow concomitantly with blood vessels. Other non-VEGF family members can also induce lymphangiogenesis and include FGF2, PDGF, and angiopoietin proteins.

Unlike with angiogenesis, the functional advantage for tumors that induce lymphangiogenesis is a matter of debate. Possibilities include lowering interstitial fluid pressure in the tumor to facilitate blood perfusion and combat hypoxia, or the growth of new lymphatics may facilitate mechanisms that contribute to angiogenesis.[100] Alternatively, lymphangiogenesis may coincidentally result from induction of angiogenesis and/or the involvement of immune cells. Part of this uncertainty results from questions regarding the degree to which intratumoral lymphatics are functional. Lymphatics can be found in a peritumoral location or reside intratumorally. Although proliferating intratumoral lymphatic vessels are observed in animal models and cancers of the head and neck and melanoma, they may collapse under high intratumoral pressure. At least one study revealed that these intratumoral lymphatics were not important in conducting metastasis, rather peritumoral lymphatics were the main route.[101] Nonetheless, mouse models have revealed that inducing lymphangiogenesis does lead to lymph node metastasis.[102,103] Once in the lymph nodes, lymphatic stromal cells are a source for EGF, IGF-1, and various chemokines.[104] Like the lung parenchyma and the bone marrow, lymph nodes secrete CXCL12, which can interact with tumor-expressing CXCR4.[68] Other chemokine receptors such as CXCR3 also play a role in lymph node metastasis.[105]

Metastasis to the regional lymph nodes is considered one of the early signs of metastatic potential and/or distant spread. A long-standing question has been whether lymphatic metastasis selects cells that have enhanced metastatic ability but has not yet spread to distant organs or whether lymph node involvement is a marker for a tumor that may have already become metastatic in general. Reasons for the former include the idea that some tumors can only intravasate into lymphatics but not directly into blood vessels because they cannot overcome higher molecular or physical barriers. Explanations for the latter include underlying molecular mechanisms that couple angiogenesis, lymphangiogenesis, and metastatic ability, resulting in synchronous dispersal. To distinguish between these possibilities, lymphangiogenesis was inhibited in a mouse model for lung cancer metastasis using a soluble VEGFR-3-immunoglobulin fusion protein that traps VEGF-C/D and inhibits VEGFR-3 signaling. This approach blocked lymph node metastasis but had no effect on lung metastasis.[106] However, in another study, blocking VEGFR-3 signaling with mammary tumors suppressed metastases to both lymph nodes and the lungs.[107] Most likely, lymphatic-dependent and -independent metastasis are both possible and dictated by underlying biological mediators and selective pressures. This would also most fit clinical data. Markers for lymphatic-dependent and -independent spread would be useful to guide whether regional lymph nodes should be addressed therapeutically or less aggressively for prognostic staging.

Early, Multiorgan Metastasis

Most cancers such as breast, prostate, and sarcoma, to name a few, demonstrate appreciable latency periods. Depending on the onset of dissemination and colonization within distant organs, this provides varying and often lengthy periods for acquiring macrometastatic-colonization genes. In contrast, some cancers, like adenocarcinomas of the lung and pancreas, have short latency periods and exhibit early systemic metastasis often to multiple organs. One explanation for short versus long periods of latency is related to origin of the cell population initially targeted for transforming and tumorigenic events. The cancer stem cell hypothesis and the role of EMT in metastasis already suggest that early progenitor cells or cells that may have played a role in developmental processes can be predisposed to activate metastasis-progression mechanisms. An example of this has been demonstrated by introducing defined oncogenic alterations into different cell types.[108] When mammary epithelial cells or fibroblasts were transformed, these cells were tumorigenic but not metastatic. In contrast, oncogenic transformation of melanocytes resulted in aggressive metastasis. This difference was because of the expression of the EMT transcription factor Slug in the melanocytes but not the

other tumor types. Thus, the transformation of certain unique cell types may predispose to early metastatic behavior and could explain certain phenomenon such as cancers of unknown primary.

Identification of genes that promote early metastasis in adenocarcinoma of the lung also supports the view that some carcinomas may not have an extensive requirement for macrometastatic-colonization functions. By using mouse models to dissect the molecular basis for lung metastasis, the existence of a WNT/TCF pathway was found capable of mediating rapid multiorgan metastasis through LEF1 and HOXB9.[109] A clinical predictor based on this pathway was associated with metastatic risk for patients with lung, but not breast, adenocarcinomas. This pathway is well characterized in stem cell and developmental biology, including EMT. Recent findings revealing that important drivers of aggressive metastasis can include developmental-related genes capable of causing genomewide changes[110,111] will likely help to uncover additional scenarios whereby macrometastatic-colonization functions play limited roles.

MICRO-RNAs AND METASTASIS

It was once thought that the effects of genes necessarily resulted from the proteins that they encode. However, as a result of developmental studies on the worm *Caenorhabditis elegans* that identified important roles for noncoding RNAs (ncRNAs), it is now appreciated that ncRNAs potentially influence cellular and organismal phenotypes on par with traditional protein-coding genes. In fact, microRNAs, which are approximately 22 nucleotide-long small ncRNAs, have been discovered to have important effects on metastasis.[112] MicroRNAs function by regulating the expression of hundreds of target genes through sequence-specific binding between the microRNA and the 3' untranslated regions of mRNAs. This engagement results in either the degradation of the target mRNA or the inhibition of protein translation. Through this action, microRNAs can influence a large number of genes. In fact, it is predicted that microRNAs preferentially interact with genes that are central to highly connected networks.[113]

MicroRNAs can function both as metastasis activators and metastasis suppressors by influencing numerous genes involved in metastasis initiation, progression, and colonization. Several microRNAs, such as miR-10b, miR-9, and members of the miR-200 family, play critical roles in EMT or EMT-related events. For example, miR-10b influences cell migration, invasion, and metastasis by repressing HOXD10, a known inhibitor of a RHOC-mediated promotility program.[114] The expression of miR-10b is under the control of the

EMT transcription factor Twist. In fact, miR-10b is essential for Twist-induced EMT and for metastasis, making miR-10b a metastasis activator. MiR-9 promotes metastasis by targeting E-cadherin, which results in β-catenin signaling and VEGF expression.[115] Accordingly, motility, invasion, angiogenesis, and metastasis ensue. MiR-200 family members also regulate EMT by inhibiting ZEB1 and ZEB2, which normally promote EMT through the suppression of E-cadherin.[116–118] Thus, in contrast to miR-10b, miR-200 family members act as metastasis suppressors. Other microRNAs such as miR-335, miR-126, miR-31, and let-7 also suppress distant spread. MiR-335 inhibits metastasis and invasion by targeting the

LMS genes *SOX4* and *TNC*, while miR-125 suppresses overall tumor growth and proliferation.[119] MiR-31 represses multiple steps in the metastatic cascade, an effect that is related to its influence on multiple metastasis genes.[120] Let-7, which is one of the most extensively studied microRNAs, interferes with both self-renewal and distant colonization, and its expression can be controlled by metastasis suppressor genes.[76,121] Numerous other microRNAs that play a role in metastasis are being rapidly identified. Interestingly, even non-microRNA ncRNAs are being identified to influence aggressive distant spread.[110] The potential for microRNAs to serve as clinical markers and/or therapeutic targets is already starting to show promise.

Selected References

The full list of references for this chapter appears in the online version.

7. Fidler IJ. The pathogenesis of cancer metastasis: the 'seed and soil' hypothesis revisited. *Nat Rev Cancer* 2003; 3:453.
8. Chambers AF, Groom AC, MacDonald IC. Dissemination and growth of cancer cells in metastatic sites. *Nat Rev Cancer* 2002;2:563.
9. Hellman S. Karnofsky memorial lecture: natural history of small breast cancers. *J Clin Oncol* 1994;12:2229.
13. Bernards R, Weinberg RA. A progression puzzle. *Nature* 2002;418:823.
14. Nguyen DX, Bos PD, Massague J. Metastasis: from dissemination to organ-specific colonization. *Nat Rev Cancer* 2009;9:274.
16. Gupta GP, Nguyen DX, Chiang AC, et al. Mediators of vascular remodelling co-opted for sequential steps in lung metastasis. *Nature* 2007;446:765.
17. Minn AJ, Gupta GP, Siegel PM, et al. Genes that mediate breast cancer metastasis to lung. *Nature* 2005;436:518.
25. Qian BZ, Pollard JW. Macrophage diversity enhances tumor progression and metastasis. *Cell* 2010;141:39.
26. Joyce JA, Pollard JW. Microenvironmental regulation of metastasis. *Nat Rev Cancer* 2009;9:239.
27. Yang L, Huang J, Ren X, et al. Abrogation of TGF beta signaling in mammary carcinomas recruits Gr-1+CD11b+ myeloid cells that promote metastasis. *Cancer Cell* 2008;13:23.
33. Thiery JP, Acloque H, Huang RY, Nieto MA. Epithelial-mesenchymal transitions in development and disease. *Cell* 2009;139:871.
34. Yang MH, Wu MZ, Chiou SH, et al. Direct regulation of TWIST by HIF-1alpha promotes metastasis. *Nat Cell Biol* 2008;10:295.
35. Wu Y, Deng J, Rychahou PG, Qiu S, Evers BM, Zhou BP. Stabilization of snail by NF-kappaB is required for inflammation-induced cell migration and invasion. *Cancer Cell* 2009;15:416.
36. Kudo-Saito C, Shirako H, Takeuchi T, Kawakami Y. Cancer metastasis is accelerated through immunosuppression during Snail-induced EMT of cancer cells. *Cancer Cell* 2009;15:195.
40. Mani SA, Guo W, Liao MJ, et al. The epithelial-mesenchymal transition generates cells with properties of stem cells. *Cell* 2008;133:704.
42. Yang J, Mani SA, Donaher JL, et al. Twist, a master regulator of morphogenesis, plays an essential role in tumor metastasis. *Cell* 2004;117:927.
44. Hermann PC, Huber SL, Herrler T, et al. Distinct populations of cancer stem cells determine tumor growth and

metastatic activity in human pancreatic cancer. *Cell Stem Cell* 2007;1:313.
45. Pantel K, Brakenhoff RH, Brandt B. Detection, clinical relevance and specific biological properties of disseminating tumour cells. *Nat Rev Cancer* 2008;8:329.
46. Husemann Y, Geigl JB, Schubert F, et al. Systemic spread is an early step in breast cancer. *Cancer Cell* 2008; 13:58.
47. Podsypanina K, Du YC, Jechlinger M, Beverly LJ, Hambardzumyan D, Varmus H. Seeding and propagation of untransformed mouse mammary cells in the lung. *Science* 2008;321:1841.
48. Psaila B, Lyden D. The metastatic niche: adapting the foreign soil. *Nat Rev Cancer* 2009;9:285.
49. Kaplan RN, Riba RD, Zacharoulis S, et al. VEGFR1-positive haematopoietic bone marrow progenitors initiate the pre-metastatic niche. *Nature* 2005;438:820.
51. Hiratsuka S, Watanabe A, Sakurai Y, et al. The S100A8-serum amyloid A3-TLR4 paracrine cascade establishes a pre-metastatic phase. *Nat Cell Biol* 2008;10:1349.
52. Erler JT, Bennewith KL, Cox TR, et al. Hypoxia-induced lysyl oxidase is a critical mediator of bone marrow cell recruitment to form the premetastatic niche. *Cancer Cell* 2009;15:35.
56. Bandyopadhyay S, Zhan R, Chaudhuri A, et al. Interaction of KAI1 on tumor cells with DARC on vascular endothelium leads to metastasis suppression. *Nat Med* 2006; 12:933.
63. Felding-Habermann B, O'Toole TE, Smith JW, et al. Integrin activation controls metastasis in human breast cancer. *Proc Natl Acad Sci U S A* 2001;98:1853.
68. Muller A, Homey B, Soto H, et al. Involvement of chemokine receptors in breast cancer metastasis. *Nature* 2001;410:50.
70. Karnoub AE, Dash AB, Vo AP, et al. Mesenchymal stem cells within tumour stroma promote breast cancer metastasis. *Nature* 2007;449:557.
71. Norton L, Massague J. Is cancer a disease of self-seeding? *Nat Med* 2006;12:875.
72. Kim MY, Oskarsson T, Acharyya S, et al. Tumor self-seeding by circulating cancer cells. *Cell* 2009;139:1315.
73. Aguirre-Ghiso JA. Models, mechanisms and clinical evidence for cancer dormancy. *Nat Rev Cancer* 2007;7: 834.
75. McAllister SS, Gifford AM, Greiner AL, et al. Systemic endocrine instigation of indolent tumor growth requires osteopontin. *Cell* 2008;133:994.
78. Schmidt-Kittler O, Ragg T, Daskalakis A, et al. From latent disseminated cells to overt metastasis: genetic analysis of systemic breast cancer progression. *Proc Natl Acad Sci U S A* 2003;100:7737.

GENERAL PRINCIPLES

81. Zhang XH, Wang Q, Gerald W, et al. Latent bone metastasis in breast cancer tied to Src-dependent survival signals. *Cancer Cell* 2009;16:67.

83. Kang Y, Siegel PM, Shu W, et al. A multigenic program mediating breast cancer metastasis to bone. *Cancer Cell* 2003;3:537.

87. Minn AJ, Kang Y, Serganova I, et al. Distinct organ-specific metastatic potential of individual breast cancer cells and primary tumors. *J Clin Invest* 2005;115:44.

88. Minn AJ, Gupta GP, Padua D, et al. Lung metastasis genes couple breast tumor size and metastatic spread. *Proc Natl Acad Sci U S A* 2007;104:6740.

89. Gupta GP, Perk J, Acharyya S, et al. ID genes mediate tumor reinitiation during breast cancer lung metastasis. *Proc Natl Acad Sci U S A* 2007;104:19506.

98. Bos PD, Zhang XH, Nadal C, et al. Genes that mediate breast cancer metastasis to the brain. *Nature* 2009;459:1005.

101. Wong SY, Haack H, Crowley D, Barry M, Bronson RT, Hynes RO. Tumor-secreted vascular endothelial growth factor-C is necessary for prostate cancer lymphangiogenesis, but lymphangiogenesis is unnecessary for lymph node metastasis. *Cancer Res* 2005;65:9789.

102. Skobe M, Hawighorst T, Jackson DG, et al. Induction of tumor lymphangiogenesis by VEGF-C promotes breast cancer metastasis. *Nat Med* 2001;7:192.

103. Stacker SA, Caesar C, Baldwin ME, et al. VEGF-D promotes the metastatic spread of tumor cells via the lymphatics. *Nat Med* 2001;7:186.

108. Gupta PB, Kuperwasser C, Brunet JP, et al. The melanocyte differentiation program predisposes to metastasis after neoplastic transformation. *Nat Genet* 2005; 37:1047.

109. Nguyen DX, Chiang AC, Zhang XH, et al. WNT/TCF signaling through LEF1 and HOXB9 mediates lung adenocarcinoma metastasis. *Cell* 2009;138:51.

110. Gupta RA, Shah N, Wang KC, et al. Long non-coding RNA HOTAIR reprograms chromatin state to promote cancer metastasis. *Nature* 2010;464:1071.

114. Ma L, Teruya-Feldstein J, Weinberg RA. Tumour invasion and metastasis initiated by microRNA-10b in breast cancer. *Nature* 2007;449:682.

116. Gregory PA, Bert AG, Paterson EL, et al. The miR-200 family and miR-205 regulate epithelial to mesenchymal transition by targeting ZEB1 and SIP1. *Nat Cell Biol* 2008;10:593.

117. Korpal M, Lee ES, Hu G, Kang Y. The miR-200 family inhibits epithelial-mesenchymal transition and cancer cell migration by direct targeting of E-cadherin transcriptional repressors ZEB1 and ZEB2. *J Biol Chem* 2008;283:14910.

118. Park SM, Gaur AB, Lengyel E, Peter ME. The miR-200 family determines the epithelial phenotype of cancer cells by targeting the E-cadherin repressors ZEB1 and ZEB2. *Genes Dev* 2008;22:894.

119. Tavazoie SF, Alarcón C, Oskarsson T, et al. Endogenous human microRNAs that suppress breast cancer metastasis. *Nature* 2008;451:147.

CHAPTER 11 CANCER STEM CELLS

JEAN C. Y. WANG AND JOHN E. DICK

A fundamental problem in cancer research is identification of the cell type capable of initiating and sustaining growth of the tumor—the cancer-initiating cell or cancer stem cell (CSC). Although it has long been known that only a fraction of cells within a tumor is capable of tumor generation upon transplantation, it has been unclear until recently whether this observed functional heterogeneity was attributable to stochastic influences or to intrinsic properties of the tumor cells. Evidence for the existence of biologically distinct CSCs, first demonstrated in a hematological malignancy and in the past 5 years in several solid tumors, has shaped a new paradigm of human cancer as a hierarchical disease whose growth is sustained by a population of CSCs. This conceptual shift has important implications not only for researchers seeking to understand mechanisms of tumor initiation and progression, but also for the development and evaluation of effective anticancer therapies.

TUMOR HETEROGENEITY

Our modern understanding of the origin of cancer can be traced to Rudolph Virchow, who in 1858 stated the heretical and revolutionary thesis *"omnis cellula e cellula,"* that all cells come from cells. Out of his early theories grew the idea that cancer cells develop from normal cells that have undergone abnormal changes, a process now called somatic mutation. Nearly 150 years later, it is now well accepted that cancer is a genetic disease that arises from the clonal expansion of a single neoplastic cell. Simplistically, cancer has been viewed as the unregulated growth of abnormal cells, with the implication that all of the cells in the tumor are proliferating uncontrollably. However, this notion is incompatible with the observation made over four decades ago that only a fraction of cells within murine lymphomas were capable of clonogenic growth when transplanted into syngeneic mice.[1] Furthermore, autotransplants of cancer cell suspensions in humans demonstrated that tumor growth occurred only after inoculation of at least 10^4 to 10^5 cells.[2] These and similar observations demonstrated that there is functional heterogeneity in the proliferative ability of cells within a tumor.

Two contrasting theories have been proposed to explain this observed heterogeneity (Fig. 11.1).[3] One view is that extrinsic factors (e.g., host resistance, growth factor concentrations, niche availability) or intrinsic factors (e.g., timing of cell cycle entry) prevent every cell from behaving in the same way. In other words, the behavior of tumor cells is unpredictable and governed by probabilities that may be influenced by any or all of these factors. The end result is that cells will appear to be heterogeneous in their proliferative capacity when tested in a functional assay. The central tenet of this stochastic model is that every cell has equal potential to initiate and sustain tumor growth, but most cells do not proliferate extensively due to the low cumulative probability of permissive events.

The alternative model is based on the biology of normal somatic tissues, many of which are arranged as hierarchies comprising cell types with different growth properties. The nonproliferating mature cells that make up the majority of these normal tissues must be continuously replenished by a pool of rapidly proliferating progenitors, which in turn are replenished by rare stem cells at the apex of the hierarchy. A key property of stem cells that distinguishes them from progenitors and allows them to maintain tissue integrity is self-renewal, whereby at cell division one or both daughter cells retain the biological properties of the parent cell. According to this model, tumors retain features of normal tissue organization, in that they are made up of distinct classes of cells that are organized hierarchically and possess intrinsically different functional capacities. The tumor hierarchy is sustained at its apex by a population of CSCs that possess the capacity to self-renew (i.e., produce more CSCs) and to recapitulate tumor heterogeneity by generating all of the various nontumorigenic cell types that compose the bulk of tumor. The essential principle of this model is that CSCs are biologically distinct from the bulk cell population, which does not possess tumor-initiating activity.

Both the stochastic and CSC models predict that only a small number of cells within a tumor will have the capacity to initiate tumor growth (i.e., to behave as CSCs); however, their underlying biological principles are very different. According to the stochastic model, the oncogenic program is operative in all cells of the tumor, thus both research to understand neoplastic processes and drug development can be directed at the bulk cell population. In contrast, the CSC model implies that CSCs are biologically distinct from the majority of cells in the tumor due to irreversible epigenetic processes that influence cell function, layered onto the common genetic aberrations present in all cells of the tumor.[4] The biological consequence of a particular cancer pathway may be different in CSCs compared to cells without tumor-initiating capacity. Thus, research must be directed at the relevant cell populations as identified through functional assays, the ultimate goal being the rational development of therapies that interfere with the oncogenic program within CSCs.

In order to test these theories and address the fundamental question of how tumor heterogeneity arises, two things are required: first, the ability to purify subpopulations of tumor cells based on physical or functional properties such as surface antigen expression or dye exclusion, and second, a functional transplantation assay to test the ability of purified cell populations to generate tumors *in vivo*, as current *in vitro* culture techniques do not reproduce the necessary microenvironment for tumor development. According to the stochastic model, the behavior of tumor cells is random and cannot be predicted; therefore, tumor-initiating activity will appear in every isolated cell fraction and cannot consistently be enriched. In contrast, the CSC model postulates that with an appropriate purification strategy, the CSCs with the capacity to initiate and sustain tumor growth *in vivo* can be identified and isolated from the bulk cells that do not have tumor-initiating activity (Fig. 11.1).

LEUKEMIA STEM CELLS

Based on the depth of knowledge gained from more than four decades of research in normal hematopoiesis, it is not surprising that identification of CSCs was first achieved in a hematological malignancy, acute myeloid leukemia (AML). This was made possible by prior detailed characterization of hematopoietic cell surface antigens and by the development of a xenotransplantation assay using severe combined immune-deficient (SCID) or nonobese diabetic (NOD)/SCID mice as recipients that allowed assessment of the ability of leukemic cells to initiate disease *in vivo*. When primary AML cells were fractionated based on expression of cell surface markers and transplanted into mice, only cells in the CD34+CD38− fraction composing less than 1% of the total blast population were able to initiate leukemic growth *in vivo*.[5,6] These leukemia stem cells (LSCs) possessed high self-renewal, as demonstrated by serial transplantation, and proliferated in the mice to produce large numbers of leukemic progenitors and nonproliferating blasts, generating a graft that recapitulated the phenotypic and functional heterogeneity of the patient's disease. These findings demonstrated that

AML, like the normal hematopoietic system, is organized as a hierarchy of functionally distinct classes of cells whose growth is sustained by a small number of LSCs, which provides the first direct evidence supporting the CSC model.

LSCs share some phenotypic characteristics with normal hematopoietic stem cells (HSCs), for example expression patterns of CD34 and CD38. However, identification of LSC-specific markers such as the interleukin-3 (IL-3) receptor alpha chain (IL-3Rα, CD123)[7] has allowed researchers to distinguish LSCs from normal HSCs. Such markers not only provide a therapeutic window for monoclonal antibody-based therapies to selectively target LSCs while sparing normal HSCs,[8] but also enable elucidation of the unique properties of LSCs. For example, recent studies have demonstrated constitutive activation of the transcription factor nuclear factor κB (NF-κB) in quiescent primitive CD34+CD38−CD123+ AML cells but not in normal CD34+CD38− cells.[9] Treatment of primitive AML cells *in vitro* with the NF-κB inhibitor parthenolide resulted in rapid induction of cell death and loss of ability to generate a leukemic graft in NOD/SCID mice, whereas normal CD34+CD38− cells were generally unaffected,[10] suggesting that NF-κB plays an important role in the survival of LSCs but not normal HSCs. PTEN is a phosphatase that negatively regulates cell proliferation and survival through the phosphatidylinositol 3-kinase (PI3K) pathway. This pathway has been implicated in the survival of human AML LSCs,[11] a finding supported by evidence that loss of PTEN in murine HSCs results in leukemia.[12,13] Notably, treatment of PTEN-deficient mice with rapamycin, which targets the PI3K effector mammalian target of rapamycin (mTOR), prevented leukemia development and restored normal function to HSCs.[12] Both NF-κB and PTEN thus represent exciting potential targets in the development of therapeutic strategies to kill AML LSCs while sparing normal HSCs.

Normal HSCs require a microenvironmental niche for maintenance of stem cell properties. If AML LSCs possess unique requirements for interaction with a supportive niche, this association could represent another therapeutic target. CD44 is a ubiquitously expressed transmembrane protein that mediates cell adhesion. Some isoforms of CD44 are highly expressed on AML blasts and are associated with poor prognosis. Treatment of AML cells *in vitro* or *in vivo* with an activating monoclonal antibody (H90) directed against CD44 resulted in killing of LSCs, as demonstrated by loss of leukemic repopulation in NOD/SCID mice, while similarly treated normal cord blood and bone marrow cells were much less affected, if at all.[14] The mechanisms underlying eradication of LSCs included interference with homing to their microenvironmental niche, loss of engraftment ability, and induction of differentiation. These findings demonstrate that the leukemogenic process does not abrogate the niche dependence of

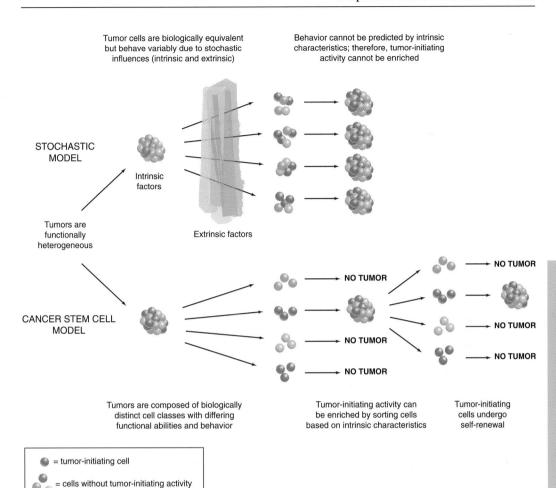

Tumor cells are biologically equivalent
but behave variably due to stochastic
influences (intrinsic and extrinsic)

Behavior cannot be predicted by intrinsic
characteristics; therefore, tumor-initiating
activity cannot be enriched

STOCHASTIC
MODEL

Intrinsic
factors

Tumors are
functionally
heterogeneous

Extrinsic factors

CANCER STEM CELL
MODEL

NO TUMOR

NO TUMOR

NO TUMOR

NO TUMOR

NO TUMOR

NO TUMOR

Tumors are composed of biologically
distinct cell classes with differing
functional abilities and behavior

Tumor-initiating activity can
be enriched by sorting cells
based on intrinsic characteristics

Tumor-initiating
cells undergo
self-renewal

= tumor-initiating cell

= cells without tumor-initiating activity

FIGURE 11.1 Models of tumor heterogeneity. Tumors are composed of phenotypically and functionally heterogeneous cells. There are two theories as to how this heterogeneity arises. According to the stochastic model, tumor cells are biologically equivalent but their behavior is influenced by intrinsic and extrinsic factors and is therefore both variable and unpredictable. Thus, tumor-initiating activity cannot be enriched by sorting cells based on intrinsic characteristics. In contrast, the cancer stem cell model postulates the existence of biologically distinct classes of cells with differing functional abilities and behavior. Only a subset of cells has the ability to initiate tumor growth; these cancer stem cells possess self-renewal and give rise to nontumorigenic progeny that make up the bulk of the tumor. This model predicts that tumor-initiating cells can be identified and purified from the bulk non-tumorigenic population based on intrinsic characteristics. (Figure originally published in Dick JE. Stem cell concepts renew cancer research. *Blood* 2008;112:4793.) © The American Society of Hematology.

LSCs and highlight a potential therapeutic target that may also be applicable to solid cancers.

CANCER STEM CELLS IN SOLID TUMORS

Breast Cancer Stem Cells

Investigations of mechanisms underlying solid tumor heterogeneity were first undertaken in human breast cancer. Al Hajj et al.[15] made single-cell suspensions of breast cancer specimens obtained from primary or metastatic sites in patients. Upon injection into the mammary fat pad of immune-deficient NOD/SCID mice, all samples studied were able to generate tumors. Thus, the NOD/SCID model provides a functional assay of the *in vivo* tumor-initiating ability of human breast cancer cells. Breast cancer cells are heterogeneous with respect to expression of a variety of surface markers, including the adhesion molecules CD24 and CD44. To test whether it would be possible to identify and isolate subpopulations enriched for tumor-initiating activity, breast cancer cells were first separated from normal hematopoietic, endothelial, mesothelial, and fibroblast cells by elimination of cells expressing lineage markers, then subfractionated based on expression of CD24 and CD44. All of the *in vivo* tumor-initiating activity was found in the CD44+CD24−/lowLineage− cell fraction, with enrichment compared to unfractionated tumor cells as judged by the cell dose required for tumor formation. CD44− and CD44+CD24+Lineage− cells, even though morphologically indistinguishable from tumor-initiating cells, did not generate tumors at injection sites. In some samples, isolation of cells expressing epithelial specific antigen (ESA) allowed further enrichment of tumor-initiating activity within the CD44+CD24−/lowLineage− population, however, ESA expression did not distinguish between tumorigenic and nontumorigenic cells in at least one sample, and therefore may not be a reliable marker for breast cancer-initiating cells. CD44+CD24−/lowLineage− tumorigenic cells could be serially propagated, demonstrating self-renewal, and gave rise not only to more CD44+CD24−/lowLineage− tumorigenic cells, but also to the phenotypically diverse nontumorigenic cells which made up the bulk of the primary tumor, thereby recapitulating the tumor's complexity and functional heterogeneity. This study was the first to isolate tumor-initiating cells from the bulk nontumorigenic population in a nonhematological malignancy, providing strong evidence that the growth of at least some types of human solid tumors is sustained by biologically distinct CSCs.

Other investigators have since shown that breast CSCs can be isolated from some patient tumors by cellular expression of aldehyde dehydrogenase (ALDH), with partial overlap with the CD44+CD24−Lineage− phenotype.[16] As few as 20 ALDH1+CD44+CD24−Lineage− cells from one patient cancer could generate tumors in NOD/SCID mice. Although highly enriched, these CSC-containing fractions are still heterogeneous, and additional CSC markers will be required for further purification. Nevertheless, identification of breast CSCs has moved cancer researchers away from studying bulk tumors and shifted their focus to understanding the biology of this subpopulation of cells. For example, Yu et al.[17] have shown that cell fractions enriched for breast CSCs have globally reduced microRNA expression compared to more differentiated cancer cells. In particular, the *let*-7 family is not expressed and increases with differentiation. Lentiviral expression of *let*-7 in Lineage−CD44+CD24− cells from patient breast cancers significantly reduced tumor formation in both primary and serially transplanted NOD/SCID mice. Insight into the biology of CSCs will be a crucial first step to develop an effective means to target them therapeutically.

Brain Cancer Stem Cells

Studies in several types of human brain cancers have clearly shown that the tumor cell population is functionally heterogeneous, in that only a fraction of cells have the ability to form tumor neurospheres when plated at low density in culture or generate tumors when transplanted *in vivo*.[18,19] As discussed above, demonstration that this heterogeneity arises from the existence of biologically distinct cell populations, rather than as a result of stochastic processes, requires isolation of tumor-initiating cells from the bulk nontumorigenic population. Singh et al.[20] reported that CD133+ cells in different types of human brain tumors possess extensive proliferative, differentiative, and self-renewal capacity *in vitro*. The development of a xenograft assay that involved injection of single-cell suspensions of human brain tumor samples into the NOD/SCID mouse brain enabled assessment of whether the CD133+ cells were capable of initiating tumor growth *in vivo*.[21] Tumors could be generated by as few as 100 CD133+ cells, while injection of up to 10^5 CD133− tumor cells did not result in tumor formation. Importantly, small numbers of viable CD133− tumor cells could be found at the injection site many weeks later, ruling out the possibility that CD133− cells did not form tumors simply because they died following transplantation. The tumors generated by CD133+ cells resembled the patient's original tumor by immunohistochemistry and consisted of a minority CD133+ and a majority CD133− cell population. CD133+ cells isolated from xenograft tumors could generate phenotypically similar tumors in secondary mice. Thus, CD133+ cells from human brain tumors possess the two key properties of CSCs: the ability to self-renew and to recapitulate tumor heterogeneity through differentiation. Interestingly, CD133 (also called prominin-1/AC133) has also been used as a marker to enrich normal human HSCs as well as stem cells in the human central nervous system, suggesting that it may be a marker of both normal and malignant stem cells.

Recently, there have been reports that CD133 may not be a universal marker of CSCs in brain cancer.[22-24] In addition, a study of neurosphere lines derived from *PTEN*-deficient human glioblastomas found that both CD133+ and CD133− cells could generate serially transplantable tumors in xenograft recipients and provided evidence that these tumors comprise a hierarchy of self-renewing CSC populations with variable tumorigenic capacity.[25] Unfortunately, these investigators were not able to study sorted cell populations directly isolated from patient tumors. Cell surface phenotype can change significantly during culture, without corresponding changes in stem cell function.[26] In addition, there is evidence that CD133 expression can vary as a function of cell cycle.[27] Thus, the results of these studies should be interpreted with caution. Nevertheless, it would not be surprising to find that the CSC phenotype is heterogeneous, even among tumors of the same histologic subtype, given the variety of genetic and epigenetic perturbations that can ultimately lead to tumor formation. These observations underscore the importance of characterizing candidate CSC populations through functional assays of their tumor-forming ability rather than relying solely on phenotypic identification.

Cancer Stem Cells in Other Solid Tumors

Two groups initially reported isolation of CD133+ tumor-initiating cells from human colon cancers.[28,29] Single-cell suspensions of primary or metastatic tumor samples were injected either under the renal capsule of NOD/SCID mice[28] or subcutaneously into SCID mice.[29] In both studies, only CD133+ and not CD133− cells, which composed the bulk of the cancers, were able to initiate tumor formation *in vivo*. Tumors could be serially propagated by reisolating CD133+ cells from xenografts and transplanting them into secondary mice. The ability to perform quantitative analysis is an essential feature of any *in vivo* assay. In one study, the frequency of colon CSCs in the bulk tumor was determined by limiting dilution analysis to be 1 in 60,000 colon cancer cells.[28] The frequency of CSCs in the CD133+ cell fraction was 1 in 262, representing a greater than 200-fold enrichment over unfractionated cells. Clearly, however, the majority of CD133+ colon cancer cells are not CSCs. As has been shown in the CD34+ cell fraction of AML,[30] there may be a hierarchy of CSCs and progenitors in the CD133+ subpopulation of colon cancer cells. Another study identified colon CSCs in the EpCAMhighCD44+CD166+ cell fraction.[31] CD44+ cells generally constituted a minority subset of the CD133+ population, thus CD44 is a marker that could potentially be used to purify the CSC-containing fraction further.

Using methodology similar to that described above, CD44+ CSCs have recently been characterized in squamous cell carcinomas of the head and neck (HNSCC),[32] adding to the rapidly growing list of human cancers in which a distinct CSC population has been identified (Fig. 11.2, Table 11.1). Significantly, in moderately to well-differentiated HNSCC in which some tissue architecture is preserved, CD44+ cells were localized to the basal layer and costained with Cytokeratin 5/14, a marker of normal squamous epithelial stem and progenitor cells, but not with the differentiation marker involucrin. Furthermore, CD44+ cells expressed much higher levels of *BMI1* than CD44− cells. *BMI1* plays an important role in the self-renewal of hematopoietic and neuronal stem cells and has been implicated in tumorigenesis.[33–35] These findings demonstrate that biological pathways likely differ between tumorigenic and nontumorigenic populations and underscore the impor-

tance of identifying and characterizing the CSCs within tumors, both for gene expression and proteomic analyses as well as therapeutic targeting.

Expression of CD44 on CSCs from both breast cancer and HNSCC suggests that this adhesion molecule may also be a marker of CSCs in other tumors of epithelial origin. Recently, Li et al.[36] showed in pancreatic adenocarcinoma that cell fractions expressing CD44, CD24, epithelial specific antigen (ESA), or a combination of these markers were enriched for tumorigenic activity, as assessed by the frequency of tumor formation following subcutaneous or intrapancreatic injection into NOD/SCID mice. The most highly enriched fraction comprised cells that express all three of these markers, with tumor formation in half of mice receiving as few as 100 CD44+CD24+ESA+ cells. However, injection of CD44−, CD24−, or ESA− cells also gave rise to tumors, albeit with lower frequency. Thus, none of the markers used in this study enabled clear separation of cells with tumor-initiating activity from the bulk nontumorigenic population. In contrast to these results, Hermann et al.[37] identified CSCs in pancreatic tumors by CD133 expression; as few as 500 freshly isolated CD133+ cells were able to generate tumors after orthotopic injection into immune-deficient mice, whereas as many as 1×10^6 CD133− cells could not.

The list of tumors in which CSC populations have been identified continues to grow (Table 11.1). There is frequent overlap in cell surface phenotype among CSCs from different tumor types, as evidenced in particular by expression of CD44 and CD133 on CSCs from epithelial tumors. Whether these are simply surrogate markers or play a functional role in CSC biology has yet to be determined.

Controversies and Future Directions

There have been a number of criticisms of the CSC model. As discussed above, characterization of CSC populations requires xenotransplantation into immune-deficient recipients. Some investigators have argued that inefficiencies of the xenotransplant system lead to underestimation of the frequency of cells with tumor-initiating ability.[38] In fact, when improvements have been made to these assay systems, for example through the use of more immune-deficient recipients such as NOD/SCID *Il2rg*$^{-/-}$ mice, the frequency of tumor initiating cells is sometimes dramatically increased, as seen recently for melanoma (greater than 4 log difference).[39,40] There are a number of issues to be considered here. First, such large increases in CSC frequency with the use of more immune-deficient recipients are not universal—for example, they have not been observed in AML[41,42,42a]—possibly reflecting variable sensitivity of tumor-initiating cells from different tumor types to residual host

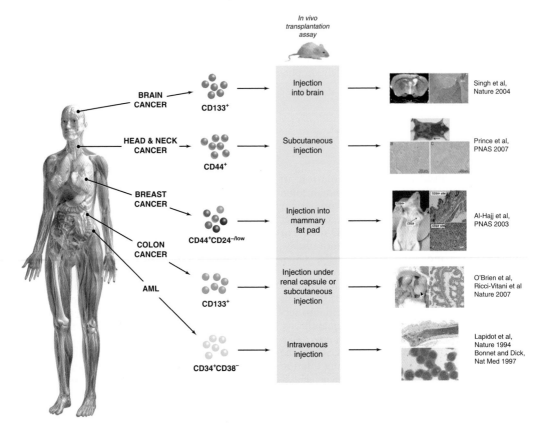

FIGURE 11.2 Identification of cancer stem cells (CSCs) in acute myeloid leukemia (AML) and solid tumors. Subfractions of tumor cells isolated from the bulk tumor population are assayed for their ability to initiate tumor growth *in vivo* using immune-deficient mice as recipients. CSCs are the only cells capable of initiating tumor growth, giving rise to more CSCs through self-renewal, and also to nontumorigenic differentiated progeny, thus recapitulating the functional heterogeneity of the original tumor. CSCs were first identified in AML and have now also been identified in several types of solid tumors (Table 11.1). (Brain cancer images adapted by permission from Macmillan Publishers Ltd: Nature (21), copyright 2004. Head and neck cancer and breast cancer images copyright 2007 (ref. 32) and 2003 (ref. 15), respectively, National Academy of Sciences, USA. Colon cancer images are from ref. 28.)

immune surveillance. Second, while human cell engraftment in xenotransplant assays is undoubtedly limited by residual elements of the recipient immune system, absence of cross-reactivity of cytokines, and other components of the host microenvironment, the low frequency of tumor-initiating cells seen in some cancers cannot be wholly explained by xenotransplantation barriers. For example, LSC frequency in two murine models of leukemia involving *MOZ-TIF* expression or *Pten* deletion was low (1 in 10^4 to 1 in 6×10^5) despite syngeneic bone marrow transplantation.[12,43] Furthermore, in contrast to the low frequency of LSCs generally seen when human AML cells are xenotransplanted, much higher LSC frequencies (on the order of 1%) have been observed in a genetically induced model of human B-cell acute lymphoblastic leukemia (ALL) that involves transplantation of human cord blood stem or progenitor cells expressing the *MLL-ENL* oncogene into

immune-deficient mice.[42,44] This frequency was comparable to that reported for a murine model of *MLL-AF9*–induced AML (1 in 150).[45] These findings indicate that CSC frequencies can vary widely in different cancers, regardless of whether they are quantified using xeno- or syngeneic transplant assays, and likely relate at least in part to the specific underlying oncogenic pathways operating within the different tumors. Third, and perhaps most important, the CSC hypothesis does not address the absolute frequency of these cells: it is not required that CSCs be rare. The CSC model, at its most fundamental level, simply proposes that the basis of functional heterogeneity within tumors is the existence of cell populations that can be distinguished from other tumor cells by their ability to initiate malignant growth *in vivo*.

It is possible that some human cancers may not follow the CSC model. For example, the high frequency (one in four) and lack of a clear isolatable

TABLE 11.1

PROSPECTIVE ISOLATION OF CANCER STEM CELLS FROM HUMAN LEUKEMIAS AND SOLID TUMORS

Tumor Type	CSC Marker	Transplantation Site	Mouse Strain	Frequency	Minimum Cell Dose for Tumor Formation	No. of Samples Engrafted	Ref.
AML	CD34+CD38−	Intravenous	SCID	1 in 2.5×10^5	2×10^5	1	5
AML	CD34+CD38−	Intravenous	NOD/SCID	0.2 to 100 per 10^6 bulk	5×10^3	7	6
Multiple myeloma	CD138−CD34−	Intravenous	NOD/SCID	NR	NA	1	114
Breast	CD44+CD24−/low	Orthotopic	NOD/SCID	5 in 10^5 bulk	10^3	8	15
Breast	CD44+CD24−	Orthotopic	NOD/SCID	NR	2×10^3	8	17
Brain	ALDH1+	Orthotopic	NOD/SCID	NR	500	4	16
Brain	CD133+	Orthotopic	NOD/SCID	NR	100	7	21
Brain	CD133+	Orthotopic	nu/nu	NR	500	2	101
Brain	A2B5+CD133±	Orthotopic	nu/nu	NR	1.5×10^4	5	24
Colon	CD133+	Kidney capsule	NOD/SCID	1 in 5.7×10^4 bulk; 1 in 262 CD133+	100	12	28
Colon	CD133+	Subcutaneous	SCID	NR	1.5×10^3	19	29
Colon	ESA+CD44+	Subcutaneous	NOD/SCID	NR	200	6	31
Colon	ESA+CD44+CD166+	Subcutaneous	NOD/SCID	NR	150	2	31
Colon	CD133+	Subcutaneous	nu/nu	NR	2.5×10^3	3	105
Head and neck	CD44+	Subcutaneous	NOD/SCID, Rag2$^{-/-}$γ$^{-/-}$	NR	5×10^3	9	32
Pancreas	CD133+	Orthotopic	NMRI-nu/nu	NR	500	7	37
Pancreas	CD44+CD24+ESA+	Orthotopic	NOD/SCID	NR	100	10	36
Lung	CD133+	Subcutaneous	SCID	NR	10^4	3	115
Liver	CD90+	Orthotopic	SCID/Beige	NR	10^3	NR	116
Melanoma	ABCB5+	Subcutaneous	NOD/SCID	1 in 10^6 bulk; 1 in 1.6×10^5 ABCB5+	10^4	4	39
Mesenchymal	Side population	Subcutaneous	NOD/SCID	NR	100	4	117

CSC, cancer stem cell; AML, acute myeloid leukemia; NOD, nonobese diabetic; SCID, severe combined immune-deficient; NR, not reported; ESA, epithelial specific antigen.

GENERAL PRINCIPLES

phenotype of tumor-initiating cells in melanoma suggest the absence of a hierarchical organization.[40] Regardless of whether a tumor contains a subpopulation of CSCs responsible for maintaining tumor growth or common tumorigenic cells with little evidence of a CSC hierarchy, all cancer cells with the ability to initiate disease must be identified and targeted therapeutically in order to achieve cure. Since the first published reports of CSCs in breast and brain cancers, there have been numerous studies of CSCs in other solid tumors, with varying degrees of robustness. When weighing evidence presented for or against the CSC hypothesis, one must consider not only the rigor of the xenotransplant assay but also experimental details such as whether cancer cells have been extensively cultured *in vitro* or passaged *in vivo*, both of which can lead to changes in function and phenotype, and whether freshly isolated cells from patients' tumors have been used versus cell lines that may not be representative of clinical disease.

Nevertheless, there is accumulating evidence that the growth of several types of human cancer is initiated and maintained by a subset of phenotypically and functionally distinct CSCs. Although the markers used to date to identify the CSC subset have enabled enrichment of this population compared to unsorted tumor cells, in all cases the enriched cell fractions are still functionally heterogeneous, containing both CSCs and their nontumorigenic progeny. One of the challenges of future research will be to obtain more purified populations of CSCs for use in molecular studies such as gene expression profiling. Novel protocols to purify cells with *in vivo* tumor-initiating capacity may combine cell surface markers with functional parameters such as Hoechst 33342 dye efflux, which identifies a "side population" of cells with high drug efflux capacity[46] or high aldehyde dehydrogenase activity.[47] Ultimately, rigorous proof for the existence of biologically distinct CSCs can only be obtained through demonstration that a single cell has the ability to self-renew and to recapitulate the entire tumor hierarchy. This will require either development of *in vivo* tumor models that support the growth of singly transplanted cells or clonal analysis techniques that enable tracking of the progeny of individually marked tumor cells *in vivo*, as demonstrated for AML LSCs.[30]

GENETIC DIVERSITY AND CLONAL EVOLUTION IN CANCER

Most of the initial studies identifying and characterizing CSCs in leukemia and solid tumors did not investigate the underlying genetic changes in cancer cells. Intratumor clonal heterogeneity has been described in many types of cancer[48] and may contribute to progression.[49] Investigators have proposed that intratumor heterogeneity arises through clonal evolution,[48] a long-standing concept in which cancer cells within a tumor acquire various mutations over time, leading to genetic drift and stepwise natural selection for the fittest, most aggressive cells, both of which drive tumor progression.[50] According to this model, the parallel growth and contraction of related but divergent subclones result in intratumor heterogeneity, and the genetic makeup of the tumor at any particular time reflects the activity of the dominant subclone(s). Recently, a number of studies have shown that phenotypically defined stem and progenitor populations in human breast cancers are clonally related but not identical.[51–53] There is now evidence from two studies in ALL[54,54a] that genetically distinct subclones that possess differing growth properties are present even at diagnosis. Examination of the genetic changes acquired by different subclones allowed reconstruction of their ancestry and provided evidence of a complex genetic architecture in ALL, with multiple subclones that are related in a branching rather than linear fashion. Importantly, the genetic diversity found in ALL patient samples was regenerated upon transplantation in immune-deficient mice, suggesting that leukemia-initiating cells are genetically diverse in this disease.

Although the existence of CSCs in most subtypes of human ALL is still under debate, based on these functional studies it may be reasonable to bring together the idea of clonal evolution driving intratumor genetic diversity and the existence of CSCs in a broader model of cancer progression, rather than viewing them as mutually exclusive concepts. Instead of being rigid, linear hierarchies that mirror normal tissue stem cell hierarchies, tumors should be thought of as genetically dynamic, comprising related but divergent subclones driven by CSCs, which are the units of evolutionary selection. On one hand, genetically distinct CSC clones may arise through changes acquired by existing CSCs. For example, the LSCs in an experimentally induced human leukemia can evolve through rearrangement of their immunoglobulin heavy chain genes.[44] On the other hand, CSCs may also arise through transformation of non-CSC populations, through acquisition of additional alterations or processes such as epithelial-mesenchymal transition (see below) (Fig. 11.3). Over time the genetic composition of the tumor may change, with different CSC-driven subclones becoming dominant or disappearing, either through natural selection based on cell-intrinsic or microenvironmental factors, or through selection by therapy. Indeed, clonal studies of matched diagnosis and relapse samples from pediatric patients with ALL have shown that relapse clones were often present as minor subpopulations at diagnosis.[55] Interestingly, therapy seemed to select for genetic abnormalities related to cell cycle regulation and B-cell development.

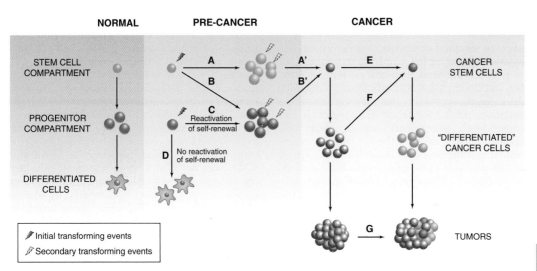

NORMAL   **PRE-CANCER**   **CANCER**

FIGURE 11.3 Models of tumor initiation and progression. Cancer stem cells (CSCs) might arise through neoplastic changes initiated in normal self-renewing stem cells, or downstream progenitors with limited or no self-renewal. Initial events in stem cells could cause (**A**) expansion of the stem cell pool and/or (**B**) expansion of downstream progenitors. Secondary events are more likely to occur in these expanded pools of target cells (**A'**, **B'**); thus, it is possible that transformation is initiated in a normal stem cell, but the final steps occur in downstream progenitors (**B→B'**). Reactivation of a self-renewal program is a central feature of oncogenic transformation of progenitors (**C**), as these short-lived cells will otherwise die or undergo terminal differentiation before enough mutations occur for full neoplastic transformation (**D**). CSCs themselves might acquire additional genetic or epigenetic changes during tumor progression (**E**), and non-CSCs can acquire CSC-like properties (**F**) through processes such as epithelial-mesenchymal transition (EMT), leading to evolution of tumor phenotype (**G**) and intratumor heterogeneity. Of note, the cell of origin debate centers around the cells and processes illustrated in the pink box, whereas CSC research focuses on characterization of cancer cell populations after they reach the green box. (Figure originally published in Wang JCY. Good cells gone bad: the cellular origins of cancer. *Trends Mol Med* 2010;16:145.)

If found to be a property of cancer in general, genetic diversity of CSCs could have important implications for the development of anticancer therapies. Regardless of their origin, CSCs are the key cells that drive tumor growth and that must therefore be eliminated in order to achieve cure. If CSCs are genetically, and as a result functionally, diverse, they could represent a moving therapeutic target. Agents that target critical molecular pathways may fail if the selected targets are not present in some CSC subclones or if others have acquired changes that bypass their dependence on the targeted pathways. The development of successful therapeutic regimens will have to take into account the genetic and functional heterogeneity of CSCs.

THE ORIGINS OF CANCER STEM CELLS

A key focus of cancer research is elucidation of the molecular changes that underlie tumor initiation and progression. Tumorigenesis is a multistep process, and CSCs can be regarded as cells that have accumulated enough genetic or epigenetic changes to become fully transformed and that possess a stem cell program. However, little is known of the order or timing of such changes or of the cellular context in which they occur. Does cancer arise through the malignant transformation of normal stem cells or of committed downstream progenitors (or both)?[56] Unfortunately, the "stem" in "cancer stem cell" has led to the frequent misconception that CSCs always arise from stem cells.[57] On the contrary, emerging evidence suggests that although some cancers may originate in normal stem cells, committed progenitors can also be initial targets for transformation.

There has been a great deal of debate over the cellular origins of cancer. A number of conceptual arguments have been invoked to support stem cells as the cell of origin. One contention is that because self-renewal is a key property of CSCs, and stem cells already possess self-renewal capacity, they would theoretically require fewer neoplastic changes in order to become fully transformed. In contrast, despite their substantial proliferative ability, progenitors do not generally retain the self-renewal capacity of stem cells. Thus to become a CSC, a progenitor must acquire mutations that reactivate the cellular self-renewal machinery. In addition, there is greater opportunity for genetic changes to accumulate in individual, long-lived stem cells compared to more mature progenitors with a limited lifespan. If a short-lived progenitor acquires a genetic mutation that does not confer increased self-renewal, that cell is likely to die or undergo terminal differentiation before enough mutations occur for full neoplastic transformation.

On the other hand, stem cells are fewer in number and divide less frequently than progenitors; therefore, the probability that they will acquire the mutations needed for cancer development is correspondingly lower. Furthermore, some have argued that stem cells are the key to tissue regeneration and the only cells in adult tissues capable of self-renewal. Thus, they might have evolved sophisticated inhibitory machinery to keep self-renewal in check as an anticancer defense.[58] If this is true, stem cells could actually be less likely to acquire mutations that affect self-renewal and proliferation or to manifest biological changes as a result of such mutations, as compared to more committed progenitors. In other words, stem cells might be under evolutionary pressure to preserve genomic integrity over promoting survival in order to prevent oncogenic transformation.

Functional Studies in Leukemia

It is problematic to make inferences regarding the cellular origins of CSCs simply by studying their surface phenotype, as disruption of normal differentiation pathways by the neoplastic process can lead to aberrant expression of lineage-associated markers. Similarly, it is difficult to draw firm conclusions by studying the lineage involvement of the neoplastic clone. For example, in chronic myeloid leukemia (CML) patients, involvement of multiple hematopoietic lineages has been taken as evidence that CML originates from a multipotent HSC, whereas lineage restriction in some AML patients has been interpreted as disease origin from a committed progenitor. However, apparent lineage restriction of the leukemic clone in AML could also result from mutations that arise in a multipotent stem cell and suppress differentiation to one or more lineages.[59] The most direct way to determine whether CSCs arise from neoplastic transformation initiated in stem cells or progenitors is to test whether oncogene expression in directly isolated, functionally validated normal stem and progenitor cell populations is able to confer *in vivo* tumor-initiating ability.

This approach has been used to study leukemic initiation in the murine hematopoietic system, facilitated by previous detailed phenotypic and functional characterization of different classes of progenitors and HSCs. One focus of investigation has been the *mixed-lineage leukemia* (MLL) gene, which undergoes fusion with a wide variety of partner genes and is associated with myeloid, lymphoid, and biphenotypic acute leukemias in both children and adults. The fusion gene *MLL-GAS7* induces mixed-lineage leukemias when expressed in murine HSCs or multipotent progen-

itors, but not in lineage-restricted progenitors.[60] In contrast, *MLL-ENL* can initiate myeloid leukemias in both self-renewing HSCs and committed myeloid progenitors,[61] although much lower numbers of transformed HSCs compared to progenitors were required for tumor initiation *in vivo*. *MLL-AF9* is also able to generate LSCs from committed granulocyte macrophage progenitors (GMPs).[45] Interestingly, when *MLL-AF9* is expressed at lower, physiologic levels in a knock-in transgenic mouse model of leukemia, HSCs and CMPs, but not GMPs, from transgenic mice are able to initiate leukemia upon transplantation into wild type recipients.[62] Compared to retrovirally transduced GMPs, GMPs from knock-in mice had 170-fold lower expression of *MLL-AF9*. These findings imply that differences in experimental transformability of HSC and progenitor populations may be related to oncogene dosage. However, the nonequivalent transformation of HSCs and committed progenitors, even by supraphysiologic levels of retrovirally driven *MLL-ENL*,[61] points to the existence of inherent differences in susceptibility between these populations.

Taken together, these findings in the murine system indicate that MLL-expressing leukemias may be initiated in either HSCs or downstream progenitors, depending on the specific fusion partner involved. This likely depends on the ability of the fusion oncogene to reactivate a self-renewal program in committed progenitors. Indeed, the LSCs generated by *MLL-AF9* expression in GMPs possessed a surface immunophenotype and global gene expression profile similar to that of normal GMPs, but also demonstrated reactivation of a subset of genes highly expressed in HSCs and associated with self-renewal.[45,63] The capacity of *MLL* fusion genes to reactivate self-renewal machinery in progenitors confers a potent transforming ability to this group of oncogenes, as evidenced by the high frequency of leukemias in NOD/SCID mice transplanted with primitive human hematopoietic cells expressing an *MLL* fusion gene[44] and the infrequency of additional detectable genetic changes in human acute lymphoblastic leukemias with *MLL* rearrangements.[64]

Conclusions drawn from studies in *MLL* leukemias may not be generalizable, as *MLL* leukemia appears to be a unique disease distinct from other subtypes of acute leukemia.[65] However, there have been a few reports of the transforming ability of other leukemia-associated oncogenes. *MOZ-TIF* can initiate AML in HSCs as well as committed progenitors, while *BCR-ABL1* did not increase self-renewal *in vitro* or initiate disease when expressed in committed progenitors, despite the induction of myeloproliferative disease in mice transplanted with *BCR-ABL1*-transduced whole bone marrow.[43] These findings suggest that *BCR-ABL1* expression in more primitive HSCs is required for disease initiation, although this was not tested directly. Nevertheless, these results are consistent with data from studies of transgenic mouse models of CML, in which BCR-ABL1 expression[66] or inactivation of JunB, a transcriptional regulator of myelopoiesis, in HSCs induces a transplantable myeloproliferative disorder, whereas JunB inactivation in more committed progenitors does not.[67] Interestingly, analysis of the JunB-deficient mice demonstrated expansion of the primitive HSC compartment as well as the GMP pool; however, the numbers of common myeloid progenitors and megakaryocytic-erythroid progenitors were similar to those of control animals, indicating that oncogenic changes in stem cells can have very specific effects in downstream progeny. Expansion or extended proliferation of progenitors may increase the risk of acquiring secondary cooperating events, resulting in progression to a fully transformed state. For example, transgenic mice that express reduced levels of the transcription factors PU.1[68] or GATA-1[69] are characterized by accumulation of an abnormal progenitor pool and a high propensity to develop acute leukemias, which in the PU.1 knockdown mice are frequently accompanied by additional chromosomal abnormalities. The mutant alleles in these engineered mice were expressed in every cell, thus it is impossible to determine whether reduced transcription factor levels would have equivalent transforming potential in the context of HSCs or progenitors. Patients with chronic phase CML have an expanded progenitor pool related at least in part to expression of BCR-ABL. Progression to blast crisis is associated with further expansion of GMPs that have activated β-catenin activity and increased self-renewal as demonstrated by in vitro replating assays.[70]

Overall, the accumulated evidence from studies in murine hematopoiesis indicates that the neoplastic changes that lead ultimately to generation of LSCs can be initiated in either normal HSCs or progenitors, depending on the ability of specific transforming events to overcome the inherent cellular barriers to transformation (Fig. 11.3). Potent oncogenes such as MLL that can reactivate self-renewal are able to transform committed progenitors, whereas less potent oncogenic changes must occur in self-renewing HSCs in order to initiate a tumorigenic program. Secondary neoplastic changes can occur within the stem cell compartment or within abnormally expanded downstream progenitor populations, ultimately resulting in the generation of LSCs. While the murine studies described above have provided significant insights, it will be important to carry out equivalent studies in the human hematopoietic system, as the processes underlying neoplastic transformation differ between mouse and man.[71]

Studies in Solid Tumors

Similar studies in solid tumors have been hampered by the lack of phenotypically and functionally defined stem and progenitor cell populations in most normal tissues. Recently, stem cells have been identified in murine[72,73] and human[74] mammary tissue and in murine prostate.[75–77] Lim et al.[78] proposed that luminal progenitors, rather than mammary stem cells, are the cell of origin for human basal breast cancers, which are associated with germline mutations in the tumor suppressor gene BRCA1, based on stronger similarity in gene expression profiles. Furthermore, the luminal progenitor population in premalignant breast tissue from BRCA1 mutation carriers is expanded and has increased growth potential in vitro. However, analogous to targeting of HSCs in CML, it is also possible that BRCA1 mutations target mammary stem cells and either drive development preferentially down the luminal lineage or have biological consequences only upon luminal differentiation. Transformation experiments of mammary cell subsets are needed to clarify this issue.

Despite the recent progress in characterizing normal cellular hierarchies in nonhematopoietic tissues, direct testing of the transformability of isolated stem and progenitor populations remains a challenge in most systems. Thus, researchers have turned to alternative methods to investigate the cell of origin in solid tumors. In brain cancer, genetic approaches have provided insights into the normal cell populations that might be targeted for transformation. Investigators used a transgenic mouse system that allows expression of oncogenes in a cell type-specific manner to show that selective expression of platelet-derived growth factor in nestin+ neural stem/progenitor cells generated oligodendrogliomas, whereas expression in GFAP+ astrocytes generated a mixture of oligodendrogliomas and oligoastrocytomas.[79] Similarly, the combined expression of activated Ras and Akt in nestin+ but not GFAP+ cells generated high-grade glioblastomas.[80] These findings suggest the existence of inherent differences in the transformability of neural cell populations but are confounded by the fact that GFAP marks neural stem cells as well as differentiated astrocytes.[81] In contrast, transduction of a constitutively active endothelial growth factor receptor mutant into either neural stem/progenitor cells or cortical astrocytes from Ink4a/Arf−/− mice gave rise to high-grade gliomas with similar latency, indicating that both cell compartments are permissive for transformation.[82] However, the isolated cell populations in this study were transduced only after a period of in vitro culture and were derived from age-mismatched animals, factors that can hamper direct comparisons of primitive and mature cell populations.

Using a different transgenic model, two groups found that activation of hedgehog (Hh) signaling, which is etiologically linked to medulloblastomas in mice and humans,[83] in both multipotent stem/progenitor cells and unilineage granule neuron precursors (GNPs), but not Purkinje neurons, generated transplantable medulloblastomas, but no tumors of other histological types.[84,85] Interestingly, Hh activation in stem/progenitor cells resulted in expansion and increased proliferation of these cells as well as committed GNPs, but caused no abnormalities in other downstream cell populations,[85] suggesting that Hh activation must occur in a lineage-specific context to manifest biological effects. The generation of medulloblastomas and no other histological tumor types is likely related to specific influences of Hh activation on target cell development, because conditional inactivation of tumor suppressor genes *p53*, *NF1*, and *Pten* (commonly mutated in human astrocytomas) in neural stem/progenitor cells generates high-grade astrocytomas.[86,87]

In the intestine, genetic lineage–tracing studies in mice have recently identified adult stem cell populations,[88–90] enabling studies of the cellular origin of intestinal tumors. Most human colorectal cancers are etiologically linked to mutations in the tumor suppressor gene *Apc*, with resultant activation of Wnt/β-catenin signaling.[91] In transgenic mouse models, rapid adenoma formation was consistently seen with conditional *Apc* deletion or expression of a stable β-catenin mutant in stem cell populations but not in more differentiated progenitors,[88,90,92] supporting a stem cell origin for intestinal tumors in the mouse. However, the findings from these transgenic models with full, constitutive β-catenin activation may not be fully applicable to human colorectal cancer, where studies have suggested that a specific degree or "dosage" of β-catenin signaling may be optimal for tumor formation,[93] as has been shown for leukemia stem/progenitor cells and *MLL* signaling. Clarification of these issues will require studies using human cells as target populations.

It is clear from these murine studies that cancers can originate in both stem cell and progenitor compartments, depending on the oncogene(s) involved, although stem and progenitor cells might differ in their inherent susceptibility to transformation. In addition, tumors generated by specific oncogenes are often phenotypically and functionally similar regardless of the cell of origin, suggesting that tumor heterogeneity in tissues is generated in large part by the differential effects of transforming events on the developmental program of the targeted cells, rather than by differences among target cells themselves. However, the results from murine studies must be confirmed in equivalent human studies using primary, functionally defined stem and progenitor cell populations. Insight into the cellular context in which the first steps of neoplastic transformation occur will be vital not only to understand how normal developmental processes become subverted during cancer initiation and progression, but also to advance our knowledge of CSC biology and facilitate the development of novel and effective therapies to eliminate these cancer-sustaining cells in patients.

EPITHELIAL-MESENCHYMAL TRANSITION

Epithelial-mesenchymal transition (EMT) is a complex molecular and cellular program involved in embryonic development whereby epithelial cells lose their differentiated characteristics and acquire a mesenchymal phenotype. There is recent evidence that EMT induction contributes to tumor progression by conferring properties such as invasiveness, the ability to metastasize, and resistance to therapy on epithelial cancer cells.[94,95] EMT induction of ras-transformed, SV40-immortalized human mammary epithelial cells (HMLEs) significantly increased their ability to generate tumors *in vivo* following subcutaneous injection into immune-deficient mice.[96] Notably, despite having undergone an EMT, transformed HMLEs did not exhibit *in vivo* tumor-initiating ability when EMT-inducing signals were removed, and the cells reverted to an epithelial phenotype when cultured further *in vitro*.[96] A number of groups have reported that EMT-inducing signals can originate from stromal cells in the tumor microenvironment.[97,98] Together, these observations suggest that in some epithelial tumors, acquisition and maintenance of CSC-like properties depend on continuous signals from the microenvironment, and support the notion that metastatic cancer cells revert to an epithelial state after dissemination and resultant loss of contact with a "tumor microenvironment." However, sustained induction of EMT might in some cases lead to irreversible, heritable epigenetic alterations that maintain the mesenchymal phenotype.[99] Such changes could have therapeutic implications, as breast cancer cells induced into EMT appear to be more resistant to standard chemotherapeutic drugs compared to control cells.[100] Furthermore, EMT of non-self-renewing cancer cell populations within a tumor could contribute to clonal evolution and intratumor heterogeneity of CSCs (Fig. 11.3). It should be noted, however, that the linkage between EMT and tumor initiation is still tenuous; a deeper understanding will require clonal assays, well-defined cell fractions, proof of self-renewal, and studies of primary tumors rather than cell lines.

CANCER STEM CELLS: TARGETED THERAPY

General Considerations

Implicit in the model of cancer as a hierarchical disease is the notion that CSCs are biologically distinct from the bulk cells in the tumor. Molecular

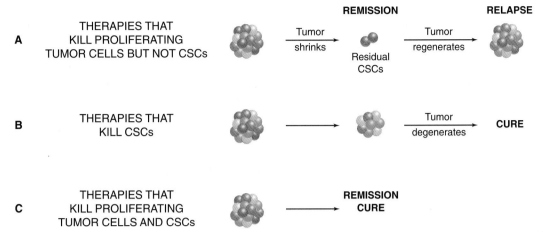

FIGURE 11.4 Development of effective anticancer therapies. **A:** Cancer stem cells (CSCs) are biologically distinct from bulk tumor cells and may not be effectively killed by conventional anticancer therapies due to properties such as quiescence or expression of drug-resistance transporters, leading to regrowth of the tumor and relapse after treatment. **B:** Ultimately, to prevent disease relapse and achieve permanent cure, the CSCs that sustain tumor growth must be eradicated. **C:** The most effective anticancer strategies will involve combination regimens that both reduce tumor bulk and kill CSCs, the latter likely best achieved through targeting of multiple critical pathways (see text). The development of new CSC-targeted therapies will require a greater understanding of the molecular pathways that drive tumor initiation and progression.

pathways for survival and response to injury may be fundamentally different in these cells compared to nontumorigenic cells. Ultimately, to prevent disease relapse and achieve permanent cure, the CSCs that sustain tumor growth must be eradicated in addition to killing the bulk cells of the tumor. However, properties of CSCs, such as quiescence or expression of drug-resistance transporters, may make them difficult to eliminate using conventional cytotoxic drugs that kill the bulk tumor cells. It will be crucial to understand the unique biology of CSCs in order to develop novel treatments that effectively target these cells (Fig. 11.4).

There are several obstacles to be overcome in the development of effective CSC-targeted therapies. Such treatments must be selective for CSCs and spare normal stem cells. There is recent evidence in AML that the pathways that regulate self-renewal in normal stem cells are not completely abolished in LSCs.[30] In other words, CSCs, although transformed, likely retain aspects of normal developmental pathways. Thus, drugs that target critical processes in CSCs, such as survival or self-renewal, may prove intolerably harmful to their normal counterparts. Furthermore, normal stem or progenitor cells may in fact be more sensitive than CSCs to the effects of chemotherapy. CSCs will likely have acquired genetic or epigenetic changes that allow them to bypass normal tumor-suppressing processes such as senescence or apoptosis in response to DNA damage. Thus, treatment with agents that normally induce senescence or apoptosis may actually provide a growth advantage to CSCs.[101] Ideally, effective therapies will target pathways that are necessary for CSC survival but not for the survival of normal stem cells.

Clinical testing of CSC-targeted therapies must take into account the relative infrequency of these cells within some tumors. Treatments that eradicate CSCs may not have significant effects on proliferation or apoptosis of the bulk of tumor cells[102] and therefore may not cause rapid tumor regression or shrinkage. There is a significant risk that agents that selectively target CSCs will be overlooked in clinical trials if assessed simply on the basis of objective tumor response. In the evaluation of CSC-targeted therapies, delay in tumor progression would be a more relevant clinical end point. In the end, the ultimate test of the effectiveness of a CSC-targeted agent is whether relapse is prevented, an end point that requires long-term follow-up. A corollary to this concept is that evaluation of toxicity toward normal stem cells should also be measured in long-term studies, in order to properly assess effects on tissue maintenance. As tumor shrinkage is not an accurate measure of the efficacy of agents that selectively kill CSCs, clinical evaluation would be greatly aided by the development of sensitive real-time imaging modalities to detect and quantify residual CSCs in patients who undergo treatment. However, such technology is currently unavailable. As discussed above, current protocols for isolating tumor cell fractions enriched in CSCs do not yield pure populations, thus it is problematic simply to correlate therapeutic effectiveness with eradication of a phenotypically

GENERAL PRINCIPLES

defined cell population. Ultimately, detection of residual CSCs with the ability to reinitiate tumor growth may depend on functional assays of tumorigenicity. However, such testing would be subject to the inherent limitations associated with *in vivo* detection of rare cells.

Resistance to Standard Therapy

The identification of CSCs in solid tumors and the development of *in vivo* assays to assess their tumorigenic properties have paved the way for studies to assess the impact of anticancer therapies on these cells. Radiation therapy for glioblastoma multiforme, an aggressive type of brain cancer, is transiently effective but is often followed by tumor recurrence or progression, implying that CSCs are not effectively eradicated. This notion is supported by recent evidence that ionizing-radiation treatment of glioblastoma grafts grown in mice leads to an increase in the proportion of CD133+ cells in the residual tumor population compared to unirradiated controls.[101] Irradiated CD133+ cells retain the ability to form heterogeneous tumors *in vivo* that can be serially propagated. *In vitro* experiments demonstrated that this radioresistance is likely due to increased activation of DNA damage checkpoint proteins and more efficient repair of DNA damage, resulting in a lower rate of apoptosis compared to CD133− cells. Intriguingly, treatment of CD133+ cells with an inhibitor of two checkpoint kinases disrupted their radioresistance, although the ability of treated cells to initiate tumor growth *in vivo* was not tested. A recent study that showed lower levels of pro-oxidants and higher expression of antioxidant genes in the CSC-enriched CD44+CD24−/lowLineage− cell population from primary human breast cancers compared to nontumorigenic cells suggests that lower levels of reactive oxygen species may also contribute to the relative radioresistance of CSCs.[103]

There have been a number of studies that indicated that CSCs may be resistant to standard chemotherapy. Following *in vitro* treatment of human pancreatic cancer cells with the nucleoside analogue gemcitabine, the CD133− population underwent apoptosis and was dramatically reduced, whereas most CD133+ cells survived, resulting in nearly 40-fold enrichment of the CD133+ fraction.[37] In addition, *in vivo* gemcitabine treatment of mice bearing pancreatic cancer cell line xenografts resulted in reduction of tumor bulk but approximately fourfold enrichment of the minority CD133+ population. These data suggest that the CSC-containing CD133+ cell population is relatively resistant to chemotherapy compared to non-CSCs. However, as discussed above, phenotypically defined populations enriched for CSCs are heterogeneous and contain non-CSCs as well. Thus, it is crucial to measure the effects of

treatment on CSCs directly through functional assays. For example, Li et al.[104] showed that human breast cancer biopsy samples obtained from patients treated with standard chemotherapy had increased percentages of CD44+CD24−/low cells and increased clonogenic efficiency *in vitro*, implying enrichment of CSCs. Importantly, posttreatment samples were twice as efficient at generating tumor xenografts when implanted into the mammary fat pads of SCID/Beige mice, confirming a functional enrichment of CSCs surviving in the treated tumors.

CD133+ human colon cancer cells are more resistant to apoptosis induced by *in vitro* treatment with 5-fluorouracil or oxaliplatin compared to CD133− cells.[105] *In vivo* oxaliplatin treatment of mice bearing colon cancer xenografts led to a reduction in tumor size but an increase in the percentage of CD133+ cells, with associated resistance of CD133+ cells to apoptosis. Cotreatment of mice with oxaliplatin plus a neutralizing antibody against IL-4 resulted in delayed tumor growth that persisted after treatment was discontinued, as well as increased apoptosis of CD133+ cells, leading to enhanced killing of these cells. These findings suggest that chemoresistance of colon CSCs may be related at least in part to autocrine IL-4 signaling, possibly through up-regulation of an antiapoptotic program.[105] Similarly, *in vivo* treatment of early passage colon cancer xenografts with cyclophosphamide led to slowing of tumor growth but enrichment of cells with a CSC phenotype and a twofold increase in CSC number measured by limiting dilution serial transplantation assays.[106] ALDH1 activity catabolizes the cytotoxic metabolites of cyclophosphamide; short hairpin RNA–mediated knockdown of ALDH1 sensitized tumors to cyclophosphamide treatment *in vivo* and reduced the frequency of CSCs in residual tumors. Thus, identification of functional pathways such as ALDH1 that are important for CSC survival can provide not only markers for isolating these cells, but potential therapeutic targets as well. Future studies using primary human tumors tested in *in vivo* functional assays will be required to determine the clinical importance of CSCs in tumor response and relapse.

Targeting the Microenvironment

Angiogenesis is a critical factor in the early stages of tumor formation as well as in tumor progression and therefore represents a potential target for anticancer treatments. Regulation of angiogenesis involves a complex interplay between tumor cells and the neovasculature. Glioblastomas, for example, express high levels of vascular endothelial growth factor (VEGF).[107] A functional interaction between brain CSCs and endothelial cells is supported by the close association of

CD133+ brain cancer cells with vascular endothelial cells *in vitro* and *in vivo*, and more importantly by the demonstration that coinjection of primary human endothelial cells enhances tumor formation by CD133+ medulloblastoma cells in immune-deficient mice.[102] Tumors initiated in mice by CD133+ cells from either primary glioblastoma biopsy specimens or xenograft cell lines are highly vascular.[107] Interestingly, treatment of xenograft tumors with bevacizumab, an antibody that neutralizes VEGF, not only potently inhibits tumor growth in mice[102,107] but also results in depletion of cells coexpressing CD133 and nestin, a marker of primitive neural cells, without directly affecting bulk tumor cell proliferation or death. Together, these results suggest that inhibition of brain tumor growth by antiangiogenic agents is mediated at least in part by disruption of a vascular niche required for maintenance of CSCs. For the most part, these experiments were done using brain cancer cell lines rather than freshly isolated tumor cells, but they nevertheless make a compelling case for further characterization and therapeutic targeting of the unique microenvironment of CSCs.

Ginestier et al.[16,108] recently showed that human breast cancer cells expressing CXCR1, a receptor that binds the proinflammatory chemokine IL-8, are present almost exclusively within the CSC-containing ALDH1+ population. IL-8 has been implicated in tumor invasion, metastasis, and self-renewal.[109,110] Treatment of orthotopically transplanted tumors in NOD/SCID mice with the CXCR1/2 inhibitor repertaxin, the standard chemotherapeutic agent docetaxel, or a combination of both drugs all resulted in impaired tumor growth. However, tumors treated with docetaxel alone showed either unchanged or increased percentage of ALDH1+ cells compared with untreated controls, whereas repertaxin treatment alone or in combination with docetaxel significantly reduced the ALDH1+ population. Importantly, upon serial transplantation, tumor cells derived from control or docetaxel-treated primary animals were able to generate tumors in secondary mice with similar efficiency, while cells from repertaxin-treated animals showed a two- to fivefold reduction in tumor growth and were only able to generate tumors at the highest injected cell dose. These findings indicate that, contrary to standard chemotherapy with docetaxel, CXCR1 blockade with repertaxin directly targets and reduces the CSC population *in vivo* and underscore the importance of directly assaying effects on CSCs rather than relying on traditional measures of efficacy such as reduction of tumor bulk.

Differentiation Therapy

Another approach to anticancer therapy is induction of differentiation of CSCs, with consequent associated loss of self-renewal capacity. This strategy has been highly successful in acute promyelocytic leukemia (APL), where the addition of retinoic acid to conventional chemotherapy has significantly improved survival rates. The demonstration that the growth of solid tumors is sustained by CSCs with the capacity to generate tumor heterogeneity implies that it should be similarly possible to drive the differentiation of CSCs in these cancers. However, the clinical development of differentiation-inducing agents to treat solid tumors has been limited to date. Bone morphogenic proteins (BMPs) are soluble factors that induce normal neural precursor cells to differentiate. BMP treatment of CD133+ glioblastoma cells *in vitro* or in immune-deficient mice results in the formation of smaller, more differentiated, less invasive tumor grafts that cannot be serially propagated in mice,[111] demonstrating the therapeutic potential of differentiation-inducing agents in brain cancer. However, the differentiation response to BMP treatment may be impaired in a subset of glioblastoma CSCs due to epigenetic silencing of BMP receptor 1B (*BMPR1B*), a feature shared with early embryonic neural stem cells.[112] Indeed, in patient-derived glioblastoma cells with reduced *BMPR1B* expression, BMP2 induced proliferation rather than differentiation. Transgenic expression of a constitutively active BMPR1B mutant in these cells followed by orthotopic injection into neonatal SCID mice resulted in higher expression of GFAP by tumor cells, impaired tumor growth, and improved host survival compared to unmanipulated tumor cells. *BMPR1B* down-regulation was found in approximately 20% of primary human glioblastomas. This elegant study not only provides insight into the role of BMPs in brain CSC biology, but highlights the existence of intertumor CSC variability, even among tumors of the same histological class. As discussed above, tumor heterogeneity is likely related in large part to differences in the underlying oncogenic changes that drive tumor growth. Thus, therapeutic approaches such as induction of differentiation may require targeting of multiple pathways and will likely need to be tailored to some degree to the biology of individual tumors. A recent unbiased RNA interference screen identified several genes whose silencing induced a "differentiation phenotype" in glioblastoma cells derived from multiple patients' tumors.[113] The strongest and most reproducible of these was *TRRAP*, which encodes an adaptor protein found in multiprotein/chromatin complexes. Knockdown of TRRAP in three different patient-derived glioblastoma lines followed by orthotopic injection into SCID mice resulted in impaired tumor growth, a more differentiated xenograft phenotype, and improved host survival compared to control cells. Future studies are required to determine the applicability and efficacy of these treatment approaches in the clinic.

GENERAL PRINCIPLES

Selected References

The full list of references for this chapter appears in the online version.

1. Bruce WR, van der Gaag H. A quantitative assay for the number of murine lymphoma cells capable of proliferation in vivo. *Nature* 1963;199:79.
2. Southam CM, Brunschwig A, Dizon Q. Autologous and homologous transplantation of human cancer. In: Brennan MJ, Simpson WL, eds. *Biological interactions in normal and neoplastic growth. A contribution to the host-tumor problem.* Boston: Little, Brown, 1962:723.
5. Lapidot T, Sirard C, Vormoor J, et al. A cell initiating human acute myeloid leukemia after transplantation into SCID mice. *Nature* 1994;367:645.
6. Bonnet D, Dick JE. Human acute myeloid leukemia is organized as a hierarchy that originates from a primitive hematopoietic cell. *Nat Med* 1997;3:730.
7. Jordan CT, Upchurch D, Szilvassy SJ, et al. The interleukin-3 receptor alpha chain is a unique marker for human acute myelogenous leukemia stem cells. *Leukemia* 2000; 14:1777.
8. Jin L, Lee EM, Ramshaw HS, et al. Monoclonal antibody-mediated targeting of CD123, IL-3 receptor alpha chain, eliminates human acute myeloid leukemic stem cells. *Cell Stem Cell* 2009;5:31.
10. Guzman ML, Rossi RM, Karnischky L, et al. The sesquiterpene lactone parthenolide induces apoptosis of human acute myelogenous leukemia stem and progenitor cells. *Blood* 2005;105:4163.
12. Yilmaz OH, Valdez R, Theisen BK, et al. Pten dependence distinguishes haematopoietic stem cells from leukaemia-initiating cells. *Nature* 2006;441:475.
14. Jin L, Hope KJ, Zhai Q, et al. Targeting of CD44 eradicates human acute myeloid leukemic stem cells. *Nat Med* 2006;12:1167.
15. Al Hajj M, Wicha MS, Benito-Hernandez A, et al. Prospective identification of tumorigenic breast cancer cells. *Proc Natl Acad Sci U S A* 2003;100:3983.
21. Singh SK, Hawkins C, Clarke ID, et al. Identification of human brain tumour initiating cells. *Nature* 2004;432: 396.
25. Chen R, Nishimura MC, Bumbaca SM, et al. A hierarchy of self-renewing tumor-initiating cell types in glioblastoma. *Cancer Cell* 2010;17:362.
28. O'Brien CA, Pollett A, Gallinger S, et al. A human colon cancer cell capable of initiating tumour growth in immunodeficient mice. *Nature* 2007;445:106.
29. Ricci-Vitiani L, Lombardi DG, Pilozzi E, et al. Identification and expansion of human colon-cancer-initiating cells. *Nature* 2007;445:111.
30. Hope KJ, Jin L, Dick JE. Acute myeloid leukemia originates from a hierarchy of leukemic stem cell classes that differ in self-renewal capacity. *Nat Immunol* 2004;5:738.
37. Hermann PC, Huber SL, Herrler T, et al. Distinct populations of cancer stem cells determine tumor growth and metastatic activity in human pancreatic cancer. *Cell Stem Cell* 2007;1:313.
38. Kelly PN, Dakic A, Adams JM, et al. Tumor growth need not be driven by rare cancer stem cells. *Science* 2007;317: 337.
40. Quintana E, Shackleton M, Sabel MS, et al. Efficient tumour formation by single human melanoma cells. *Nature* 2008;456:593.
42. Kennedy JA, Barabe F, Poeppl AG, et al. Comment on "Tumor growth need not be driven by rare cancer stem cells." *Science* 2007;318:1722.
42a. Ishizawa K, Rasheed ZA, Karisch R, et al. Tumor-initiating cells are rare in many human tumors. *Cell Stem Cell* 2010;7:279.
43. Huntly BJ, Shigematsu H, Deguchi K, et al. MOZ-TIF2, but not BCR-ABL, confers properties of leukemic stem cells to committed murine hematopoietic progenitors. *Cancer Cell* 2004;6:587.

44. Barabe F, Kennedy JA, Hope KJ, et al. Modeling the initiation and progression of human acute leukemia in mice. *Science* 2007;316:600.
45. Krivtsov AV, Twomey D, Feng Z, et al. Transformation from committed progenitor to leukaemia stem cell initiated by MLL-AF9. *Nature* 2006;442:818.
48. Marusyk A, Polyak K. Tumor heterogeneity: causes and consequences. *Biochim Biophys Acta* 2010;1805:105.
54. Notta F, Mullighan CG, Wang JCY, et al. Evolution of human BCR-ALB1 lymphoblastic leukaemia-initiating cells. *Nature In Press.*
54a. Anderson K, Lutz C, van Delft FW, et al. Genetic variegation of clonal architecture and propagating cells in leukaemia. *Nature* 2010 doi:10.1038/nature09650.
60. So CW, Karsunky H, Passegue E, et al. MLL-GAS7 transforms multipotent hematopoietic progenitors and induces mixed lineage leukemias in mice. *Cancer Cell* 2003;3:161.
61. Cozzio A, Passegue E, Ayton PM, et al. Similar MLL-associated leukemias arising from self-renewing stem cells and short-lived myeloid progenitors. *Genes Dev* 2003;17: 3029.
62. Chen W, Kumar AR, Hudson WA, et al. Malignant transformation initiated by Mll-Af9: gene dosage and critical target cells. *Cancer Cell* 2008;13:432.
63. Somervaille TC, Cleary ML. Identification and characterization of leukemia stem cells in murine MLL-AF9 acute myeloid leukemia. *Cancer Cell* 2006;10:257.
67. Passegue E, Wagner EF, Weissman IL. JunB deficiency leads to a myeloproliferative disorder arising from hematopoietic stem cells. *Cell* 2004;119:431.
70. Jamieson CH, Ailles LE, Dylla SJ, et al. Granulocyte-macrophage progenitors as candidate leukemic stem cells in blast-crisis CML. *N Engl J Med* 2004;351:657.
78. Lim E, Vaillant F, Wu D, et al. Aberrant luminal progenitors as the candidate target population for basal tumor development in BRCA1 mutation carriers. *Nat Med* 2009; 15:907.
79. Dai C, Celestino JC, Okada Y, et al. PDGF autocrine stimulation dedifferentiates cultured astrocytes and induces oligodendrogliomas and oligoastrocytomas from neural progenitors and astrocytes in vivo. *Genes Dev* 2001;15: 1913.
80. Holland EC, Celestino J, Dai C, et al. Combined activation of Ras and Akt in neural progenitors induces glioblastoma formation in mice. *Nat Genet* 2000;25:55.
82. Bruggeman SW, Hulsman D, Tanger E, et al. Bmi1 controls tumor development in an Ink4a/Arf-independent manner in a mouse model for glioma. *Cancer Cell* 2007;12:328.
84. Schuller U, Heine VM, Mao J, et al. Acquisition of granule neuron precursor identity is a critical determinant of progenitor cell competence to form Shh-induced medulloblastoma. *Cancer Cell* 2008;14:123.
85. Yang ZJ, Ellis T, Markant SL, et al. Medulloblastoma can be initiated by deletion of Patched in lineage-restricted progenitors or stem cells. *Cancer Cell* 2008;14:135.
90. Zhu L, Gibson P, Currle DS, et al. Prominin 1 marks intestinal stem cells that are susceptible to neoplastic transformation. *Nature* 2009;457:603.
92. Barker N, Ridgway RA, van Es JH, et al. Crypt stem cells as the cells-of-origin of intestinal cancer. *Nature* 2009;457: 608.
96. Mani SA, Guo W, Liao MJ, et al. The epithelial-mesenchymal transition generates cells with properties of stem cells. *Cell* 2008;133:704.
100. Gupta PB, Onder TT, Jiang G, et al. Identification of selective inhibitors of cancer stem cells by high-throughput screening. *Cell* 2009;138:645.
101. Bao S, Wu Q, McLendon RE, et al. Glioma stem cells promote radioresistance by preferential activation of the DNA damage response. *Nature* 2006;444:756.
102. Calabrese C, Poppleton H, Kocak M, et al. A perivascular niche for brain tumor stem cells. *Cancer Cell* 2007; 11:69.

104. Li X, Lewis MT, Huang J, et al. Intrinsic resistance of tumorigenic breast cancer cells to chemotherapy. *J Natl Cancer Inst* 2008;100:672.

105. Todaro M, Alea MP, Di Stefano AB, et al. Colon cancer stem cells dictate tumor growth and resist cell death by production of interleukin-4. *Cell Stem Cell* 2007;1: 389.

106. Dylla SJ, Beviglia L, Park IK, et al. Colorectal cancer stem cells are enriched in xenogeneic tumors following chemotherapy. *PLoS One* 2008;3:e2428.

107. Bao S, Wu Q, Sathornsumetee S, et al. Stem cell-like glioma cells promote tumor angiogenesis through vascular endothelial growth factor. *Cancer Res* 2006;66:7843.

108. Ginestier C, Liu S, Diebel ME, et al. CXCR1 blockade selectively targets human breast cancer stem cells in vitro and in xenografts. *J Clin Invest* 2010;120:485.

111. Piccirillo SG, Reynolds BA, Zanetti N, et al. Bone morphogenetic proteins inhibit the tumorigenic potential of human brain tumour-initiating cells. *Nature* 2006;444:761.

112. Lee J, Son MJ, Woolard K, et al. Epigenetic-mediated dysfunction of the bone morphogenetic protein pathway inhibits differentiation of glioblastoma-initiating cells. *Cancer Cell* 2008;13:69.

113. Wurdak H, Zhu S, Romero A, et al. An RNAi screen identifies TRRAP as a regulator of brain tumor-initiating cell differentiation. *Cell Stem Cell* 2010;6:37.

CHAPTER 12 BIOLOGY OF PERSONALIZED CANCER MEDICINE

RAJU KUCHERLAPATI

It is well established that cancer is a genetic disease. At the genetic level cancer cells are different from their precursor cells. It is understood that a series of genetic changes are necessary for a normal cell to begin the process of transformation, eventually leading to cancer. Cancers can be generally classified into sporadic cancers and those that result from a genetic predisposition. Some individuals in the population inherit specific mutations in particular genes that predispose them to certain types of cancers. Although these individuals are born with a mutation in a predisposition gene, they do not develop tumors until later in life; and it is now well understood that, besides the inherited predisposition gene mutation, additional genetic changes are required for the cells in these individuals to become tumors. In sporadic cases a randomly acquired somatic mutation or another type of genetic change in a gene that is critical for the normal regulation of growth in the appropriate cell type might initiate a series of events that eventually leads to tumor formation. In addition to genetic mutations, changes in copy number of individual genes or subsets of genes; chromosomal aberrations including translocations, insertions, deletions and inversions; and changes in expression patterns of genes as well as epigenetic changes also play critical roles in tumor susceptibility, tumor initiation, and progression. Understanding all of the important genetic and genomic changes in each cancer type will help in accurate diagnosis and prognosis and increase the ability to stratify the patient populations to help assess the most optimal treatments for each patient. The use of such genetic and genomic information to determine treatment decisions is referred to as *personalized medicine*. Knowledge about the genetic and genomic changes that accompany cellular transformation and the events that are critical for initiation and maintenance of the cancerous state is increasing at a rapid pace. Because most cancers are clonal in origin and because it is possible to obtain an adequate amount of tumor material from tumor biopsies or resections, it is now possible to examine and document the genetic and genomic changes in tumor cells very accurately. As a result,

understanding of the genetic and genomic changes in cancer is significantly greater than many other human diseases. This knowledge allows implementation of the principles of personalized medicine into clinical management of cancer patients. This chapter will consider examples of how cancer genetics and genomics are affecting the ability to manage cancer patients.

CANCER PREDISPOSITION

There is a large body of evidence that indicates that certain families have a higher incidence of a particular cancer. Epidemiological studies reveal that family members descendant from individuals who developed cancer, especially at a younger age, have a higher risk of developing cancer. This was followed by studies of families where the predisposition to develop cancer was found to be inherited. Another line of evidence that reveals the genetic basis for cancer came from studies of twins. Monozygotic twins have the same genetic composition, while dizygotic twins have a 50% probability of sharing an identical copy of any gene. The fact that there is a higher concordance of cancer incidence in monozygotic twins but not in dizygotic twins provides additional critical evidence for the genetic basis of cancer.[1] Studies during the past half century have established not only the familial predisposition of cancer but also to identified several genes that are involved in cancer predisposition. That knowledge, in turn, helps to explain the genetic processes and mechanisms that lead to cancer and to develop tests to identify individuals at risk for certain types of cancers.

There are several examples of gene mutations that are responsible for cancer predisposition. Cancers that show a familial predisposition include childhood retinoblastoma, colorectal cancer, early onset breast cancer, and several types of renal cancer, among many others. One cancer type where there is a large amount of information about familial predisposition is colorectal cancer (CRC).[2] CRC is one of the most common cancers, and it is estimated that as many 875,000 new cases of CRC are diagnosed every year in the world. The greater accessibility of the colon and rectum to detect or follow the cancer as well as the relative ease of obtaining biopsies facilitate study of this cancer.

CRC can be classified into familial cases and sporadic cases. Various estimates of the relative proportions of these two categories of CRC have been made and in some estimates the familial cases represent 10% of all CRCs, while other estimates place this number to be 25% or more.[3] Several genes that are involved in familial cases have been identified and are discussed in the sections that follow.

FAMILIAL ADENOMATOUS POLYPOSIS

Individuals with familiar adenomatous polyposis (FAP) are born normally and develop hundred to thousands of benign colonic polyps during their early adulthood. Unless these tumors are detected and treated (usually by surgery), one or more of them may develop into adenocarcinomas that can metastasize. Family studies revealed that this predisposition was inherited in an autosomal dominant fashion, and individuals who have inherited the susceptibility allele almost always exhibit the phenotype (near 100% penetrance). Linkage analysis revealed that the gene for FAP is located on human chromosome 5. Positional cloning has enabled the cloning of the gene that was designated as adenomatous polyposis coli (APC).[4,5] APC is a classic tumor suppressor gene, and inactivation or modification of both copies of the gene is necessary for the initiation of CRC development.

APC plays an important role not only in the relatively rare cases of FAP but also in a majority of sporadic CRC. Most of the sporadic colorectal tumors are also the result of the inactivation of both copies of the APC gene, but unlike FAP, where one copy is already mutated in the germline, in sporadic cases both copies are sequentially mutated in somatic colonic epithelial cells.[6] This observation explains the earlier onset of tumors and the abundance of tumors in FAP patients.

Since FAP is inherited in an autosomal dominant fashion and since individuals with FAP are born with a mutation in the APC gene, when an individual with FAP is identified it is recognized that all of the immediate family members are at risk to carry the mutant allele. The siblings of the affected individual are at 50% risk, and other relatives would also be at risk depending on the nature of familial relationship. Because the diagnosis of FAP is unambiguous, genetic testing is not always conducted. It is most desirable to sequence the germline DNA of the affected individual to identify the mutation, inform the relatives of their risk, and

recommend the testing for the specific mutation as appropriate.

LYNCH SYNDROME

Another predisposition to CRC is Lynch syndrome (LS), named after Henry Lynch who first described this syndrome.[7] LS is also inherited as an autosomal dominant disorder, and individuals who inherit a disease allele develop CRC at an earlier age than sporadic CRC but later than FAP patients. The manifestation of colorectal neoplasms in individuals with this syndrome is less severe than in FAP patients, with the development of a few tumors later in life.

It was noted that the LS tumors have a unique feature in that they show genetic instability as revealed by expansion or contraction of the length of microsatellites.[8-10] Based on these observations these tumors are classified as microsatellite instable (MSI+). This knowledge of microsatellite instability plays an important role in discovering the genes important for LS. The first gene that was responsible for a subset of LS cases was found to be a human gene that has homology to a bacterial gene that is necessary for repairing single nucleotide mismatches and small insertions or deletions that result from errors in DNA replication.[11,12] This gene was designated Mut S homolog 2 (MSH2). MSH2 encodes a protein that is required for recognition and repair of DNA mismatches. It was later discovered that mutations in other genes that encode members of the mismatch repair complex also cause LS. In addition to MSH2 the genes that encode other members of this complex that are now known to be involved are Mut L homolog 1 (MLH1), Mut S homolog 6 (MSH6), postmeiotic segregation 2 (PMS2), and Mut L homolog 3 (MLH3). Mutations in all of these genes are now implicated in colon cancer susceptibility.[11,13-18]

Relatives of LS patients are also at increased risk to carry the mutant gene and, therefore, for CRC. As is the case for FAP it would be desirable to establish the specific mutation that causes LS and test the immediate relatives to establish or rule out the presence of the specific mutation in their germline. The presence or absence of mismatch repair proteins, especially MLH1, can also be detected by immunological methods, and individuals whose tumors do not have a detectable level of MLH1 are excellent candidates for testing of their germline; if a germline mutation in the gene is detected, informing that patient's immediate relatives and testing them for the specific mutation may be warranted.

The precise incidence of LS in the population has been difficult to assess. Because individuals with LS develop fewer tumors and later in life than those with FAP, they are more difficult to distinguish from sporadic cases, and, therefore, testing for LS has not become routine. According to some studies the incidence of LS among patients with colorectal neoplasms is as high as 3%.[19] These results suggest that examination of all colorectal tumors for its MSI status and testing for mismatch repair gene mutations in individuals whose tumors are MSI+ may help identify individual at risk with a greater efficiency.[20,21]

OTHER POLYPOSIS SYNDROMES

There are other syndromes that are relatively rare that predispose individuals to CRC risk. These include Peutz-Jeghers syndrome, juvenile polyposis, and Cowden's disease. Genes that are involved in these syndromes have been identified and include *LKB1*, *SMAD4*, *BMPR1A*, and *PTEN*. Although all of the syndromes mentioned above are inherited in a dominant fashion, mutations in *MYH*, a homolog of an excision repair gene in *Escherichia coli*, cause a tumor predisposition but in a recessive fashion (de la Chapelle[22] gives a detailed review).

ASSOCIATION STUDIES

Most of the genetic mutations in genes described above result in CRC with high penetrance. This raises the question if there are other genes where mutations or variants cause a predisposition to CRC but with lower penetrance. Studies of sibling pairs that are concordant or discordant for CRC as well as association studies have identified regions of the genome or single nucleotide polymorphisms (SNP) that may be important in CRC susceptibility. One such polymorphism is that located on human chromosome 8. In an initial study Zanke et al.[23] examined a large cohort of individuals who had large bowel cancer and an equal number of controls for associations with genes or variants in the genome. In this study they identified SNPs at 8q24, which shows significant association with susceptibility to colon cancer. This region was also shown to be responsible for susceptibility to several other cancers.[24,25] Additional follow-up studies confirmed and extended these observations, implicating other regions of the genome in susceptibility to colon cancer among "sporadic" cancer cases.[26] Like several other SNP variants that have been shown to be associated with complex diseases, the SNPs at 8q24 also lie in a region that is not known to harbor any genes. However, Pomerantz et al.[27] were able to show that this variant is functionally important in regulating the expression of the cellular oncogene c-myc that is located a few hundred kilobases away from the variant. This group also showed that variants at 8q24 that are known to be involved in other solid tumors also act through their action on the myc oncogene.[28] These results suggest that it might be possible to identify individuals within the general population that show susceptibility to several different solid tumors. Identification of such susceptible individuals may, in turn, help in more careful monitoring or other interventions, which may lead to prevention of the cancers.

BREAST CANCER

Susceptibility to early onset breast cancer has been extensively studied. It was recognized that certain families have a high incidence of breast and ovarian cancers. Careful examination of these families revealed that the predisposition to these cancers is inherited in an autosomal dominant fashion. Genetic linkage analysis revealed that, at least in some families, this trait is linked to markers on human chromosome 17.[29] When positional cloning approaches became available, it was determined that mutations in a gene on this chromosome were found to be responsible for this predisposition.[30,31] That gene was designated *BRCA1* (BReast CAncer-1). In other families a second gene, *BRCA2*, located on chromosome 13, was found to be involved in the cancer predisposition. Women who inherit a mutation either in *BRCA1* or *BRCA2* are at high risk for development of breast or ovarian cancer. Mutations in these genes can be inherited or they could result from new mutational events. If an individual with mutations in either *BRCA1* or *BRCA2* has been identified, it would be important to assess if other members in their family are at risk. If inherited, since the mutations are dominant acting, each of the immediate relatives (siblings) would have a 50% risk of carrying the same mutation and therefore would also be at high risk for developing cancer. Individuals with known pathogenic mutations may elect prophylactic mastectomy and oophorectomy or careful surveillance to detect tumors at their earliest stage.

Testing individuals at high risk for breast cancer or colon cancer is a common practice. If an individual tests positive for a pathogenic mutation, it is prudent to test for the presence of the same mutation in that individual's immediate relatives and manage them based on the results.

It is estimated that only a fraction of women that carry a pathogenic mutation in *BRCA1* or *BRCA2* are detected. Detection of these mutations well in advance of the time at which they would develop their first breast or ovarian tumor would have significant positive implications for their health. A relatively simple way of identifying individuals at risk is through the use of family history. Several family history tools are available, and one that was developed by the surgeon general of the United States is easily accessible and free of charge on the U.S. Department of Health and Human Services Web site (search for "My Family Health Portrait Tool"). Algorithms that can assess relative risk have been developed, and depending on these risk predictions, appropriate individuals may be recommended to undergo genetic testing.

EARLY DETECTION

It is well established that the long-term survival of patients, whose tumors were diagnosed at early stages, are significantly greater than those whose tumors are detected at a later stage. For example, the long-term survival of patients whose colonic tumors were detected at stage I is 95%, while it is only 5% when the tumors are detected at stage IV.

There are different methods for early detection of cancers. For colon cancer detection, colonoscopies are recommended for all individuals over the age 50. Palpation of the prostate is a routine procedure during annual medical examinations. Mammograms are useful in detecting at least a significant portion of breast tumors. Some of these methods are expensive and patient compliance is not adequately high. Alternative strategies for detection of cancer at early stages are in development.

One approach to identify such markers was used by Faca et al.[32] In this study, a murine model for pancreatic cancer was used as a starting point. These mice reliably develop pancreatic tumors during specific periods of their life. Plasma samples from these mice at different stages of tumor development were sampled and analyzed for their protein composition using proteomic approaches. Several proteins that were found to be overexpressed during early stages of cancer were examined in the blood from 30 newly diagnosed patients with pancreatic cancer and an appropriate set of 30 controls. This approach enabled them to identify a panel of five proteins that was able to discriminate pancreatic cancer cases from matched controls in blood specimens obtained as much as 12 months prior to the diagnosis of pancreatic cancer. Similar approaches enabled identification of protein markers that are important for ovarian and colon cancers.[33,34]

The reason why tumor-specific markers can be detected in the circulating system prior to clinical diagnosis of disease is not well understood. It is possible that some tumor cells die, releasing their contents into circulation. Alternatively, some subsets of tumor cells escape their original site and are in circulation. Such cells are referred to as circulating tumor cells (CTC). Escape of tumor cells from their source of origin and entering the circulation is, of course, an important step in metastasis. Methods to detect CTC have advanced significantly in the past few years. It has been long known that tumor cells may express novel proteins on their cell surface. Although antibodies against many of these proteins are available, purification of circulating tumors cells proved to be difficult. However, many of the solid tumors are derived from epithelial cells, and such cells are not normally part of the circulation. Therefore, epithelial cell markers can be used as capture agents. This approach, together with the development of novel flow cells that allow for slow and gentle movement of cells through a substrate coated with the appropriate antibodies, is now shown to be a suitable method for capturing these rare circulating tumor cells.[35] The availability of intact cells will allow more detailed molecular examination of tumor cells, which could prove to be powerful in early diagnosis. It is important, however, to understand how well these circulating cells reflect the state of the tumor at its initial location. The ability to isolate circulating tumor cells has significant implications for our ability to understand the nature of the tumor and to devise appropriate interventions for the patients.

TUMOR CLASSIFICATION AND PATIENT STRATIFICATION

Assessment of the molecular origins of tumors and the molecular profiles of the tumors has important implications for accurate diagnosis, determination of the prognosis, and treatment decisions for a patient. Methodologies for assessing such features are rapidly evolving.

Early methods of tumor classification were based on cytogenetic methods in hematological malignancies. The first of chromosomal translocations that was identified as important in human cancer is the t(9;22)(q34;q11) associated with chronic myelogenous leukemia (CML).[36] Because the discovery was made from investigators from Philadelphia, this rearranged chromosome has been designated the Philadelphia chromosome. During the past 40 years hundreds of such translocations have been described in many different malignancies, and more than 300 different genes have been implicated in these abnormalities. For example, in acute myeloid leukemia 267 balanced rearrangements have been described.[37] These translocations sometimes result in inappropriate activation of genes or the creation of novel fusion genes, with novel functions resulting in cancer. The nature of these translocations is critical for accurate diagnosis and in several cases for targeted therapies. Although a majority of these translocations are described in hematological malignancies, several such translocations have been described in solid tumors, and it is now clear that such translocations are also common in most, if not all, solid tumors.[38,39] As is the case for hematological malignancies, specific translocations would not only help classify the tumors but also may provide novel targets for drug development. One such example is the EML-ALK4 translocation in lung cancer.[38]

Diagnosis of tumors can also be made on the basis of the gene expression profiles of the tumor.

An example is the distinction between Burkitt's lymphoma and large B-cell lymphoma. These two disorders are treated differently, and, therefore, it is important to distinguish between them accurately. The diagnosis of Burkitt's lymphoma is largely based on morphologic findings, immunological data, and cytogenetic features. Diffuse large B-cell lymphoma and Burkitt's lymphoma have some overlapping clinical features. In addition, Burkitt's lymphoma has the t(8;14) translocation that results in the activation of the myc oncogene, but this translocation is also present in a subset of diffuse large B-cell lymphoma. Examination of Burkitt's lymphoma cases and large B-cell lymphoma samples by global gene expression profile analysis enabled the identification of a panel of genes whose expression profiles can distinguish the two categories with a very high level of accuracy.[40]

Some novel tests based on the patterns of gene expression profiling have been developed, and intensive efforts for additional tests are currently under way. An example of a type of test that was developed was one to predict the recurrence of cancer in women with tamoxifen-treated, node-negative breast cancer.[41] RNA extracted from paraffin-embedded sections of breast tumors from women who were enrolled in a clinical trial to study the effects of tamoxifen treatment were examined for expression of a panel of 21 genes. Based on the analysis of the data the investigators were able to translate the data into a recurrence score. It is likely that similar efforts with either gene expression profiles or protein expression profiles of tumors will result in identification of marker sets that can be used for accurate diagnosis and prognosis of many tumor types.

Efforts to use comprehensive genomic data for tumor diagnosis and stratification are proving to be extremely valuable. An example is the examination of human glioblastomas.[42] In this study several groups of investigators examined tumor samples from human glioblastomas and the corresponding normal DNA from the same patients for changes in gene and genomic copy number, gene expression profiles, and the mutational status of a large number of genes. Based on this comprehensive analysis this group of investigators was able to classify the tumors and assess the pathways that are deregulated in this cancer type. Similar types of efforts are under way for many other cancer types.

Other investigations have focused on a comprehensive examination of genetic changes in tumor cells and tumor tissue. These efforts have examined all of the coding regions of the tumor genome and in some cases the complete genomes of tumors.[43–46]

TREATMENT

As the understanding of the genetic and genomic changes that are responsible for tumor progression increases, it is becoming possible to understand the particular genetic changes and biochemical pathways that are modified in tumor cells. This knowledge, in turn, helps determine which patients are most likely to benefit from which drugs. There are several excellent examples of this feature and others are emerging rapidly. Some of these are briefly described below.

One of the first examples of a targeted therapy is for CML. In 1960 Nowell and Hungerford[47] described a marker chromosome in a human leukemia. In 1973 Rowley[48] defined this marker chromosome, designated the Philadelphia chromosome, to be the result of a translocation involving human chromosomes 9 and 22. It was later shown that this specific translocation results in a novel fusion gene product that involves a break point cluster region (BCR) and an oncogene that is homologous to the Abelson murine leukemia virus (ABL). The fusion product, designated BCR-ABL, is a tyrosine kinase and is expressed only in these tumor cells. It has been shown that the formation of this fusion gene is sufficient for the cells to become transformed. Mutational analysis of the fusion gene revealed that the loss of function of this protein leads to loss of its oncogenic activity. These observations led to the development of a specific inhibitor for this fusion protein. The drug, originally designated STI571, now imatinib, was found to be efficacious in preclinical studies. Clinical studies with this drug revealed that the drug that is orally administered is relatively safe and as many as 98% of the CML patients showed hematologic response in as little as 4 weeks of drug administration.[49,50] Additional studies showed that the drug's effects favorably compare with standard therapy for newly diagnosed CML patients. This is the current choice of drug for CML that is diagnosed to have the Philadelphia chromosome.

A second example of targeted therapy is for a subset of breast cancer patients. A subset of breast cancers (20% to 30%) are known to have amplification of a growth factor receptor gene, ERBB2 (HER2). Women whose breast cancers have a high level of expression of this gene have a shortened survival. It has been shown that the amplification of the HER2 gene is directly involved in the pathogenesis. Therefore, it was considered that development of inhibitors of this protein, which is expressed on the surface of the tumor cells, might provide an approach to treat these breast cancer patients. Several antibodies directed against this target were found to bind this target with high affinity and inhibit their proliferation. A humanized murine monoclonal antibody was developed as a therapeutic agent. This drug, trastuzumab, was found to be relatively safe, and its administration resulted in better disease-free progression and higher rates of overall response compared to chemotherapy alone. Combination of chemotherapy and trastuzumab improved the outcomes even more.[51,52] Based on these clinical trails the drug was approved and is currently the standard of therapy for patients whose breast tumors have amplification of HER2.

The role of genetic changes in drug response was well described in non–small cell lung cancer (NSCLC). Until the early part of this century the most widely used treatment for NSCLC has been chemotherapy, which results in a small increase in survival and is associated with several adverse effects. It was known that these lung cancer cells express higher levels of epidermal growth factor (EGFR) as compared to normal lung cells. EGFR is a member of a class of transmembrane signaling proteins. In the presence of its ligand, epidermal growth factor, the receptor dimerizes, resulting in phosphorylation of tyrosine in the intracellular domain and leading to a cascade of events that promote cell growth. One of the drugs that was developed to inhibit this tyrosine kinase activity is gefitinib. Treatment of patients with gefitinib resulted in variable responses among individuals with lung cancer. In early clinical trials individuals from Japan had better responses than those from the United States, and female never-smokers were better responders among both ethnic groups. In the United States the response rates were less than 20%, and the response did not correlate with EGFR levels as measured by immunohistochemistry. To understand the basis for this variable response, one group hypothesized that mutations in a receptor tyrosine kinase may be responsible for drug response.[53] To test this hypothesis they obtained tumor DNA samples from tumors prior to treatment and examined the DNA for mutations in the activation loops of 47 receptor kinase genes. A small number of tumors had heterozygous mutations in the EGFR gene. A more comprehensive examination revealed heterozygous missense and deletion mutations in a region corresponding to proximity of the adenosine triphosphate (ATP) binding cleft and the target of the drug gefitinib. Tumor DNA from patients who responded to the drug, obtained prior to initiation of treatment, had a mutation in EGFR in all responders, while only 1 of 61 nonselected patients had such a mutation. They were also able to show that lung caner cell lines that carried one of the mutations responded to low doses of gefitinib and also inhibited the autophosphorylation of the EGFR protein.

A second group of investigators reasoned that since the drug targets EGFR, mutations in that gene might be responsible for the differential effect of the drug.[54] To test this hypothesis they examined the biopsy samples from patients who later showed responses to gefitinib. These studies revealed that of the nine samples examined, eight had genetic changes in the region of the gene corresponding to the intracellular domain of the protein. The nature of the mutations detected were also point mutations, leading to a change in amino acid and deletions that resulted in loss of a few amino acids of the protein. No such mutations were detected in other tumor types, and the changes were found to be somatic. Using transient transfection of the mutant version of the gene into mammalian cells revealed that the mutations led to hyperactivation of the protein and to better responses to the drug at lower concentrations.

Both of these studies and another study published soon after[55] revealed that in NSCLC, the target of the drug gefitinib acquires certain somatic mutations, some of which result in activation of the protein. It is those patients whose EGFR has acquired one of these activation mutations who respond to the drug. These observations paved the way for the development of a molecular diagnostic test to identify patients who might be better responders to the tyrosine kinase inhibitors gefitinib and erlotinib.

To clinically assess if selection of patients whose lung tumors had an activation mutation would respond better to a tyrosine kinase inhibitor, several clinical trials were conducted. Although the trail designs and the number of patients in each trial varied, the general schema of several clinical trials was to examine the tumor DNA for EGFR mutations and assess their response rates and progression-free survival as well as long-term survival benefits of the drug.

In one study Mok et al.[56] compared the effectiveness of chemotherapy versus gefitinib treatment in patients with lung cancer. In a phase 3 study, they randomly assigned treatment-naive patients to receive gefitinib or chemotherapy. They observed that in the cohort who had EGFR mutations both the response rates as well as progression-free survival were better in the mutation-positive group. Interestingly, in the mutation-negative cohort chemotherapy yielded better response rates and better progression-free survival. These trial results suggest that patient stratification based on EGFR status and treatment with a tyrosine kinase inhibitor for mutation-positive patients and chemotherapy for mutation-negative patients would yield optimal response rates.

DEVELOPMENT OF RESISTANCE TO TYROSINE KINASE INHIBITORS

Despite the fact that individuals whose tumors have an activation mutation in EGFR respond better to tyrosine kinase inhibitors and such treatment leads to longer survival, all patients appear to relapse and tumor begins to grow again. To understand the basis for this relapse Kobayashi et al.[57] obtained a biopsy sample from a relapsed patient and examined the status of the EGFR gene in the sample prior to treatment and the sample after relapse. Using direct DNA sequencing and sequencing of cDNA prepared from the tumor RNA sample, they observed that the relapsed tumor contained a novel mutation in the *EGFR* gene that resulted in a T790M mutation. Using molecular biological methods the investigators showed that the presence of this mutation in the background of an original responsive mutation rendered the EGFR protein 100 times more resistant to the drug. When they tested cells carrying the resistant allele with four commercial EGFR inhibitors, they found that an irreversible inhibitor of EGFR strongly inhibited EGFR function at relatively low concentrations. This observation suggested that periodic genetic monitoring of the tumor prior to treatment and at the time of relapse might help in the choice of the most appropriate drug or treatment for the patient.

ALTERNATIVE MECHANISMS OF RESISTANCE

It was observed that some individuals whose tumors have activating mutations in the *EGFR* gene do not respond to tyrosine kinase inhibitors. It is noted that some of these tumors have mutations in *KRAS*.[58-60] Activation of the EGFR-mediated signaling pathway involves the activation of the RAS-Map kinase pathway. Thus the product of RAS acts downstream of EGFR. Therefore, it is reasonable that independent activation of the downstream target renders the status of *EGFR* irrelevant to growth phenotype of these cells. These results form the basis for testing NSCLC for both *EGFR* and *KRAS* mutations. Patients who are most likely to respond to EGFR tyrosine kinase inhibitors would be those whose tumors have an activating mutation in *EGFR* and are wild type for *KRAS*.

Role of KRAS Mutations in Other Epidermal Growth Factor Receptor Inhibitors

Patients with colorectal cancer who failed chemotherapy were administered an antibody against EGFR, cetuximab. Although treatment with this monoclonal antibody resulted in improved overall survival, the disease progressed in more than 50% of the patients. Since a subset of colorectal tumors were known to have activating mutations in KRAS, a downstream component of EGFR signaling cascade, it is reasonable to assume that the *KRAS* mutations might render the treatment with cetuximab ineffective. This hypothesis was directly tested in a clinical trial. Patients who did not receive prior EGFR inhibitor treatment were randomized to receive cetuximab plus best supportive care or best supportive alone. Tumor samples, when available, were assessed for the status of *KRAS*. Approximately 40% of both groups had *KRAS* activation mutations. Patients with wild type *KRAS* tumors had better overall survival, better progression-free survival, and significantly better response rates than supportive care alone.[61] Similar results were obtained with the use of another monoclonal antibody against EGFR, panitumumab.[62] Based on these studies the U.S. Food and Drug Administration has changed the label for both drugs to require genetic testing of the *KRAS* prior to administration of either of these antibody drugs.

BRAF INHIBITORS

The RAS-Map kinase pathway is activated in a number of different tumor types. Efforts to identify small molecule inhibitors that can effectively inhibit this pathway have been under way for many years. There are different genetic changes that could result in the activation of this pathway.

EGFR amplification, mutations in the *EGFR* gene, mutations in a member of the *RAS* gene family, or certain mutations in *BRAF* are some of the examples of how this activation is accomplished. Efforts to target BRAF have been significantly successful.

Melanomas are capable of metastasis, and there are few effective therapies for metastatic melanoma. It was discovered that in melanomas as many as 40% to 60% may carry an activation mutation in *BRAF*. Interestingly, nearly 90% of the *RAF* mutations in this cancer involve codon 600, which results in a substitution of glutamic acid to valine (V600E). Two drugs, PLX4032 and PLX4720 (Plexxikon, Roche Pharmaceuticals, South San Francisco, California), effectively inhibit this modified protein in *in vitro* studies. Based on these encouraging data, clinical trials were conducted to assess the clinical efficacy of one of these drugs. In the initial dose escalation study the testing for the genetic status of *BRAF* was not a requirement, while in an extension study only those patients with an activation mutation in *BRAF* were included. In the dose escalation study a substantial number of patients were positive for the *BRAF* mutation. A substantial number (61%) of the patients responded to the drug, and all of the individuals whose tumors had *BRAF* mutations were among the responders, while patients without the mutation did not show a response.[63]

In the extension phase of the study only patients with the V600E mutation were treated with drug and remarkably 81% of them responded. The responses were durable and involved all metastatic sites of the tumor. The overall survival in this population is being assessed in a phase 3 trial. If these trials are successful it would benefit the patients to conduct testing for the status of *BRAF* and treat those who have the BRAF activation with this inhibitor. *BRAF* mutations are also detected in other tumor types, and the mutations detected in these tumors include V600E. Therefore, it is possible that this or other BRAF inhibitors will find widespread use in many tumor types.

The importance of genetic testing prior to treatment with BRAF inhibitors is underscored by studies that indicate that treatment of BRAF-negative melanoma patients with an RAF inhibitor may result in activation of the MAP kinase pathway and is therefore contraindicated.[64,65]

THE FUTURE

As the knowledge about the genetic changes that lead to the initiation and progression of cancer increases, so too the ability to choose the most appropriate drug to which the tumor will respond is also increasing. Understanding of the genetic and genomic changes in cancer has been fueled by new high-throughput technologies and large-scale approaches. During the past few years the ability to detect copy number changes, chromosomal aberrations, gene expression profile changes, global methylation changes, and DNA sequence changes has dramatically improved. More recently a significant reduction in the cost of DNA sequencing is also fueling efforts to sequence large sets of genes, whole exomes, and even whole genome sequencing from tumors and, when available, their corresponding normal samples. All of these results are increasing the understanding of the biology of cancer, but they are also increasing the ability to stratify patients and to choose the most appropriate drug or treatment based on the genetic composition of the tumor and the patient.

An illustrative example of the types of information that can be obtained from such large-scale studies can be found in the results on human glioblastomas published by two groups.[66,67] The Cancer Genome Atlas Research Network[42] analyzed copy number changes, expression profile changes, and methylation changes and sequenced a subset of genes in the genome in a large number of glioblastoma multiforme and compared them with normal samples obtained from the same patients. Parsons et al.[43] examined the coding sequence of more than 22,000 genes in 22 samples. They also examined copy number changes and expression profiles in these tumor samples. These studies identified a number of genes that were not previously implicated in gliomagenesis, most notably *NF1* and *IDH1*. The results also provided important clues about how glioblastoma multiforme acquire resistance to the alkylating agent temozolomide. Similar types of studies in other cancers have been published.

CHANGING FACE OF PERSONALIZED MEDICINE

As the information about critical genetic and genomic changes in many different cancers is accumulating, it is becoming possible to incorporate this information into patient treatment. The types of changes can be illustrated from the changes in treatment of lung cancer. The importance of *EGFR* and *KRAS* testing in making decisions about the suitability of tyrosine kinase inhibitors was described earlier in this chapter. A subset of lung tumors have mutations in the *BRAF* gene and, based on the results from clinical studies of melanoma patients, highly specific BRAF inhibitors might be the choice treatment for these patients. A subset of tumors have ErbB2 amplification, which is a common event in breast cancers, and patients whose breast tumors have this amplification respond well to trastuzumab. Clinical trials to evaluate the efficacy of using trastuzumab in lung cancer patients with ErbB2 amplification are under way. A subset of lung tumors also has activation mutations in one of several genes, leading to an activation of the PI3K pathway. There are several drugs, some of which are already approved for clinical use, that are effective inhibitors of this pathway, and these are excellent candidates with which to treat this group of patients. Another subset of patients has a unique translocation that involved the *EML* and *ALK4* genes. It has been shown that lung cancer patients with tumors that bear this translocation respond well to a new tyrosine kinase inhibitor crizotinib.[66]

Other NSCLC tumors have amplification in the oncogene *MET*. Inhibitors against this target and its ligand hepatocyte growth factor are in development, and some of them are being tested for their efficacy to treat lung cancer patients in clinical trials. Therefore, it is highly likely that in the near future tumors from patients diagnosed with NSCLC will be tested for the status of a battery of genes that include *EGFR*, *RAS*, *RAF*, *ErbB2*, *Met*, and the presence of the EML-ALK4 translocation to determine the most optimal treatment for each patient. Such efforts are already in place at several academic medical centers. A list of examples of genetic changes that could affect treatment decisions is presented in Table 12.1.

SUMMARY

The understanding of the genetic and genomic differences among individuals that affect cancer susceptibility and the genetic and genomic changes that are critical for the initiation and progression of cancer is increasing at a rapid pace. The rapid decrease in the cost of DNA sequencing and other

TABLE 12.1

EXAMPLES OF GENETIC CHANGES TO FACILITATE TREATMENT DECISIONS

Genetic Change	Indication
BCR-ABL translocation	Chronic myelogenous leukemia
ErbB2 amplification	Certain breast cancers
EGFR mutations	Sensitivity to tyrosine kinase inhibitors in NSCLC
EGFR mutations	Resistance to tyrosine kinase inhibitors in NSCLC
K-RAS	Resistance to tyrosine kinase inhibitors in NSCLC
K-RAS	Resistance to EGFR antibodies in colon cancer
B-RAF	Sensitivity to B-RAF inhibitors in melanoma
EML-ALK4 translocation	Sensitivity to ALK4 inhibitors
RAS-MAPK pathway members	Sensitivity to drugs that inhibit RAS-MAPK pathway
PTEN, AKT and PI3 kinase	Sensitivity to drugs that inhibit the AKT and PI kinase pathways
BRCA1 and BRCA2	Sensitivity to PARP inhibitors
HGF and MET mutations or amplification	Sensitivity to HGF and MET inhibitors
Mutations in genes in the angiogenesis pathway	Sensitivity to angiogenesis inhibitors

EGFR, epidermal growth factor receptor; NSCLC, non–small cell lung cancer; PARP, poly(adenosine diphosphate-ribose) polymerase; PI3, phosphatidylinositol 3; HGF, hepatocyte growth factor; MET, mesenchymal-to-epithelial transition.

genomic analysis is fueling this increase in knowledge. This new knowledge is helping in accurate prediction, early detection, and prognosis of cancer. Genetic differences among individuals and somatic changes during the development of cancer are also important in determining the appropriate treatment strategies for each patient. The use of genetic and genomic information is referred to as personalized medicine, which has the ability to transform the practice of oncology.

Selected References

The full list of references for this chapter appears in the online version.

1. Lichtenstein P, Holm NV, Verkasalo PK, et al. Environmental and heritable factors in the causation of cancer—analyses of cohorts of twins from Sweden, Denmark, and Finland. *N Engl J Med* 2000;343:78.
2. Ashley DJ. Oesophageal cancer in Wales. *J Med Genet* 1969;6:70.
3. St. John DJ, McDermott FT, Hopper JL, et al. Cancer risk in relatives of patients with common colorectal cancer. *Ann Intern Med* 1993;118:785.
4. Nishisho I, Nakamura Y, Miyoshi Y, et al. Mutations of chromosome 5q21 genes in FAP and colorectal cancer patients. *Science* 1991;253:665.
5. Kinzler KW, Nilbert MC, Su LK, et al. Identification of FAP locus genes from chromosome 5q21. *Science* 1991;253 (5020):661.
6. Nakamura Y, Nishisho I, Kinzler KW, et al. Mutations of the adenomatous polyposis coli gene in familial polyposis coli patients and sporadic colorectal tumors. *Princess Takamatsu Symp* 1991;22:285.
7. Lynch HT, Krush AJ. Heredity and adenocarcinoma of the colon. *Gastroenterology* 1967;53:517.
8. Parsons R, Li GM, Longley MJ, et al. Hypermutability and mismatch repair deficiency in RER+ tumor cells. *Cell* 1993; 75:1227.
9. Aaltonen LA, Peltomäki P, Leach FS, et al. Clues to the pathogenesis of familial colorectal cancer. *Science* 1993;260:812.
10. Powell SM, Zilz N, Beazer-Barclay Y, et al. APC mutations occur early during colorectal tumorigenesis. *Nature* 1992; 359:235.

11. Leach FS, Nicolaides NC, Papadopoulos N, et al. Mutations of a mutS homolog in hereditary nonpolyposis colorectal cancer. *Cell* 1993;75:1215.
12. Fishel R, Lescoe MK, Rao MR, et al. The human mutator gene homolog MSH2 and its association with hereditary nonpolyposis colon cancer. *Cell* 1993;75:1027.
13. Papadopoulos N, Nicolaides NC, Wei YF, et al. Mutation of a MutL homolog in hereditary colon cancer. *Science* 1994;263:1625.
14. Bronner CE, Baker SM, Morrison PT, et al. Mutation in the DNA mismatch repair gene homologue hMLH1 is associated with hereditary non-polyposis colon cancer. *Nature* 1994;368:258.
15. Nicolaides NC, Papadopoulos N, Liu B, et al. Mutations of two PMS homologues in hereditary nonpolyposis colon cancer. *Nature* 1994;371:75.
16. Miyaki M, Konishi M, Tanaka K, et al. Germline mutation of MSH6 as the cause of hereditary nonpolyposis colorectal cancer. *Nat Genet* 1997;17:271.
17. Lipkin SM, Wang V, Jacoby R, et al. MLH3: a DNA mismatch repair gene associated with mammalian microsatellite instability. *Nat Genet* 2000;24:27.
18. Loukola A, Vilkki S, Singh J, Launonen V, Aaltonen LA. Germline and somatic mutation analysis of MLH3 in MSI-positive colorectal cancer. *Am J Pathol* 2000;157:347.
19. Aaltonen LA, Salovaara R, Kristo P, et al. Incidence of hereditary nonpolyposis colorectal cancer and the feasibility of molecular screening for the disease. *N Engl J Med* 1998;338:1481.
20. Loukola A, Salovaara R, Kristo P, et al. Microsatellite instability in adenomas as a marker for hereditary nonpolyposis colorectal cancer. *Am J Pathol* 1998;155:1849.

21. Salovaara R, Loukola A, Kristo P, et al. Population-based molecular detection of hereditary nonpolyposis colorectal cancer. *J Clin Oncol* 2000;18:2193.
22. de la Chapelle A. Genetic predisposition to colorectal cancer. *Nat Rev Cancer* 2004;4:769.
23. Zanke BW, Greenwood CM, Rangrej J, et al. Genome-wide association scan identifies a colorectal cancer susceptibility locus on chromosome 8q24. *Nat Genet* 2007;39:989.
24. Al Olama AA, Kote-Jarai Z, Giles GG, et al. Multiple loci on 8q24 associated with prostate cancer susceptibility. *Nat Genet* 2009;41:1058.
25. Gudmundsson J, Sulem P, Gudbjartsson DF, et al. Genome-wide association and replication studies identify four variants associated with prostate cancer susceptibility. *Nat Genet* 2009;41:1122.
26. Tenesa A, Farrington SM, Prendergast JG, et al. Genome-wide association scan identifies a colorectal cancer susceptibility locus on 11q23 and replicates risk loci at 8q24 and 18q21. *Nat Genet* 2008;40:631.
27. Pomerantz MM, Ahmadiyeh N, Jia L, et al. The 8q24 cancer risk variant rs6983267 shows long-range interaction with MYC in colorectal cancer. *Nat Genet* 2009;41:882.
28. Ahmadiyeh N, Pomerantz MM, Grisanzio C, et al. 8q24 prostate, breast, and colon cancer risk loci show tissue-specific long-range interaction with MYC. 2010 *Proc Natl Acad Sci U S A* 2010;107:9742.
29. Hall JM, Lee MK, Newman B, et al. Linkage of early-onset familial breast cancer to chromosome 17q21. *Science* 1990;250:1684.
30. Miki Y, Swensen J, Shattuck-Eidens D, et al. A strong candidate for the breast and ovarian cancer susceptibility gene BRCA1. *Science* 1994;266:66.
31. Futreal PA, Liu Q, Shattuck-Eidens D, et al. BRCA1 mutations in primary breast and ovarian carcinomas. *Science* 1994;266:120.
32. Faca VM, Song KS, Wang H, et al. A mouse to human search for plasma proteome changes associated with pancreatic tumor development. *PLoS Med* 2008;5:e123.
33. Pitteri SJ, JeBailey L, Faça VM, et al. Integrated proteomic analysis of human cancer cells and plasma from tumor bearing mice for ovarian cancer biomarker discovery. *PLoS One* 2009;4:e7916.
34. Hung KE, Faça V, Song K, et al. Comprehensive proteome analysis of an Apc mouse model uncovers proteins associated with intestinal tumorigenesis. *Cancer Prev Res* 2009;2:224.
35. Nagrath S, Sequist LV, Maheswaran S, et al. Isolation of rare circulating tumour cells in cancer patients by microchip technology. *Nature* 2007;450(7173):1235.
37. Mitelman F, Johansson B, Mertens F. The impact of translocations and gene fusions on cancer causation. *Nat Rev Cancer* 2007;7(4):233.
38. Soda M, Choi YL, Enomoto M, et al. Identification of the transforming EML4-ALK fusion gene in non-small-cell lung cancer. *Nature* 2007;448:561.
39. Tomlins SA, Laxman B, Dhanasekaran SM, et al. Distinct classes of chromosomal rearrangements create oncogenic ETS gene fusions in prostate cancer. *Nature* 2007;448:595.
40. Dave SS, Fu K, Wright GW, et al. Lymphoma/Leukemia Molecular Profiling Project. Molecular diagnosis of Burkitt's lymphoma. *N Engl J Med* 2006;354:2431.
41. Paik S, Shak S, Tang G, et al. A multigene assay to predict recurrence of tamoxifen-treated, node-negative breast cancer. *N Engl J Med* 2004;351(27):2817.
42. Cancer Genome Atlas Research Network. Comprehensive genomic characterization defines human glioblastoma genes and core pathways. *Nature* 2008;455:1061.
43. Parsons DW, Jones S, Zhang X, et al. An integrated genomic analysis of human glioblastoma multiforme. *Science* 2008;321:1807.
44. Jones S, Zhang X, Parsons DW, et al. Core signaling pathways in human pancreatic cancers revealed by global genomic analyses. *Science* 2008;321:1801.
45. Pleasance ED, Cheetham RK, Stephens PJ, et al. A comprehensive catalogue of somatic mutations from a human cancer genome. *Nature* 2010;463:191.
46. Mardis ER, Ding L, Dooling DJ, et al. Recurring mutations found by sequencing an acute myeloid leukemia genome. *N Engl J Med* 2009;361:1058.
47. Nowell P, Hungerford D. A minute chromosome in human chronic granulocytic leukemia *Science* 1960;132:1497.
48. Rowley JD. A new consistent chromosomal abnormality in chronic myelogenous leukemia. *Nature* 1973;243:290.
49. Druker BJ, Talpaz M, Resta DJ, et al. Efficacy and safety of a specific inhibitor of the BCR-ABL tyrosine kinase in chronic myeloid leukemia. *N Engl J Med* 2001;344:1031.
50. Druker BJ, Sawyers CL, Kantarjian H, et al. Activity of a specific inhibitor of the BCR-ABL tyrosine kinase in the blast crisis of chronic myeloid leukemia and acute lymphoblastic leukemia with the Philadelphia chromosome. *N Engl J Med* 2001;344:1038.
51. Slamon DJ, Leyland-Jones B, Shak S, et al. Use of chemotherapy plus a monoclonal antibody against HER2 for metastatic breast cancer that overexpresses HER2. *N Engl J Med* 2001;344:783.
52. Arteaga CL. ErbB-targeted therapeutic approaches in human cancer. *Exp Cell Res* 2003;284:122.
53. Paez JG, Jänne PA, Lee JC, et al. EGFR mutations in lung cancer: correlation with clinical response to gefitinib therapy. *Science* 2004;304:1497.
54. Lynch TJ, Bell DW, Sordella R, et al. activating mutations in the epidermal growth factor receptor underlying responsiveness of non-small-cell lung cancer to gefitinib. *N Engl J Med* 2004;350:2129.
56. Mok TS, Wu YL, Thongprasert S, et al. Gefitinib or carboplatin-paclitaxel in pulmonary adenocarcinoma. *N Engl J Med* 2009;361:947.
61. Karapetis CS, Khambata-Ford S, Jonker DJ, et al. K-ras mutations and benefit from cetuximab in advanced colorectal cancer. *N Engl J Med* 2008;359:1757.
63. Flaherty KT, Puzanov I, Kim KB, et al. Inhibition of mutated, activated BRAF in metastatic melanoma. *N Engl J Med* 2010;363:809.

GENERAL PRINCIPLES

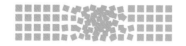

CHAPTER 13 TARGETED THERAPY WITH SMALL MOLECULE KINASE INHIBITORS

CHARLES L. SAWYERS

In 2001 the first tyrosine kinase inhibitor, imatinib, was approved for clinical use in chronic myeloid leukemia (CML). The spectacular success of this first-in-class agent ushered in a transformation in cancer drug discovery from efforts that were largely based on novel cytotoxic chemotherapy agents to an almost exclusive focus on molecularly targeted agents across the pharmaceutical and biotechnology industry and academia. This chapter summarizes this remarkable decade of progress with the focus on the concepts underlying this paradigm shift as well as the considerable challenges that remain (Tables 13.1 and 13.2). Readers in search of more specific details on individual drugs and their indications should consult the relevant disease-specific chapters elsewhere in this volume as well as references cited within this chapter. Readers should also note that the epidermal growth factor receptor (EGFR) and human epidermal growth factor receptor 2 (HER2) tyrosine kinases covered here have also been successfully targeted by monoclonal antibodies that engage these proteins at the cell surface. These drugs, often referred to as biologics rather than small molecule inhibitors, are covered in other chapters. The chapter is organized around kinase targets rather than diseases and, intentionally, has a historical flow to make certain thematic points and illustrate the broad lessons that have been and continue to be learned through the clinical development of these exciting agents.

Perhaps the most stunning discovery from the clinical trials of the ABL kinase inhibitor imatinib was the recognition that tumor cells acquire exquisite dependence on the BCR-ABL fusion oncogene, created by the Philadelphia chromosome translocation.[1] Although this may seem intuitive at first glance, consider the fact that the translocation arises in an otherwise normal hematopoietic stem cell whose survival is regulated by a complex array of growth factors and interactions with the bone marrow microenvironment. While BCR-ABL clearly gives this cell a growth advantage that, over years, results in the clinical phenotype of CML, there was no reason to expect that these cells would depend on BCR-ABL for their survival when confronted with an inhibitor. In the absence of BCR-ABL, these tumor cells could presumably rely on the marrow microenvironment for their survival, just like their normal nontransformed neighbors. Thus, it seemed more likely that by shutting down the driver oncogene, BCR-ABL inhibitors would halt the progression of CML but not eliminate the pre-existing tumor cells. But in fact, CML progenitors are eliminated after just a few months of anti-BCR-ABL therapy, indicating they are dependent on the driver oncogene for their survival and have "forgotten" how to return to normal. This phenomenon, subsequently documented in a variety of human malignancies, is colloquially termed "oncogene addiction."[2] Although the molecular basis for this addiction remains to be defined, the notion of finding an Achilles' heel for each cancer has captivated the cancer research community, spawning a broad array of efforts to elucidate the molecular identity of these targets and discover relevant inhibitors.

EARLY SUCCESSES: TARGETING CANCERS WITH WELL-KNOWN KINASE MUTATIONS

From the beginning, clinical trials of imatinib were restricted to patients with Philadelphia chromosome–positive CML. For what seem like obvious reasons, there was never any serious discussion about treating patients with Philadelphia chromosome–negative leukemia because the assumption was that only patients with the BCR-ABL fusion gene would have a chance of responding. This was clearly a wise decision because hematologic response rates approached 90% and cytogenetic remissions were seen in nearly half of the patient in the early phase studies.[3] It was obvious the drug worked and imatinib was approved in record time. Unwittingly, the power of genome-based patient selection was demonstrated in the clinical development of the very first kinase inhibitor. It has

TABLE 13.1

APPROVED KINASE INHIBITORS

Target	Drug	Approved Indications	Anticipated Future Indications[a]
BCR-ABL	Imatinib Dasatinib Nilotinib	Chronic myeloid leukemia Philadelphia chromosome positive acute lymphoid leukemia	
KIT	Imatinib Sunitinib	Gastrointestinal stromal tumor	
PDGFRα/β	Imatinib	Chronic myelomonocytic leukemia (with TEL-PDGFRβ fusion) Hypereosinophilic syndrome (with PDGFRβ fusion) Dermatofibrosarcoma protuberans	
HER2	Lapatinib	Her2+breast cancer	
EGFR	Gefitinib Erlotinib	Lung adenocarcinoma (with EGFR mutation, although not required for initial approval)	
VEGFR	Sorafenib Sunitinib	Kidney cancer Hepatocellular carcinoma (sorafenib only)	Hepatocellular carcinoma (sunitinib) Pancreatic neuroendocrine tumors (sunitinib) Thyroid cancer (sorafenib)
TORC1 (mTOR)	Sirolimus (rapamycin) Everolimus Temsirolimus	Kidney cancer	Mantle cell lymphoma Endometrial cancer

[a]Indications are considered "anticipated" based on data from randomized phase 2 trials that led to initiation of phase 3 registration studies.

taken a decade for this lesson to be fully learned. Today the much larger clinical experience with an array of different kinase inhibitors across many tumor types has led to a much better understanding of the principles that dictate oncogene addiction that, in retrospect, were staring researchers in the face. Foremost among them is the notion that tumors with somatic mutation or amplification of a kinase drug target are much more likely to be dependent on that target for survival. Hence, a patient whose tumor has such a mutation is much more likely to respond to treatment with the appropriate inhibitor.

After CML, the next example to illustrate this principle was gastrointestinal stromal tumor (GIST), which is associated with mutations in the KIT tyrosine kinase receptor or, more rarely, in the platelet-derived growth factor receptor (PDGFR).[4,5] Serendipitously, imatinib inhibits both KIT and PDGFR; therefore, the clinical test of KIT inhibition in GIST followed quickly on the heels of the success in CML.[6] In retrospect, the rapid progress made in these two diseases was based, in part, on the fact that the driver molecular lesion (BCR-ABL

or KIT mutation, respectively) is present in nearly all patients who are diagnosed with these two diseases. The molecular analysis merely confirmed the diagnosis that was made using standard clinical and histological criteria. Consequently, clinicians could identify the patients most likely to respond based on clinical criteria rather than rely on an elaborate molecular profiling infrastructure to prescreen patients. Consequently, clinical trials evaluating kinase inhibitors in CML and GIST accrued quickly and the therapeutic benefit became clear almost immediately.

The notion that molecular alteration of a driver kinase determines sensitivity to a cognate kinase inhibitor was further validated during the development of the dual EGFR/HER2 kinase inhibitor lapatinib. Clinical trials of this kinase inhibitor were conducted in women with advanced HER2-positive breast cancer based on earlier success in these same patients with the monoclonal antibody trastuzumab that targets the extracellular domain of the HER2 kinase. Lapatinib was initially approved in combination with the cytotoxic agent capecitabine for women with resistance to

TABLE 13.2

UNAPPROVED KINASE INHIBITORS WITH CLEAR EVIDENCE OF CLINICAL ACTIVITY

Target	Drug	Clinical Development Path	Clinical Trial Stage	Other Potential Indications
BRAF	PLX4032 GSK2118436	BRAF mutant melanoma	Phase 3 Phase 1	Thyroid cancer Colon cancer
ALK	PF02341066	ALK mutant lung cancer	Phase 3	ALK-positive anaplastic lymphoma ALK-mutant neuroblastoma
JAK2	INCB018424 TG101348	Myelofibrosis	Phase 3 Phase 2	Polycythemia vera Essential thrombocytosis
FLT3	Midostaurin (PKC412) AC220	FLT3 mutant acute myeloid leukemia	Phase 1 Phase 2	FLT3 mutant acute lymphoid leukemia
MEK	AZD6244 GSK1120212	BRAF mutant melanoma	Phase 2 Phase 1	Combination therapy with PI3K pathway inhibitors (many tumor types) or RAF inhibitors (BRAF mutant melanoma)
RET	Vandetanib (AZD6474) Sorafenib XL184 motesanib (AMG706)	Thyroid cancer	Phase 3 Phase 3 Phase 3 Phase 2	Combination with chemotherapy (lung cancer, motesanib phase 3 trial)[a]
VEGFR	Axitinib (AG013736) Tivozanib (AV951) Pazopanib (GW786034)	Kidney cancer	Phase 3 Phase 3 Phase 3	Combination therapy with TORC1 inhibitors (in kidney cancer) Hepatocellular carcinoma

[a]Based on the success of chemotherapy in combination with the VEGF antibody bevacizumab in several tumor types, several VEGFR inhibitors and RET inhibitors (which have activity against VEGFR) have been evaluated in chemotherapy combinations in lung cancer and colon cancer. Most trials have failed in the phase 3 setting.

trastuzumab,[7] then was subsequently approved for frontline use in metastatic breast cancer in combination with chemotherapy or hormonal therapy, depending on estrogen-receptor status. A key ingredient that enabled the clinical development of lapatinib was the routine use of HER2 gene amplification testing in the diagnosis of breast cancer, pioneered during the development of trastuzumab several years earlier. This widespread clinical practice allowed rapid identification of those patients most likely to benefit. If lapatinib trials had been conducted in unselected patients, the clinical signal in breast cancer would likely have been missed.

The Serendipity of Unexpected Clinical Responses

In contrast to the logical development of imatinib and lapatinib in molecularly defined patient populations, the EGFR kinase inhibitors gefitinib and erlotinib entered the clinic without the benefit of such a focused clinical development plan. Although considerable preclinical data implicated EGFR as a cancer drug target, there was little insight into which patients were most likely to benefit. The first clue that EGFR inhibitors would have a role in lung cancer came from the recognition, by several astute clinicians, of remarkable responses in a small fraction of patients with lung adenocarcinoma.[8] Further studies revealed the curious clinical circumstance that those patients most likely to benefit tended to be never smokers, women, and those of Asian ethnicity.[9] Clearly there was a strong clinical signal in a subgroup of patients who could perhaps be enriched based on these clinical features, but it seemed that a unifying molecular lesion must be present. Three academic groups simultaneously converged on the answer. Mutations in the *EGFR* gene were detected in the 10% to 15% of patients with lung adenocarcinoma who had radiographic responses.[10–12] It may seem surprising that mutations in a gene as highly visible as *EGFR* and in such a prevalent cancer had not been detected earlier. But the motivation to search aggressively for *EGFR* mutations was not there until the clinical responses were seen. Perhaps even more surprising was the failure of the pharmaceutical company sponsors of the two most advanced compounds, gefitinib and erlotinib, to embrace this important discovery and refocus future clinical development plans on patients with *EGFR* mutant lung adenocarcinoma.

Clinical development of cytotoxic agents has always proceeded empirically. Typically, small numbers of patients with different cancers are treated in "all comer" phase 1 studies (no enrichment for subgroups) with the goal of eliciting a clinical signal in at least one tumor type. A single agent response rate of 20% to 30% in a disease-specific phase 2 trial can justify a randomized phase 3 registration trial where the typical end point for drug approval is time to progression or survival. Cytotoxics are also typically evaluated in combination with existing standard of care treatment (typically approved chemotherapy agents) with the goal of increasing the response rate or enhancing the duration of response.

The clinical development of gefitinib and erlotinib followed the cytotoxic model. Both drugs had similarly low but convincing single agent response rates (10% to 15%) in chemotherapy-refractory advanced lung cancer. Indeed, gefitinib was originally granted accelerated approval by the U.S. Food and Drug Administration (FDA) in 2003 based on the impressive nature of these responses, contingent on the completion of formal phase 3 studies with survival end points.[13] The sponsors of both drugs therefore conducted phase 3 registration studies in patients with chemotherapy-refractory advanced stage lung cancer but without prescreening patients for EGFR mutation status. (In fairness, these trials were initiated prior to the discovery of EGFR mutations in lung cancer.) Erlotinib was approved in 2004 on the basis of a modest survival advantage over placebo (the BR.21 trial); however, gefitinib failed to demonstrate a survival advantage in essentially the same patient population.[14,15] This difference in outcome was surprising since the two drugs have highly similar chemical structures and biological properties. Perhaps the most important difference in the two trials was drug dose. Erlotinib was given at the maximum tolerated dose, which produces a high frequency of rash and diarrhea. Both side effects are presumed "on target" consequences of EGFR inhibition since EGFR is highly expressed in skin and gastrointestinal epithelial cells. In contrast, gefitinib was dosed slightly lower to mitigate these toxicities, with the rationale that responses should not be compromised since clinical responses were clearly documented at lower doses.

In parallel with the single agent phase 3 trials in chemotherapy-refractory patients, both gefitinib and erlotinib were studied as upfront therapy for advanced lung cancer to determine if either would improve the efficacy of standard "doublet" (carboplatin/paclitaxel or gemcitabine/cisplatin) chemotherapy when all three drugs were given in combination. These trials, termed INTACT-1 and INTACT-2 (gefitinib with either gemcitabine/cisplatin or with carboplatin/paclitaxel) and TRIBUTE (erlotinib with carboplatin/paclitaxel) collectively enrolled over 3,000 patients.[16–18] Excitement in the oncology community was high based on the clear single agent activity of both EGFR inhibitors. But both trials were spectacular failures—neither drug showed any benefit over chemotherapy alone. The emerging data on *EGFR* mutations in the 10% to 15% of patients who responded to single agent *EGFR* inhibitor therapy provided a logical explanation. Only a small fraction of patients enrolled in these phase 3 trials had a chance of benefit since the clinical signal from those whose tumors had *EGFR* mutations was diluted by all the patients whose tumors had no *EGFR* alterations, many of whom benefited from chemotherapy.

The convergence of the *EGFR* mutation discovery with these clinical trial results will be remembered as a remarkable time in the history of targeted cancer therapies, not just for the important role of these agents as lung cancer therapies but for the delays in studying whether *EGFR* genotype should drive treatment selection. Perhaps the most egregious error came from a retrospective analysis of tumors from patients treated in the BR.21 trial that concluded that *EGFR* mutations did *not* predict for a survival advantage.[19] (*EGFR* gene amplification *was* associated with survival but only in univariate analysis.) This conclusion was concerning because less than 30% of patients on the trial had tissue available for EGFR mutation analysis, raising questions about the adequacy of the sample size. Furthermore, the *EGFR* mutation assay used by the authors was subsequently criticized because a significant number of the *EGFR* mutations reported in these patients were in residues not previously found by others who had sequenced thousands of tumors. Many of these mutations were suspected to be an artifact of working from formalin-fixed biopsies. (Formalin fixed, paraffin-embedded tissue samples present special challenges for nucleic acid analysis that can be avoided if the tissue is fresh frozen at the time of acquisition or can be overcome with additional controls.)

More recently, clinical investigators in Asia, where a greater fraction of lung cancers (roughly 30%) are positive for *EGFR* mutations, addressed the question of whether mutations predict for clinical benefit in a prospective trial. In this study known as IPASS, gefitinib was clearly superior to standard doublet chemotherapy as frontline therapy for patients with advanced *EGFR* mutation-positive lung adenocarcinoma.[20] Conversely, *EGFR* mutation–negative patients fared much worse with gefitinib and benefited from chemotherapy. In addition, *EGFR* mutation–positive patients had a more favorable overall prognosis regardless of treatment, indicating that *EGFR* mutation is also a prognostic biomarker. The IPASS trial serves as a compelling example of a properly designed (and executed) biomarker-driven clinical trial. Although the rationale for this clinical development strategy had been demonstrated years earlier with BCR-ABL in leukemia, KIT in GIST, and HER2 in breast cancer, it was difficult to derail the empiric approach that had been used for decades in developing cytotoxic agents.

Platelet-Driven Growth Factor Receptor Leukemias and Sarcoma

The discovery of *EGFR* mutations in lung cancer (motivated by dramatic clinical responses in a subset of patients treated with EGFR kinase inhibitors) is the most visible example of the power of bedside-to-bench science, but it is not the only (or the first) such example from the kinase inhibitor era. Shortly after the approval of imatinib for CML in 2001, two case reports documented dramatic remissions in patients with hypereosinophilic syndrome (HES), a blood disorder characterized by prolonged elevation of eosinophil counts and subsequent organ dysfunction from eosinophil infiltration, when treated with imatinib.[21,22] Although HES resembles myeloproliferative diseases such as chronic myeloid leukemia, the molecular pathogenesis of HES was completely unknown at the time. Reasoning that these clinical responses must be explained by inhibition of a driver kinase, a team of laboratory-based physician scientists quickly searched for mutations in the three kinases known to be inhibited by imatinib (ABL, KIT, and PDGFR). ABL and KIT were quickly excluded, but the *PDGFRα* gene was targeted by an interstitial deletion that fused the upstream FIP1L1 gene to PDGFRα.[23] FIP1L1-PDGFRα is a constitutively active tyrosine kinase, analogous to BCR-ABL, and also inhibited by imatinib. As with *EGFR*-mutant lung cancer, the molecular pathophysiology of HES was discovered by dissecting the mechanism of response to the drug used to treat it.

The HES/FIP1L1-PDGFRα story serves as a nice bookend to an earlier discovery that the t(5,12) chromosome translocation, found rarely in patients with chronic myelomonocytic leukemia, creates the TEL-PDGFRβ fusion tyrosine kinase.[24] Similar to HES, treatment of patients with t(5,12) translocation-positive leukemias with imatinib has also proven successful.[25] A third example comes from dermatofibrosarcoma protuberans, a sarcoma characterized by a t(17,22) translocation that fuses the *COL1A* gene to the gene for *PDGFB ligand* (not the receptor). COL1A-PDGFB is onco-genic through autocrine stimulation of the normal PDGFR in these tumor cells. Patients with dermatofibrosarcoma protuberans respond to imatinib therapy because it targets the PDGFR, just one step downstream from the oncogenic lesion.[26]

Exploiting the New Paradigm: Searching for Other Kinase-Driven Cancers

The benefits of serendipity notwithstanding, the growing number of examples of successful kinase inhibitor therapy in tumors with mutation or amplification of the drug target begged for a more rational approach to drug discovery and development. In 2002, the list of human tumors known to have mutations in kinases was quite small. Due to advances in automated gene sequencing, it became possible to ask whether a much larger fraction of human cancers might also have such mutations through a brute force approach. To address this question comprehensively, one would have to sequence all of the kinases in the genome in hundreds of samples of each tumor type. Several early pilot studies demonstrated the potential of this approach by revealing important new targets for drug development. Perhaps the most spectacular was the discovery of mutations in the BRAF kinase in over half of patients with melanoma, as well as in a smaller fraction of colon and thyroid cancers[27] Another was the discovery of mutations in the Janus-associated tyrosine kinase 2 (*JAK2*) in nearly all patients with polycythemia vera, as well as a significant fraction of patients with myelofibrosis and essential thrombocytosis.[28-30] A third example was the identification of *PIK3CA* mutations in a variety of tumors, with the greatest frequencies in breast, endometrial, and colorectal cancers.[31] *PIK3CA* encodes a lipid kinase that generates the second messenger phosphatidyl inositol 3-phosphate (PIP3). PIP3 activates growth and survival signaling through the AKT family of kinases as well as other downstream effectors. Coupled with the well-established role of the PTEN (phosphatase and tensin homologue) lipid phosphatase in dephosphorylating PIP3, the discovery of *PIK3CA* mutations focused tremendous attention on developing inhibitors at multiple levels of this pathway, as discussed further below.

Each of these important discoveries—BRAF, JAK2, PIK3CA—came from relatively small efforts (less than 100 tumors) generally focused on resequencing only those exons that coded for regions of kinases where mutations had been found in other kinases (typically the juxtamembrane and kinase domains). These restricted searches were largely driven by cost. In 2006, a comprehensive effort to sequence all of the exons in all kinases in 100 tumors could easily exceed several million dollars. Financial support for such projects could not be obtained easily through traditional funding agencies as the risk/reward ratio was considered too high. Furthermore, substantial infrastructure for sample acquisition, microdissection of tumor from normal tissue, nucleic acid preparation, high throughput automated sequencing, and computational analysis of the resulting data were essential. Few institutions were equipped to address these challenges. In response, the National Cancer Institute in the United States (in partnership with the National Human Genome Research Institute) and an international group known as the International Cancer Genome Consortium (ICGC) launched large-scale efforts to sequence the complete genomes of thousands of cancers. By 2010 the U.S. effort (called The Cancer Genome Atlas [TCGA]) had completed an analysis of glioblastoma[32] and ovarian cancer and had launched efforts in lung, kidney, endometrial, and other cancers. The international consortium had committed to sequencing 25,000 tumors representing 50 different cancer subtypes.[33] Both groups stipulated immediate release of all sequence information to the research community free of charge so that the entire scientific community could learn from the data. These grand-scale projects were possible due to a dramatic decline in sequencing costs. Discussions just a few years earlier about which genes (or regions of genes) to include in such projects were no longer necessary. The cost of complete exome (all exons from all genes in the human genome—not just kinases) and complete genome (all DNA) resequencing had fallen to about $5,000 per sample.

Rounding Out the Treatment of Myeloproliferative Disorders: JAK2 and Myelofibrosis

Taken together with the BCR-ABL translocation in chronic myeloid leukemia and FIP1L1-PDGFRα in HES, the discovery of *JAK2* mutations in polycythemia, essential thrombocytosis, and myelofibrosis provided a unifying understanding of myeloproliferative disorders as diseases of abnormal kinase activation. JAK family kinases are the primary effectors of signaling through inflammatory cytokine receptors and had therefore been considered compelling targets for anti-inflammatory drugs. But the JAK2 mutation discovery immediately shifted these efforts toward developing JAK2 inhibitors for myeloproliferative disorders. Since most patients have a common JAK2 V617F mutation, these efforts could rapidly focus on screening for activity against a single genotype. Progress has been rapid. Two compounds (INCB018424 and TG101348) were active in phase 2 studies in myelofibrosis, one of which has already progressed to a randomized phase 3 trial.[34,35] Myelofibrosis was selected as the initial

indication (instead of essential thrombocytosis or polycythemia vera) because the time to registration is expected to be shortest. Currently there are no approved treatments for myelofibrosis and shrinkage in spleen size can be used as an end point for drug approval. Successful trials in myelofibrosis will likely lead to studies in essential thrombocytosis and polycythemia vera.

BRAF Mutant Melanoma: Several Missteps before Finding the Right Inhibitor

As with JAK2 mutations in myeloproliferative disorders, the discovery of *BRAF* mutations in patients with melanoma launched widespread efforts to find potent BRAF inhibitors. One early candidate was the drug sorafenib, which had been optimized during drug discovery to inhibit RAF kinases. (Sorafenib also inhibits vascular endothelial growth factor receptor [VEGFR], which led to its approval in kidney cancer as discussed later in this chapter.) Despite the compelling molecular rationale for targeting BRAF, clinical results of sorafenib in melanoma were extremely disappointing and reduced enthusiasm for pursuing BRAF as a drug target.[36] In hindsight, this concern was completely misguided. Sorafenib dosing is limited by toxicities that preclude achieving serum levels in patients that potently inhibit RAF (but are sufficient to inhibit VEGFR). In addition, patients were enrolled without screening for *BRAF* mutations in their tumors. Although the frequency of *BRAF* mutations in melanoma is high, the inclusion of patients without *BRAF* mutation diluted the chance of seeing any clinical signal. In short, the clinical evaluation of sorafenib in melanoma was poorly designed to test the hypothesis that BRAF is a therapeutic target. The danger is that negative data from such clinical experiments can slow subsequent progress. It is critical to know the pharmacodynamic properties of the drug and the molecular phenotype of the patients being studied when interpreting the results of a negative study.

The fact that RAF kinases are intermediate components of the well-characterized RAS/MAP kinase pathway (transducing signals from RAS to RAF to MEK to ERK) raised the possibility that tumors with BRAF mutations might respond to inhibitors of one of these downstream kinases (Fig. 13.1). Preclinical studies revealed that tumor cell lines with BRAF mutation were exquisitely sensitive to inhibitors of the downstream kinase MEK.[37] Sorafenib, in contrast, does not show this profile of activity.[38] Thus, proper preclinical screening would have revealed the shortcomings of sorafenib as a BRAF inhibitor. Curiously, cell lines with mutation or amplification of *EGFR* or *HER2*, which function upstream in the pathway, were insensitive to MEK inhibition. Even tumor

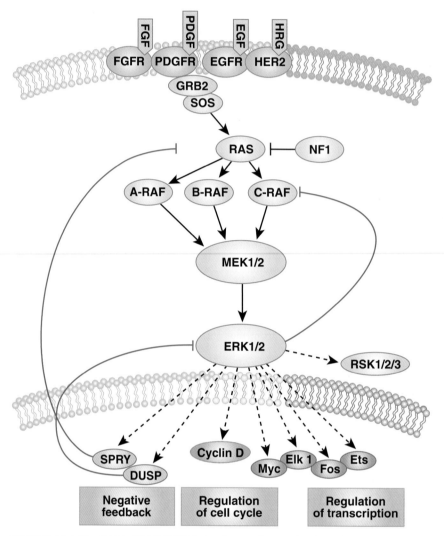

FIGURE 13.1 The RAS-RAF-MEK-ERK signaling pathway. The classical mitogen-activated protein kinase (MAPK) pathway is activated in human tumors by several mechanisms, including the binding of ligand to receptor tyrosine kinases (RTK), mutational activation of an RTK, by loss of the tumor suppressor NF1, or by mutations in RAS, BRAF, and MEK1. Phosphorylation and thus activation of ERK regulates transcription of target genes that promote cell cycle progression and tumor survival. The ERK pathway contains a classical feedback loop in which the expression of feedback elements such as SPRY and DUSP family proteins are regulated by the level of ERK activity. Loss of expression of SPRY and DUSP family members due to promoter methylation or deletion is thus permissive for persistently elevated pathway output. In the case of tumors with mutant BRAF, pathway output is enhanced by impaired upstream feedback regulation. (From ref. 114, with permission.)

lines with RAS mutations were variably sensitive. In short, the preclinical data made a strong case that MEK inhibitors should be effective in *BRAF* mutant melanoma but not in other subtypes. The reason that *HER2, EGFR*, and *RAS* mutant tumors were not sensitive to MEK inhibitors is explained, at least in part, by the existence of negative feedback loops that modulate the flux of signal transduction through MEK.[39]

In parallel with the generation of these preclinical findings, clinical trials of several MEK inhibitors were initiated. Patients with various cancers were enrolled in the early studies but there was a strong bias to include melanoma patients. Significant efforts were made to demonstrate MEK inhibition in tumor cells by measuring the phosphorylation status of the direct downstream substrate ERK using immunohistochemical analysis of biopsies from patients with metastatic disease. Phase 1 studies of the two earliest compounds in clinical development (PD325901 and AZD6244) documented reduced phospho-ERK staining at multiple dose levels in several patients on whom baseline and treatment biopsies were obtained.[40,41]

These pharmacodynamic studies, while well intentioned, were not quantitative enough to document the magnitude of MEK inhibition in these patients. Furthermore, clinical responses were observed in a few patients with BRAF mutant melanoma. Armed with this confidence, a randomized phase 2 clinical trial of AZD6244 was conducted in advanced melanoma, with the chemotherapeutic agent temozolomide (approved for glioblastoma) as the comparator arm. Clinical development of PD325901 was discontinued because of safety concerns about ocular and neurologic toxicity. Disappointingly, patients receiving AZD6244 had no benefit in progression-free survival when compared to temozolomide-treated patients, raising further concerns about the viability of BRAF as a drug target.[42] Closer examination of the data revealed that clinical responses were, indeed, seen in patients receiving AZD6244. The fact that *BRAF* mutation status was not required for study entry likely diminished the clinical signal in the AZD6244 arm, a lesson learned from the EGFR inhibitor trials in lung cancer. In addition, the results in the control group were better than expected and reflect greater activity of temozolomide in melanoma than previously believed.

All doubts about BRAF as a target vanished in 2009 to 2010 when dramatic clinical responses were observed with a novel BRAF inhibitor PLX4032. Like sorafenib, this compound was optimized to inhibit RAF but with an additional focus on mutant BRAF. PLX4032 differs dramatically from sorafenib because it potently inhibits BRAF without the additional broad range of activities that sorafenib has against other kinases like VEGFR.[43] The greater selectivity of PLX4032 relative to sorafenib resulted in much greater tolerability such that it could be given at high doses while avoiding significant toxicity. The early days of PLX4032 clinical development were plagued by challenges in maximizing the oral bioavailability of the drug.[44] Consequently, the initial phase 1 clinical trial was temporarily halted to develop a novel formulation (the coingredients in the drug capsule or tablet that improve solubility and absorption through the gastrointestinal tract). Much higher serum levels were obtained in patients who received the new PLX4032 formation and, shortly thereafter, complete and partial responses were observed in about 80% of the melanoma patients with *BRAF* mutant tumors. Strikingly, no activity was observed in patients whose tumors were wild type for *BRAF*.[45,46] The data were so compelling that PLX4032 was immediately advanced to a phase 3 registration trial. Similarly impressive responses in *BRAF* mutant melanoma patients were observed in a phase 1 trial of another, even more potent RAF inhibitor GSK2118436,[47] providing further proof that BRAF is an important cancer target.

The PLX4032 and GSK2118436 data also provide insight into why sorafenib and the early MEK inhibitor trials failed to demonstrate activity. One lesson is the critical importance of achieving adequate target inhibition. Clinical responses with PLX4032 were observed only after the drug was reformulated to achieve substantially higher serum levels. Reductions in phospho-ERK staining (as documented by immunohistochemistry) were documented in the earlier trials but, in retrospect, the assays were not sensitive enough to distinguish between modest (approximately 50%) kinase inhibition versus more complete BRAF or MEK inhibition. Efficacy in preclinical models is significantly improved using doses that give greater than 80% inhibition, and the human trial data suggest that this degree of pathway blockade is also required for a high clinical response rate.[46] Interestingly, investigators conducting a phase 1 clinical trial with a third MEK inhibitor, GSK1120212, have reported a high response rate (approximately 40%) in BRAF-mutant melanoma patients. These data appear to be substantially better than those observed with the earlier MEK inhibitors, although not as impressive as with PLX4032.[48] There is speculation that this newer MEK inhibitor inhibits MEK more completely that the earlier generation compounds, but this remains to be demonstrated in patients. Collectively, these experiences illustrate the critical need for quantitative pharmacodynamic assays to measure target inhibition early in clinical development. A second lesson is the importance of genotyping all patients for mutation or amplification of the relevant drug target. Not only does this ensure that a sufficient number of patients with the biomarker of interest are included in the study, the results also provide compelling evidence early in clinical development in support (or not) of the preclinical hypothesis.

Getting It Right: ALK and Lung Cancer

The development of the ALK inhibitor crizotinib (PF02341066), which is currently under evaluation in a phase 3 registration trial in lung cancer, illustrates how an unexpected signal obtained in a small number of patients can quickly shift a program in an entirely new direction with a high probability of success. The key ingredient is this story is a familiar one—a strong molecular hypothesis backed up by clinical response data in a small number of carefully selected patients. Crizotinib emerged from a drug discovery program at Pfizer focused on finding inhibitors of the MET receptor tyrosine kinase and entered the clinic with this target as its lead indication.[49] As discussed above with imatinib, essentially all kinase inhibitors have activity against other targets (so-called off target activities), which can sometimes prove to be advantageous. Off target activities are typically discovered by screening compounds against a large panel of kinases to establish profiles of relative selectivity against the intended target. Off target activity, potency, and pharmaceutical properties (bioavailability, half-life) are all factors that influence the decision of which compound to advance to clinical development. The primary off target activity of crizotinib is against the ALK tyrosine kinase.

ALK was first identified as a candidate driver oncogene in 1994 through the cloning of the t(2,5) chromosomal translocation associated with anaplastic large cell lymphoma, which creates the NPM-ALK fusion gene.[50] This discovery, together with the demonstration that NPM-ALK causes lymphoma in mice, made a compelling case for ALK as a drug target in this disease. But there was limited interest in developing ALK inhibitors because this particular lymphoma subtype is rare and most commonly found in children. Companies are generally reluctant to develop drugs solely for pediatric indications because of complexities related to dose selection and additional regulatory guidelines. Efforts to streamline this development process are under way.

In 2007, another ALK fusion gene called EML4-ALK was discovered in a small fraction of patients with lung adenocarcinoma, with an estimated frequency of 1% to 5%.[51] This discovery did not immediately capture the attention of drug developers, but several academic groups that had already begun testing lung cancer patients seen at their institutions for EGFR mutations simply added an EML4-ALK fusion test to the screening panel. Astute clinical investigators participating in the phase 1 trial of crizotinib, which was designed to include patients with a broad array of advanced cancers, were aware of the off target ALK activity and enrolled several lung cancer patients with EML4-ALK fusions in the study. These patients had remarkably dramatic responses.[52] This serendipitous finding in a few ALK-positive patients was confirmed in a larger cohort, resulting in the initiation of a phase 3 study in ALK-positive lung cancer, just 2 years after the discovery of the EML4-ALK fusion. Crizotinib is also being evaluated in other diseases associated with genomic alterations in ALK, including large cell anaplastic lymphoma, neuroblastoma,[53] and inflammatory myofibroblastic sarcoma.[54]

Extending the Model to RET Mutations in Thyroid Cancer

Subsets of patients with papillary or medullary thyroid cancer have activating mutations or translocations targeting the RET tyrosine kinase receptor, raising the question of whether RET inhibitors might have a role in this disease.[55] Although no drugs specifically designed to inhibit RET have entered the clinic, four compounds with off target activity against RET (vandetanib, sorafenib, motesanib, and XL184) have all shown single agent activity in phase 2 thyroid cancer studies.[56–60] Three are currently under evaluation in phase 3 registration trials, one of which (vandetanib) has recently reported improved progression-free survival. Because all four compounds also inhibit VEGFR, it is unclear whether the clinical benefit observed in these studies is explained by inhibition of RET, VEGFR, or both. Unlike the crizotinib trials in ALK-positive lung cancer, enrollment in these registration studies was not restricted to patients with RET mutations. In addition to the fact that thyroid cancer patients are not routinely screened for these mutations, the primary reason for including all comers in these studies is that clinical responses are observed in a larger fraction of patients than can be accounted for based on the suspected frequency of RET mutation. Responses in patients without RET mutation (if they occur) might be explained by mutations in other genes in the RAS-MAP kinase pathway such as BRAF or HRAS, which are found in a substantial fraction of patients and are typically nonoverlapping with RET alterations.[55] Clearly, detailed genotype–response correlations, as demonstrated in lung cancer and melanoma, will clarify the role of these mutations in predicting response to these drugs. Thyroid cancer is also a compelling indication for the BRAF and MEK inhibitors discussed above in melanoma.

FLT3 Inhibitors in Acute Myeloid Leukemia

Shortly after the success of imatinib, the receptor tyrosine kinase FLT3 emerged as a compelling drug candidate based on the presence of activating mutations in about one-third of patients with acute myeloid leukemia (AML).[61] Laboratory studies documented that FLT3 alleles bearing these mutations, which occur as internal tandem duplications (ITDs) of the juxtamembrane domain or point mutation in the kinase domain, function as driver oncogenes in mouse models, giving phenotypes analogous to BCR-ABL.[62] As with RET in thyroid cancer, no compounds had been specifically optimized to target FLT3, but several drugs with off target FLT3 activity were redirected to AML. Disappointingly, the first three of the compounds tested (midostaurin, lestaurtinib, sunitinib) showed only marginal single agent activity in relapsed AML patients, even in those with FLT3 mutations.[63–65] Despite the strong molecular rationale for FLT3 as a driver lesion, questions were raised about the viability of FLT3 as a drug target. Pharmacodynamic studies showed evidence of FLT3 kinase inhibition in tumor cells, but the magnitude and duration of these effects were difficult to quantify, raising the possibility of inadequate target inhibition.[63] Indeed, the dose of all three compounds was limited by toxicities believed to be independent of FLT3. A more pessimistic interpretation was that FLT3, although presumably important for initiation of AML, was no longer required for tumor maintenance due to the accumulation of additional driver genomic alterations. If true, even complete FLT3 blockade with a highly selective inhibitor would be expected to fail. But this view was not supported by the fact that clinical responses were observed in the somewhat analogous situation of single agent ABL kinase inhibitor treatment of chronic myeloid leukemia in blast crisis, where BCR-ABL is just one of many additional genomic alterations that contributes to disease progression yet complete remissions are observed in many patients.

Despite this pessimism about FLT3 as a viable drug target, two drugs are now advancing toward drug registration trials. Midostaurin, one of the early compounds that showed disappointing single agent activity in relapsed AML, is being evaluated in a randomized phase 3 trial for newly diagnosed AML combined with standard induction chemotherapy. A single arm phase 2 study showed higher and more durable remission rates in FLT3 mutant patients when compared to historical controls.[66] The second compound, AC220, is a next generation FLT3 inhibitor with greater potency and specificity and with impressive single agent activity in *FLT3*-mutant relapsed AML—precisely the population where midostaurin and others failed.[67,68] It is not clear if this success is due to more potent FLT3 inhibition in patients since detailed pharmacodynamic studies are not yet available. Assuming these compounds prove successful in AML, it will be important to examine their activity in the rare cases of pediatric acute lymphoid leukemia associated with *FLT3* mutation. Although testing is still inconclusive on FLT3 inhibitors, the failure of early compounds in AML is reminiscent of the failures of early RAF and MEK inhibitors in melanoma. Collectively, these examples emphasize the importance of using optimized compounds to test a molecularly based hypothesis in patients and to focus enrollment on those patients with the relevant molecular lesion.

Kidney Cancer: Targeting the Tumor and the Host

A recurring theme in this chapter is the critical role of driver kinase mutations in guiding the development of kinase inhibitors. Ironically, four kinase inhibitors have been approved for kidney cancer over the past 5 years in a tumor type with no known kinase mutations. The most common molecular alteration in kidney cancer is loss of function in the Von Hippel-Lindau (*VHL*) tumor suppressor gene, resulting in activation of the

hypoxia inducible factor[66] pathway.[69] As a consequence of *VHL* loss, which normally targets hypoxia-induced factor (HIF) proteins for proteosomal degradation, HIF1α and HIF2α are constitutively active transcription factors that function as oncogenes through activation of an array of downstream target genes. Among these is the angiogenesis factor VEGF, which is secreted by HIF-expressing cells and promotes the development and maintenance of tumor neovasculature. HIF-mediated secretion of VEGF by tumor cells likely explains the highly vascular histopathology of clear cell renal carcinoma. All three currently approved angiogenesis inhibitors (the monoclonal antibody bevacizumab targeting VEGF and the kinase inhibitors sorafenib and sunitinib targeting its receptor VEGFR) have single agent clinical activity in clear cell carcinoma.[70–72] The high specificity of bevacizumab for VEGF leaves little doubt that the activity of this drug is explained by antiangiogenic effects. In contrast, the off target activities of sorafenib and sunitinib include several kinases expressed in kidney tumor cells, stroma, and inflammatory cells (PDGFR, RAF, RET, FLT3, and others). Interestingly, the primary effect of bevacizumab in kidney cancer is disease stabilization, whereas sorafenib and sunitinib have substantial partial response rates. This raises the question of whether the superior antitumor activity of the VEGFR kinase inhibitors is due to concurrent inhibition of other kinases. However, partial responses rates with next generation VEGFR inhibitors (axitinib, pazopanib, and tivozanib), all of which have greater potency and selectivity for VEGFR, are similarly high and reinforce the importance of VEGFR as the critical target in kidney cancer.[73–75] Molecular characterization of tumors from these patients should clarify the mechanism by which each of these inhibitors exerts antitumor activity, particularly if drug-resistant kinase domain mutations are found in any of the targets at relapse.

Two inhibitors of the mammalian target of rapamycin (mTOR) kinase (temsirolimus and everolimus) are also approved for advanced renal cell carcinoma.[76,77] Both temsirolimus and everolimus are known as rapalogs since both are chemical derivatives of the natural product sirolimus (rapamycin). Sirolimus was approved more than 10 years ago to prevent graft rejection in transplant recipients based on its immunosuppressive properties against T cells. Sirolimus also has potent antiproliferative effects against vascular endothelial cells and, on that basis, is incorporated into drug eluting cardiac stents to prevent coronary artery restenosis following angioplasty.[78] Rapalogs differ from other kinase inhibitors discussed in this chapter in that they inhibit the kinase through an allosteric mechanism rather than by targeting the mTOR kinase domain. Because rapalogs also inhibit the growth of cancer cell lines from different tissues of origin, clinical trials were initiated to study their potential role as anticancer agents in a broad range of tumor types. Based on responses in a few phase 1 patients with different tumor types (including kidney cancer), exploratory phase 2 studies were conducted in several diseases. Single agent activity of temsirolimus was observed in a phase 2 kidney cancer study[79] then confirmed in a phase 3 registration trial.[76] The phase 3 everolimus trial, which was initiated after temsirolimus, was noteworthy because clinical benefit was demonstrated in patients who had progressed on the VEGFR inhibitors sorafenib or sunitinib.[77]

In parallel with the empirical clinical development of rapalogs, various laboratories explored the molecular basis for mTOR dependence in cancer cells. mTOR functions at the center of a complex network that integrates signals from growth factor receptors and nutrient sensors to regulate cell growth and size (Fig. 13.2). It does so, in part, by controlling the translation of various mRNAs with complex 5′ untranslated regions into protein. mTOR exists in two distinct complexes known as TORC1 and TORC2. Rapalogs only inhibit the TORC1 complex, which is largely responsible for downstream phosphorylation of targets such as S6K1/2 and 4EBP1/2, which regulate protein translation.[80] The TORC2 complex contributes to activation of AKT by phosphorylating the important regulatory serine residue S473 and is unaffected by rapalogs.

Two hypotheses have emerged to explain the clinical activity of rapalogs in kidney cancer. The antiproliferative activity of these compounds against endothelial cells suggests an antiangiogenic mechanism and is consistent with the clinical activity of the VEGFR inhibitors. But rapalogs also inhibit the growth of kidney cancer cell lines in laboratory models where the effects on tumor angiogenesis have been eliminated. Interestingly, mRNAs for HIF1/2 are among those whose translation is impaired by rapalogs, and this effect has been implicated as the primary mechanism of rapalog activity in kidney cancer xenograft models.[81] As with the VEGFR inhibitors, detailed molecular annotation of tumors from responders and nonresponders will shed light on these issues.

Other Potential Indications for Mammalian Target of Rapamycin Inhibitors

The fact that rapalogs inhibit the growth of cancer cell lines and xenografts from different tumor types raised hopes for a broad role in cancer, but clinical trials of rapalogs outside of kidney cancer have generally been disappointing. Two exceptions are mantle cell lymphoma and endometrial cancer, where convincing single agent activity has led to ongoing drug registration trials.[82–85] Mantle cell lymphoma is characterized by a chromosome translocation that results in constitutive expression of the cell cycle regulatory protein cyclin D1, which functions as a driver oncogene in this disease. Rapalogs inhibit translation of cyclin D1 mRNA in laboratory models, analogous to the inhibition of HIF1/2 translation by rapalogs observed in VHL-mutant kidney cancer models. Endometrial cancers often have mutations in one of several genes in the PI3K pathway (PTEN, PIK3CA, PIK3R1), any one of which causes pathway activation. Because mTOR functions downstream of PI3K, tumors with these mutations should, in theory, respond to rapalogs. Many studies of cell lines, xenografts, and genetically engineered mouse models have linked PI3K pathway activation to increased sensitivity to rapalogs.[86,87] In fact, endometrial hyperplasia in mice with heterozygous loss of Pten is completely reversible by temsirolimus treatment.[88] As with kidney cancer, molecular annotation of the tumors from the mantle cell lymphoma and endometrial cancer patients on these trials is essential to address these questions.

It is unclear why rapalogs have failed in other tumor types. One likely explanation is the concurrence of PI3K pathway mutations with alterations in other pathways that mitigate sensitivity to rapalogs. Another possibility is the disruption of negative feedback loops regulated by mTOR that inhibit signaling from upstream receptor tyrosine kinases. Rapalogs paradoxically *increase* signaling through PI3K due to loss of this negative feedback. A primary consequence is *increased* AKT activation, which signals to an array of downstream substrates that can enhance cell proliferation and survival (other than TORC1, which remains inhibited by rapalog) (Fig. 13.2). This problem might be overcome by combining rapalogs with an inhibitor of an upstream kinase in the feedback loop, such as the insulin-like growth factor receptor (IGFR), to block this undesired effect of rapalogs on PI3K activation.[89] Alternatively, this feedback-mediated activation could, in theory, prevent use of inhibitors of PI3K itself or of the TORC2 complex that activates AKT.

TARGETING THE PI3K PATHWAY DIRECTLY

Mutations or copy number alterations (amplification or deletion of oncogenes or tumor suppressor genes) in PI3K pathway genes (PIK3CA, PIK3R1, PTEN, AKT1, and others) are among the most common abnormalities in cancer. Consequently, intensive efforts at many pharmaceutical companies have been devoted to the discovery of small molecule inhibitors targeting kinases in the PI3K pathway. Inhibitors of PI3K-, AKT-, and ATP-competitive (rather than allosteric) inhibitors of mTOR that target both the TORC1 and TORC2

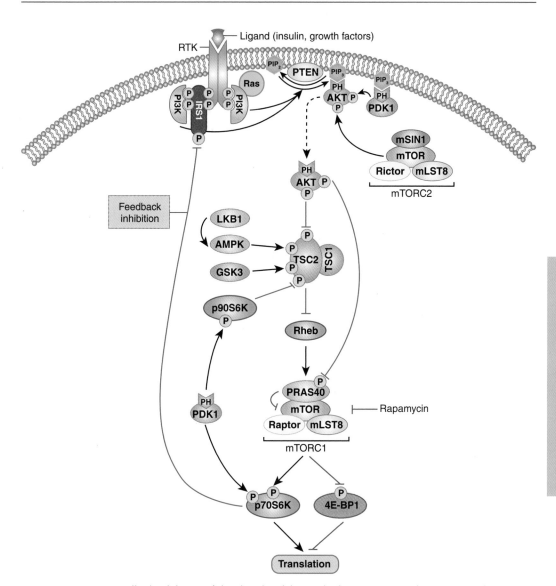

FIGURE 13.2 Feedback inhibition of the phosphatidylinositol 3-kinase (PI3K) pathway. Activated AKT regulates cellular growth through mammalian target of rapamycin (mTOR), a key player in protein synthesis and translation. mTOR forms part of two distinct complexes known as mTORC1 (which contains mTOR, Raptor, mLST8, and PRAS40) and mTORC2 (which contains mTOR, Rictor, mLST8, and mSIN1). mTORC1 is sensitive to rapamycin and controls protein synthesis and translation, at least in part, through p70S6K and eukaryotic translation initiation factor 4E–binding protein 1 (4E-BP1). AKT phosphorylates and inhibits tuberous sclerosis complex 2 (TSC2), resulting in increased mTORC1 activity. AKT also phosphorylates PRAS40, thus relieving the PRAS40 inhibitory effect on mTOR and the mTORC1 complex. mTORC2 and 3-phosphoinositide-dependent kinase (PDK1) phosphorylate AKT on Ser473 and Thr308, respectively, rendering it fully active. mTORC1-activated p70S6K can phosphorylate insulin receptor substrate 1 (IRS1), resulting in inhibition of PI3K activity. In addition, PDK1 phosphorylates and activates p70S6K and p90S6K. The latter has been shown to inhibit TSC2 activity through direct phosphorylation. Conversely, LKB1-activated AMP-activated protein kinase (AMPK) and glycogen synthase kinase 3 (GSK3) activate the TSC1/TSC2 complex through direct phosphorylation of TSC2. Thus, signals through PI3K as well as through LKB1 and AMPK converge on mTORC1. Inhibition of mTORC1 can lead to increased insulin receptor–mediated signaling, and inhibition of PDK1 may lead to activation of mTORC1 and may, paradoxically, promote tumor growth. (From ref. 115, with permission.)

TABLE 13.3

COMPOUNDS IN CLINICAL DEVELOPMENT THAT TARGET THE PI3K PATHWAY

Compound	Target	Company	Clinical Trial Stage
BEZ235	PI3K & mTOR	Novartis	Phase 2
BKM120	PI3K	Novartis	Phase 1
SF1126	PI3K family	Semafore	Phase 1
GSK1059615B	PI3K & mTOR	GSK	Phase 1
XL765	PI3K & mTOR	Exelixis	Phase 2
XL147	PI3K	Exelixis	Phase 2
GDC0941	PI3K alpha	Genentech	Phase 1
PX-866	PI3K	Oncothyreon	Phase 1
VQD-002 (triciribine)	pan-AKT	VioQuest	Phase 1
GSK690693	pan-AKT	GSK	Phase 1
MK-2206	AKT	Merck	Phase 2
Perifosine (KRX-0401)	pan-AKT	Keryx	Phase 2
Everolimus (RAD001)	TORC1 (mTOR)	Novartis	Approved
Temsirolimus (CCI779)	TORC1 (mTOR)	Wyeth	Approved
Rapamycin (Rapamune)	TORC1 (mTOR)	Wyeth	Approved
AZD8055	TORC1/2 (mTOR)	AstraZeneca	Phase 1
OSI-027	TORC1/2 (mTOR)	OSI	Phase 1
INK-128	TORC1/2 (mTOR)	Intellikine	Phase 1

complex are all in clinical development (Table 13.3). Phase 1 clinical trials have, in general, established that the pathway can be efficiently targeted without serious toxicity other than easily manageable effects on glucose metabolism (anticipated based on the importance of PI3K signaling in insulin signaling). Unfortunately, there has been no evidence to date of dramatic single agent clinical activity with any of these agents. To be fair, most compounds are still in a very early clinical development stage and have been evaluated without enriching for patients with PI3K pathway mutations.

Conducting a PI3K pathway mutation-enriched trial is challenging because no single tumor type has such a high frequency of mutations that it becomes the obvious disease for early clinical development (in contrast to BRAF in melanoma). A compelling case can be made for PIK3CA mutant breast or endometrial cancer, but these trials are not straightforward because PIK3CA mutations in breast cancer are associated with good prognosis disease that is often cured by standard therapy.[90] A further complication is the fact that mutations in the PI3K pathway can occur in one of many different genes in the pathway (PIK3CA, PIK3R1, PTEN, AKT1, etc.) and sometimes in combination.[91] Treatment response may vary depending on the type of mutation; therefore, lumping patients with different PI3K pathway mutations into the same trial may complicate data interpretation. Indeed, tumor cell lines with PIK3CA mutation respond differently to a PI3K pathway inhibitor compared to those with PTEN loss.[92] There are also technical challenges in developing an assay to determine mutation status for genes like PTEN, which can be inactivated by point mutation, deletion, or transcriptional silencing. The success or failure of these drugs as single agents should become clear in the next few years based on the outcome of many phase 2 studies that are currently under way.

COMBINATIONS OF KINASE INHIBITORS

Preclinical studies indicate that combinations of kinase inhibitors are required to realize their full potential as anticancer agents. The most common rationale is to address the problem of concurrent mutations in different pathways that alleviate dependence on a single driver oncogene. The best examples are cancers with mutations in both the RAS/MAP kinase pathway (RAS or BRAF) and the PI3K pathway (PIK3CA or PTEN). In mouse models, such doubly mutant tumors fail to respond to single agent treatment with either an AKT inhibitor or a MEK inhibitor. However, combination treatment can give dramatic regressions.[93] Similarly, genetically engineered mice that develop KRAS-driven lung cancer respond only to combination therapy with a PI3K inhibitor and a MEK inhibitor.[94] Several combination therapy trials combining different PI3K pathway and RAS/MAP kinase pathway inhibitors have recently been initiated.

Many of the tumor types discussed in this chapter *do* respond to treatment with a single agent kinase but relapse despite continued inhibitor therapy. Research into the causes of "acquired" kinase inhibitor resistance has revealed two primary mechanisms: novel mutations in the kinase domain of the drug target that preclude inhibition, or "bypass" of the driver kinase signal by activation of a parallel kinase pathway. In both cases, the solution is combination therapy to prevent the emergence of resistance. An elegant demonstration of this approach comes from CML where resistance to imatinib is primarily caused by mutations in the BCR-ABL kinase domain.[95,96] The second-generation ABL inhibitors dasatinib and nilotinib are effective against most imatinib-resistant BCR-ABL mutants and were initially approved as single agent therapy for imatinib-resistant chronic myeloid leukemia.[97,98] Very recently, both drugs have proven superior to imatinib in upfront treatment of chronic myeloid leukemia, due to increased potency and fewer mechanisms of acquired resistance.[99–101] However, one BCR-ABL mutation called T315I is resistant to all three drugs. A novel ABL kinase inhibitor AP24534 that blocks T315I has shown promising activity in a phase 1 clinical trial that included CML patients with the T315I mutation.[102,103] If AP24534 proves successful, a two drug combination of AP24534 with either dasatinib or nilotinib would likely shut off all mechanisms of relapse, analogous to triple drug highly active antiretroviral therapy (HAART) for human immunodeficiency virus (HIV). Analogous approaches should also be successful in other diseases such as EGFR-mutant lung cancer and KIT-mutant GIST where acquired resistance to the front-line kinase inhibitor is also associated with mutations in the target kinase.[104,105]

The clinical development of kinase inhibitor combinations to prevent acquired resistance is straightforward. Since the frontline drug is already approved, success would be determined by an improvement in response duration using the combination. The situation is more complex when two experimental compounds (e.g., a PI3K pathway inhibitor and a MEK inhibitor) are combined, neither of which shows significant single agent activity. Current regulatory guidelines require a four arm study that compares each single agent to the combination and to a control group in order to obtain approval of the combination. This design can discourage drug developers as well as patients from moving forward because it requires a large sample size, and it requires that 75% of the patients be assigned to treatment arms that are expected to be inactive. In response to growing preclinical evidence supporting the unique activity of certain combinations, these guidelines are now under revision. A more challenging issue may be optimization of the dose and schedule needed to safely combine two investigational drugs. Much like the development of combination chemotherapy several decades ago, it may be important to select compounds with nonoverlapping toxicities to allow sufficient doses of each drug to be achieved. Investigators may also need to adopt higher toxicity thresholds.

SPECULATIONS ON THE FUTURE ROLE OF KINASE INHIBITORS IN CANCER MEDICINE

The role of genomics in predicting response to kinase inhibitor therapy is now irrefutable. As the number of kinase driver mutations continues to grow, the field is likely to move away from the current strategy of a "companion diagnostic" for each drug. Rather, comprehensive mutational profiling platforms that query each tumor for hundreds of potential cancer mutations are more likely to emerge as the diagnostic platform. Only a small number of mutations are "actionable" in 2010 (meaning the presence of a mutation defines a treatment decision), but this number will undoubtedly grow. In addition, the presence or absence of concurrent mutations will guide decisions about combination therapies.

More effort must be devoted to manipulating the dose and schedule of kinase inhibitor therapy to maximize efficacy and minimize toxicity. To date all kinase inhibitors have been developed based on the assumption that 24/7 coverage of the target is required for efficacy. Consequently, most compounds are optimized to have a long serum half-life (12 to 24 hours). Phase 2 doses are then selected based on the maximum tolerated dose determined with daily administration. But a recent clinical trial of the ABL inhibitor dasatinib in CML indicates that equivalent antitumor activity can be achieved with intermittent therapy.[106] By giving larger doses intermittently, higher peak drug concentrations were achieved that resulted in equivalent and possibly superior efficacy.[107] Similar results were observed in laboratory studies of EGFR inhibitors in EGFR-mutant lung cancer. Clinically robust, quantitative assays of target inhibition are needed to hasten progress in this area.

Although the focus of this chapter is kinase inhibitors, the themes developed here should apply broadly to inhibitors of other cancer targets. Early clinical results with inhibitors of the G-protein coupled receptor smoothened (SMO) in patients with metastatic basal cell carcinoma or medulloblastoma establish that the driver mutation hypothesis extends beyond kinase inhibitors. SMO is a component in the hedgehog pathway that is constitutively activated in subsets of patients with basal cell carcinoma and medulloblastoma due to mutations in the hedgehog ligand binding receptor Patched-1. Treatment with the SMO inhibitor GDC-0449 led to impressive responses in basal cell carcinoma and medulloblastoma patients whose tumors had Patched-1

GENERAL PRINCIPLES

mutations.[108,109] Other novel cancer targets are emerging from cancer genome sequencing projects. Somatic mutations in the Krebs cycle enzyme isocitrate dehydrogenase (*IDH1/2*) were found in subsets of patients with glioblastoma and acute myeloid leukemia.[110–112] Mutations in enzymes involved in chromatin remodeling were recently found in kidney cancer.[113] Drug discovery programs are already under way to find inhibitors of several of these mutant enzymes. Kinase inhibitors are just the first wave of molecularly targeted drugs ushered in through understanding of the molecular underpinnings of cancer cells. There is much more to follow.

Selected References

The full list of references for this chapter appears in the online version.

1. Sawyers CL. Shifting paradigms: the seeds of oncogene addiction. *Nat Med* 2009;15(10):1158.
2. Weinstein IB. Cancer. Addiction to oncogenes—the Achilles heal of cancer. *Science* 2002;297(5578):63.
3. Druker BJ, Talpaz M, Resta DJ, et al. Efficacy and safety of a specific inhibitor of the BCR-ABL tyrosine kinase in chronic myeloid leukemia. *N Engl J Med* 2001;344(14):1031.
4. Hirota S, Isozaki K, Moriyama Y, et al. Gain-of-function mutations of c-kit in human gastrointestinal stromal tumors. *Science* 1998;279(5350):577.
6. Demetri GD, von Mehren M, Blanke CD, et al. Efficacy and safety of imatinib mesylate in advanced gastrointestinal stromal tumors. *N Engl J Med* 2002;347(7):472.
7. Geyer CE, Forster J, Lindquist D, et al. Lapatinib plus capecitabine for HER2-positive advanced breast cancer. *N Engl J Med* 2006;355 (26):2733.
8. Kris MG, Natale RB, Herbst RS, et al. Efficacy of gefitinib, an inhibitor of the epidermal growth factor receptor tyrosine kinase, in symptomatic patients with non-small cell lung cancer: a randomized trial. *JAMA* 2003;290(16):2149.
10. Paez JG, Jänne PA, Lee JC, et al. EGFR mutations in lung cancer: correlation with clinical response to gefitinib therapy. *Science* 2004; 304(5676):1497.
11. Lynch TJ, Bell DW, Sordella R, et al. Activating mutations in the epidermal growth factor receptor underlying responsiveness of non–small-cell lung cancer to gefitinib. *N Engl J Med* 2004;350(21):2129.
12. Pao W, Miller V, Zakowski M, et al. EGF receptor gene mutations are common in lung cancers from "never smokers" and are associated with sensitivity of tumors to gefitinib and erlotinib. *Proc Natl Acad Sci U S A* 2004;101 (36):13306.
14. Shepherd FA, Rodrigues Pereira J, Ciuleanu T, et al. Erlotinib in previously treated non-small-cell lung cancer. *N Engl J Med* 2005;353(2):123.
19. Tsao MS, Sakurada A, Cutz JC, et al. Erlotinib in lung cancer—molecular and clinical predictors of outcome. *N Engl J Med* 2005;353(2):133.
20. Mok TS, Wu YL, Thongprasert S, et al. Gefitinib or carboplatin-paclitaxel in pulmonary adenocarcinoma. *N Engl J Med* 2009;361(10):947.
23. Cools J, DeAngelo DJ, Gotlib J, et al. A tyrosine kinase created by fusion of the PDGFRA and FIP1L1 genes as a therapeutic target of imatinib in idiopathic hypereosinophilic syndrome. *N Engl J Med* 2003;348(13):1201.
27. Davies H, Bignell GR, Cox C, et al. Mutations of the BRAF gene in human cancer. *Nature* 2002;417(6892):949.
28. Baxter EJ, Scott LM, Campbell PJ, et al. Acquired mutation of the tyrosine kinase JAK2 in human myeloproliferative disorders. *Lancet* 2005;365(9464):1054.
29. James C, Ugo V, Le Couédic JP, et al. A unique clonal JAK2 mutation leading to constitutive signalling causes polycythaemia vera. *Nature* 2005;434(7037):1144.
30. Levine RL, Wadleigh M, Cools J, et al. Activating mutation in the tyrosine kinase JAK2 in polycythemia vera, essential thrombocythemia, and myeloid metaplasia with myelofibrosis. *Cancer Cell* 2005;7(4):387.

31. Samuels Y, Wang Z, Bardelli A, et al. High frequency of mutations of the PIK3CA gene in human cancers. *Science* 2004;304(5670):554.
37. Solit DB, Garraway LA, Pratilas CA, et al. BRAF mutation predicts sensitivity to MEK inhibition. *Nature* 2006;439 (7074):358.
45. Flaherty KT, Puzanov I, Kim KB, et al. Inhibition of mutated, activated BRAF in metastatic melanoma. *N Engl J Med* 2010;363(9):809.
46. Bollag G, Hirth P, Tsai J, et al. Clinical efficacy of a RAF inhibitor needs broad target blockade in BRAF-mutant melanoma. *Nature* 2010;467:596.
51. Soda M, Choi YL, Enomoto M, et al. Identification of the transforming EML4-ALK fusion gene in non-small-cell lung cancer. *Nature* 2007;448(7153):561.
61. Sawyers CL. Finding the next Gleevec: FLT3 targeted kinase inhibitor therapy for acute myeloid leukemia. *Cancer Cell* 2002;1(5):413.
67. Zarrinkar PP, Gunawardane RN, Cramer MD, et al. AC220 is a uniquely potent and selective inhibitor of FLT3 for the treatment of acute myeloid leukemia (AML). *Blood* 2009;114(14):2984.
70. Yang JC, Haworth L, Sherry RM, et al. A randomized trial of bevacizumab, an anti-vascular endothelial growth factor antibody, for metastatic renal cancer. *N Engl J Med* 2003;349(5):427.
71. Escudier B, Eisen T, Stadler WM, et al. Sorafenib in advanced clear-cell renal-cell carcinoma. *N Engl J Med* 2007;356(2):125.
72. Motzer RJ, Hutson TE, Tomczak P, et al. Sunitinib versus interferon alfa in metastatic renal-cell carcinoma. *N Engl J Med* 2007;356(2):115.
76. Hudes G, Carducci M, Tomczak P, et al. Temsirolimus, interferon alfa, or both for advanced renal-cell carcinoma. *N Engl J Med* 2007;356(22):2271.
77. Motzer RJ, Escudier B, Oudard S, et al. Efficacy of everolimus in advanced renal cell carcinoma: a double-blind, randomised, placebo-controlled phase III trial. *Lancet* 2008; 372(9637):449.
81. Thomas GV, Tran C, Mellinghoff IK, et al. Hypoxia-inducible factor determines sensitivity to inhibitors of mTOR in kidney cancer. *Nat Med* 2006;12(1):122.
82. Hess G, Herbrecht R, Romaguera J, et al. Phase III study to evaluate temsirolimus compared with investigator,s choice therapy for the treatment of relapsed or refractory mantle cell lymphoma. *J Clin Oncol* 2009;27(23):3822.
86. Neshat MS, Mellinghoff IK, Tran C, et al. Enhanced sensitivity of PTEN-deficient tumors to inhibition of FRAP/mTOR. *Proc Natl Acad Sci U S A* 2001;98(18):10314.
87. Majumder PK, Febbo PG, Bikoff R, et al. mTOR inhibition reverses Akt-dependent prostate intraepithelial neoplasia through regulation of apoptotic and HIF-1-dependent pathways. *Nat Med* 2004;10(6):594.
88. Podsypanina K, Lee RT, Politis C, et al. An inhibitor of mTOR reduces neoplasia and normalizes p70/S6 kinase activity in Pten+/- mice. *Proc Natl Acad Sci U S A* 2001;98 (18):10320.
89. O,Reilly KE, Rojo F, She QB, et al. mTOR inhibition induces upstream receptor tyrosine kinase signaling and activates Akt. *Cancer Res* 2006;66 (3):1500.

93. She QB, Halilovic E, Ye Q, et al. 4E-BP1 is a key effector of the oncogenic activation of the AKT and ERK signaling pathways that integrates their function in tumors. *Cancer Cell* 2010;18(1):39.

94. Engelman JA, Chen L, Tan X, et al. Effective use of PI3K and MEK inhibitors to treat mutant Kras G12D and PIK3CA H1047R murine lung cancers. *Nat Med* 2008; 14(12):1351.

95. Gorre ME, Mohammed M, Ellwood K, et al. Clinical resistance to STI-571 cancer therapy caused by BCR-ABL gene mutation or amplification. *Science* 2001;293(5531):876.

96. Shah NP, Nicoll JM, Nagar B, et al. Multiple BCR-ABL kinase domain mutations confer polyclonal resistance to the tyrosine kinase inhibitor imatinib (STI571) in chronic phase and blast crisis chronic myeloid leukemia. *Cancer Cell* 2002;2(2):117.

97. Shah NP, Tran C, Lee FY, et al. Overriding imatinib resistance with a novel ABL kinase inhibitor. *Science* 2004;305 (5682):399.

98. Talpaz M, Shah NP, Kantarjian H, et al. Dasatinib in imatinib-resistant Philadelphia chromosome-positive leukemias. *N Engl J Med* 2006; 354(24):2531.

99. Kantarjian H, Shah NP, Hochhaus A, et al. Dasatinib versus imatinib in newly diagnosed chronic-phase chronic myeloid leukemia. *N Engl J Med* 2010;362(24): 2260.

100. Sawyers CL. Even better kinase inhibitors for chronic myeloid leukemia. *N Engl J Med* 2010;362(24):2314.

101. Saglio G, Kim DW, Issaragrisil S, et al. Nilotinib versus imatinib for newly diagnosed chronic myeloid leukemia. *N Engl J Med* 2010;362(24):2251.

104. Pao W, Miller VA, Politi KA, et al. Acquired resistance of lung adenocarcinomas to gefitinib or erlotinib is associated with a second mutation in the EGFR kinase domain. *PLoS Med* 2005;2(3):e73.

105. Antonescu CR, Besmer P, Guo T, et al. Acquired resistance to imatinib in gastrointestinal stromal tumor occurs through secondary gene mutation. *Clin Cancer Res* 2005; 11(11):4182.

106. Shah NP, et al. Intermittent target inhibition with dasatinib 100 mg once daily preserves efficacy and improves tolerability in imatinib-resistant and -intolerant chronic-phase chronic myeloid leukemia. *J Clin Oncol* 2008;26(19): 3204.

107. Shah NP, Kasap C, Weier C, et al. Transient potent BCR-ABL inhibition is sufficient to commit chronic myeloid leukemia cells irreversibly to apoptosis. *Cancer Cell* 2008;14 (6):485.

GENERAL PRINCIPLES

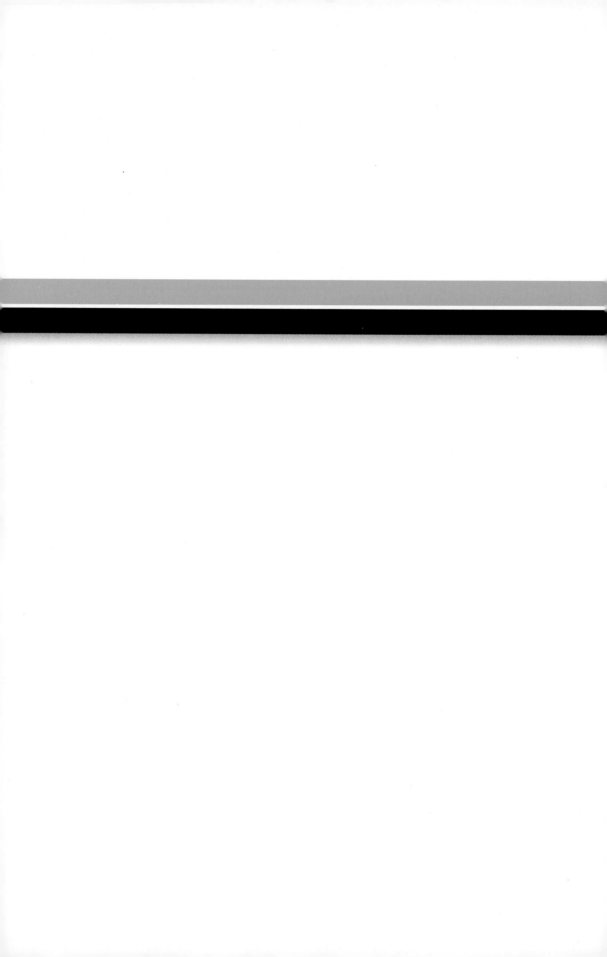

PART TWO

MOLECULAR BIOLOGY OF INDIVIDUAL CANCERS

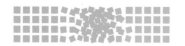

CHAPTER 14 HEAD AND NECK CANCERS

NISHANT AGRAWAL, JOSEPH CALIFANO, AND PATRICK HA

Research regarding head and neck squamous cell carcinoma (HNSCC) has shifted from the detection of individual gene mutations and deletions to detailing the complex interactions of networks of genes altered by genetic alterations, including sequence alterations, chromosomal aberrations, epigenetic modifications, microRNA changes, and even mitochondrial mutations. High throughput, whole-genome–based discovery approaches that have been successful in other tumor types are currently being employed in the study of HNSCC.

With improved understanding of HNSCC has come the solidification of several different mechanisms of carcinogenesis. Although the majority of these cancers still come from mutagenic environmental exposures, namely tobacco (smoking or chewing) and use of betel products, the rise in prevalence of oropharyngeal cancer in the United States is largely related to human papillomavirus (HPV) type 16. With the different etiologies of cancer development, we have seen distinctions in clinical behavior and thus can directly see how the underlying molecular mechanisms may have important clinical implications.

In this chapter, we highlight some of the newer developments in HNSCC research that have special relevance to clinical therapeutics. As we further understand the underlying genetic basis of this disease, we can transition this knowledge into developing targeted therapy and refine treatment paradigms. These data are by no means comprehensive, as the expansion in detailed knowledge regarding HNSCC biology has dramatically expanded.

GENETIC SUSCEPTIBILITY

Despite the well-established association between HNSCC and smoking, heavy ethanol use, and betel use, the overall incidence of HNSCC remains relatively low. Thus, there must be elements of genetic susceptibility that predispose certain patients to disease progression while in others there is relative resistance to cancer formation. Several case-control studies have demonstrated that first-degree relatives of patients with HNSCC were 3.5- to 3.8-fold more likely to also

develop HNSCC even when controlling for factors such as age, gender, ethnicity, tobacco, and alcohol use.[1–3] Likewise, HNSCC patients were found to be 3.8 times more likely to develop a second primary tumor if one or more first-degree relatives suffered from upper aerodigestive tract cancer.[4]

These familial susceptibilities provide evidence that there are likely underlying genetic mechanisms that preclude one to cancer formation. However, direct evidence of heritable HNSCC syndromes is rare. The most common direct, genetic association with HNSCC exists with Fanconi anemia, a rare, autosomal recessive disease associated with aplastic anemia, congenital anomalies, and a predisposition for cancer development, especially head and neck and anogenital squamous cell carcinoma.[5] There has been suggestion that one of the mechanisms of cancer development in Fanconi anemia is HPV-related, but recent studies show that the precise mechanism of susceptibility remains unknown and that the presence of high-risk HPV viruses in Fanconi anemia–related HNSCC is variable.[6] There have also been associations with HNSCC and other syndromes such as Lynch-II, Bloom, xeroderma pigmentosum, ataxia telangiectasia, and Li-Fraumeni,[7] all of which have specific genetic aberrations that link them to cancer. The fact that a consistent genetic mechanism remains elusive in HNSCC highlights its heterogeneity.

Building on the link between these known syndromes and gene alterations, investigators have looked to other genetic polymorphisms, such as single nucleotide polymorphisms (SNPs), to evaluate whether patterns of HNSCC susceptibility can be detected. It is important to note that it is generally not known what the exact differential function is of these SNPs and whether they have a direct link toward carcinogenesis. Many of the single-institution studies also suffer from smaller sample sizes and lack the ability to control for the potential ethnic or geographic variability inherent in these polymorphisms.

The general families of gene alterations have focused on carcinogen-detoxifying mechanisms (cytochrome p450 members [CYP], glutathione-S-transferases [GSTs], alcohol and ethanol dehydrogenases [ADH and ALDH]), DNA damage repair, nucleotide excision repair enzymes (NER), excision repair cross-complementing rodent repair deficiency complementation genes (ERCC), x-ray repair complementing defective repair in Chinese hamster cells (XRCC), and RecA homolog, *Escherichia coli* (Rad51), inflammation/angiogenesis (cyclooxygenase-2 [COX-2], hypoxia-inducible factors [HIF], cytokines), apoptosis, cell cycle, and many other pathways salient to cancer formation.

Larger cooperative studies, across institutions, help to further refine the most important polymorphisms and provide the greatest evidence for their role in carcinogenesis. A cooperative European group (ARCAGE) surveyed 115 polymorphisms in 62 selected genes in a cohort of 1,511 cases and 1,457 controls.[8] Several genes showed promise (*CYP2*, murine double-minute 2 [*MDM2*], and tumor necrosis factor [*TNF*]), but there still remains work to be done in looking at the mechanisms and applicability of these markers. Another multinational study pooled patient samples from several institutions and used a cohort of over 3,000 HNSCC patients along with over 5,000 controls and discovered a protective effect from two of the studied ADH polymorphisms.[9]

Despite the numerous studies looking at these relationships, the effects of polymorphic variants seem to be quite modest, and there are often conflicting studies reported on the same polymorphisms, underscoring the complexity of HNSCC as well as the role of these DNA changes. Further study to validate the previously studied SNPs with a relationship to HNSCC as well as mechanistic confirmation of an altered function would help to further our understanding of carcinogenesis. With newer technology, there will be an opportunity to perform further genome-wide screens to discover new targets as well in an effort to make sense of the complicated pathway associations that these SNPs have in the context of specific patient variables.

MOLECULAR NETWORKS ALTERED IN HNSCC

Tumorigenesis in the head and neck is the result of multiple genetic and epigenetic alterations of molecular pathways in the squamous epithelium.[10,11] The progression of head and neck cancer is thought to result from multistep alterations in tumor suppressor genes and oncogenes.[10,12–18] A variety of genetic changes have been reported for squamous cell carcinomas (SCCs) including loss of heterozygosity or amplification of specific chromosomal regions, although tumor suppressor genes have not been characterized for most of the regions that are commonly lost in HNSCC. Nevertheless, several signaling pathways have been implicated and are described in the following sections (Table 14.1).

MOLECULAR BIOLOGY OF INDIVIDUAL CANCERS

TABLE 14.1

COMMON GENETIC ALTERATIONS IN HEAD AND NECK SQUAMOUS CELL CARCINOMA

Alteration	Frequency	Comments
p16 inactivation	70%	Via homozygous deletion and less frequently promoter methylation
p53 mutation	50%	Predominantly mutation
High-risk HPV integration	25%	Found predominantly in oropharyngeal sites
EGFR axis alteration	80%–90%	Via amplification, overexpression, and downstream target activation
PI3-K/AKT/mTOR	>40%	
(DIME-6), ATM, p15, TIMP-3, MGMT, RARB-2, DAP-K, E-cadherin, cyclin A1, RASSF1A, CDKN2A, CDH1, and DCC	Variable, up to 60% (DCC)	Inactivated by promoter hypermethylation
HIF-1α	60%	Proliferation, angiogenesis
VEGF and other angiogenic pathways	Variable	
E-cadherin, matrix metalloproteinases	Variable	Invasion, anoikis, and metastasis
TKTL1, cancer testes antigens	50%	Protooncogenes activated by promoter hypomethylation

HPV, human papillomavirus; EGFR, epidermal growth factor receptor; DCC, deleted in colon cancer; HIF-1α, hypoxia-inducible factor-1-α; VEGF, vascular endothelial growth factor; TKTL1, tansketolase-like-1.

P16/p53/Cyclin D

Loss of 9p21, resulting in inactivation of the *p16* gene, is the most common genetic alteration in the progression of head and neck cancer.[19,20] P16 is an inhibitor of cyclin-dependent kinase (CDK), which is intimately involved in G1 cell-cycle regulation. Phosphorylation and inactivation of pRb by unbridled CDK4 and CDK6 enable cells to escape senescence. Loss of chromosome 9p21 occurs in the majority of invasive tumors and is also present at a high frequency in the earliest definable lesions, including dysplasia and carcinoma *in situ*.[19] Loss of p16 appears necessary for immortalization of keratinocytes.[21] Loss of p16 protein has been observed in most advanced premalignant lesions.[22] In addition to deletions and point mutations, p16 is also inactivated by methylation of the 5′CpG region.[23] This methylation is associated with complete block of *p16* transcription and appears to be a common mechanism for p16 inactivation. The notion that p16 inactivation is directly involved in the progression of primary tumors has been strengthened. Lack of p16 protein was detected by immunostaining in most primary invasive lesions, and tumors with absent p16 protein contained a homozygous deletion, methylation, or point mutation of p16.[24]

Loss of *p53* on chromosomal region 17p13 and subsequent point mutation within the remaining allele is another critical step in tumor progression. Inactivation of *p53* now represents the best-described and most common genetic change in all of human cancer.[25] Initially by analysis of exons 5-8, *p53* mutations were observed in approximately 50% of head and neck tumors.[26,27] The *p53* gene can be inactivated by a large variety of distinct mutations and more thorough sequence analyses of exons 2-11, a *p53* mutation rate of almost 80% has been observed in head and neck tumors.[28] *p53* normally halts cell-cycle progression in the setting of DNA damage and induces apoptosis with inadequate DNA repair. *p53* mutations result in a progression from preinvasive to invasive lesions, while increasing the probability of further progression. If 17p loss or *p53* mutation is present in early lesions, the chance of progression to cancer within 10 years approaches 80% (33-fold relative risk). In a large definitive collaborative group study, disruptive *p53* mutations were an independent prognostic marker and predicted a worse outcome in surgically resected primary tumors.[29]

Carcinogens in tobacco and alcohol have a causal role as the prevalence of *p53* mutations is greater in patients who smoke and drink alcohol.[30] HPV16- and HPV18-induced SCC of the oropharynx is more common in nonsmokers and is not associated with *p53* mutations. Instead, the viral oncoprotein E6 promotes the accelerated, ubiquitin-mediated, degradation of *p53*.

Amplification of chromosome region 11q13 containing cyclin D1 is seen in approximately one-third of head and neck tumors.[31] The role of cyclin *D1* in the progression of human cancer is now well established and constitutive activation of oncogene cyclin D1 has been shown to confer a growth advantage in SCCs.[32] Other tumor suppressor genes, including *Rb* and *p16*, are negative regulators of the *cyclin D1* pathway and often are inactivated in human neoplasms. Cyclin *D1* amplification is independent of *p16* inactivation in head and neck cancers.[33]

PI3-K/AKT/mTOR

Mutation in the PI3-K signaling pathway are found in up to 30% of all human cancers, and activation of the PI3-K/AKT/mTOR pathway has also been implicated in tumorigenesis of HNSCC.[34] Mutations of the PI3-K network have shown to confer a growth advantage, transforming capacity, and drug resistance.[35] The PI3-K family is divided into three different classes based on structure and substrate specificity. Class I PI3-Ks are heterodimers of a p85 regulatory subunit and a p110 catalytic subunit, which is mutated in many cancers. The class I PI3-Ks are activated by tyrosine kinase receptors, including epidermal growth factor receptor (EGFR) and oncogenic proteins, and lead to the production of the lipid second messenger, phosphatidylinositol 3-phosphatase (PIP3), which in turn facilitates phosphorylation and subsequent activation of AKT. The PI3-K pathway also leads to activation of the serine/threonine kinase, mammalian target of rapamycin (mTOR), which in turn phosphorylates p70S6K, a kinase that modulates protein synthesis.

Invasion/Metastasis

Metastasis is a complicated, multistep process in which selective pressures select for a clone of malignant cells selected to survive in a distant, permissive environment. The multistep process includes angiogenesis, altered cellular adhesion, cellular motility, disruption of the base membrane/extracellular matrix, and anchorage-independent proliferation.

Up-regulation of hypoxia-inducible factor 1-α (HIF-1α), induced by intratumor hypoxia, has been documented in invasive HNSCC and correlates with progression to a more invasive and aggressive phenotype.[36,37] HIF-1α is a master regulator of oxygen homeostasis and activates genes involved in angiogenesis, glucose metabolism, cell survival, invasion, cell renewal, and immortalization.[38–40]

The vascular endothelial growth factor (VEGF) pathway is critical in angiogenesis in HNSCC. Increased expression of VEGF and its receptors is regulated by HIF-1α–dependent and -independent pathways, both of which converge on the PI3-K/AKT pathway.

Diminished cell-to-cell adhesion, through down-regulation of cellular adhesions molecules such as E-cadherin, is integral to invasion.[41,42] In addition to cell-to-cell adhesion mediated by cadherins, integrins that mediate cell-to-extracellular matrix interaction also play a fundamental role in tumor cells gaining access to the angiolymphatic system.[43] Laminins, which are extracellular glycoproteins, are one of the ligands for integrins. Laminin 5 is overexpressed in invasive fronts, is associated with poorer prognosis, and downstream activates mitogen-activated protein kinase, which leads to cell survival and proliferation.[44–51] In addition to altered cell adhesion, migration mediated by the Rho family of GTPases is an important step in the multistep process of metastasis.[52] Cancer cells also actively disrupt the base membrane through the proteolytic activity of zinc-dependent endopeptidases, matrix metalloproteinases (MMPs), to disseminate. MMPs degrade most components of the base membrane, including collagen. Evasion from anchorage-dependent survival is a feature of metastatic HNSCC, and anoikis resistance is crucial in the process of metastasis as a defense against microenvironmental death stimuli. E-cadherin has been implicated in conferring anoikis resistance in HNSCC by physically associating with a number of signaling effectors such as PI3K and EGFR.[53,54]

Epidermal Growth Factor Receptor

The *EGFR* is one of the best-studied oncogenes in HNSCC. This receptor tyrosine kinase belongs to the ErbB family of cell surface receptors and has many downstream signaling targets associated with carcinogenesis. Once phosphorylated, the receptor can signal via the MAPK, Akt, ERK, and Jak/STAT pathways (Fig. 14.1). These pathways are related to cellular proliferation, apoptosis, invasion, angiogenesis, and metastasis.[55–57] Expression of *EGFR* is a normal finding in many tissues including the dermis, gastrointestinal tract, and kidneys. However, dysfunction of this receptor and its associated pathways occurs in most epithelial cancers[55] and 80% to 90% of HNSCC specifically.[9,56] The story of *EGFR* is promising in that our understanding of its molecular biology has led directly to clinically beneficial targeted therapies and its use as a marker and prognosticator of disease.

Initially, EGFR was first found to be up-regulated in HNSCC cell lines and in a high percentage of primary HNSCC.[58–60] Further study showed that histopathologically normal mucosa adjacent to cancer had a high degree of overexpression[61] and that the up-regulation of EGFR occurs in the transition from dysplasia to HNSCC.[62] Now it is well known that elevated levels of expression predict a worse disease-free and cause-specific survival.[63] Studies looking at copy number amplification have also been shown to be associated with poorer prognosis in HNSCC. One study has demonstrated that the overexpression of *EGFR* is a biomarker for an improved response to therapy and could serve as a predictive marker to separate patients into different arms of therapeutic trials.[64]

In addition to serving as a marker for prognosis, EGFR axis alterations are currently under investigation as markers for response to treatment and as therapeutic targets. Several strategies exist for targeting the EGFR pathway including the use of specific tyrosine kinase inhibitors (TKIs), monoclonal antibodies blocking receptor dimerization, and antisense oligodeoxynucleotides or siRNA blocking mRNA expression.

Cetuximab is one of the most well studied monoclonal antibodies directed against EGFR. A recently published phase 3 clinical trial examined the effects of this drug in conjunction with radiotherapy in the treatment of locoregionally advanced HNSCC. This study demonstrated an overall survival benefit (49 vs. 29 months) and increased duration of locoregional control (24.4 vs. 14.9 months) in the cetuximab plus radiotherapy arm versus the arm receiving radiotherapy alone. This was the first randomized study showing a survival benefit with an EGFR targeting agent in locally advanced HNSCC.[65,66] Conversely, the TKI gefitinib has shown no survival benefit for recurrent or metastatic HNSCC.[66,67] There are, however, several phase 1 and 2 trials under way studying the concomitant use of chemoradiation with gefitinib and two other TKIs (erlotinib and lapatinib) in the treatment of HNSCC.[68] There are several other studies currently investigating the role of EGFR targeting agents, three of which are mentioned here. The first trial is evaluating gefitinib plus docetaxel versus placebo on recurrent or metastatic disease. The second trial is examining the role of cetuximab as an adjuvant to cisplatin and 5-fluorouracil therapy in recurrent/metastatic disease. The last notable trial is studying cetuximab as an adjuvant to radiotherapy and cisplatin treatment for locally advanced disease.[66] A shortcoming of all these clinical trials is that they fail to incorporate the presence of *EGFR*-activating mutations, *EGFR* gene copy number, or both, into their primary analyses, although both of these factors have recently emerged as predictors of efficacy.[66] However, retrospective analysis of these factors within the context of prospective therapeutic trials should provide some information.

As mentioned previously, increased *EGFR* expression correlates with a poor prognosis; conversely, the presence of activating somatic mutations in the EGFR-TK domain have been shown to be a positive predictor for a patient's response to treatment. These mutations, which are present

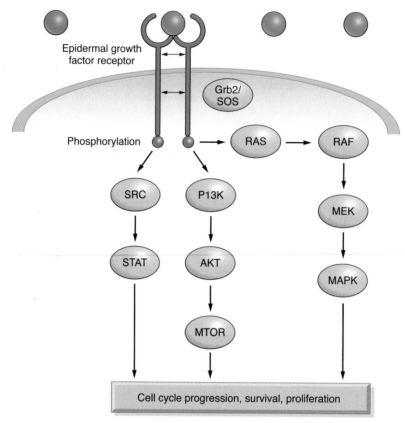

Epidermal growth factor receptor

Grb2/ SOS

Phosphorylation

RAS → RAF

SRC   P13K   MEK

STAT   AKT   MAPK

MTOR

Cell cycle progression, survival, proliferation

FIGURE 14.1 Cell-cycle progression, survival, and proliferation.

in ~10% of NSCLC[69,70] and 1% to 7% in non–small cell lung cancer (HNSCC),[71,72] correlated with prolonged survival in patients with advanced NSCLCs treated with chemotherapy regardless of EGFR-TKI.[73] Several other studies in NSCLCs did show that *EGFR* mutations were predictive of survival in patients treated with EGFR-TKIs.[74–76] Multiple clinical trials are under way to evaluate the use of EGFR-TKIs in chemotherapy-naive patients with advanced NSCLC and *EGFR*-activating mutations.[66,77,78] Both gefitinib and erlotinib have demonstrated response rates of 75% to 82%.[66,77,78] It is yet to be determined whether the same correlation and response to therapy will be found in HNSCC with *EGFR*-activating mutations.

Human Papillomavirus in HNSCC

Although it is well known that tobacco and alcohol are the two primary environmental risk factors associated with the development of HNSCC, it is now recognized that HPV infection plays an important role in the pathogenesis of a unique subset of oropharyngeal HNSCCs.[79–85] These tumors primarily emerge from the lingual and palatine tonsils in the oropharynx.[80,83,86–91] HPV-related HNSCC has distinguished itself as a separate entity with an improved prognosis and response to therapy from non-HPV–related HNSCC. It has also been proposed that it is the reason for the increasing incidence of oropharyngeal HNSCC relative to all other anatomic sites in the head and neck. This section will first briefly review what is known about the molecular biology of HPV as this topic is covered in other chapters within this edition, and then move on to how HPV-related HNSCC affects everyday clinical practice.

HPV is an ~7.9-kb, nonenveloped, double-stranded, circular DNA virus that has a specific tropism for squamous epithelium.[92] Although the sequences for over 320 different types of HPV have been identified, HPV-16 and -18 are the two types most pertinent to the development of HNSCC. The E6 and E7 oncoproteins contained within the viral genome, if overexpressed, are able to disrupt the function of *Rb* and *p53*, well-known tumor suppressor genes, leading to development of a malignant phenotype (Fig. 14.2).[93] It is now established that histopathologically, HPV-positive tumors tend to have a poorly differentiated and frequently basaloid histology that often

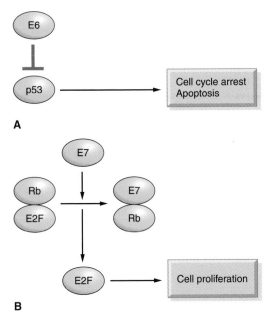

FIGURE 14.2 **A:** E6 binds p53, targets it for degradation, and promotes cell-cycle progression. **B:** E7 binds Rb and releases E2F, which promotes cellular proliferation.

lacks keratin.[79,80,85,94] Researchers have also discovered that human keratinocytes expressing E6 and E7 genes from HPV-16 become immortal,[95] as do oral epithelial cells.[96–98]

In a recent meta-analysis, HPV genomic DNA was detected in approximately 26% of all HNSCC by sensitive polymerase chain reaction–based methods.[99] However, in the majority of studies, 50% or more of oropharyngeal tumors contained the HPV genome.[100] A multinational study conducted by the International Agency for Research on Cancer (IARC), only 18% of oropharyngeal tumors were HPV-positive, indicating that this proportion likely varies by geography.[101] Regardless of the study population, high-risk HPV-16 accounts for the overwhelming majority (90% to 95%) of HPV-positive tumors.[99]

Our knowledge of HPV and its causal relationship with oropharyngeal cancer has improved our ability to diagnose and locate disease in patients with occult primary tumors.[102] Tonsillectomy has been shown in retrospective analyses to identify the primary site of cervical metastases as the contralateral or ipsilateral tonsil in approximately 10% and 30% of cases, respectively.[103–106] Therefore, HPV-related cancer is a distinct established entity that can be reliably diagnosed.

On average, patients with HPV-positive HNSCC are approximately 5 years younger than HPV-negative HNSCC patients, with equal distribution among the sexes.[90,107–110] HPV-positive HNSCC is more likely than HPV-negative HNSCC to occur in the nonsmoker and nondrinker.[80,81,88,89] Risk factors

for HPV-related HNSCC include a high lifetime number of vaginal-sex partners (26 or more), a high lifetime number of oral-sex partners (6 or more),[111] and seropositivity for HPV-16 viral capsid protein antibodies,[82] which carries a 15-fold increased risk for HNSCC. In a study restricted to patients with oropharyngeal cancers, nonsmokers were approximately 15-fold more likely to have a diagnosis of HPV-positive HNSCC than smokers.[112]

Our knowledge of the HPV status of our patients' tumors also improves our ability to provide an accurate prognosis. Patients with HPV-positive tumors have improved prognosis when compared with patients with HPV-negative tumors in the majority of studies, with as much as 60% to 80% reduction in risk of dying from their cancer when compared with the HPV-negative patient after controlling for other risk factors.[80,108,112–115] The reason for the improved survival is unclear; however, improved radiation responsiveness, immune surveillance to viral antigens, and the absence of field cancerization in these patients who tend to be nonsmokers have been postulated as possibilities. In addition, E6-related degradation of *p53* in HPV-positive cancers may not be functionally equivalent to HPV-negative *p53* mutations, and therefore HPV-positive tumors may have an intact apoptotic response to radiation and chemotherapy.

Therapeutic implications of an HPV-positive diagnosis are an active area of investigation. The Eastern Cooperative Oncology Group is studying the impact of HPV presence on oropharyngeal organ-preservation therapy. It is believed that HPV-HNSCC will perform better than HPV-negative HNSCC. A clinical trial of an HPV-16–specific therapeutic vaccine is also currently being evaluated. The vaccine is administered in the adjuvant setting and is intended to enhance the cytotoxic T-cell response to the HPV-16 oncoproteins.[116] With regard to prevention, a prophylactic vaccine composed of the HPV-16 viral capsid protein has recently been shown to prevent persistent HPV-16 infection and the development of cervical dysplasia.[117,118] However, the clinical trials have not included an evaluation of the impact of the vaccine on oral HPV infection. The vaccine does have the potential to have an impact on HNSCC incidence because the current vaccines are targeted to HPV-16 and there are animal models that demonstrate a protective effect and a reduction in the development of HPV-related oral lesions.

Possible future diagnostic tests that would likely have high specificity but low sensitivity for a diagnosis of HPV-associated HNSCC will include the detection of HPV-16 DNA in plasma,[119] which can be used for surveillance. Other screening tests like fluorescence *in situ* hybridization (FISH) on Papanicolaou smears obtained directly from tumors and HPV-16 E6 and E7 seroreactivity are other tests currently being tested.

MOLECULAR BIOLOGY OF INDIVIDUAL CANCERS

EPIGENETICS

Regulation of gene expression by DNA methylation was first recognized in development, where the coordinated expression and silencing of genes needs to take place in an organized fashion.[120] As a novel mechanism of gene regulation, it was quickly proposed that epigenetic control of tumor suppressor genes could be an important mechanism of carcinogenesis.[121,122] To date, methylation has been primarily considered as a mechanism of tumor suppressor gene inactivation, and one of the earliest genes to be characterized as being epigenetically controlled was the retinoblastoma gene. Primary tissue analysis showed that 10% of the retinoblastomas analyzed were hypermethylated at the Rb promoter[123] in the absence of any other mutations. In recent years, new assays such as sodium bisulfite treatment of DNA, which converts nonmethylated cytosines to uracil and methylation-sensitive quantitative polymerase chain reaction, have further advanced our ability to evaluate the methylation status of tissue samples.[124–126] With these advances, many different tumor suppressor genes in various tumor types have been shown to be down-regulated by methylation. The utilization of comprehensive whole-genome profiling approaches to promoter hypermethylation has identified novel putative tumor suppressor genes silenced by promoter hypermethylation. These *in vitro* techniques employ treatment of cultured cells with pharmacologic demethylating agents and subsequent expression array analysis with validation of tumor suppressor gene targets.[127]

Promoter hypermethylation of p16 is a frequent event in HNSCC and this mechanism of gene silencing accounts for the low levels of expression.[23,24,123,128,129] Thus, Knudsen's two-hit hypothesis could include promoter hypermethylation as one of the "hits" along with the more traditional sequence mutation or chromosomal deletion.

Studies of promoter methylation have uncovered many other putative tumor suppressor genes in HNSCC including lhx-6 (*DIME-6*), *ATM, p15, TIMP-3, MGMT, RARB-2, DAP-K,* E-cadherin, cyclin A1, *RASSF1A, CDKN2A, CDH1,* and *DCC*. These genes are known to function in pathways that control cell-cycle progression, apoptosis, cell-cell adhesion, DNA repair, and tumor invasion.[130–141] With the advent of new molecular techniques and whole-genome screening strategies, the list of tumor suppressor genes that are silenced through promoter hypermethylation continues to grow at a rapid pace. For instance, in the relatively young field of microRNA research, it has been demonstrated that those microRNAs having tumor-suppressor function also undergo DNA methylation-associated silencing in cancer.[137,142,143]

LOSS OF HETEROZYGOSITY AND RISK OF MALIGNANT PROGRESSION

Premalignant lesions of the head and neck are often characterized by large patches of clonally related precursors, often demonstrating dysplastic changes. Increased risk of progression to malignancy is also associated with prior head and neck cancer, advanced histologic grade, and evidence of genetic instability including chromosomal loss and aneuploidy. Those patients with moderate or severe dysplasia are noted to have a risk of progression to malignancy of approximately 60%, in a study with median 7-year follow up. Likewise, a prior history of head and neck cancer resulted in a similar 60% risk of progression in the same study.[6] Approximately 40% of patients with mild dysplasia or hyperplasia combined with 3p or 9p loss of heterozygosity demonstrated progression to malignancy within 5 years.

Selected References

The full list of references for this chapter appears in the online version.

1. Foulkes WD, Brunet JS, Sieh W, Black MJ, Shenouda G, Narod SA. Familial risks of squamous cell carcinoma of the head and neck: retrospective case-control study. *BMJ* 1996;313:716.
6. van Zeeburg HJ, Snijders PJ, Wu T, et al. Clinical and molecular characteristics of squamous cell carcinomas from Fanconi anemia patients. *J Natl Cancer Inst* 2008; 100:1649.
12. Califano J, van der Riet P, Westra W, et al. Genetic progression model for head and neck cancer: implications for field cancerization. *Cancer Res* 1996;56:2488.

16. Mao L, Lee JS, Fan YH, et al. Frequent microsatellite alterations at chromosomes 9p21 and 3p14 in oral premalignant lesions and their value in cancer risk assessment. *Nat Med* 1996;2:682.
23. Reed AL, Califano J, Cairns P, et al. High frequency of p16 (CDKN2/MTS-1/INK4A) inactivation in head and neck squamous cell carcinoma. *Cancer Res* 1996;56: 3630.
28. Poeta ML, Manola J, Goldwasser MA, et al. TP53 mutations and survival in squamous-cell carcinoma of the head and neck. *N Engl J Med* 2007;357:2552.
36. Hoogsteen IJ, Marres HA, Bussink J, van der Kogel AJ, Kaanders JH. Tumor microenvironment in head and neck squamous cell carcinomas: predictive value and clinical

relevance of hypoxic markers. A review. *Head Neck* 2007;29:591.

41. Mandal M, Myers JN, Lippman SM, et al. Epithelial to mesenchymal transition in head and neck squamous carcinoma: association of Src activation with E-cadherin down-regulation, vimentin expression, and aggressive tumor features. *Cancer* 2008;112:2088.

55. Kalyankrishna S, Grandis JR. Epidermal growth factor receptor biology in head and neck cancer. *J Clin Oncol* 2006;24:2666.

64. Bonner JA, Harari PM, Giralt J, et al. Radiotherapy plus cetuximab for squamous-cell carcinoma of the head and neck. *N Engl J Med* 2006;354:567.

78. Andl T, Kahn T, Pfuhl A, et al. Etiological involvement of oncogenic human papillomavirus in tonsillar squamous cell carcinomas lacking retinoblastoma cell cycle control. *Cancer Res* 1998;58:5.

79. Gillison ML, Koch WM, Capone RB, et al. Evidence for a causal association between human papillomavirus and a subset of head and neck cancers. *J Natl Cancer Inst* 2000; 92:709.

80. Hafkamp HC, Speel EJ, Haesevoets A, et al. A subset of head and neck squamous cell carcinomas exhibits integra-tion of HPV 16/18 DNA and overexpression of p16INK4A and p53 in the absence of mutations in p53 exons 5-8. *Int J Cancer* 2003;107:394.

81. Mork J, Lie AK, Glattre E, et al. Human papillomavirus infection as a risk factor for squamous-cell carcinoma of the head and neck. *N Engl J Med* 2001;344:1125.

82. Schwartz SM, Daling JR, Doody DR, et al. Oral cancer risk in relation to sexual history and evidence of human papillomavirus infection. *J Natl Cancer Inst* 1998;90: 1626.

110. D'Souza G, Kreimer AR, Viscidi R, et al. Case-control study of human papillomavirus and oropharyngeal cancer. *N Engl J Med* 2007;356:1944.

120. Feinberg AP, Vogelstein B. Hypomethylation of ras oncogenes in primary human cancers. *Biochem Biophys Res Commun* 1983;111:47.

127. El-Naggar AK, Lai S, Clayman G, et al. Methylation, a major mechanism of p16/CDKN2 gene inactivation in head and neck squamous carcinoma. *Am J Pathol* 1997; 151:1767.

140. Ha PK, Califano JA. Promoter methylation and inactivation of tumour-suppressor genes in oral squamous-cell carcinoma. *Lancet Oncol* 2006;7:77.

CHAPTER 15 LUNG CANCER

JACOB KAUFMAN, LEORA HORN, AND DAVID P. CARBONE

Lung cancer tumorigenesis is a multistep process of transformation from normal bronchial epithelium to overt lung cancer. Various molecular events that result in gain or loss of function cause dysregulation of key genetic pathways involved in cellular proliferation, differentiation, apoptosis, migration, invasion, and other processes characteristic of the malignant phenotype. Mutations, including single nucleotide substitution or deletion, and translocation, deletion, or amplification of larger portions of genetic material may result from environmental factors, inherited susceptibility, or random events. Many genes are involved in tumorigenesis of both small cell lung cancer (SCLC) and non–small cell lung cancer (NSCLC) (Table 15.1, Fig. 15.1), but there are also unique genetic aberrations associated with each tumor type. Following the development of overt cancer, continued accumulation of genetic abnormalities influences the processes of invasion, metastases, and resistance to cancer therapy. Identification of the nature and frequency of these molecular abnormalities is necessary to determine their clinical implications (e.g., associations with smoking, histological type, stage, survival, response to therapy) and define their clinical utility for prevention and early diagnosis of lung cancer, as well as for the development of therapeutic targets.

SUSCEPTIBILITY TO LUNG CANCER: GENETIC SUSCEPTIBILITY AND CARCINOGENS IN TOBACCO SMOKE

Tobacco use is the most important environmental factor associated with the development of lung cancer. Approximately 85% of lung cancer occurs in current or former smokers, which corresponds to a greater than tenfold increase in risk of lung cancer compared to never-smokers. Cigarette smoke contains more than 60 known carcinogens, 20 of which have been convincingly shown to cause lung tumors in laboratory animals or humans.[1] Of these, polycyclic aromatic hydrocarbons, such as benzo(a)pyrene, tobacco-specific nitrosamines, such as 4-(methylnitrosamino)-1-(3-pyridyl)-1-butanone (NNK), and aromatic amines, such as 4-aminobiphenyl, appear to have an important role in cancer causation. Nitrosamines such as NNK induce lung tumors, primarily adenomas and adenocarcinomas, in mice independent of the route of administration. Among the polycyclic aromatic hydrocarbons, benzo(a)pyrene is the most extensively tested and the first to be detected in tobacco smoke. Its role in cancer tumorigenesis is well described, and its diol epoxide metabolite has been implicated as the cause of mutation in the *TP53* gene.[2] One of the carcinogenic effects of tobacco smoke in the lung is the formation of DNA adducts, leading to errors in DNA replication and resulting mutations. DNA adducts have been identified in the bronchial tissue of patients with lung cancer. In current smokers, adduct levels correlate with the amount of tobacco smoke exposure.[3,4] Smoking cessation for at least 5 years results in adduct levels similar to nonsmokers.[4] In addition, in former smokers, age at smoking initiation has been inversely associated with levels of DNA adducts, suggesting that prevention of smoking in adolescence is of utmost importance in decreasing lung cancer risks.

Although tobacco use can account for the majority of lung cancers, most chronic smokers still do not develop lung cancer. Differences in inherent susceptibility may be related to variations in carcinogen metabolizing enzymes, DNA repair mechanisms, chromosome fragility, and other homeostatic mechanisms. Among genes for carcinogen-metabolizing enzymes, polymorphisms in the cytochrome P-450 genes *CYP1A1*, *CYP2D6*, and *CYP2E1* and in mu-class glutathione S-transferase (*GSTM1*) have received the most attention. Although studies have suggested that there may be a modest association of *GSTM1* null polymorphism with lung cancer, knowledge of the state of single candidate genes may not be adequate to predict lung cancer risk due to the complexity of carcinogen metabolism, gene–gene and gene–environment interactions, and the relatively

TABLE 15.1

MOST FREQUENTLY ACQUIRED MOLECULAR ABNORMALITIES IN LUNG CANCER

Abnormalities	Small Cell Lung Cancer	Non–Small Cell Lung Cancer
Microsatellite instabilities	~35%	~22%
Autocrine loops	GRP/GRP receptor; SCF/KIT	TGF-α/EGFR; heregulin/ERBB2; HGF/MET
RAS point mutation	<1%	15%–20%
EGFR mutation	<1%	<10% (West), ~40% (Asia)
EML4-ALK	0%	3%–7%
MYC family overexpression	15%–30%	5%–10%
p53 inactivation	~90%	~50%
RB inactivation	~90%	15%–30%
p16^{INK4A} inactivation	0%–10%	30%–70%
LKB1 inactivation	~40%–60% (IHC)	20%–40%
Frequent allelic loss	3p, 4p, 4q, 5q, 8p, 10q, 13q, 17p, 22q	3p, 6q, 8p, 9p, 13p, 17p, 19q
Telomerase activity	~100%	80%–85%
BCL2 expression	75%–95%	10%–35%

EGFR, epidermal growth factor receptor; GRP, gastrin-releasing peptide; HGF, hepatocyte growth factor; RB, retinoblastoma protein; SCF, stem cell factor; TGF-α, transforming growth factor-α; IHC, immunohistochemistry.

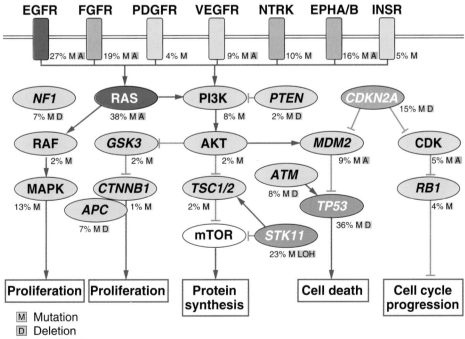

FIGURE 15.1 Significantly mutated pathways in lung adenocarcinomas. Genetic alterations in lung adenocarcinoma frequently occur in genes of the mitogen-activated protein kinase (MAPK) signaling, p53 signaling, Wnt signaling, cell cycle, and mammalian target of rapamycin (mTOR) pathways. Oncoproteins are indicated in pink to red and tumor suppressor proteins are shown in light to dark blue. The darkness of the colors is positively correlated to the percentage of tumors with genetic alterations. Frequency of genetic alterations for each of these pathway members in 188 tumors is indicated. (From Macmillan Publishers Ltd, ref. 113, copyright 2007, with permission.).

small effect of an individual gene. In addition to inherent susceptibility to the carcinogenic effects of tobacco smoke, large genome-wide association studies have identified lung cancer susceptibility loci at 15q25, 5p15, and 6p21.[5,6] In particular, polymorphisms in and around nicotinic cholinergic receptors at chromosome 15q25 appear to correlate with messenger RNA (mRNA) and protein expression of these receptors as well as functional changes in the calcium ion channel of the A5 nicotine receptor; these differences confer susceptibility to smoking behaviors.[7]

Researchers are optimistic that molecular epidemiology will help identify individuals at the highest risk of developing lung cancer. Such information, in addition to the smoking history, will be of great value in new lung cancer screening trials and in chemoprevention trials to identify persons at highest risk of developing lung cancer.

MOLECULAR CHANGES IN PRENEOPLASIA

Before lung cancer is clinically recognizable, a series of morphologically distinct changes (hyperplasia, metaplasia, dysplasia, and carcinoma in situ) are thought to occur. Whether one cell of origin leads to all histological variants is unclear. It is believed that dysplasia and carcinoma *in situ* represent true preneoplastic changes. These sequential changes found within squamous cell cancers that arise from central bronchi have long been recognized. Although the exact cell of origin for lung cancer is unknown, it is thought that type II epithelial cells have the capacity to give rise to lung adenocarcinomas, while cells of neuroendocrine origin are likely precursors of SCLC.

It is evident that preneoplastic cells contain several genetic abnormalities identical to some of the abnormalities found in overt lung cancer cells. For squamous cell cancers, immunohistochemical analysis has confirmed abnormal expression of protooncogenes (cyclin D1) and tumor suppressor genes (TSGs) (p53).[8] Allelotyping of precisely microdissected, preneoplastic foci of cells shows that 3p allele loss is currently the earliest known change, suggesting that one or more 3p TSGs may act as gatekeepers for lung cancer pathogenesis.[9] This is followed by 9p, 8p, and 17p allele loss and p53 mutation. Even histologically normal bronchial epithelium has been shown to have genetic losses. Similarly, atypical alveolar hyperplasia, the potential precursor lesion of adenocarcinomas, can harbor Kristen rat sarcoma viral oncogene homolog (*KRAS*) mutations and allele losses of 3p, 9p, and 17p.[10] Other genetic alterations, such as inactivation of *LKB1*, whose germline mutations cause Peutz-Jeghers syndrome, have also been implicated in the development of adenocarcinoma. These observations are consistent with the multistep model of carcinogenesis and a field cancerization process, whereby the whole tissue region is repeatedly exposed to carcinogenic damage (tobacco smoke) and is at risk for development of multiple, separate foci of neoplasia.[11]

Although all types of lung cancers have associated molecular abnormalities in their normal and preneoplastic lung epithelium, SCLC patients in particular appear to have multiple genetic alterations occurring in their histologically normal-appearing respiratory epithelium. Molecular changes have been found not only in the lungs of patients with lung cancer but also in the lungs of current and former smokers without lung cancer. These molecular alterations are thus important targets for use in the early detection of lung cancer and for use as surrogate biomarkers in following the efficacy of lung cancer chemoprevention. In this regard, it appears that the smoking-damaged respiratory epithelium has thousands of clonal patches, each containing clones of cells with 3p and other allele loss abnormalities.[12] The challenge is to identify not only the prevalence and temporal sequence of molecular lesions in lung preneoplasia, but to determine which are rate limiting and indispensable and thus represent potential candidates for intermediate biomarker monitoring and therapeutic efforts.

GENETIC AND EPIGENETIC ALTERATIONS IN LUNG CANCERS

Genomic Instability and DNA Repair Genes

Similar to other epithelial tumors, lung cancer cells typically display chromosomal instability—both numeric abnormalities (aneuploidy) of chromosomes and structural cytogenetic abnormalities.[13] Allele loss on chromosome 3p is thought to be among the earliest genetic change occurring in both NSCLC and SCLC.[14] In addition, nonreciprocal translocations and recurrent losses involving 1p, 4p, 4q, 5q, 6p 6q, 8p, 9p, 11p, 13q, 17p, 18q, and 22q may occur, representing changes in known and potential tumor suppressor genes.[15] Polysomies or regions of gene amplifications also occur and often involve protooncogenes such as epidermal growth factor receptor (*EGFR*) and myelocytomatosis viral oncogene homolog (*MYC*).[16,17] Simple reciprocal translocations are uncommonly observed in lung cancer, although translocations that give rise to BRD4-NUT,[18] CRCT1-MAML2,[19] SLC34A2–ROS,[20] and EML4-ALK[21] fusion proteins have been reported, and for the case of EML4-ALK this has been shown to drive the development and proliferation of tumors. Alterations in microsatellite polymorphic repeat sequences are found in 35% of SCLC and 22% of NSCLC.[22] The underlying mechanism for this chromosomal instability has not yet been discovered.

The most powerful tumor surveillance mechanism is involved in DNA damage response and repair of errors in DNA replication.[23] The DNA glycosylase 8-Oxo guanine (OGG1) specifically excises the oxidatively damaged mutagenic base 8-hydroxyguanine, which causes G:C→T:A transversions frequently found in lung cancer. Lung adenocarcinoma spontaneously develops in Ogg1 knockout mice and 8-hydroxyguanine accumulates in their genomes.[24,25] Individuals with low OGG activity have a greatly increased risk of developing lung cancer. Polymorphisms in other DNA repair genes *ERCC1*, *XRCC1*, *ERCC5/XPG*, and *MGMT/AGT* have been correlated with reduction of polyaromatic hydrocarbon DNA adduct formation as well as with lower lung cancer risks in case-control studies. High expression of excision repair cross-complementation gene-1 (ERCC1) is associated with decreased response to platinum-based chemotherapy, but in contrast, overexpression of ERCC1 correlates with better overall prognosis in NSCLC,[26] reflecting improved repair of lethal DNA damage by platinum, on the one hand, and greater DNA stability with less aggressive disease course, on the other. Similarly, ribonucleotide reductase M1 (RRM1) overexpression correlates with better *de novo* prognosis but resistance to gemcitabine. Assays of both ERCC1 and RRM1 are commercially available and are marketed as tools to guide cytotoxic therapy in NSCLC; treatment based on these assays has not yet been prospectively validated, but may prove important.

PROTOONCOGENES, GROWTH FACTOR SIGNALING, AND GROWTH FACTOR TARGETED THERAPIES

EGFR and *KRAS* are the two most commonly mutated protooncogenes in lung adenocarcinomas; these mutations appear to be mutually exclusive. EGFR is a transmembrane tyrosine kinase, which, when activated by binding with one of its ligands, members of the EGF family, stimulates cell proliferation. When mutated, EGFR tyrosine kinase is constitutively activated, resulting in uncontrolled proliferation, invasion, and metastasis. Coexpression of EGFRs and their ligands, especially transforming growth factor-α, by lung cancer cells indicates the presence of an autocrine (self-stimulatory) growth factor loop. Activating *EGFR* mutations are observed in approximately 10% of North American and European populations and 30% to 50% of Asian populations[27–32]

and are significantly more common in never-smokers (100 or less cigarettes per lifetime) or light former smokers (quit 1 year or more ago and less than ten-pack per year smoking history). The leucine to arginine substitution at position 858 (L858R) in exon 21 and short in-frame deletions in exon 19 are the most common mutations seen in adenocarcinomas of the lung. These mutations result in prolonged activation of the receptor and downstream signaling through phosphorylated Akt, in the absence of ligand stimulation of the extracellular domain. *EGFR* mutations are both prognostic for response rate to chemotherapy and survival irrespective of therapy and are predictive of response to specific inhibitors of the EGFR tyrosine kinase—gefitinib and erlotinib.[31,33,34] *EGFR* mutations are found almost exclusively in adenocarcinomas and occur much more frequently in tumors from never-smokers, women, and in Asian populations, explaining the increased clinical response to gefitinib noted in these subpopulations before the association with *EGFR* mutation was discovered.[31,33,34] A recent review by Rosell et al.[32] suggested patients with adenocarcinoma who are never or light remote smokers, especially women and Asians, should be screened for the presence of an *EGFR* mutation. The IPASS (Iressa Pan-Asia Study) trial demonstrated an improved outcome with up-front treatment with gefitinib compared with chemotherapy for patients with *EGFR* mutation, but on the other hand, much worse outcome compared with chemotherapy in patients with wild type *EGFR*.[35,36] Previous suggestions that *EGFR* gene amplification by detected by fluorescence *in situ* hybridization (FISH) or immunohistochemistry may correlate with response to therapy with an EGFR tyrosine kinase inhibitor[28] have not been corroborated. Cetuximab, a human murine chimeric immunoglobulin G subclass-1 (IgG-1) antibody that binds to the extracellular domain of EGFR and affects ligand-induced phosphorylation and degradation has been evaluated in patients with NSCLC. Contrary to data from colon cancer studies, neither expression of nor mutations in EGFR or KRAS appear to predict response or survival to this agent.[37]

ERBB2 (formerly human epidermal growth factor receptor 2 [HER2]/neu) is also a member of the erbB receptor family, along with *EGFR*. The ERBB2 receptor is unusual in that it does not interact with the EGF ligand family; its activation depends on heterodimerization with other erbB receptors following ligand binding. *ERBB2* mutations have been detected with low frequency in lung adenocarcinomas.[30] Similar prevalence of gene amplification of *ERBB2* can be observed.[38] A meta-analysis suggested that overexpression of ERBB2 is a poor prognostic indicator for survival in NSCLC.[39] Several clinical trials examining trastuzumab (Herceptin), a recombinant humanized monoclonal antibody against ERBB2, as a single agent or in combination with chemotherapy, have failed to demonstrate a survival benefit.[40] A new generation of dual irreversible EGFR/ERBB2 inhibitors is under development. These agents form a covalent bond with CYS-733 in EGFR and may be effective in patients with resistance to reversible EGFR tyrosine kinase inhibitors.[41]

c-KIT belongs to the PDGF/c-Kit receptor tyrosine kinase family that results in activation of the Janus-associated tyrosine kinase/signal transducers and activators of transcription (JAK-STAT), phosphoinositide 3-kinase (PI3K), and mitogen-activated protein kinase (MAPK) pathways important in cell growth and differentiation. Along with its ligand, stem cell factor (SCF), it is preferentially expressed in many SCLCs and is thought to have prognostic implications.[42–45] Activation of this putative autocrine loop may also mediate chemoattraction and may provide a growth advantage in tumor cells. Although the c-KIT tyrosine kinase inhibitor imatinib reduces cell proliferation and induces cell death in several preclinical SCLC models,[46] it failed to demonstrate any objective response in clinical trials.[47–49] Another receptor tyrosine kinase, c-MET and its ligand, hepatocyte growth factor (HGF), play an important role in fetal lung development. Coexpression of this putative loop is observed in both NSCLC and SCLC. High HGF levels have also been associated with a poor outcome in resectable NSCLC patients; furthermore, elevated expression of MET is associated with resistance to EGFR targeted therapy,[50] and improvement in patient outcome has recently been reported when monoclonal antibodies inhibiting MET are combined with erlotinib.[51] The insulin-like growth factor receptor 1 (IGFR1) signaling pathway plays an important role in cancer growth and progression and has been associated with resistance to therapy. IGFR1 monoclonal antibodies and small molecule inhibitors are currently in clinical testing in patients with NSCLC. A phase 3 clinical trial of figitumumab (CP-751871) was closed early due to excess toxicities, including treatment-related deaths, in the experimental arm, so the possible role of these agents in the treatment of NSCLC remains to be determined.

In addition to protooncogene products, other growth stimulatory loops are found in lung cancer. The best known is that governed by gastrin-releasing peptide and other bombesin-like peptides, together with their receptors, which participate in lung development and repair and promote SCLC growth in cell culture via an autocrine loop. Immunohistochemical studies showed that gastrin-releasing peptide is expressed in 20% to 60% of SCLC but less frequently in NSCLCs. Although this loop is a possible therapeutic target, a phase 1 clinical trial of the anti–gastrin-releasing peptide monoclonal antibody 2A11 did not result in an objective antitumor response in patients with lung cancer.[52]

Other signaling pathways historically linked to embryonic development likely to be relevant for lung carcinogenesis include the Sonic hedgehog (Shh) and Notch signaling pathways. Extensive activation of the hedgehog pathway has been demonstrated within the airway epithelium during repair of acute airway injury and in a subset of SCLC.[53] Notch 3 has been found to be overexpressed in about 40% of lung cancers. Inhibition of this pathway in vitro has resulted in the loss of tumor phenotypes.[54] Clinical trials are under way to determine whether targeting these pathways has any clinical utility.

As downstream effectors are required for intracellular transduction of incoming growth factor or receptor signals, it is not surprising that proteins important in cytoplasmic signal transduction cascades are also implicated in carcinogenesis. Mutation of KRAS is the most frequently reported alteration in the downstream EGFR signaling pathways. The RAS gene family, in particular KRAS, can be activated by point mutations at codons 12 or 13 in exon 2 in approximately 20% to 30% of NSCLCs, with 90% of the RAS mutations observed in lung adenocarcinomas and with approximately 85% of the KRAS mutations affecting codon 12.[55] KRAS mutations are rarely observed in SCLCs. Transgenic mice with oncogenic Kras alleles that are activated by spontaneous recombination events in the whole animal are highly predisposed to early onset lung cancer, further supporting the hypothesis that KRAS mutation is an early oncogenic event in lung cancer.[56] Interestingly, the remaining wild type Ras allele appears to function as a potential tumor suppressor, because mice susceptible to the chemical induction of lung tumors frequently lose wild type Kras2 during lung tumor progression.[57] KRAS mutations more commonly occur in patients with a significant smoking history.[58] Approximately, 70% of KRAS mutations are G→T transversions, with the substitution of glycine by either cysteine or valine. Similar G→T transversions are observed in the mutated p53 gene, representing similar DNA damage as a result of bulky DNA adducts caused by the polycyclic hydrocarbons and nitrosamines in tobacco smoke. This observation provides further evidence for a causative role for tobacco smoke in KRAS mutations. In a meta-analysis of 3,779 lung cancer patients, 18.4% of whom had KRAS mutations detected by polymerase chain reaction (PCR), mutant KRAS was associated with worse prognosis in adenocarcinoma but not in squamous histology.[59] However, a prospective study failed to show a survival difference correlated with KRAS mutation in advanced NSCLC.[60] Although the oncogenicity of aberrant KRAS mutation appears to be well established, all attempts to inhibit mutant KRAS have failed to demonstrate objective responses in clinical trials, including attempts to prevent binding to the inner cell membrane by inhibiting farnesyltransferase or geranylgeranyl-transferase.[61]

Direct downstream effectors of RAS are the RAF1 and BRAF protooncogenes. Unlike *RAS*, mutations in the RAF1 gene have not been detected in human lung cancers. Its role is complex, as growth arrest of SCLC by activated RAF1 suggests that it has a TSG-like function, and one copy of *RAF1* is frequently lost in lung cancer.[62] Although *BRAF*, another member of the RAF family, is commonly mutated in malignant melanomas and colon cancers, mutations in this gene are found in fewer than 5% of lung cancers.

Activation of nuclear protooncogene products, such as those encoded by the myc family genes (*MYC, MYCN,* and *MYCL*) is often the end point for many signaling cascades. MYC, when heterodimerized with MAX, functions as a transcription factor, and this functional complex is necessary for normal cell cycle progression and differentiation, as well as programmed cell death. *MYC* gene amplification or transcriptional dysregulation is often observed in SCLC and to a lesser degree in NSCLC. One member of the *MYC* family is amplified in 18% of SCLC tumors and 31% of cell lines, compared to 8% of NSCLC tumors and 20% of cell lines. Amplification appears more frequently in SCLC patients previously treated with chemotherapy, giving rise to the "variant" subtype of SCLC, and its presence correlates with adverse survival.[63] There are no MYC-specific drugs in development.

EML4-ALK fusion protein is a recently identified activating oncogenic driver of lung adenocarcinomas occurring in less than 5% of all NSCLC. It is formed by fusion of the N-terminal portion of the protein encoded by the echinoderm microtubule-associated protein-like 4 (*EML4*) gene with the intracellular signaling portion of the receptor tyrosine kinase encoded by the anaplastic lymphoma kinase (*ALK*) gene, resulting from a t(2;5) translocation.[21] Multiple *EML4-ALK* variants have been identified in lung cancer.[64-67] Similar to EGFR mutations, *EML4-ALK* fusions appear to occur almost exclusively in adenocarcinomas, specifically with acinar histology, in never or former light smokers.[65,68-70] *EML4-ALK* fusions do not occur in tumors with mutations in *EGFR* or *KRAS*, and patients appear to be of younger age compared to patients with *EGFR* mutations.[70] A variety of methods are currently being used to assess for the presence of the *EML4-ALK* fusion, including immunohistochemistry, FISH, and reverse transcription PCR (RT-PCR), however, each method has its own attributes and flaws and none has been adopted to date as a standard for testing. Several novel selective inhibitors of ALK kinase are in clinical development. A trial of crizotinib (PF-02341066), a dual MET/ALK inhibitor, in heavily pretreated patients with tumors that harbor the ALK fusion protein has resulted in a 57% response rate and 72% 6-month progression-free survival (PFS) with median PFS not reached at the time of report.[71] Phase 2 and 3 trials with this agent are currently under way.

TUMOR SUPPRESSOR GENES AND GROWTH SUPPRESSION

A number of TSGs have been identified that inhibit lung tumorigenesis or suppress key phenotypes in developed lung carcinomas. Germline mutations in some TSGs such as LKB1, *p53*, and *RB1* give rise to inherited tumor syndromes; however, somatic loss of TSGs within sporadic cancers is more commonly seen. Such genes can be lost through multiple mechanisms, such as inactivating mutations, chromosomal loss, methylation, or overexpression of other proteins that inhibit the suppressive gene's expression or activity. Many classical tumor suppressors, such as the three identified above, have been identified by decades of work examining genes involved in human-inherited cancer syndromes and elucidating their role in sporadic cancers. Many additional suppressor gene candidates have been identified as a result of profiling large numbers of tumors for loss of heterozygosity (LOH) using high-resolution comparative genomic hybridization systematically to look for recurrent regions of chromosomal loss. Results are expected in the next few years from whole genome sequencing of hundreds of tumors to identify novel mutations.

p53 Pathway

The *p53* gene, located at chromosome 17p13, is crucial for maintaining genomic integrity in the face of cellular stress from DNA damage through gamma and ultraviolet irradiation, carcinogens, and chemotherapy. It is the most frequently mutated TSG in human malignancies, and mutations affect approximately 90% of SCLCs and 50% of NSCLCs. In NSCLCs, p53 alterations occur more frequently in squamous cell (51%) and large cell (54%) carcinoma than adenocarcinomas (39%).[72] p53 mutations have been linked to poorer prognosis retrospectively; however, they were not shown to correlate with survival in a prospective randomized clinical trial.[60,73] Most p53 mutations are G→T transversions, which correlate with cigarette smoking. A major cigarette smoke carcinogen, benzo(a)pyrene, selectively forms adducts at *p53* mutational hot spots.[2] The Li-Fraumeni syndrome of inherited germline *p53* mutation may also lead to increased susceptibility to lung cancer in adults; this risk is magnified by tobacco smoking, as carriers who smoked had a

3.16-fold higher risk for lung cancer than non-smokers.[74] The majority of missense mutations occur in the DNA-binding domain of the protein, and five of the six most prevalently mutated sites are arginine residues that are involved with electrostatic interactions with DNA strands.[75] Missense mutations prolong the half-life of the p53 protein, leading to increased protein levels detectable with immunohistochemistry. Also, because p53 exerts its cellular actions as a tetramer, mutant forms of the protein appear to exert dominant negative effects on wild type p53 and have also been shown to inhibit the function of p63 and p73 family members.[76]

In addition to mutational or deletional loss of p53, other regulatory components of the p53 pathway are altered in lung cancer, including the ataxia-telangiectasia (ATM) gene, the p53 binding protein MDM2, and the p14^{ARF} tumor suppressor. ATM and the related protein ATR are tumor suppressive serine/threonine kinases that activate cell cycle checkpoints in response to DNA damage and ultimately activate and stabilize p53.[77] Although ATR and the downstream checkpoint kinases (CHEK) are mutated in less than 1% of lung adenocarcinomas, ATM has been found to have deleterious mutations in 7% of lung adenocarcinomas; these mutations were largely mutually exclusive with p53 mutations, likely indicating that mutations in both genes would have redundant effects, especially since it has been shown that gain-of-function mutations in p53 can inactivate ATM.[78,79] Conversely, the MDM2 oncogene product negatively regulates p53 by binding its transcriptional activation domain, inducing its nuclear export, and by polyubiquitinating p53, marking it for proteasomal degradation.[80] Abnormal overexpression of MDM2 is found in NSCLC, where it is amplified in a significant number of tumors. MDM2 activity is inhibited by other tumor suppressor genes in the p53 pathway, including ATM and also the p14^{ARF} tumor suppressor gene, which is often lost in lung cancer.[81]

When p53 is functional, it is activated by phosphorylation in response to cellular stress (e.g., DNA damage). Once activated, p53 strongly induces the expression of other tumor suppressor genes that control cell cycle checkpoints (e.g., p21$^{WAF1/CIP1}$), apoptosis (BAX), DNA repair (GADD45), and angiogenesis (thrombospondin).[82] p53 activation has also been found to alter microRNA expression and maturation,[83] and some effects of p53 are mediated by the induced expression of the microRNA miR-34.[84] The high frequency of p53 loss across the entire spectrum of human tumors is a strong testament to its importance in inhibiting tumor development and growth. Restoring p53 activity in tumors is effective in halting their growth and could represent an effective therapy, although development of this strategy is challenging.[85] Several gene therapy clinical trials have been reported in which lung cancers are treated by intratumoral injection (endobronchially or by computed tomography–guided needle injection), introducing a wild type p53 gene using retroviral or adenoviral vectors. Future therapeutic gains may come from combining gene and conventional therapies, but this approach may be limited to locoregional disease control.[86] Other strategies have been developed to restore p53 activity without attempting to reintroduce the entire gene into tumor cells. These include the use of small molecule inhibitors of the MDM2–p53 interface that prevent the degradation of wild type p53 and the use of peptides and small molecules that are intended to restore wild type conformation to mutated p53.[85,87] Immunologic targeting of cancer with vaccines is a different strategy that is potentially nontoxic and specific. Such a strategy takes advantage of novel protein sequences that result from p53 mutations, which can potentially be recognized as foreign epitopes by cytotoxic T cells mounting an immune response against a tumor. Vaccination of patients with advanced cancer with a custom vaccine corresponding to their tumor's mutation in p53 or RAS has demonstrated the generation of mutant oncogene specific immune responses associated with prolonged survival.[88] A trial of p53 vaccination in SCLC produced measurable increases in tumor-specific immune response that was associated with improved outcome and response to therapy in some patients.[89,90]

CYCLINS AND CELL CYCLE REGULATORY PATHWAYS

p16^{INK4A} is a cyclin-dependent kinase (CDK) inhibitor important for the integrity of the G_1 checkpoint. Loss of p16^{INK4A} frees CDKs from inhibition, permitting constitutive phosphorylation of retinoblastoma (RB) protein and inactivation of its growth suppressive function. Approximately 40% of primary NSCLCs lose p16^{INK4A}, located on chromosome 9p21, making it the most common component of the p16^{INK4A}–cyclin D1–CDK4–RB pathway to be inactivated in NSCLC. Other CDK inhibitors are also lost at a lower prevalence in NSCLC, and the RB gene is mutated or lost in a significant minority of cases.[79] In contrast, a strikingly different pattern of pathway dysregulation is observed in SCLC, in which abnormalities in p16 are rarely observed but RB itself is nearly always abnormal. Although p16^{INK4A} point mutations in NSCLCs were observed in only 14% of tumors, homozygous deletions or aberrant promoter methylation are common mechanisms for p16^{INK4A} inactivation.[22] Indeed, aberrant p16^{INK4A} methylation is a frequent, early preneoplastic event in the pathogenesis of squamous cell carcinomas.[91] Furthermore, p16^{INK4A} and p14^{ARF} are alternative splice forms of RNA transcripts from the same DNA locus. p14[ARF] is also a tumor suppressor gene and functions to stabilize p53. Thus, alteration at the $p16^{INK4A}$ locus may not only abrogate $p16^{INK4A}$ function but also disrupt p53 pathway through $p14^{ARF}$.[92]

In the absence of inhibitory regulation by the CDK inhibitors, cyclins and their catalytic partners, the CDKs, phosphorylate the retinoblastoma protein, a growth-suppressive nuclear phosphoprotein located on chromosomal region 13q14. When in its active, unphosphorylated form, RB binds and inactivates proteins such as transcription factor E2F-1 preventing G_1/S transition. Mutations of one *RB* allele together with loss of the other wild type *RB* allele are frequently observed in SCLC. The RB protein is absent or structurally abnormal in more than 90% of SCLCs and 15% to 30% of NSCLCs. Lung-targeted, conditional deletion of *Rb* and *p53* in mice leads to development of SCLC that recapitulated that observed in humans.[93] Although the *p16* and *RB* tumor suppressive components of this pathway are frequently lost in lung cancer, the growth promoting cyclin and CDK components of the pathway are often overexpressed and cyclin D1, cyclin E1, and CDK4 have each been shown to be amplified in a subset of lung cancers[94] and are overexpressed by immunohistochemical evaluation.

LKB1, AMPK, mTOR Pathway

LKB1 is a serine/threonine kinase that serves as a "master regulator" of several key intracellular pathways through phosphorylation of downstream regulatory kinases. Its tumor suppressive role became apparent when it was discovered that inherited mutations in *LKB1* gave rise to a rare autosomal dominant polyposis/cancer susceptibility disease, Peutz-Jeghers syndrome. This disease is characterized by the development of many hamartomas polyps throughout the intestinal tract, abnormalities in mucocutaneous pigmentation, and a 20-fold increase in lifetime risk for cancer, including gastrointestinal, breast, and pancreatic neoplasia.[95,96] Subsequent to this discovery it was found that *LKB1* is somatically mutated and deleted in a range of other carcinomas, most prevalently in non–small cell lung carcinoma, where approximately 20% to 30% of adenocarcinomas exhibit *LKB1*.[97–99] Squamous cell and large cell lung carcinomas also exhibit *LKB1* loss, but at a lower frequency, and immunohistochemical analysis revealed absent LKB1 expression in two-thirds of SCLC.[100] In a mouse model, tumors rapidly develop when conditional *Lkb1* knockout was combined with conditional expression of oncogenic *Kras*, using inhaled adenovirus-expressing Cre recombinase. High penetrance and multiple tumors per animal were noted. More than half of the incident tumors are associated with metastases. Additionally, whereas most other mouse models of lung tumorigenesis (e.g., oncogenic *Kras* with conditional *p53* deletion) cause only lung adenocarcinomas, more than half of the tumors that result from *Kras* with conditional *Lkb1* deletion showed squamous or mixed histology, and large cell histology was also observed.[98]

LKB1 regulates a key metabolic checkpoint through its phosphorylation of the AMP activated protein kinase AMPK. AMPK is sensitive to conditions of hypoxia and nutrient deprivation; under these conditions, AMPK is phosphorylated by LKB1, resulting in suppression of tumor growth and metabolic activity by direct phosphorylation of metabolic enzymes and by activation of the tuberous sclerosis complex tumor suppressors, which block activation of the mammalian target of rapamycin (mTOR) pathway.[101] In tumors that have lost LKB1, this growth suppressive checkpoint is defunct. Resultant tumors show elevated activity of the mTOR pathway and may be selectively dependent on this pathway for growth, and pharmacologic activation of AMPK may also be a therapeutic target in these cancers.[102,103] Metformin, an oral hypoglycemic drug commonly used for diabetes, activates AMPK and has been found to inhibit proliferation and colony formation *in vitro*.[104] Retrospective analyses demonstrate reduced incidence of cancer among diabetics treated with metformin.[105–107] In addition, metformin treatment for diabetes is associated with higher rates of complete response among neoadjuvantly treated breast cancer patients.[108] Although metformin appears to require functional LKB1 in order to effect AMPK activation, other compounds have been identified that circumvent this requirement. Thus, direct pharmacologic reactivation of the downstream tumor suppressive functions of AMPK may be a viable therapeutic strategy for LKB1 deficient tumors.

In addition to its role in regulating the AMPK metabolic checkpoint, LKB1 has many other distinct roles dependent on other downstream effector kinases, such as salt-inducible kinase, NUAK, and microtubule-affinity regulating kinase. These actions play a role in regulating a variety of cellular phenotypes important to cancer, such as cellular motility and transcriptional regulation, and LKB1 has been shown to exert profound effects in maintaining cellular polarity.[109,110] However, the relative importance of these various phenotypes in the biology of LKB1-deficient lung cancers is poorly understood.

Other Putative Tumor Suppressors

Several other genes that are less well characterized than the tumor suppressor genes detailed above have been identified as targets of recurrent mutational inactivation, chromosomal loss, and epigenetic repression in lung cancer. These candidate suppressor genes are often identified as regions of copy number loss or LOH that occur in multiple tumors in large genome-wide studies of chromosomal architecture in lung cancer. Further experimentation is required to elucidate which molecular pathways and cellular phenotypes are affected and to define the functional importance of these candidates. Common regions of genomic loss surround the chromosomal regions of classical tumor suppressors *CDKN2A*, *CDKN2B*, *LKB1*, and *RB1* (in SCLC). Other areas of recurrent loss in NSCLC occur at 9p23, 3p14.2, 3p21.3 16q23.1, 2q21.2, 4q35, 5q12.1, and 13q12.11.[94] Many of these regions are also altered in SCLC, although there are fewer data available for this tumor type. Areas of deletion may encompass many genes in any individual tumors. Determining the functional roles of each individual gene can be challenging. However, peak regions can be identified that are most frequently included in the deleted region across multiple tumors, and key genes are thought to be most likely to be included in these regions. Furthermore, integrating multiple types of data can reveal genes that are somatically inactivated by methylation or mutation, in addition to chromosomal loss; these are also likely to be the key suppressive genes within a deleted region. Of genes included in the regions listed above, missense mutations have been identified in *PTPRD* (9p23), *LRP1B* (2q21.2), *BLU* (3p21.3), and WWOX (16q23.1).[111,112] Experimental reexpression of candidate genes has been shown to inhibit proliferation in tumor cell lines for many of these putative tumor suppressors, including *PTPRD*, *LRP1B*, *WWOX* (16q23.1), *FHIT* (3p14.2), *SMARCA4* (19p13.2), *PTEN* (10q23), and *RASSF1*, *FUS1*, *BLU*, and *SEMA3B* (3p21.3).[113,114] However, for most of these candidates the biological implications of gene loss in a tumor is uncertain. More research devoted to these targets is required to further elucidate the roles they may play in lung cancer biology with the goal of identifying driver pathways that may become activated in the absence of particular TSGs and may thus be effective targets for therapeutic intervention.

OTHER BIOLOGIC ABNORMALITIES IN LUNG CANCER

Cellular Immortality Resulting from Increased Telomerase Activity

Cellular senescence is mainly regulated by telomerase, a ribonucleoprotein enzyme responsible for maintaining telomere length by *de novo* synthesis of telomeres and elongation of existing telomeres.

The human telomerase reverse transcriptase (hTERT) catalytic subunit is the major determinant of telomerase activity *in vitro* and *in vivo*. During normal cell division, telomere shortening leads to cell senescence and thus governs normal cell mortality. Telomerase reverse transcriptase maintains telomere ends via the synthesis of TTAGG nucleotide repeats. Telomerase activation is considered mandatory for tumor cells to escape senescence and contributes to immortalization and cancer pathogenesis. For example, immortalization of primary human airway epithelial cells can be achieved by the successive introduction of the simian virus SV40 early region and *hTERT*.[115] Malignant transformation is seen when these immortalized cells are transfected by an activated *RAS* oncogene. Approximately 100% of SCLCs and 80% to 85% of NSCLCs have been demonstrated to express high levels of telomerase activity. Furthermore, hTERT gene amplification occurs in 57% of NSCLCs, suggesting that this pathway is commonly targeted in lung cancer.[116] The prognostic significance of hTERT expression or activity remains controversial, although a recent study demonstrated that the copy number of serum *hTERT* mRNA was independently correlated with tumor size, tumor number, presence of metastasis, likelihood of recurrence, and smoking.[117] Furthermore, elevated telomerase activity and hTERT levels have been associated with worse disease-free and overall survival in patients with stage I NSCLC.[118] In preneoplastic lesions, telomerase activity or expression of its RNA component, or both, are observed *in situ* in lesions with the expression proportional to the severity of histology grade, supporting a temporal role for telomerase activation during lung preneoplasia.[119] Thus, telomerase activity or expression can be used as a potential biomarker to detect premalignant as well as tumor cells. For these reasons, there is much interest in developing antitelomerase drugs as new therapeutics. GV1001 and HR2882 are telomerase peptide vaccines that are being evaluated in clinical trials in patients with NSCLC.[120]

Deregulation of Apoptosis

Loss of normal apoptosis commonly occurs in many cancer types and is associated with expansion of viable cells and the development of resistance to chemotherapy and radiation therapy. Many members of both the mitochondrial (intrinsic) and the death receptor (extrinsic) apoptotic signaling pathways are found to be abnormal in lung cancer. A member of the intrinsic pathway, the antiapoptotic gene *BCL2* originally described in follicular lymphomas, is abnormally overexpressed in SCLC (75% to 95%) and some NSCLCs (25% of squamous cell carcinoma and approximately 10% of adenocarcinoma).[121–123]

BCL2 expression was associated with good prognosis in NSCLC.[124] Cytotoxicity of many chemotherapeutic agents is induced through the BCL2 apoptotic pathway; overexpression of BCL2 is associated with increased resistance to these agents.[125,126] Given the role of BCL2 in suppressing apoptosis and in reducing the efficacy of chemotherapy and radiotherapy, considerable effort is being made to develop BCL2-targeted therapeutics in combination with chemotherapy. In early phase 1 studies in patients with SCLC, *BCL2* antisense was found to be well tolerated when combined with chemotherapy.[127] However, randomized phase 2 trials found no difference in outcome compared with that of chemotherapy alone.[128] Despite these discouraging results, a new class of oral BCL2 antagonists is current being developed.

In the extrinsic pathway, death receptors are members of the tumor necrosis factor (TNF) receptor gene superfamily that consists of more than 20 proteins with a broad range of biological functions, including regulation of cell death and survival, differentiation, or immune regulation. The best-characterized death receptor, Fas (CD95), and its ligand (FasL) have also been implicated in lung cancer. In general, lung cancers express FasL but not the receptor. However, as T cells express Fas, one model that may help explain the resistance of lung cancer cells to immune surveillance involves the clonal deletion of immune T cells that would otherwise be directed against lung cancer antigens by this Fas–FasL interaction. Both caspase-8 and caspase-10 expression appears to be decreased in lung cancer. Homozygous deletion or methylation of *CASP8* gene has been observed in SCLC cell lines, with 79% demonstrating loss of expression.[129] Polymorphisms in the promoter region of caspase-9 have been shown to contribute to risk of lung cancer development.[130] Inhibitors of apoptosis (IAPs) impede cell death through caspase function, especially caspase-3 and -7. IAPs also inhibit apoptosis via modulation of the transcription of nuclear factor κB. One of the best-known members of this class of protein is survivin. Its expression is high in tumor but nearly nonexistent in adult normal tissue. Suppression of survivin has been shown to sensitize lung cancer cells to radiation, suggesting that it can be a potential target for intervention.[131]

Invasion, Metastasis, and Angiogenesis

Investigation of the molecular mechanisms of invasion and metastasis has yielded a variety of candidate genes, including cell adhesion molecules such as the cadherins, integrins, and CD44. The E-cadherin–catenin complex is critical for intercellular adhesiveness and maintenance of normal and malignant tissue architecture. Epigenetically reduced expression of this complex in malignant disease is associated with tumor invasion, metastasis, and unfavorable prognosis in lung cancer. Another family of adhesion molecules are the integrins. Integrin α_3 has been shown to be important for normal lung development and diminished expression correlated with a poor prognosis of patients with lung adenocarcinoma. Specific isoforms of CD44 may also be associated with lung cancer metastasis. Matrix metalloproteinases (MMPs) are zinc-dependent proteases that belong to a family of endopeptidases, which degrade the extracellular matrix and basement membrane, necessary first steps in angiogenesis. Increased expression of MMPs has been strongly implicated in tumor growth, invasion, and metastasis. MMP2 and MMP9 have been associated with poorer prognosis. However, despite its established role in invasion and metastasis, many randomized phase 3 trials of MMP inhibitors have failed to demonstrate a survival benefit in patients with advanced lung cancer.[132] This is perhaps related to the lack of specificity of these inhibitors and recent findings that some MMPs actually inhibit tumor growth.[133] Many of the genes that confer invasive and metastatic phenotypes are coordinately regulated by transcription factors such as ZEB and SNAIL, which can be activated by several stimuli, especially the actions of transforming growth factor-beta.[134] It has recently been shown that a key set of microRNAs of the miR-200 family plays a crucial role in regulating this phenotype.[135] The stimuli that regulate tumor cell invasiveness are often generated or influenced by surrounding stromal or inflammatory cells, and as such, the invasive phenotype seems to be quite plastic, complex, and highly dependent on the context of the tumor microenvironment.[136]

Angiogenesis, the formation of new blood capillaries, is necessary for a tumor mass to grow beyond a few millimeters in size. The angiogenic switch results from perturbation in the balance between inducers and inhibitors, both of which are produced by tumor and host cells. Vascular endothelial growth factor (VEGF), basic fibroblast growth factor (bFGF), and angiogenic cytokines, such as interleukin-8, have all been implicated in lung cancer.[137] Furthermore, high microvessel density (MVD) and VEGF overexpression are predictive of poor outcome. Thus, tumor angiogenesis has become a major new therapeutic target for lung cancer.[138] Clinical trials in lung cancer with agents targeting angiogenesis have shown great promise and have demonstrated that the addition of bevacizumab, the humanized monoclonal antibody to VEGF, to chemotherapy prolongs progression-free survival in phase 3 clinical trials, although improvements in overall survival were not always observed.[139–141]

CANCER STEM CELL HYPOTHESIS

The cancer stem cell hypothesis proposes that a self-renewing undifferentiated stem cell population that comprises a small fraction of the total tumor burden gives rise to more numerous and more differentiated progeny that populate the tumor.[142] Among the characteristics reported to distinguish stem-like cell from cells constituting the bulk of tumors include the potential for supporting the continued growth of the local tumor mass, for seeding metastases throughout the body, and resistance to cytotoxic therapies that allow the residual viable stem cells to repopulate the tumor after treatment. Because of their resistance to treatment and potential for seeding distant metastatic disease, the study of cancer stem cell and development of strategies effectively to eradicate all residual stem cells is of critical importance in cancer treatment.

Cancer stem-like cells can be isolated from a variety of tumor types using antibodies to unique cell surface proteins. They are capable of forming xenograft tumors at a high frequency after injection into immunocompromised mice. Empirically selected surface markers have been used to isolate putative stem cells from human breast cancer, glioblastoma multiforme, colon cancer, and other carcinomas, and these cells have demonstrably greater potential for xenograft formation than do unselected tumor cells. The resulting tumors recapitulate the histological appearance of the primary tumor as well as the heterogeneous expression of various surface and intracellular molecular markers.[142]

Putative lung progenitor cells have been described as cells that reside at the bronchoalveolar duct junction that express both Clara cell and pneumocyte markers or as lung resident cells of hematopoietic origin that express CD133.[143,144] These cells have not been conclusively shown to be lung adult stem cell populations but are intriguing and have been shown to be involved in repair of lung tissue after injury and may be involved in cancer development. In lung tumors, CD133[145-148] and other commonly used markers of stem-like tumor cells—Hoechst dye efflux and aldehyde dehydrogenase activity[149]—have been shown to identify subsets of tumor cells that display characteristics consistent with the cancer stem cell hypothesis. CD133 has been shown to segregate with template DNA in lung cells undergoing asymmetric cell division.[150] However, conflicting reports suggest that CD133 may not define a specific subset of cells, as interconversion between CD133+ and CD133− populations is observed, and CD133 expression may be associated with specific stages of cell cycle progression[151]; furthermore, some studies show no association between CD133 expression and propensity to initiate tumors.[152] The cancer stem cell hypothesis has other important gray areas as well; it is not yet certain whether a consistent developmental hierarchy would exist for every individual tumor or only in certain cases; whether or not lineage differentiation in a tumor can be a reversible; and which basic properties should be required to define a stem-like phenotype in a given population of cells. A highly increased propensity for xenograft formation is one of the most convincing features that can be demonstrated experimentally for proposed cancer stem-like cells. However, even the reliability of this evidence is called into question by the observation that a much higher rate of tumor formation is observed when mouse tumor lines are propagated in isogenic immunocompetent mice, which raises the possibility that the xenograft initiation phenotype may be related to the ability to adapt to the tissue environment of an immunocompromised mouse, rather than a general property of enhanced tumor formation.[153]

Nevertheless, the balance of evidence from diverse tumor types favors the hypothesis that stem-like cells are present within tumors and may play a key role in certain aspects of tumor biology. Furthermore, developmental pathways that are proposed to be important in governing cancer stem cell biology may be important oncogenic drivers of proliferation and invasion for unselected tumor cell populations in certain subsets of tumors, and are important avenues of research in their own right. For instance, the activity of particular genes—achaete-scute complex homologue 1[148] and OCT4 transcription factors[146]—have been implicated in regulating this subset of lung tumor cells. Given the far-reaching implications of the cancer stem cell hypothesis, and especially the concept that targeting developmental pathways cancer stem cells or in particular subsets of cancer could represent an important therapeutic strategy, these complex and exciting areas warrant further study in lung cancer.

GENOMIC ANALYSIS OF LUNG CANCER

In recent years technological advances in high-throughput sequencing approaches have enabled the comprehensive analyses of gene expression, copy number alterations, mutations, and other genetic perturbations across a large number of tumors. A number of studies have employed cDNA microarray chips to profile transcriptional expression in large sets of tumors. The largest such study of 443 lung adenocarcinomas from four institutions determined that clusters of coexpressed genes were consistently associated with patient outcome.[154] Prognostic profiles have been derived in several independent studies, although it is unclear how reproducible their associations are when applied to independent datasets. Associations with patient prognosis and response to treatment are potentially useful as an adjunct to classical staging approaches to help inform clinical decision making. For instance, when treating early stage tumors, adjuvant treatment may be more likely to benefit patients with a poor prognostic profile; whereas, a good prognostic profile could justify avoidance of adjuvant therapy. Although gene expression profiling of breast cancers has been validated and are widely used for making adjuvant treatment decisions, so far gene expression assays in lung cancer have not been validated prospectively as a useful guide for treatment planning.

Beyond prognostic associations, global approaches to the study of lung cancer have great potential as discovery tools that can increase the understanding of cancer biology and the molecular mechanisms underlying key cancer phenotypes. Arguably the most important outcome of such studies will be the identification of subsets of tumors whose biology can be affected by interventions targeted against key dysregulated genes or pathways. Hypotheses regarding such relationships can be derived from statistical associations between patterns of transcriptional regulation, copy number alterations, and mutations and tumor characteristics such as proliferative rate, tendencies for invasion and metastasis, response to therapy, and survival. Several large studies have already begun in search of clinically important genetic patterns. High-resolution analysis of copy number alterations has led to the identification of chromosomal regions that are frequently amplified or deleted in subsets of lung cancer encompassing regions containing key oncogenes and tumor suppressor genes such as *EGFR*, *KRAS*, *myc*, *p53*, and *LKB1*, as well as other candidate genes whose importance may become apparent after further study.[79,94] Microarray data from large cohorts of patients may reveal coordinately regulated sets of genes potentially associated with underlying dysregulation of particular pathways or cellular phenotypes. Such gene sets can be subjected to computational analyses to discover the biological and clinical significance (e.g., elucidation of specific oncogenic pathways, regulation of a transcription factors) *inter alia*. Furthermore, a greater depth of understanding may arise from coordinated analysis of multiple types of data from the same samples, greatly adding to the ability to interpret the significance of these data. For example, gene expression profiling has been carried out on tumors that have additionally been characterized by comparative genomic hybridization and extensive mutational sequencing[112,155] or by microRNA expression profiling.[156] It then becomes apparent that common mutations such *p53* and *EGFR*, as well as regions of amplification and deletion, are consis-

tently associated with altered expression of particular sets of genes.

A special case regarding the value of confluence of multiple types of data is seen with the analysis of large panels of lung cancer cell lines. Complete microarray expression profiling of the available lung cancer cell lines is complemented by independent knowledge of chromosomal changes, sequencing of mutations in common and novel cancer-associated genes, and profiling of microRNA expression, characterization of promoter methylation patterns and protein expression, and other molecular data. These molecular data can then be integrated with phenotypic observations such as sensitivity to targeted or cytotoxic therapies,[157-159] pathway activation,[160] or response to various perturbations.[161] High throughput approaches have also been applied to genetic perturbations using short interfering RNA screens and to drug treatment of cell lines, and these data can give additional detail regarding functional significance of particular genes.[162,163] Discovery efforts in cell lines may then generate hypotheses that can be applied back to enhance the understanding of data from primary tumors. For instance, expression profiles altered by oncogenic HRAS have been shown to be similar to profiles observed in lung cancer patients with *KRAS* mutations.[160] Profiles thought to be associated with activation of PI3K seem to be up-regulated in normal bronchial epithelia from smokers with cancer compared with smokers without cancer.[164] However, caution must be taken in generating these signatures and interpreting published associations, since a particular set of genes may be nonspecifically associated with the phenotype of interest, or the association may only be observed in the context of the *in vitro* system used in the experiments.

Global analysis of cancer biology is now poised to make an important step forward as massively parallel sequencing technologies become less expensive and more widespread. These technologies enable the sequencing of entire cancer genomes, allowing comprehensive determination of somatic mutations, polymorphisms, alternative splicing events, and chromosomal fusions. When this has been applied to a sufficient number of lung cancer samples, recurrent genetic alterations should become evident that may represent pharmaceutical targets or may highlight deregulated pathways where therapeutic intervention could be effective. The Cancer Genome Atlas represents a large-scale implementation of this strategy, and when it is complete it will combine gene expression, copy number alterations, single nucleotide polymorphisms, methylation status, microRNA expression, and mutation sequencing into a single compendium of data from several hundred clinically annotated tumors from multiple sites, including squamous cell lung carcinoma.

MOLECULAR BIOLOGY OF INDIVIDUAL CANCERS

MOLECULAR TOOLS IN THE LUNG CANCER CLINIC

The understanding of the molecular genetic changes in lung cancer pathogenesis is advancing rapidly. Many genetic abnormalities identified in lung cancer are common to other human cancers, while others appear more specific for lung cancer, perhaps because of characteristics of the cells of origin and the unique nature of carcinogen exposure. Where their biochemical function is known, the proteins rendered abnormal appear to fall into several growth regulatory pathways.[160] Thus, understanding of the fundamental workings and diverse molecular drivers of lung cancer is becoming clearer. A substantial effort has been made to translate the current scientific knowledge of these abnormalities from the bench to the bedside in order to improve patient outcomes. These approaches fall into three general categories:

1. Development of early detection tools to identify primary and recurrent disease to enable effective early treatment. Because lung cancer eventually develops in only one of ten cigarette smokers, the identification of persons with a genetic susceptibility to lung cancer should allow targeting and intensification of smoking cessation, early detection, and chemoprevention efforts. To date screening trials applied to smokers at high risk for the development of lung cancer, including the use of spiral computed tomography scans, have not been documented to decrease mortality. The identification of genetic epidemiologic markers and acquired respiratory genetic alterations may help to identify the most at-risk individuals for screening and chemoprevention trials.

2. Development of new cancer-specific therapies based on knowledge of genetic abnormalities. These may include replacing or pharmacologically reactivating mutant tumor suppressor genes, development of new drugs targeting activated protooncogenes, interfering with autocrine or paracrine growth stimulatory loops, and inhibiting angiogenesis, metastasis, and antiapoptotic. Some new therapies may be highly effective as single agents in some patients. However, it is likely that for many patients combinations of two or more targeted or cytotoxic agents will be required to maximize clinical benefit; and determining the optimal combination of therapy for a given patient will be an additional challenge in the field.

3. Identification of prognostic and predictive biomarkers, such as the *EGFR* mutation and *ALK-EML4* fusion, previously described, that predict the response to specific therapies and prognosticate outcomes. Such tools will play an increasingly important role in selecting optimal treatment strategies as the number of molecularly targeted therapies expands.

Selected References

The full list of references for this chapter appears in the online version.

6. Truong T, Hung RJ, Amos CI, et al. Replication of lung cancer susceptibility loci at chromosomes 15q25, 5p15, and 6p21: a pooled analysis from the International Lung Cancer Consortium. *J Natl Cancer Inst* 2010;102:959.

11. Braakhuis BJ, Tabor MP, Kummer JA, Leemans CR, Brakenhoff RH. A genetic explanation of Slaughter's concept of field cancerization: evidence and clinical implications. *Cancer Res* 2003;63:1727.

12. Park IW, Wistuba, II, Maitra A, et al. Multiple clonal abnormalities in the bronchial epithelium of patients with lung cancer. *J Natl Cancer Inst* 1999;91:1863.

15. Virmani AK, Gazdar AF. Tumor suppressor genes in lung cancer. *Methods Mol Biol* 2003;222:97.

21. Soda M, Choi YL, Enomoto M, et al. Identification of the transforming EML4-ALK fusion gene in non–small cell lung cancer. *Nature* 2007;448:561.

32. Rosell R, Moran T, Queralt C, et al. Screening for epidermal growth factor receptor mutations in lung cancer. *N Engl J Med* 2009;361:958.

40. Swanton C, Futreal A, Eisen T. Her2-targeted therapies in non–small cell lung cancer. *Clin Cancer Res* 2006;12:4377s.

44. Potti A, Moazzam N, Ramar K, et al. CD117 (c-KIT) overexpression in patients with extensive-stage small-cell lung carcinoma. *Ann Oncol* 2003;14:894.

51. Schiller JH, Akerley WL, Brugger W, et al. Results from ARQ 197-209: a global randomized placebo-controlled phase II clinical trial of erlotinib plus ARQ 197 versus erlotinib plus placebo in previously treated EGFR inhibitor-naive patients with locally advanced or metastatic non–small cell lung cancer (NSCLC). *J Clin Oncol* 2010;28: (abst LBA7502).

59. Mascaux C, Iannino N, Martin B, et al. The role of RAS oncogene in survival of patients with lung cancer: a systematic review of the literature with meta-analysis. *Br J Cancer* 2005;92:131.

62. Ravi RK, Weber E, McMahon M, et al. Activated Raf-1 causes growth arrest in human small cell lung cancer cells. *J Clin Invest* 1998;101:153.

65. Koivunen JP, Mermel C, Zejnullahu K, et al. EML4-ALK fusion gene and efficacy of an ALK kinase inhibitor in lung cancer. *Clin Cancer Res* 2008;14:4275.

68. Inamura K, Takeuchi K, Togashi Y, et al. EML4-ALK lung cancers are characterized by rare other mutations, a TTF-1 cell lineage, an acinar histology, and young onset. *Mod Pathol* 2009;22:508.

80. Klein C, Vassilev LT. Targeting the p53-MDM2 interaction to treat cancer. *Br J Cancer* 2004;91:1415.

84. Raver-Shapira N, Marciano E, Meiri E, et al. Transcriptional activation of miR-34a contributes to p53-mediated apoptosis. *Molecular Cell* 2007;26:731.

88. Carbone DP, Ciernik IF, Kelley MJ, et al. Immunization with mutant p53- and K-ras-derived peptides in cancer patients: immune response and clinical outcome. *J Clin Oncol* 2005;23:5099.

89. Antonia SJ, Mirza N, Fricke I, et al. Combination of p53 cancer vaccine with chemotherapy in patients with extensive stage small cell lung cancer. *Clin Cancer Res* 2006; 12:878.

91. Belinsky SA, Nikula KJ, Palmisano WA, et al. Aberrant methylation of p16(INK4a) is an early event in lung cancer and a potential biomarker for early diagnosis. *Proc Natl Acad Sci U S A* 1998;95:11891.

92. Zhang Y, Xiong Y, Yarbrough WG. ARF promotes MDM2 degradation and stabilizes p53: ARF-INK4a locus deletion impairs both the Rb and p53 tumor suppression pathways. *Cell* 1998;92:725.

97. Carretero J, Medina PP, Pio R, Montuenga LM, Sanchez-Cespedes M. Novel and natural knockout lung cancer cell lines for the LKB1/STK11 tumor suppressor gene. *Oncogene* 2004;23:4037.

100. Amin RMS, Hiroshima K, Iyoda A, et al. LKB1 protein expression in neuroendocrine tumors of the lung. *Pathol Int* 2008;58:84.

102. Mahoney CL, Choudhury B, Davies H, et al. LKB1/KRAS mutant lung cancers constitute a genetic subset of NSCLC with increased sensitivity to MAPK and mTOR signalling inhibition. *Br J Cancer* 2009;100:370.

106. Evans JMM, Donnelly LA, Emslie-Smith AM, Alessi DR, Morris AD. Metformin and reduced risk of cancer in diabetic patients. *BMJ* 2005;330:1304.

109. Baas AF, Kuipers J, van der Wel NN, et al. Complete polarization of single intestinal epithelial cells upon activation of LKB1 by STRAD. *Cell* 2004;116:457.

117. Miura N, Nakamura H, Sato R, et al. Clinical usefulness of serum telomerase reverse transcriptase (hTERT) mRNA and epidermal growth factor receptor (EGFR) mRNA as a novel tumor marker for lung cancer. *Cancer Sci* 2006; 97:1366.

118. Marchetti A, Pellegrini C, Buttitta F, et al. Prediction of survival in stage I lung carcinoma patients by telomerase function evaluation. *Lab Invest* 2002;82:729.

120. Brunsvig PF, Aamdal S, Gjertsen MK, et al. Telomerase peptide vaccination: a phase I/II study in patients with non–small cell lung cancer. *Cancer Immunol Immunother* 2006;55:1553.

121. Adams JM, Cory S. The Bcl-2 apoptotic switch in cancer development and therapy. *Oncogene* 2007;26:1324.

122. Pezzella F, Turley H, Kuzu I, et al. Bcl-2 protein in non–small cell lung carcinoma. *N Engl J Med* 1993;329:690.

129. Shivapurkar N, Reddy J, Matta H, et al. Loss of expression of death-inducing signaling complex (DISC) components in lung cancer cell lines and the influence of MYC amplification. *Oncogene* 2002;21:8510.

130. Park JY, Park JM, Jang JS, et al. Caspase 9 promoter polymorphisms and risk of primary lung cancer. *Hum Mol Genet* 2006;15:1963.

142. Jordan CT, Guzman ML, Noble M. Cancer stem cells. *N Engl J Med* 2006;355:1253.

143. Germano D, Blyszczuk P, Valaperti A, et al. Prominin-1/CD133+ lung epithelial progenitors protect from bleomycin-induced pulmonary fibrosis. *Am J Respir Crit Care Med* 2009;179:939.

144. Kim CFB, Jackson EL, Woolfenden AE, et al. Identification of bronchioalveolar stem cells in normal lung and lung cancer. *Cell* 2005;121:823.

149. Jiang F, Qiu Q, Khanna A, et al. Aldehyde dehydrogenase 1 is a tumor stem cell-associated marker in lung cancer. *Mol Cancer Res* 2009;7:330.

150. Pine SR, Ryan BM, Varticovski L, Robles AI, Harris CC. Microenvironmental modulation of asymmetric cell division in human lung cancer cells. *Proc Natl Acad Sci U S A* 2010;107:2195.

158. Sos ML, Fischer S, Ullrich R, et al. Identifying genotype-dependent efficacy of single and combined PI3K- and MAPK-pathway inhibition in cancer. *Proc Natl Acad Sci U S A* 2009;106:18351.

162. Luo J, Emanuele MJ, Li D, et al. A genome-wide RNAi screen identifies multiple synthetic lethal interactions with the Ras oncogene. *Cell* 2009;137:835.

163. Whitehurst AW, Bodemann BO, Cardenas J, et al. Synthetic lethal screen identification of chemosensitizer loci in cancer cells. *Nature* 2007;446:815.

164. Gustafson AM, Soldi R, Anderlind C, et al. Airway PI3K pathway activation is an early and reversible event in lung cancer development. *Sci Transl Med* 2010; 2:26ra25.

MOLECULAR BIOLOGY OF INDIVIDUAL CANCERS

CHAPTER 16 ESOPHAGUS AND STOMACH CANCERS

ANIL K. RUSTGI

This chapter will deal with the molecular biology of esophageal and gastric cancers. There are several key aspects in the elucidation of the genetic basis of esophageal and gastric cancers through molecular biology approaches. These include, but are not limited to, new insights into underlying pathogenesis, possibilities for risk stratification and prognosis, correlations with traditional pathology classification schemes, development of new diagnostics, and potential applications in imaging and therapy. In considering the genetic underpinnings of esophageal and gastric cancers, or for any cancer, critical appraisal is required of oncogenes, tumor suppressor genes, and DNA mismatch repair genes as they modulate, either positively or negatively, growth factor receptor–mediating signaling cascades, transcription of target genes, and cell-cycle progression. These molecular networks conspire to influence cellular behaviors, such as proliferation, differentiation, apoptosis, senescence, and response to stress and injury. The exquisite equilibrium that is the signature of normal cellular homeostasis is perturbed in uncontrolled cell growth, resulting in eventual evolution of premalignant stages and malignant transformation. However, the time required for malignant transformation varies, depending on cellular- and tissue-specific context, and is affected by environmental factors.

The salient features of tumorigenesis and acquisition of the malignant phenotype that are required, as described by Hanahan and Weinberg,[1] include growth signal autonomy, ability to surmount antigrowth signals, evasion of apoptosis, unlimited replicative ability, angiogenesis, and invasion and metastatic potential. More recently, the role of inflammation in carcinogenesis has gained much attention.

MOLECULAR BIOLOGY OF ESOPHAGEAL CANCER

The vast majority of esophageal cancers are of two subtypes: esophageal squamous cell cancer (ESCC) and esophageal adenocarcinoma (EAD). ESCC is preceded by squamous dysplasia, whereas EAD is preceded by Barrett's esophagus or incomplete intestinal metaplasia of the normal squamous epithelium of the esophagus (Fig. 16.1). Barrett's esophagus undergoes transition from low-grade and high-grade dysplasia before converting into EAD. ESCC and EAD have common and divergent genetic features as manifest by alterations in canonical oncogenes and tumor suppressor genes in somatic cells of tumors (Table 16.1). However, inherited predisposition to ESCC is rare, as described in tylosis palmaris et plantaris. Although the gene mutation for tylosis has remained elusive, the region of allelic deletion is on chromosome 17p.[2] Similarly, there is no classic syndrome that distinguishes familial Barrett's esophagus or familial EAD. That being said, studies continue to analyze families with Barrett's esophagus in an effort to identify relevant genes or single-nucleotide polymorphisms. It is estimated that about 7% of patients with Barrett's esophagus may have a family history. As a separate consideration, ESCC or EAD does not appear to emerge from infectious etiologies, although a small subset of ESCC is associated with human papillomavirus in some endemic regions of the world.

The Epidermal Growth Factor Receptor

The epidermal growth factor receptor (EGFR) family of receptor tyrosine kinases stimulates a number of signal transduction cascades (e.g., *Ras/Raf/MEK/ERK, PI3K/AKT*) that regulate diverse cellular processes, such as proliferation, differentiation, survival, migration and adhesion.[3] These signaling pathways are important in normal cellular homeostasis, but aberrant activation of the EGFR members are crucial in esophageal carcinogenesis. This family of receptors comprises EGFR (also referred to as *erbB1*), *erbB2, erbB3*, and *erbB4*. The receptors have the ability to homo- or heterodimerize on engagement with one of several ligands: TGF (transforming growth factor)-α, EGF (epidermal growth factor), amphiregulin, heparin-binding EGF-like growth factor, betacellulin, and epiregulin. Tyrosine phosphorylation of homo- or heterodimers of EGFRs creates docking sites for

Normal esophagus → Squamous dysplasia → Squamous cell cancer

Normal esophagus → Intestinal metaplasia → Low-grade dysplasia → High-grade dysplasia → Adenocarcinoma

FIGURE 16.1 Progression of stages in esophageal squamous cell cancer and esophageal adenocarcinoma.

signaling proteins or adapter proteins. EGFR is commonly overexpressed in early-stage esophageal cancer, and overexpression correlates with a poor prognosis.[4–7] EGFR overexpression is typically due to increased engagement with ligands and decreased turnover. However, mutation of a tyrosine residue in the cytoplasmic domain is rare. Increased expression of TGF-α and EGF has been detected in Barrett's esophagus, EAD, and ESCC.[8–12] EGFR overexpression may predict a poor response to chemoradiotherapy[13,14] and is associated with decreased survival in patients with squamous cell carcinoma.[13] Furthermore, EGFR overexpression was associated with recurrent disease and diminished overall survival in patients undergoing esophagectomy for ESCC.[14,15] In contrast to EGFR, it is not clear if *erbB2* overexpression is consistently found either in ESCC or EAD.

Cyclin D1 and *p16INK4a*

The mammalian cell cycle is regulated exquisitely by cyclins, cyclin-dependent kinases (CDK), and cyclin-dependent kinase inhibitors (CDKi such as p15, p16, p21, and p27). During G1 phase, the cyclin D1 oncogene complexes with either CDK4 or CDK6 to phosphorylate the retinoblastoma (pRb) tumor suppressor protein and, in so doing, relieves the negative regulatory effect of pRb, allowing the E2F family of transcription factors to propel the cell cycle toward the G_1/S phase transition.[16] Toward the late G_1 phase, cyclin E complexes with CDKs to phosphorylate p107, which is related to pRb, and liberate more E2F members to navigate the cell cycle into S phase. As with EGFR, cyclin D1 overexpression is found in premalignant lesions, such as esophageal squamous dysplasia or Barrett's

esophagus, and the majority of early-stage ESCC or EAD.[17,18] Additionally, cyclin D1 overexpression correlates with poor outcomes and survival as well as poor response to chemotherapy.[19,20]

Although cyclin D1 overexpression accounts for cyclin D1 dysregulation, other mechanisms include mutations in cyclin D1 and mutations in Fbx4, which is the E3 ligase for cyclin D1, thereby preventing degradation of cyclin D1 in the cytoplasm and reimportation into the nucleus, where it exerts its oncogenic effects.[21]

In a similar vein, *p16INK4a* is an early genetic alteration, via promoter hypermethylation, point mutation, or allelic deletion, in Barrett's esophagus and EAD, but interestingly, a late event in ESCC. Loss of heterozygosity of 9p21, the locus for both p16 and p15, has been demonstrated with high frequency in both dysplastic Barrett's epithelium and Barrett's adenocarcinoma (90% and more than 80% of cases, respectively).[22,23] Promoter hypermethylation, which prevents tumor suppressor function by blocking transcription, has been documented and correlates with the degree of dysplasia in Barrett's esophagus. It is present in up to 75% of specimens with high-grade dysplasia and is found in almost 50% of patients with adenocarcinoma of the esophagus.[24] Point mutations of p16 in ESCC have been found and promoter hypermethylation has been noted in up to 50% of these tumors.[25,26] *Rb* gene mutation is not found in either type of esophageal neoplasm, but allelic loss of 13q where the locus of the *Rb* gene resides is found in up to 50% of patients with Barrett's adenocarcinoma and squamous cell carcinoma.[18,27] This can correlate with diminished or loss of pRb protein in Barrett's esophagus with dysplasia, EAD, and ESCC.[28,29]

p53 Tumor Suppressor Gene

p53 is one of the most commonly mutated genes in human cancer.[22–24] *p53* (molecular weight approximately 53 kDa) is a tumor suppressor that interrupts the G1 phase to evaluate and permit repair of damaged DNA, which may arise from environmental exposure (e.g., irradiation, ultraviolet light) or cellular stress.[30] In the face of irreparable damage, *p53* induces apoptosis. The *p53* transcription factor binds DNA to activate or suppress a large repertoire of target genes.[31] *p53* mutations induce loss of cell-cycle checkpoints and promote genomic instability. The majority of *p53* mutations occur in the DNA-binding region, and more than 80% of them are missense mutations resulting in loss of wild type

TABLE 16.1

COMMON MOLECULAR GENETIC ALTERATIONS OBSERVED IN ESOPHAGEAL AND GASTRIC CANCERS

Oncogenes
  Epidermal growth factor receptor (*EGFR*)
  Cyclin D1
Tumor suppressor genes
  P16INK4a
  p53
  E-cadherin
DNA mismatch repair genes (*hMLH1*, *hMSH2*)
  Mismatch repair instability

p53 function.[32] Wild type *p53* has a short half-life and is difficult to detect by immunohistochemistry; mutation in *p53* results in stabilization of the protein and allows for easier detection by immunohistochemistry.

Detection of mutated p53 protein by immunohistochemistry has been demonstrated with increasing frequency during histologic progression from Barrett's esophagus (5%) through dysplasia (65% to 75%) to frank adenocarcinoma (up to 90%).[33–36] Thus, *p53* mutation or loss of heterozygosity appears early in Barrett's esophagus and EAD. Both mutant p53 protein detected by immunohistochemistry and specific *p53* gene mutations detected by genomic sequencing have been identified in 40% to 75% of patients with ESCC.[37–40] The presence of a *p53* point mutation correlates with response to induction chemoradiotherapy and predicted survival after esophagectomy in patients with either ESCC or EAD.[41]

Telomerase Activation

Maintenance of telomere length allows DNA replication to be sustained indefinitely. Aberrant expression of telomerase has been observed in most esophageal cancers examined to date.[42] Morales et al.[43] observed increased telomerase expression in 100% of adenocarcinoma and Barrett's esophagus cases with high-grade dysplasia. Telomerase activation is important, but alternative mechanisms to maintain the length of telomeres may operate in these cancers as well.[44]

Tumor Invasion and Metastasis

Loss of cell-cell adhesion can lead to both invasion and metastases. Alterations in expression of E-cadherin, a cell-cell adhesion molecule, or its associated catenins disrupt cell-cell interactions, which results in the potential for tumor progression.[45] Reduced expression of E-cadherin has been correlated with progression from Barrett's esophagus to dysplasia and finally to adenocarcinoma, and also observed in ESCC.[46,47]

Models of ESCC and EAD

Advances in diagnosis and therapy of esophageal neoplasms will ultimately be fostered through cell lines, xenotransplantation mouse models, surgically based rodent models, and genetically engineered mouse models. There is a vast array of cell lines established from primary and metastatic human esophageal cancers that allow perturbation of gene expression to gauge effects on cellular behavior. Recently, organotypic (three-

dimensional) cell culture models, which mimic human tissue, have revealed that the combination of EGFR and mutant *p53* results in transformation of human esophageal epithelial cells immortalized with hTERT.[48] A classic rodent model involves total gastrectomy followed by esophagojejunostomy.[49] This creates a milieu whereby the esophagus is exposed to high concentrations of bile ("nonacid reflux") with the development of Barrett's esophagus and EAD. In transgenic mice in which cyclin D1 is targeted to the esophagus, esophagi reveal evidence of dysplasia that evolves into squamous cell cancer on crossbreeding the mice with *p53* haploinsufficiency or loss.[50] Rodents have also been treated with nitrosamines to yield esophageal papillomas and ESCC.[51,52]

The underlying fate switch between ESCC and EAD may be influenced as well by the expression and function of "lineage"-specific transcriptional factors as demonstrated through functional genomics. To that end, *SOX2*, found to be part of an amplicon on chromosome 3q26.33 in human ESCC, fosters growth of these cancers. This may have implications in the therapy of human ESCC.[53]

MOLECULAR BIOLOGY OF GASTRIC CANCER

The most common type of gastric cancer is adenocarcinoma, of which there are two subtypes: intestinal and diffuse. They are distinguished by different anatomic locations within the stomach, variable clinical outcomes, and different pathogenesis. The intestinal type of sporadic gastric adenocarcinoma has a hallmark progression from normal gastric epithelium to chronic atrophic gastritis (typically due to *Helicobacter pylori* infection) to intestinal metaplasia (which has some overlapping but also different features than intestinal metaplasia of Barrett's esophagus) to dysplasia to cancer (Fig. 16.2). Diffuse-type gastric adenocarcinoma is even more invasive and aggressive in its behavior, has overlap with lobular-type breast cancer, and may be highlighted by loss of E-cadherin.

Inherited Susceptibility

Case-control studies have observed consistent, up to threefold, increases in risk for gastric cancer among relatives of patients with gastric cancer.[54,55] Studies of monozygotic twins have even shown a slight trend toward increased concordance of gastric cancers compared with dizygotic twins.[56,57] Large families with an autosomal dominant,

Normal gastric mucosa → Chronic atrophic gastritis → Intestinal metaplasia → Low-grade dysplasia → High-grade dysplasia → Adenocarcinoma

FIGURE 16.2 Progression of stages in intestinal-type gastric adenocarcinoma.

highly penetrant inherited predisposition for the development of gastric cancer are rare. However, early-onset diffuse gastric cancers have been described and linked to the *E-cadherin/CDH1* locus on chromosome 16q and associated with mutations in this gene.[58] This seminal finding has been confirmed in other studies with gastric cancers at a relatively high (67% to 83%) penetrant rate.[59–62] Thus, E-cadherin mutation testing should be considered in the appropriate clinical setting. In fact, prophylactic gastrectomy should be considered strongly in families with germ line E-cadherin mutation even without gross mucosal abnormalities by endoscopic examination of the stomach.[63]

Lynch syndrome or hereditary nonpolyposis colon cancer involves germ line mutations of DNA mismatch repair genes.[64] Gastric adenocarcinoma may be observed in some families with Lynch syndrome. Gastric cancers have also been noted to occur in patients with familial adenomatous polyposis and Peutz-Jeghers syndrome.

The Role of *Helicobacter pylori* Infection and Other Host-Environmental Factors

As a commensal organism, *H. pylori* infection is widely prevalent throughout the world. Despite its classification by the World Health Organization as a class I carcinogen, infection with *H. pylori* does not typically lead to gastric cancer. This underscores the importance of other factors, such as virulence, environmental, and host factors, as well as genetic polymorphisms (e.g., in interleukin-1β, a potent inhibitor of acid secretion).[65] The blood group A phenotype has been reported to be associated with gastric cancers.[66,67] *H. pylori* may adhere to the Lewis blood group antigen, indicating a factor for increased risk for gastric cancer.[68] Small variant alleles of a mucin gene, *Muc1*, were found to be associated with gastric cancer patients when compared with a blood donor control population.[69] Epstein-Barr virus infection has been noted in a certain type of gastric carcinoma (lymphoepithelioid type), although the importance of this is unclear.[70]

Molecular Genetic Alterations

In contrast to ESCC, EAD, pancreatic cancer, and colon cancer in which certain oncogenes and tumor suppressor genes are altered with high frequency, such degree of alteration is not observed in sporadic gastric cancers. A reasonably prevalent alteration is microsatellite instability, the result of changes in DNA mismatch repair genes (Table 16.1). Microsatellite instability and associated alterations of the *TGF*-beta *II receptor*, *IGFRII*, *BAX*, *E2F-4*, *hMSH3*, and *hMSH6* genes are found in a subset of gastric carcinomas.[71–75] Microsatellite instability has been found in 13% to 44% of sporadic gastric carcinomas.[76] A high degree of microsatellite instability occurs in gastric cancers of the intestinal type, reduced involvement of lymph nodes, enhanced lymphoid infiltration, and better prognosis.[77] This is reminiscent of colon cancers associated with Lynch syndrome.

The *p53* tumor suppressor gene is consistently altered in most gastric cancers.[78] In a study of the promoter region of p16 in gastric cancers, a significant number (41%) exhibited CpG island methylation.[79] Many cases with hypermethylation of promoter regions displayed the phenotype with a high degree of microsatellite instability and multiple sites of methylation, including the *hMLH1* promoter region.[80]

Many sporadic diffuse gastric cancers display altered E-cadherin, a transmembrane, calcium-dependent adhesion molecule important in epithelial cell homophilic and heterophilic interactions. E-cadherin may be down-regulated in gastric carcinogenesis (especially diffuse gastric adenocarcinoma) by point mutation, allelic deletion, or promoter methylation.[81,82] In addition, during epithelial-mesenchymal transition, E-cadherin transcription can be silenced by transcriptional factors such as Snail and Slug. However, it is not clear if epithelial-mesenchymal transition is an important process in gastric carcinogenesis, as is believed to be the case, for example, in breast cancer.

Alterations in a number of other oncogenes and tumor suppressor genes have been described in a very small subset of gastric cancers by polymerase chain reaction–based or immunohistochemical analysis, but the variability in methods and lack of uniformity in quality control make these observations less compelling. As with esophageal cancer, high-throughput assays, such as single-nucleotide polymorphism arrays, chromosomal genomic hybridization (to assess chromosomal gains and losses) arrays, gene expression profiling through microarrays, and tissue- and plasma-based proteomics may unravel molecular signatures (and even specific genes and/or pathways) that define subtypes of gastric cancers, different stages of gastric cancers, and correlations with clinical outcomes.

MOLECULAR BIOLOGY OF INDIVIDUAL CANCERS

Models of Gastric Cancer

Genetically engineered mouse models of gastric cancer have emerged in rapid fashion in recent years, indicating that activated Wnt signaling and induced downstream effectors, *p53* inactivation, *APC* gene inactivation, *Smad4* gene inactivation, and gastrin are critical factors.[83–87] Gastric cancers in these protean mouse models are facilitated by concomitant infection with *Helicobacter*.[88,89] Furthermore, recruitment of bone marrow stem cells may augment the effects of *Helicobacter* infection during gastric carcinogenesis.[90]

Recently, it has been demonstrated that overexpression of interleukin-1β in mice results in gastric inflammation and cancer, with concomitant recruitment of immature myeloid cells (also referred to as *myeloid-derived suppressor cells*).[91]

Selected References

The full list of references for this chapter appears in the online version.

1. Hanahan D, Weinberg RA. The hallmarks of cancer. *Cell* 2000;100:57.
3. Schlessinger J. Cell signaling by receptor tyrosine kinases. *Cell* 2000;103(2): 211.
5. Torzewski M, Sarbia M, Verreet P, et al. The prognostic significance of epidermal growth factor receptor expression in squamous cell carcinomas of the oesophagus. *Anticancer Res* 1997;17(5B):3915.
8. Jankowski J, McMenemin R, Hopwood D, et al. Abnormal expression of growth regulatory factors in Barrett's oesophagus. *Clin Sci (Lond)* 1991;81: 663.
10. Jankowski J, Hopwood D, Wormsley KG. Flow-cytometric analysis of growth-regulatory peptides and their receptors in Barrett's oesophagus and oesophageal adenocarcinoma. *Scand J Gastroenterol* 1992;27:147.
12. Yacoub L, Goldman H, Odze RD. Transforming growth factor-alpha, epidermal growth factor receptor, and MiB-1 expression in Barrett's-associated neoplasia: correlation with prognosis. *Mod Pathol* 1997;10:105.
13. Itakura Y, Sasano H, Shiga C, et al. Epidermal growth factor receptor overexpression in esophageal carcinoma: an immunohistochemical study correlated with clinicopathologic findings and DNA amplification. *Cancer* 1994; 74:795.
17. Arber N, Lightdale C, Rotterdam H, et al. Increased expression of the cyclin D1 gene in Barrett's esophagus. *Cancer Epidemiol Biomarkers Prev* 1996;5:457.
19. Shamma A, Doki Y, Shiozaki H, et al. Cyclin D1 overexpression in esophageal dysplasia: a possible biomarker for carcinogenesis of esophageal squamous cell carcinoma. *Int J Oncol* 2000;16:261.
20. Sarbia M, Bektas N, Muller W, et al. Expression of cyclin E in dysplasia, carcinoma, and nonmalignant lesions of Barrett esophagus. *Cancer* 1999;86: 2597.
21. Barbash O, Zamfirova P, Lin DI, et al. Mutations in Fbx4 inhibit dimerization of the SCF(Fbx4) ligase and contribute to cyclin D1 overexpression in human cancer. *Cancer Cell* 2008;14(1):68.
22. Barrett MT, Sanchez CA, Galipeau PC, et al. Allelic loss of 9p21 and mutation of the CDKN2/p16 gene develop as early lesions during neoplastic progression in Barrett's esophagus. *Oncogene* 1996;13:1867.
24. Klump B, Hsieh CJ, Holzmann K, et al. Hypermethylation of the CDKN2/p16 promoter during neoplastic progression in Barrett's esophagus. *Gastroenterology* 1998;115:1381.
25. Xing EP, Nie Y, Wang LD, et al. Aberrant methylation of p16INK4a and deletion of p15INK4b are frequent events in human esophageal cancer in Linxian, China. *Carcinogenesis* 1999;20:77.
26. Maesawa C, Tamura G, Nishizuka S, et al. Inactivation of the CDKN2 gene by homozygous deletion and de novo methylation is associated with advanced stage esophageal squamous cell carcinoma. *Cancer Res* 1996;56:3875.
28. Coppola D, Schreiber RH, Mora L, et al. Significance of Fas and retinoblastoma protein expression during the progression of Barrett's metaplasia to adenocarcinoma. *Ann Surg Oncol* 1999;6:298.
29. Ikeguchi M, Oka S, Gomyo Y, et al. Clinical significance of retinoblastoma protein (pRB) expression in esophageal squamous cell carcinoma. *J Surg Oncol* 2000;73:104.
33. Hamelin R, Flejou JF, Muzeau F, et al. TP53 gene mutations and p53 protein immunoreactivity in malignant and premalignant Barrett's esophagus. *Gastroenterology* 1994;107: 1012.
35. Younes M, Lebovitz RM, Lechago LV, et al. p53 protein accumulation in Barrett's metaplasia, dysplasia, and carcinoma: a follow-up study. *Gastroenterology* 1993;105:1637.
37. Gaur D, Arora S, Mathur M, et al. High prevalence of p53 gene alterations and protein overexpression in human esophageal cancer: correlation with dietary risk factors in India. *Clin Cancer Res* 1997;3:2129.
38. Kato H, Yoshikawa M, Miyazaki T, et al. Expression of p53 protein related to smoking and alcoholic beverage drinking habits in patients with esophageal cancers. *Cancer Lett* 2001;167:65.
40. Taniere P, Martel-Planche G, Saurin JC, et al. TP53 mutations, amplification of P63 and expression of cell cycle proteins in squamous cell carcinoma of the oesophagus from a low incidence area in Western Europe. *Br J Cancer* 2001;85:721.
41. Ribeiro U Jr, Finkelstein SD, Safatle-Ribeiro AV, et al. p53 sequence analysis predicts treatment response and outcome of patients with esophageal carcinoma. *Cancer* 1998;83:7.
43. Morales CP, Lee EL, Shay JW. In situ hybridization for the detection of telomerase RNA in the progression from Barrett's esophagus to esophageal adenocarcinoma. *Cancer* 1998;83:652.
44. Opitz OG, Suliman Y, Hahn WC, et al. Cyclin D1 overexpression and p53 inactivation immortalize primary oral keratinocytes by a telomerase-independent mechanism. *J Clin Invest* 2001;108(5):725.
45. Christofori G, Semb H. The role of the cell-adhesion molecule E-cadherin as a tumour-suppressor gene. *Trends Biochem Sci* 1999;24:73.
47. Takeno S, Noguchi T, Fumoto S, et al. E-cadherin expression in patients with esophageal squamous cell carcinoma: promoter hypermethylation, Snail overexpression, and clinicopathologic implications. *Am J Clin Pathol* 2004; 122(1):78.
48. Okawa T, Michaylira CZ, Kalabis J, et al. The functional interplay between EGFR overexpression, hTERT activation, and p53 mutation in esophageal epithelial cells with activation of stromal fibroblasts induces tumor development, invasion, and differentiation. *Genes Dev* 2007;21(21): 2788.
50. Opitz OG, Harada H, Suliman Y, et al. A mouse model of human oral-esophageal cancer. *J Clin Invest* 2002;110: 761.

51. Siglin JC, Khare L, Stoner GD. Evaluation of dose and treatment duration on the esophageal tumorigenicity of N-nitrosomethylbenzylamine in rats. *Carcinogenesis* 1995;16(2):259.

53. Bass AJ, Watanabe H, Mermel CH, et al. SOX2 is an amplified lineage-survival oncogene in lung and esophageal squamous cell carcinomas. *Nat Genet* 2009;41(11):1238.

58. Guilford P, Hopkins J, Harraway J, et al. E-cadherin germline mutations in familial gastric cancer. *Nature* 1998; 392:402.

59. Gayther SA, Gorringe KL, Ramus SJ, et al. Identification of germ-line E-cadherin mutations in gastric cancer families of European origin. *Cancer Res* 1998;58:4086.

62. Pharoah PD, Caldas C. Incidence of gastric cancer and breast cancer in CDH1 (E-cadherin) mutation carriers from hereditary diffuse gastric cancer families. *Gastroenterology* 2001;121:1348.

63. Lewis FR, Mellinger JD, Hayashi A, et al. Prophylactic total gastrectomy for familial gastric cancer. *Surgery* 2001;130 (4):612.

64. Chung DC, Rustgi AK. The hereditary nonpolyposis colorectal cancer syndrome: genetics and clinical implications. *Ann Intern Med* 2003;138(7):560.

65. El Omar EM, Rabkin CS, Gammon MD, et al. Increased risk of noncardiac gastric cancer associated with proinflammatory cytokine gene polymorphisms. *Gastroenterology* 2003;124:1193.

69. Silva F, Carvalho F, Peixoto A, et al. MUC1 polymorphism confers increased risk for intestinal metaplasia in a Colombian population with chronic gastritis. *Eur J Hum Genet* 2003;11(5):380.

70. Lee HS, Chang MS, Yang HK, Lee BL, Kim WH. Epstein-Barr virus-positive gastric carcinoma has a distinct protein expression profile in comparison with Epstein-Barr virus-negative carcinoma. *Clin Cancer Res* 2004;10(5): 1698.

71. Kim SJ, Bang YJ, Park JG, et al. Genetic changes in the transforming growth factor beta (TGF-beta) type II receptor gene in human gastric cancer cells: correlation with sensitivity to growth inhibition by TGF-beta. *Proc Natl Acad Sci U S A* 1994;91:8772.

72. Yamamoto H, Sawai H, Perucho M. Frameshift somatic mutations in gastrointestinal cancer of the microsatellite mutator phenotype. *Cancer Res* 1997;57:4420.

76. Seruca R, Santos NR, David L, et al. Sporadic gastric carcinomas with microsatellite instability display a particular clinicopathologic profile. *Int J Cancer* 1995;64:32.

77. dos Santos NR, Seruca R, Constancia M, et al. Microsatellite instability at multiple loci in gastric carcinoma: clinicopathologic implications and prognosis. *Gastroenterology* 1996;110:38.

80. Toyota M, Ahuja N, Suzuki H, et al. Aberrant methylation in gastric cancer associated with the CpG island methylator phenotype. *Cancer Res* 1999;59:5438.

82. Grady WM, Willis J, Guilford PJ, et al. Methylation of the CDH1 promoter as the second genetic hit in hereditary diffuse gastric cancer. *Nat Genet* 2000;26:16.

83. Taketo MM. Wnt signaling and gastrointestinal tumorigenesis in mouse models. *Oncogene* 2006;25(57):7522.

84. Fox JG, Dangler CA, Whary MT, et al. Mice carrying a truncated Apc gene have diminished gastric epithelial proliferation, gastric inflammation, and humoral immunity in response to *Helicobacter felis* infection. *Cancer Res* 1997; 57(18):3972.

85. Teng Y, Sun AN, Pan XC, et al. Synergistic function of Smad4 and PTEN in suppressing forestomach squamous cell carcinoma in the mouse. *Cancer Res* 2006;66(14):6972.

86. Watson SA, Grabowska AM, El-Zaatari M, Takhar A. Gastrin—active participant or bystander in gastric carcinogenesis? *Nat Rev Cancer* 2006;6(12): 936.

87. Wang TC, Dangler CA, Chen D, et al. Synergistic interaction between hypergastrinemia and *Helicobacter* infection in a mouse model of gastric cancer. *Gastroenterology* 2000;118(1):36.

88. Rogers AB, Taylor NS, Whary MT, et al. *Helicobacter pylori* but not high salt induces gastric intraepithelial neoplasia in B6129 mice. *Cancer Res* 2005;65(23):10709.

89. Cai X, Carlson J, Stoicov C, et al. *Helicobacter felis* eradication restores normal architecture and inhibits gastric cancer progression in C57BL/6 mice. *Gastroenterology* 2005;128 (7):1937.

90. Houghton J, Stoicov C, Nomura S, et al. Gastric cancer originating from bone marrow-derived cells. *Science* 2004;306(5701):1568.

91. Tu S, Bhagat G, Cui G, et al. Overexpression of interleukin-1beta induces gastric inflammation and cancer and mobilizes myeloid-derived suppressor cells in mice. *Cancer Cell* 2008;14(5):408.

MOLECULAR BIOLOGY OF INDIVIDUAL CANCERS

CHAPTER 17 PANCREAS CANCER

SCOTT E. KERN AND RALPH H. HRUBAN

Pancreatic ductal adenocarcinoma is a genetic disease. This perspective is supported by reproducible patterns of genetic mutations that accumulate during tumorigenesis. These patterns indicate the operation of a selective process favoring the emergence of specific constellations of genetic changes. Individuals who inherit a mutant form of certain genes have an increased risk of developing pancreatic cancer. According to this genetic theory, most pancreatic cancers share a common foundation of genetic mutations disrupting specific cellular regulatory controls. These shared abnormalities are responsible for the processes of growth, invasion, and metastasis in individual patients.

Four categories of mutated genes play a role in the pancreatic tumorigenesis: oncogenes, tumor-suppressor genes, genome-maintenance genes, and tissue-maintenance genes (summarized in Table 17.1). Some of these mutations are germ line, for example, they are transmitted within a family. Genetic mutations acquired during life, termed *somatic mutations*, contribute to tumorigenesis within a tissue but are not passed to offspring.

Very recently, techniques were developed to sequence all of the genes of individual cancers. Whole-exomic sequencing of pancreatic ductal cancers revealed an average of 63 somatic mutations per tumor.[1] Most of these mutations undoubtedly were nonfunctional "passenger" mutations, each mutated at a low frequency and not contributing to tumorigenesis. Indeed, most passenger mutations might arise as a normal aspect of tissue aging before tumorigenesis begins.[2] Smoking is associated with a doubling of the risk for pancreatic cancer, and remarkably is also associated with a 40% increase of the prevalence of low-frequency mutations in the cancers.[3] A subset of the mutations, however, is responsible for "driving" the neoplastic process in the ducts and is the focus here.

Telomere abnormalities and signs of chromosome instability are the most common alterations in pancreatic neoplasia. Four genes are mutated in most pancreatic cancers: the *KRAS*, *p16/CDKN2A*, *TP53*, and *SMAD4* genes. Other genetic abnormalities are seen at a much lower frequency, including mutations in the genes *BRCA2*, *PALB2*, *FANCC*, *FANCG*, *FBXW7*, *BAX*, *RB1*, the TGFβ (transforming growth factor-beta) receptors *TGFBR1* and *TGFBR2*, the activin receptors *ACVR1B* and *ACVR2*, *MKK4*, *STK11*, *GUCY2F*, *NTRK3*, *EGFR*, and cationic trypsinogen, alterations in the mitochondrial genome, amplifications, various chromosomal deletions, inactivation of DNA mismatch-repair genes, and rarely the presence of the Epstein-Barr virus genome as an episome.

Knowing the genes mutated in a cancer can have direct clinical impact. For example, many cancers occur from an inherited mutation, and these patients and their families could benefit from genetic counseling.[4–7] A distinct morphologic subtype of pancreatic cancer, the medullary cancer, can suggest such an inherited mutation.[8,9] Another example includes the analysis of the genetic alterations in precursors to invasive pancreatic neoplasia, which has indicated that most carcinomas arise by a process of progressive intraductal tumorigenesis.[10] Epigenetic changes in DNA methylation and in gene expression are also highly specific for the cancerous cells and can serve as diagnostic markers.

COMMON MOLECULAR CHANGES

Telomere shortening is the earliest and most prevalent genetic change identified in the precursor lesions.[11] Telomere shortening is thought to predispose to chromosome fusion (translocations) and the mis-segregation of genetic material during mitosis.[12] Later during tumorigenesis, telomerase is reactivated,[13,14] moderating the telomere erosive process while permitting continued chromosomal instability.[15]

The *KRAS* gene mediates signals from growth factor receptors and other signaling inputs (Fig. 17.1). The mutations convert the normal Kras protein (a protooncogene) to an oncogene, causing the protein to become overactive in transmitting the growth factor-initiated signals.[16] *KRAS* is mutated in over 90% of conventional pancreatic

TABLE 17.1

GENETIC PROFILE OF PANCREATIC CARCINOMA

Gene	Gene Locations	Frequency in Cancers (%)	Timing During Tumorigenesis[a]	Mutation Origin
Oncogenes				
KRAS	12p	95	Early-mid	Som.
BRAF	7q	4		Som.
AKT2	19q	10–20		Som.
GUCY2F		3		Som.
NTRK3		1		Som.
EGFR		1		Som.
EBV genome		<1		
Tumor Suppressors/Genome-Maintenance Genes				
p16	9p	>90	Mid-late	Som. > Germ.
TP53	17p	75	Late	Som.
SMAD4	18q	55	Late	Som.
BRCA2/PALB2	13q/16p	8	Late	Germ. > Som.
FANCC/FANCG	9q/9p	3		Germ. or Som.
MAP2K4	17p	4		Som.
LKB1/STK11	19p	4		Som. > Germ.
ACVR1B	12q	2		Som.
TGFBR1	9q	1		Som.[b]
MSI⁻/TGFBR2	3p	1		Som.[b]
MSI⁺/TGFBR2	3p	4		Som. > Germ.[c]
ACVR2	2q	4		Som. > Germ. [c]
BAX	19q	4		Som. > Germ. [c]
MLH1	3p	4		Som. > Germ. [c]
FBXW7/Cyclin E dereg.	4q	6		Som.[d]
Tissue-Maintenance Genes				
PRSS1	7q	<1	Prior	Germ.

Som., (prevalence of) somatic mutation or methylation; Germ., (prevalence of) germ line mutation.
[a]Stage of appearance of the genetic changes during the intraductal precursor phase of the neoplasm, where known. For BRCA2, most mutations are inherited, but the loss of the second allele is reported only in a single advanced pancreatic intraepithelial neoplasm.
[b]Single examples of homozygous deletion of the TGFBR1 gene and TGFBR2 gene have been identified in MSI-negative pancreatic cancer.
[c]In MSI-positive tumors, the mismatch repair defect is usually somatic in origin; the TGFBR2, ACVR2, and BAX alterations are somatic.
[d]A single example of homozygous mutation of the FBXW7 gene is reported in a series having a 6% prevalence of cyclin E overexpression. Cyclin E amplification is reported to date only in cell lines.

ductal carcinomas.[17] The first genetic change in the ducts is probably not (or not always) a KRAS gene mutation, for the prevalence of this mutation is highest in the more advanced lesions (Table 17.1).[18,19] KRAS is one of a family of RAS genes that can harbor mutations in human cancers. The other RAS genes include NRAS and HRAS, although it is possible that only KRAS is mutated in pancreatic carcinomas.

As one of the most commonly mutated genes in pancreatic cancer, Ras is an attractive target for the development of gene-specific therapies, and an understanding of the normal biology of the Ras protein should help in the development of these Ras targeted therapies. The Ras proteins require an attachment to the plasma membrane for activity.

For many proteins, including Ras, a hydrophobic prenyl group is essential for the attachment. Either farnesyl (15-carbon) or geranylgeranyl (20-carbon) makes a covalent thioether linkage at a cysteine residue located near the C-terminal end of Ras proteins, termed the CAAX motif. Working mostly in artificial legacy models of the HRAS oncogene (rather than the more widely available but experimentally less tractable natural KRAS-mutant cancer cell lines), the farnesylation reaction was readily inhibited by various means; in these models, the Ras protein was rendered inactive and often accompanied by cytotoxicity limited to the mutant cells.

Although many types of compounds capable of blocking the farnesyltransferase enzyme were

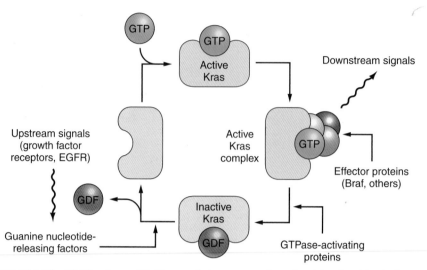

FIGURE 17.1 The *KRAS* pathway. *KRAS* normally integrates and regulates signals arising in the growth factor receptors that are passed to *KRAS* using the Grb2 and the Sos1 nucleotide exchange factor. The active GTP-bound form of *KRAS* recruits effector proteins such as Raf1 and Braf, in turn stimulating the downstream mitogen-activated protein kinases such as MEK and ERK and activating certain transcription factors. The EGF receptor can be overexpressed and occasionally mutated to provide inappropriately strong upstream signals, and the BRAF protein can be activated by point mutation, but more often in pancreatic cancer the Kras protein is mutated. These latter mutations impair the GAP (GTPase-activating protein)-stimulated reaction that normally returns Kras to the inactive state.

developed as drugs, they have not been successful anticancer agents. There are many reasons for this. Although Hras protein is linked predominantly through farnesyl groups, the Kras protein can be alternately prenylated by geranylgeranyl linkages. Unfortunately, the latter type of linkage is thought to be critical for a wider number of cellular proteins, and for fear of excessive toxicity, geranylgeranyl linkages have not usually been considered as an attractive drug target. Kras protein also appears to bind more tightly than Hras to the farnesyltransferase enzyme, requiring higher drug concentrations.[16] Additionally, the artificial models usually employed the engineered overexpression of the Ras protein, a situation in which the unattached Ras proteins would serve as a dominant-negative inhibitor, binding the necessary interacting proteins and sequestering them in the cytoplasm to ensure the inactivation of all three Ras pathways. Such a concentration-driven mechanism would presumably not occur under the normal levels of Ras proteins present in human cancers.[20] Indeed, it is proposed that the limited efficacy of farnesyltransferase inhibitors observed in some experimental models and in clinical trials may be attributable to a cellular target not yet identified.[21] Attention has turned to compounds that target the downstream mediators, such as Raf and Mek protein kinase inhibitors.

The Smad pathway mediates signals initiated on the binding of the extracellular proteins TGFβ

and activin to their receptors (Fig. 17.2). These signals are transmitted to the nucleus by the Smad family of related genes, including *SMAD4 (DPC4)*.[22] Smad protein complexes bind specific recognition sites on DNA and cause the transcription of certain genes.[23] Mutations in the *SMAD4* gene are found in nearly half of pancreatic carcinomas, including both homozygous deletions and intragenic mutations combined with loss of heterozygosity (LOH).[24] Other Smad genes are also mutated occasionally.[1]

Homozygous deletions and mutation/LOH affecting the *TGFβ* receptor genes are seen in a few pancreatic cancers.[25] A more common abnormality, in pancreatic as well as in other tumor types, is the underexpression of TGFβ receptors, which results in cellular resistance to the usual suppressive effects of the TGFβ ligand.[26]

The *p16/RB1* pathway is a key control of the cell division cycle (Fig. 17.3). The retinoblastoma protein (Rb1) is a transcriptional regulator and regulates the entry of cells into S phase. A complex of cyclin D and a cyclin-dependent kinase (Cdk4 and Cdk6) phosphorylates and thereby regulates Rb1. The p16 protein is a Cdk-inhibitor that binds Cdk4 and Cdk6.[27–29] Virtually all pancreatic carcinomas suffer a loss of *p16* function, through homozygous deletions, mutation/LOH, or promoter methylation of the *p16/CDKN2A* gene associated with a lack of gene expression.[30,31] In addition, inherited mutations of the *p16/CDKN2A* gene cause a familial melanoma/pancreatic cancer

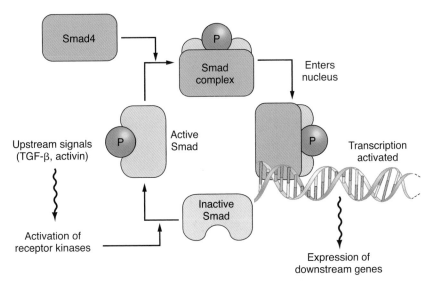

FIGURE 17.2 The transforming growth factor-beta (TGFβ)/Activin/Smad pathway. Dimeric kinase receptors of the TGFβ superfamily respond to extracellular ligands, causing phosphorylation of one or more of the receptor-associated Smad proteins and leading them to complex with the unphosphorylated common Smad, Smad4. This complex binds to specific DNA sequences and works with other transcription factors to stimulate gene expression. Mutations in pancreatic cancer can inactivate either partner of the dimeric receptors that respond to extracellular TGFβ or activin. More commonly, however, mutations and large deletions in the *SMAD4* gene destabilize its protein product or ablate gene expression.

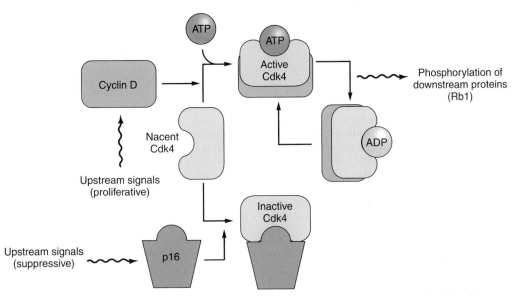

FIGURE 17.3 The *p16/RB1* pathway. *p16* binds to, inhibits, and thereby controls the availability of the cyclin-dependent kinases Cdk4 and Cdk6 (not shown). When activated by binding to cyclin D, these kinases phosphorylate and thereby inactivate the Rb1 tumor suppressor protein. The activity of *p16* is controlled in a complex manner, through changes in gene expression and by displacement reactions involving other similar kinase inhibitor proteins. *p16* mutations and deletions are nearly ubiquitous in pancreatic cancer, resulting in dysregulation of these cyclin-dependent kinases that regulate the cell division cycle.

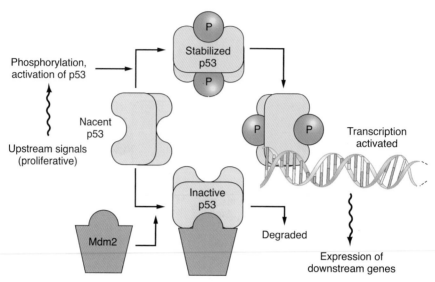

FIGURE 17.4 The *p53* pathway. Many modes of control affect *p53* activity, one of which is shown in the diagram. Stresses such as DNA damage result in phosphorylation of *p53*, preventing its degradation by an Mdm2-directed pathway. When stabilized, *p53* binds to specific DNA sequences and activates the transcription of many genes, including Mdm2 as part of a negative feedback loop. When *p53* is mutated, it fails to bind effectively to DNA to activate transcription. Because Mdm2 then lacks its transcriptional stimulus from *p53*, mutant but inactive p53 proteins are usually expressed at very high levels.

syndrome known as familial atypical multiple mole melanoma.[32–36] Occasional pancreatic cancers have inactivating mutations of the *RB1* gene.[37]

The protein product of the *TP53* gene binds to specific sites of DNA and activates the transcription of certain genes that control the cell division cycle and apoptosis.[38,39] Tp53 protein, normally a short-lived protein, becomes phosphorylated and stabilized after DNA damage and other cellular stresses (Fig. 17.4). In about 75% of pancreatic cancers the *TP53* gene has point mutations that inhibit the ability of p53 to bind DNA, or occasionally other types of inactivating mutation.[40–42]

Most human carcinomas have chromosomal instability (CIN), which produces changes in chromosomal copy numbers or aneuploidy.[43] Most pancreatic cancers have complex karyotypes including deletions of whole chromosomes and subchromosomal regions.[44–46] CIN is the process that causes most of the tumor deletions (LOH).[47] A few percent of pancreatic carcinomas, however, do not have significant gross or numerical chromosomal changes and instead have a different form of genetic instability; they have defects in DNA mismatch repair, producing high mutation rates at sites of simple repetitive sequences termed *microsatellites*.[8,9,48–51] The pattern of genetic damage in these carcinomas differs considerably from the pattern in carcinomas with CIN. The type II TGFβ and activin receptors (*TGFBR2*) and (*ACVR2*), as well as the *BAX* gene have a repetitive sequence within their coding regions, and biallelic inactivating mutations of

these sequences are seen in many microsatellite instability (MIN) pancreatic cancers.[25,51–54]

There are also alterations in pancreatic carcinomas, some probably being important to tumorigenesis, that are not attributed to genetic mutations. These include expression of telomerase,[13,14] underexpression of TGFβ receptors,[26] overexpression of the growth-stimulating HER2/neu cell surface receptor,[55–58] a constitutive elevation of RelA and hedgehog pathway activities.[55,56] Some of these activities are proposed to be attractive as therapeutic targets, although supportive clinical evidence is not yet available. Pancreatic carcinomas also have reproducible alterations in gene expression, such as overexpression of the proteins mesothelin and prostate stem cell antigen that currently can serve as diagnostic aids in the histopathologic interpretation of biopsies and surgical resections.[57–59] The epigenetic patterns of gene hypermethylation in pancreatic cancers are considered promising for developing additional diagnostic markers for analysis of pancreatic secretions and for noninvasive diagnostic screening.[59]

The dominating genetic patterns previously described are altered among other diagnostic categories of pancreatic neoplasia. The precursor lesions, termed *PanIN* (pancreatic intraepithelial neoplasia), in their most advanced stage, closely resemble the genetic patterns of the conventional invasive ductal carcinomas. The intraductal papillary mucinous neoplasms, the mucinous cystic neoplasms, acinar cell carcinomas, neuroendocrine carcinomas, pancreatoblastomas, and solid pseudopapillary neoplasms, however, diverge significantly from the patterns of PanINs and typical invasive ductal carcinomas. Notable differences are the *PIK3CA* mutations present in some intraductal papillary mucinous neoplasms and the colloid carcinomas that can derive from them,[60] the *CTNNB1* (beta-catenin) mutations present in virtually all solid pseudopapillary neoplasms[61] and pancreatoblastomas,[62] and the *MEN1* mutations in many neuroendocrine neoplasms.[63]

LOW-FREQUENCY GENETIC CHANGES

The causative genes of *Fanconi anemia* play a role in human tumorigenesis. The *BRCA2* gene represents Fanconi complementation group D1 and is thought to aid DNA strand repair.[64] Because of this function, it is perhaps best to categorize *BRCA2* as a genome-maintenance gene rather than a standard tumor suppressor. As much as 7% of apparently "sporadic" pancreatic cancers (more, in instances of familial aggregation) harbor an inactivating intragenic inherited mutation of one copy of the *BRCA2* gene, accompanied by LOH.[1,2,66] The *PALB2* gene represents Fanconi group N, and its protein product functions by binding the Brca2 protein.[65] Three percent of familial pancreatic cancers had a germ line inactivating mutation of *PALB2*, and in a tumor studied in depth, the other copy was inactivated by a somatic mutation,[1,66,67] The *FANCC* and *FANCG* genes have somatic or germ line mutations in some pancreatic cancer patients, again with loss of the wild type allele in the cancer.[68] The known hypersensitivity of Fanconi cells to interstrand DNA-crosslinking agents, such as cisplatin, melphalan, and mitomycin C, has led to the hypothesis that pancreatic cancers with Fanconi pathway genetic defects should be especially susceptible to treatment with such agents.[69–72] Occasional complete remissions of pancreatic cancer have been reported with therapies that included DNA cross-linkers,[73–77] and there are recent reports of prolonged responses using such agents in patients having *BRCA2* mutations.[78,79] Cells made experimentally deficient for Fanconi genes are also hypersensitive to certain nongenotoxic compounds,[80] and patients having *BRCA2*-mutant cancers other than pancreatic cancer are reported to respond to therapeutic drug inhibition of the poly (ADP-ribose) polymerase enzyme, which normally becomes activated to facilitate DNA strand repair.[81] These opportunities are beginning to be explored clinically in pancreatic cancer.

BRCA1 gene mutations are not found in unselected pancreatic cancers or pancreatic cancer families.[82] Nonetheless, pancreatic cancers do occur in carriers of *BRCA1* inactivating mutations.[83,84] In these persons, the relatively high rate of LOH affecting the other *BRCA1* copy indicates that a loss of *BRCA1* function likely plays a role in tumorigenesis within these patients.[83]

The *mitochondrial genome* is mutated in a majority of pancreatic cancers.[85–87] These mutations most likely represent genetic drift, and perhaps do not directly contribute to the process of tumorigenesis.[87] Such mutations, however, could potentially serve as a diagnostic target because of the large number of copies of the mitochondrial genome in human carcinoma cells.[86,87]

The *MAP2K4* (*MKK4*) gene participates in a stress-activated protein kinase pathway.[81,82] It is stimulated by various influences, including chemotherapy, and its downstream effects include apoptosis and cellular differentiation. The *MKK4* gene is inactivated by homozygous deletions or mutation/LOH in about 4% of pancreatic cancers.[88,89] Experimental loss of one or both copies of the *MKK4* gene in cancer cells reduces Jun kinase activation and JUN expression; this is a rare example of a tumor-suppressor pathway affected by gene dosage. Such gene dose-dependent effects could rationalize the high rate of loss of chromosomal arm 17p affecting 90% of pancreatic cancers and more than half of the *TP53*-wild type cancers.[90]

Germ line mutations of the *STK11* (*LKB1*) gene, a serine-threonine kinase, are responsible for the Peutz-Jeghers syndrome (PJS).[91,92] PJS was anecdotally associated with pancreatic cancer.[93] A follow-up study examined lifetime risk, finding nearly a third of PJS patients to develop pancreatic cancer.[94] Sporadic pancreatic cancers, independent of PJS, also lose the gene by homozygous deletion or by somatic mutation/LOH in about 4% of cases.[95]

Kinase oncogenes are mutated at low frequency, including the *GUCY2F*, *EGFR*, and *NTRK3* genes.[91,92] This class of mutations is important in that these mutations can be targeted with antikinase drugs.[93]

Gene amplification also occurs in pancreatic cancer. Amplified regions include the *AKT2* gene within an amplicon on chromosome 19q, involving about 10% to 20% of cases studied.[94–96] About 6% of pancreatic cancers overexpress the oncogene, *CCNE1* (cyclin E). Two mechanisms have been demonstrated, cyclin E gene amplification and the genetic inactivation of the *FBXW7* (*AGO*) gene, which normally serves to degrade cyclin E during the normal phases of the cell division cycle.[1,96]

The patterns of *chromosomal deletion* in pancreatic cancer are complex. In one study, from 1.5% to 32% of all tested loci, in different cancers, had a deletion.[97] For most lost regions, we know of no particular tumor-suppressor genes targeted by the deletions. Conversely, in some regions known to harbor tumor-suppressor genes, the known mutated genes do not justify the high observed prevalence rates of LOH unless gene dose-dependent effects are postulated (90). Individual homozygous deletions are found at some additional genetic locations, again without a definitive target gene yet identified for most of these events.[98]

Defects in DNA mismatch repair (MIN) are seen in some pancreatic cancers. These cancers typically have a medullary histologic phenotype[8] and mutations of the type II TGFβ (*TGFBR2*) and activin (*ACVR2*) receptor genes.[25,52,53] They can also have mutations of the proapoptotic *BAX* gene[51] and of the growth factor pathway mediator *BRAF* gene (affecting the same pathway, presumably, as mutations of the *KRAS* gene).[8,9,51,96] The MIN tumors do not have the propensity for large chromosomal alterations and gross aneuploidy.[15,99] In a study of four cases of pancreatic cancers having MIN, all lacked expression of the Mlh1 protein.[9] Not all cancers with a medullary phenotype have MIN. Yet, medullary pancreatic carcinomas as a whole have a number of clinical and genetic differences as compared to those with conventional histologic appearance; the carcinomas have pushing rather than infiltrative borders, the *KRAS* gene often is wild type, and there is often a family history of malignancy.[5,6,47] A reported case of *Epstein-Barr virus (EBV)*–associated pancreatic cancer[9] had a medullary phenotype with heavy lymphocytic infiltration. Because of its distinctive features, it is advisable to separately designate the medullary category in the reporting of all clinical, genetic, and pathologic studies of pancreatic cancer.

Inherited mutations of the *cationic trypsinogen* (*PRSS1*) gene prevent the inactivation of prematurely activated trypsin within the ducts, causing a familial form of severe early-onset acute pancreatitis.[100] Some affected kindred have a cumulative risk of pancreatic cancer that approaches 40% by the time the affected individuals reach 60 years of age.[101] This cancer diathesis falls in a unique category of cancer susceptibility, in that the predisposition emanates from genetic alterations of a tissue-maintenance gene, one that is neither an oncogene, a tumor- suppressor gene, nor a genome-maintenance gene.

In summary, pancreatic cancer is fundamentally a genetic disease. An understanding of the genes altered in pancreatic cancer has led to a better understanding of the familial aggregation of pancreatic cancer, and, it is hoped, will lead to novel gene-specific targeted therapies for this deadly form of cancer.

Selected References

The full list of references for this chapter appears in the online version.

1. Jones S, Zhang X, Parsons DW, et al. Core signaling pathways in human pancreatic cancers revealed by global genomic analyses. *Science* 2008;321:1801.
4. Goggins M, Schutte M, Lu J, et al. Germline *BRCA2* gene mutations in patients with apparently sporadic pancreatic carcinomas. *Cancer Res* 1996;56:5360.
6. Murphy KM, Brune KA, Griffin C, et al. Evaluation of candidate genes MAP2K4, MADH4, ACVR1B, and BRCA2 in familial pancreatic cancer: deleterious BRCA2 mutations in 17%. *Cancer Res* 2002;62:3789.
8. Goggins M, Offerhaus GJA, Hilgers W, et al. Adenocarcinomas of the pancreas with DNA replication errors (RER+) are associated with apparently wild-type K-ras and characteristic histopathology: poor differentiation, a syncytial growth pattern, and pushing borders suggest RER+. *Am J Pathol* 1998;152:1501.
10. Hruban RH, Wilentz R, Kern SE. Genetic progression in the pancreatic ducts. *Am J Pathol* 2000;156:1821.
13. Hiyama E, Kodama T, Shinbara K, et al. Telomerase activity is detected in pancreatic cancer but not in benign tumors. *Cancer Res* 1997;57:326.
17. Almoguera C, Shibata D, Forrester K, et al. Most human carcinomas of the exocrine pancreas contain mutant c-K-ras genes. *Cell* 1988;53:549.
18. Caldas C, Hahn SA, Hruban RH, et al. Detection of K-ras mutations in the stool of patients with pancreatic adenocarcinoma and pancreatic ductal hyperplasia. *Cancer Res* 1994;54:3568.
24. Hahn SA, Schutte M, Hoque ATMS, et al. DPC4, a candidate tumor-suppressor gene at 18q21.1. *Science* 1996;271:350.
26. Baldwin RL, Friess H, Yokoyama M, et al. Attenuated ALK5 receptor expression in human pancreatic cancer: correlation with resistance to growth inhibition. *Int J Cancer* 1996;67:283.
30. Caldas C, Hahn SA, da Costa LT, et al. Frequent somatic mutations and homozygous deletions of the p16 (MTS1) gene in pancreatic adenocarcinoma. *Nature Genetics* 1994;8:27.
34. Whelan AJ, Bartsch D, Goodfellow PJ. Brief report: a familial syndrome of pancreatic cancer and melanoma with a mutation in the CDKN2 tumor-suppressor gene. *N Engl J Med* 1995;333:975.
41. Redston MS, Caldas C, Seymour AB, et al. p53 mutations in pancreatic carcinoma and evidence of common involvement of homocopolymer tracts in DNA microdeletions. *Cancer Res* 1994;54:3025.
47. Hahn SA, Seymour AB, Hoque ATMS, et al. Allelotype of pancreatic adenocarcinoma using a xenograft model. *Cancer Res* 1995;55:4670.
48. Ionov Y, Peinado MA, Malkhosyan S, et al. Ubiquitous somatic mutations in simple repeated sequences reveal a new mechanism for colonic carcinogenesis. *Nature* 1993;363:558.
66. Jones S, Hruban RH, Kamiyama M, et al. Exomic sequencing identifies PALB2 as a pancreatic cancer susceptibility gene. *Science* 2009;324:217.
81. Fong PC, Boss DS, Yap TA, et al. Inhibition of poly(ADP-ribose) polymerase in tumors from BRCA mutation carriers. *N Engl J Med* 2009;361:123.
83. Al-Sukhni W, Rothenmund H, Borgida AE, et al. Germline BRCA1 mutations predispose to pancreatic adenocarcinoma. *Hum Genet* 2008;124:271.
88. Su GH, Hilgers W, Shekher M, et al. Alterations in pancreatic, biliary, and breast carcinomas support MKK4 as a genetically targeted tumor-suppressor gene. *Cancer Res* 1998;58:2339.
94. Giardiello FM, Brensinger JD, Tersmette AC, et al. Very high risk of cancer in familial Peutz-Jeghers syndrome. *Gastroenterology* 2000;119:1447.
95. Su GH, Hruban RH, Bova GS, et al. Germline and somatic mutations of the STK11/LKB1 Peutz-Jeghers gene in pancreatic and biliary cancers. *Am J Pathol* 1999;154:1835.
101. Lowenfels AB, Maisonneuve P, DiMagno EP, et al. Hereditary pancreatitis and the risk of pancreatic cancer. International Hereditary Pancreatitis Study Group. *J Natl Cancer Inst* 1997;89:442.

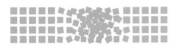

CHAPTER 18 LIVER CANCER

SNORRI S. THORGEIRSSON AND JOE W. GRISHAM

Hepatocellular carcinoma (HCC) is one of the most common cancers worldwide, accounting for at least 600,000 deaths annually.[1] Although most frequent in southeast Asia and sub-Sahara Africa, the incidence and mortality rates of HCC have doubled in the United States and Europe in the past four decades and are expected to double again during the next 10 to 20 years.[2] As the incidence of HCC has increased, the age distribution of HCC has shifted toward relatively younger ages.[2] These observations make it clear that liver cancer is a major heath problem in the United States and Europe.

The etiologic agents responsible for the majority of HCC are known (e.g., infections with hepatitis B and C viruses [HBV and HCV], ethanol abuse), and additional causes are being identified (e.g., obesity, type 2 diabetes, nonalcoholic fatty liver disease).[3] Furthermore, the liver diseases that are associated with increased risk of HCC and the cellular alterations that precede HCC have been identified.[4–6] Research into the molecular pathogenesis of HCC currently focuses on the interrelationship of abnormal genomics and consequent alterations in molecular signaling pathways. Implicit in this research is the goal to integrate new data with clinicopathologic aspects of HCC in order to uncover new diagnostic, treatment, and prevention strategies.

Recent introduction of DNA microarray-based technologies makes it possible to measure simultaneously the expression of tens of thousands of genes in a tissue under a variety of conditions (reviewed in ref. 7). High-throughput microarray-based technologies and the recent advent of the next generation of whole genome DNA sequencers offer a unique opportunity to define the descriptive characteristics (i.e., "phenotype") of a biological system in terms of the genomic readout (e.g., gene expression, coding mutations, insertions and deletions in DNA, copy number variations and chromosomal translocations). Integrated views of biological systems have caused a paradigm shift in biological research methods, that is, from classic reductionism to systems biology.[8] Fundamental to the systems approach to the study of diseased biological systems is the hypothesis that disease processes are driven by aberrant regulatory networks of genes and proteins that differ from the normal counterparts. Application of multiparametric measurements promises to transform current approaches to diagnosis and therapy, providing the foundation for predictive and preventive personalized medicine.[8]

In this chapter we discuss the application of high-throughput genomic technologies to characterize HCC.

ALLELIC IMBALANCE IN LIVER CANCER

Chromosomal aberrations in tumors are regarded traditionally as evidence of gene deregulation and genome instability, and their detection may facilitate the identification of crucial genes and regulatory pathways that are perturbed in diseases. Several powerful analytical tools are currently available for analyzing chromosomal aberrations (reviewed in ref. 9). Comparative genomic hybridization (CGH), in particular array CGH, enables high-throughput analysis of DNA copy number and yields comprehensive information applicable to determining the molecular pathogenesis of human HCC. Meta-analysis of CGH studies of chromosome aberrations in human HCC shows that specific chromosomal gains and losses correlate with etiology and histologic grade (Table 18.1).[10] In HCC the most frequent amplifications of genomic material involve 1q (57.1%), 8q (46.6%), 6p (22.3%), and 17q (22.2%), whereas losses are most common in 8p (38%), 16q (35.9%), 4q (34.3%), 17p (32.1%), and 13q (26.2%). Deletions of 4q, 16q, 13q, and 8p correlate with HBV infection and lack of HCV infection. Chromosomes 13q and 4q are significantly underrepresented in poorly differentiated HCC, and gains of 1q correlate with other high-frequency alterations.[11] Amplifications and deletions often occur on chromosome arms at sites of oncogenes (e.g., *MYC* on 8q24) and tumor suppressor genes (e.g., *RB1* on 13q14), as well as at several loci that contain genes with known and/

MOLECULAR BIOLOGY OF INDIVIDUAL CANCERS

TABLE 18.1

FREQUENCIES IN CHROMOSOMAL ABERRATION IN HUMAN HEPATOCELLULAR CARCINOMA[a]

Chromosome	p-Arm Loss (%)	Gain (%)	High Frequency	Genes	q-Arm Loss (%)	Gain (%)	High Frequency	Genes
1	15.4	5.2	—	—	0.6	**57.1**	q21.1–q44	WNT14, FASL
2	1.4	7.1	—	—	2.9	8	—	—
3	3.9	5	—	—	1.9	8.8	—	—
4	10.6	6	—	—	**34.3**	1.7	q21.1–q35	LEF1, CCNA
5	1.7	13.6	—	—	7.8	11.1	—	—
6	1	**22.3**	—	PIM1, CDKN1A	15	7.9	—	—
7	0.9	15	—	—	3.1	16.8	—	—
8	**38**	4.6	p21.1–p22	FZD3, PLK3	1.9	**46.6**	q22.1–q24.3	MYC, WISP1
9	14	3.3	—	—	11.1	2.9	—	—
10	2.7	8.3	—	—	11.1	4.1	—	—
11	5.4	4.3	—	—	10.2	9.4	—	—
12	6.5	2.4	—	—	2.9	6.9	—	—
13	0	0	—	—	**26.2**	7.4	q14.1–q22	RB1, BRCA3
14	0	0	—	—	11.3	4.1	—	—
15	0	0	—	—	5.4	4.6	—	—
16	16.8	3.4	—	—	**35.9**	1.8	q12.1–q24	SIAH1, CDH1
17	**32.1**	2.9	p13	p53, HIC1	3.7	**22.2**	q23–q25	AXIN2, TIMP2
18	4.1	5.5	—	—	10.8	5	—	—
19	6.9	5	—	—	3.8	10.4	—	—
20	2	14.9	—	—	0.9	18.6	—	—
21	0	0	—	—	8.8	2.2	—	—
22	0	0	—	—	6.4	2.8	—	—
X	5	11.2	—	—	4.5	15	—	—
Y	5.1	2.3	—	—	5.6	2.3	—	—

[a]Summary of 785 different comparative genomic hybridization analyses of human hepatocellular carcinoma. Frequencies more than 20% are highlighted in bold. Region of highest frequency of imbalance on respective chromosomal arms are highlighted in bold. Examples of known tumor-relevant genes located on respective chromosomal high-frequency region are shown.
(Modified from ref. 10, with permission.)

or suspected oncogenic functions (e.g., FZD3, WISP1, SIAH-1, and AXIN2, all of which modulate the WNT signaling pathway). In this metaanalysis, etiology and poor differentiation of HCC correlated with specific genomic alterations. In preneoplastic dysplastic nodules (DNs), amplifications are most frequent in 1q and 8q, whereas deletions occur in 8p, 17p, 5p, 13q, 14q, and 16q.[11] Gain of 1q appears to be an early event developing in DN, possibly predisposing affected cells to acquire additional chromosomal aberrations.

Bioinformatic analysis of CGH data was recently used to develop a progression model for human HCC.[11] Based on an evolutionary tree constructed from statistically significant CGH events, three subgroups of patients with different patterns of HCC progression were identified. The subgroups reflect the extent of tumor progression as indicated by the number of chromosomal aberrations, tumor stage, tumor size, and disease outcome. Gains of 1q21-23 and 8q22-24 appear to be early genomic events in development of HCC and gain of 3q22-24 a late genomic event, the latter associated with tumor recurrence and poor survival. The HCC progression model uncovered chromosomal imbalances associated with clinical pathologic characteristics of the disease and explained a significant part of the variations in clinical outcome among the HCC patients.[11]

These two studies illustrate the power of CGH analysis to identify the functional significance of genomic alterations in human HCC. Nevertheless, because CGH only analyzes genomic DNA, additional studies are required to measure and integrate data on global gene expression to confirm the roles of candidate genes. This can be accomplished by adapting the expression imbalance map method and array CGH analysis (reviewed in ref. 12). This approach was recently applied to human HCC.[13] Using regional pattern recognition approaches, the authors discovered the most probable copy number-dependent regions and 50 potential driver genes (Table 18.2). At each step of the gene selection process, the functional relevance of the selected genes was evaluated by estimating the prognostic significance of the selected genes. Further validation using small interference RNA-mediated knockdown experiments showed proof-of-principle evidence for the potential driver roles of the genes in HCC progression (i.e., *NCSTN* and *SCRIB*). In addition, systemic prediction of drug responses implicated the association of the 50 genes with specific signaling molecules (*mTOR*, *AMPK*, and *EGFR*). It was concluded that the application of an unbiased and integrative analysis of multidimensional genomic data sets can effectively screen for potential driver genes and provides novel mechanistic and clinical insights into the pathobiology of HCC.

It seems inevitable that new and improved array designs for both CGH and gene expression and the advent of whole genome sequencing combined with better software for statistical analysis of the data will continue to emerge.

CLASSIFICATION AND PROGNOSTIC PREDICTION OF HEPATOCELLULAR CARCINOMA

The application of microarray technologies to characterize tumors on the basis of global gene expression has had a significant impact on both basic and clinical oncology.[7] The goal of tumor microarray studies generally includes discovery of subsets of tumors (class discovery), which enables diagnostic classification (class comparison), prediction of clinical outcome (class prediction), and mechanistic analysis. Verification and validation of the primary results are essential for discovery of oncogenic pathways and identification of therapeutic targets (for technical details on microarray analysis see Chapter 2 and ref. 7). Analysis of global gene expression in selected tumors has successfully classified them into homogeneous groups and predicted the clinical outcome and survival (reviewed in ref. 7).

The goal of all staging systems is to separate patients into homogeneous prognostic groups to permit the selection of the most appropriate therapy for each group. Although much work has been devoted to establishment of prognostic models for HCC by using clinical information and pathologic classification,[6] many issues still remain unresolved. For example, a staging system that reliably separates patients into homogeneous early and intermediate-to-advanced HCC groups

with respect to prognosis does not exist. This is of particular importance because the natural course of early HCC is unknown, and the natural progression of intermediate and advanced HCC is known to be quite variable.[6] Because the accuracy of imaging techniques is rapidly evolving and affording detection of early HCC,[14] the inability to predict the prognosis of these early lesions poses a therapeutic dilemma. Although the accurate pathologic diagnosis of high-grade DNs and early HCC is currently difficult, it is likely that many HCC evolve from DN.[15]

A new insight on the transition of DN into early HCC was recently obtained.[16] A gene expression profiling on cirrhotic (regenerative) and DNs as well as early HCC was performed, and 460 differentially expressed genes were detected between DN and early HCC. Functional analysis of the significant gene set identified the *MYC* oncogene as a plausible driver gene for malignant conversion of the dysplastic nodules. In addition, gene set enrichment analysis revealed global activation of the *MYC* up-regulated gene set in early HCC versus dysplasia. Presence of the *MYC* signature significantly correlated with increased expression of *CSN5* gene as well as with higher overall transcription rate of genes located in the 8q chromosome region. Furthermore, a classifier constructed from *MYC* target genes could robustly discriminate early HCC from high- and low-grade DNs. Importantly, this study identified unique expression patterns associated with the transition of high-grade DNs into early HCC and demonstrated that activation of the *MYC* transcription signature is strongly associated with the malignant conversion of pre-neoplastic liver lesions.

Many studies on HCC gene expression profiling, as well as several reviews, have appeared during the last 5 years.[17] Interpretation of molecular profiling studies of HCC poses more challenges than other human tumors, mainly because of the complex pathogenesis of this cancer.[5] HCC arises in diverse settings ranging from infection with HBV or HCV, to chronic metabolic diseases as varied as diabetes, nonalcoholic fatty liver disease, and hemochromatosis. These different diseases represent complex assortments of genetic and epigenetic aberrations as well as altered molecular pathways.[5,6] Nevertheless, because of its extraordinary power of resolution, global gene expression profiling currently offers the most appropriate technology to resolve the complex molecular pathogenesis of HCC. Indeed, gene expression profiling of HCC has already generated impressive data sets that represent a remarkable progress toward the elucidation of the molecular pathogenesis of HCC, and may ultimately improve diagnosis and outcome prognosis for HCC patients.[17]

A class discovery approach applying hierarchical clustering of gene expression data from human HCC[18] revealed two subclasses of HCC that are strongly associated with survival of the

TABLE 18.2

LIST OF 50 POTENTIAL DRIVER GENES[a]

Chr.	Cytoband	Gene Symbol	Correlation Coefficient	Correlation P-value	Copy Numbers	mRNA (Mean)	Chr.	Cytoband	Gene Symbol	Correlation Coefficient	Correlation P-value	Copy Numbers	mRNA (Mean)
chr1	q21.3	C1orf43	0.693	4.17E-03	0.366	0.324	chr8	q22.2	POLR2K	0.706	3.25E-03	0.291	0.805
chr1	q21.3	HAX1	0.668	6.47E-03	0.314	0.083	chr8	q22.3	NCALD	0.712	9.42E-03	0.086	0.204
chr1	q21.3	ADAR	0.803	3.14E-04	0.187	0.546	chr8	q22.3	RRM2B	0.788	8.23E-04	0.182	0.198
chr1	q22	CCT3	0.724	2.28E-03	0.313	1.084	chr8	q22.3	AZIN1	0.805	2.94E-04	0.205	0.271
chr1	q23.1	CD1C	0.716	2.70E-03	0.164	-0.432	chr8	q24.12	TAF2	0.659	7.56E-03	0.159	0.556
chr1	q23.2	NCSTN	0.668	6.48E-03	0.147	0.486	chr8	q24.13	DERL1	0.754	1.15E-03	0.209	0.224
chr1	q31.3	CFHR2	0.733	1.88E-03	0.106	-1.513	chr8	q24.13	ZHX1	0.672	8.49E-03	0.193	-0.08
chr1	q42.12	PYCR2	0.795	1.17E-03	0.201	0.751	chr8	q24.13	TATDN1	0.814	3.92E-04	0.229	0.654
chr6	p21.31	C6orf107	0.655	8.04E-03	0.198	0.075	chr8	q24.13	NDUFB9	0.754	1.15E-03	0.152	0.466
chr6	q16.3	CCNC	0.737	2.61E-03	-0.046	-0.315	chr8	q24.13	KIAA0196	0.678	5.46E-03	0.136	0.414
chr6	q22.31	MAN1A1	0.668	6.49E-03	-0.146	-1.293	chr8	q24.3	TSTA3	0.68	5.25E-03	0.153	0.401
chr6	q22.31	SERINC1	0.678	5.48E-03	-0.156	-0.825	chr8	q24.3	SCRIB	0.717	2.64E-03	0.163	1.102
chr7	q22.1	EPHB4	0.743	5.65E-03	0.286	0.189	chr8	q24.3	HSF1	0.654	8.12E-03	0.129	0.736
chr7	q22.1	CUTL1	0.73	1.99E-03	0.275	0.081	chr8	q24.3	KIFC2	0.677	7.76E-03	0.218	0.141
chr8	p22	PCM1	0.649	8.82E-03	-0.23	-0.225	chr16	q23.1	KARS	0.899	5.16E-06	0.012	0.072
chr8	p21.1	ELP3	0.745	2.23E-03	-0.204	-0.122	chr19	p13.12	ILVBL	0.914	1.86E-06	0.167	-0.253
chr8	p21.1	HMBOX1	0.771	7.57E-04	-0.204	-0.055	chr19	p13.12	BRD4	0.769	2.13E-03	0.163	0.209
chr8	q21.13	MRPS28	0.771	7.75E-04	0.087	-0.072	chr19	p13.12	WIZ	0.739	1.64E-03	0.163	0.463
chr8	q22.1	KIAA1429	0.699	3.76E-03	0.206	0.332	chr19	p13.12	CYP4F11	0.68	5.24E-03	0.109	-0.891
chr8	q22.1	UQCRB	0.676	5.67E-03	0.096	0.628	chr19	p13.12	RAB8A	0.722	2.38E-03	0.289	-0.081
chr8	q22.1	PTDSS1	0.818	1.96E-04	0.154	0.365	chr19	p13.11	FAM32A	0.769	8.09E-04	0.346	0.15
chr8	q22.1	PGCP	0.666	6.74E-03	0.041	0.388	chr19	p13.11	C19orf42	0.735	6.49E-03	0.3	0.366
chr8	q22.1	MTDH	0.669	6.37E-03	0.245	0.282	chr19	p13.11	MYO9B	0.825	1.75E-03	0.291	0.096
chr8	q22.2	STK3	0.686	4.78E-03	0.096	0.184	chr19	q12	CCNE1	0.76	1.62E-03	0.363	0.174
chr8	q22.2	COX6C	0.799	3.54E-04	0.172	0.508	chr19	q12	C19orf2	0.791	4.45E-04	0.069	0.437

[a]See ref. 13 for details.

patient. In this study, several independent prediction algorithms determined whether gene expression patterns could be used to predict survival. HCC patients were randomly divided into two equal groups, that is, a training set that was used to develop the HCC classifiers and a validation set that was used to evaluate the test. All the classifiers successfully separated patients with shorter survival from patients who survived longer. Gene expression patterns strongly associated with patient survival, and the reproducibility of these gene expression-based predictors, were robust. Moreover, application of a Cox regression model identified genes whose expression was highly correlated with the length of survival. Survival-associated genes could also be used for highly accurate subclass prediction without the application of sophisticated prediction models. The knowledge-based annotation of the survival genes provided insight into the underlying biological differences between the two subclasses of HCC.[18] Among several biological groups of the survival genes, the cell-proliferation group was the best predictor of an unfavorable outcome of the disease. Expression of proliferating cell nuclear antigen, a typical cell-proliferation marker, and cell cycle regulators such as *CDK4*, *CCNB1*, *CCNA2*, and *CKS2* was greater in the poor survival subclass (cluster A). Not surprisingly, many genes that were more highly expressed in the poor survival subclass had antiapoptotic functions. Higher expression of genes involved in ubiquitination and sumoylation also characterized the poor survival subclass. Enhanced activation of ubiquitin-dependent protein degradation may account for deregulation of cell cycle control and faster cell proliferation in the poor survival subclass. This study demonstrates that gene expression profiling can identify previously unrecognized, clinically relevant subclasses of HCC in a robust and reproducible manner.

Using a similar approach, Boyault et al.[19] further refined the transcriptome classification of HCC. Unsupervised transcriptome analysis identified six robust subgroups of HCC (G1-G6) associated with clinical and genetic characteristics of the tumors. G1 tumors had low HBV copy number and overexpressed genes controlled by parental imprinting in fetal liver. G2 tumors included HCC infected with a high copy number of HBV and mutations in *PIK3CA* and *TP53*. Specific activation of the AKT pathway was detected in both groups. G3 tumors were characterized by *TP53* mutations and overexpression of genes controlling the cell cycle. G4 was a heterogeneous subgroup of tumors that included both HCC and hepatocellular adenomas with *TCF1* mutations. G5 and G6 tumors contained β-catenin mutations that activate the WNT pathway. These results emphasize the genetic diversity of human HCC and provide specific identifiers for classifying the tumors. Also, this new classification shows that WNT and AKT pathways are activated in about 50% of the tumors, suggesting attractive potential therapeutic targets. Most recently Hoshida et al.[20] performed a meta-analysis of gene expression profiles in data sets from eight independent patient cohorts across the world. A total of 603 patients were analyzed, representing the major etiologies of HCC (hepatitis B and C) collected from Western and Eastern countries. Three robust HCC subclasses (termed S1, S2, and S3) were observed, each correlated with clinical parameters such as tumor size, extent of cellular differentiation, and serum alpha-fetoprotein levels. An analysis of the components of the signatures indicated that S1 reflected aberrant activation of the WNT signaling pathway, S2 was characterized by proliferation as well as MYC and AKT activation, and S3 was associated with hepatocyte differentiation. Functional studies indicated that the WNT pathway activation signature characteristic of S1 tumors was not simply the result of β-catenin mutation but rather was the result of transforming growth factor-β activation, thus representing a new mechanism of WNT pathway activation in HCC. These experiments establish the first attempt to develop consensus classification framework for HCC based on gene expression profiles and highlight the power of integrating multiple data sets to define a robust molecular taxonomy of the disease.

The transcriptomic analyses have also been used to address lineage heterogeneity of HCC. The two major adult liver cancers are HCC and cholangiocarcinoma (CC). The existence of combined hepatocellular-cholangiocarcinoma (CHC), a histopathologic intermediate form between HCC and CC, suggests phenotypic overlap between these tumors. Woo et al.[21] applied an integrative oncogenomic approach to address the clinical and functional implications of the overlapping phenotype between these tumors. By performing gene expression profiling of human HCC, CHC, and CC, the authors identified a novel HCC subtype, that is, cholangiocarcinoma-like HCC (CLHCC), which expressed cholangiocarcinoma-like traits (CC signature). Similar to CC and CHC, CLHCC showed an aggressive phenotype with shorter recurrence-free and overall survival. In addition, CLHCC coexpressed embryonic stem cell-like expression traits (ES signature) suggesting its derivation from bipotent hepatic progenitor cells. By comparing the expression of CC signature with previous ES-like, hepatoblast-like, or proliferation-related traits, the authors demonstrated that the prognostic value of the CC signatures was independent of the expression of those signatures (Fig. 18.1). These data suggest that the acquisition of cholangiocarcinoma-like expression traits plays a critical role in the heterogeneous progression of HCC.

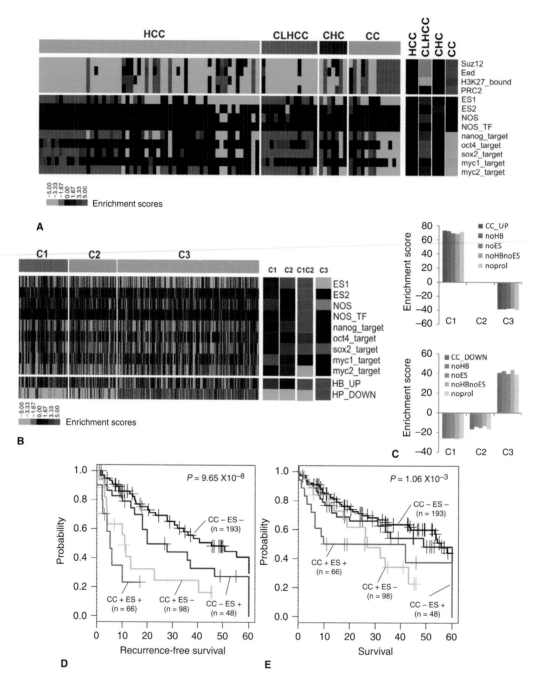

FIGURE 18.1 Comparison of the CC signature (cholangiocarcinoma-like traits) with ES signatures (embryonic stem cell-like expression traits). **A:** The enrichment of ES signatures and polycomb target gene sets in C1 and C2 classes in HCCcomp. The enrichment scores of ES signatures without proliferation signature (noprol; right bar). **B:** Bar plots for the enrichment scores of the CC_UP (**top**) and CC_DOWN (**bottom**) signatures and the CC_UP and CC_DOWN signatures subtracted by ES (noES), HB (noHB), or ES and HB (noESnoHB) signatures. **C:** The enrichment ES signatures in six independent data sets are shown. For each data set, the group enrichment in C1 and C2 tumors is indicated in the right bars ($P < .05$). **D:** Kaplan-Meier plots analyses for RFS (**left**) and OS (**right**) based on the expression status of CC and ES signatures in the integrated Laboratory of Experimental Carcinogenesis and Seoul National University data sets (n = 209). The CC+represents C1 tumors, and ES+ represents the tumors that express ES1 signature. RFS, recurrence-free survival; OS, overall survival. For details, see ref. 21. (From ref. 21, with permission.)

COMPARATIVE FUNCTIONAL GENOMICS

Despite the fact that transgenic and knockout mouse models have greatly enhanced the understanding of human cancers, in most cases we still rely on casual correlation between human and mouse models owing to lack of methods for direct comparisons.[22] Based on the neutral theory of molecular evolution, it is possible to identify both protein coding sequences and functional noncoding sequences in a genome.[22] Because regulatory elements of evolutionarily related species are conserved, it is likely that gene expression signatures reflecting similar phenotypes in different species could be also conserved. Based on this hypothesis, cross-comparison of global gene expression data from human HCC and mouse models of HCC has been undertaken to identify aberrant phenotypes that reflect evolutionarily conserved molecular pathways. Lee et al.[23] integrated gene expression data from human and transgenic mouse models of liver cancer. Hierarchical clustering analysis of integrated and standardized datasets revealed that HCC induced in mice by *Myc*, *E2f1*, and the combination of *Myc/E2f1* transgenes had the highest similarity with those of the better survival group of human HCC. However, the expression patterns in HCC induced by *Myc/Tgfa* transgenes or by the chemical carcinogen diethylnitrosamine were most similar to those of the poor survival group of human HCC. The results suggest that these mouse models might recapitulate the molecular patterns of the two subclasses of human HCC. In contrast, gene expression patterns of HCC from Acox1-/- and ciprofibrate-treated mice, in which development of HCC was driven by peroxisome proliferation in the liver, were least similar to those observed in either subclass of human HCC. These results suggest that the molecular pathways underlying hepatocarcinogenesis induced by peroxisome proliferation in mice are not frequent in humans.[23]

The similarity of gene expression profiles between human and mouse models is in good agreement with the phenotypic characteristics of the tumors,[23] that is, the human tumors with increased proliferation, decreased apoptosis, and worse prognosis pair with mouse models with the same features. The fact that these findings were first uncovered by unsupervised methods and later validated by supervised methods suggests that the underlying principles in gene expression changes are conserved between mouse and human HCC. These results strongly support the hypothesis that well-defined gene expression signatures from experimental conditions or animal models can be used to stratify human cancer patients into more homogeneous groups based on molecular similarity. The unique molecular identities of each subclass of HCC uncovered by comparative analysis of a genomewide survey of gene expression from human and animal models will facilitate the development of new therapeutic strategies.

Recent studies in different human tumors have provided further insights into how comparison of gene expression patterns from human and mouse tumors may permit the direct identification of common aberrant molecular pathways.[24,25] Comparison of gene expression profiles from a *Myc*-driven mouse prostate cancer model and human prostate cancer enabled Ellwood-Yen et al.[24] to identify a conserved expression module of human genes that corresponded to *Myc* signature genes defined in the mouse model. The *Myc* signature genes permitted the definition of a subset of *MYC*-like human cancers that are probably driven by *MYC* amplification or other mechanisms of *MYC* pathway activation. In a similar study, Sweet-Cordero et al.[25] detected a *KRAS2* gene expression signature by comparing a *KRAS2*-mediated mouse model of lung cancer with human lung cancer. It should be noted that when the investigators examined gene expression data from human lung adenocarcinomas alone, no statistically significant gene expression pattern correlated with *KRAS2* mutation status between wild type and mutated *KRAS2* tumors. The authors were able to identify a gene expression signature that reflected the *KRAS2* mutation in human adenocarcinomas only by comparing gene expression in tumors from humans and mice.

Functional genomics has the potential power to identify the cell of origin of cancer and the cellular pathway by which cancer subsequently evolves. This notion was recently tested in HCC.[26] Because HCC can originate from both adult hepatocytes and hepatic progenitor cells, our experimental strategy involved the integration of gene expression data generated from rat fetal hepatoblasts and adult hepatocytes with expression data from human HCC and mouse HCC models.[26] Patients with HCC that shared a gene expression pattern with fetal hepatoblasts had a poor prognosis. The gene expression program that distinguished this subtype from other types of HCC included markers of hepatic oval cells, suggesting that this HCC subtype may arise from hepatic progenitor cells. Furthermore, analyses of gene networks in these tumors showed that activation of AP-1 transcription factors in this newly identified HCC subtype might have a key role in tumor development.

CONCLUSION AND PERSPECTIVE

DNA microarray technology has provided an extraordinary opportunity for integrative analysis of the cancer transcriptome. Array-based gene expression profiling not only has advanced our understanding of cancer biology, but has begun to influence decisions in clinical oncology and ultimately may allow for the development of more effective therapies. The power of gene expression profiling of HCC can be further enhanced by cross-comparison analysis of multiple gene expression data sets from human HCC and the rich database of HCC in animal models.[22] The success of these new analytical approaches, comparative and/or integrative functional genomics, suggests that integration of independent data sets will enhance our ability to identify robust predictive markers. For example, a model to predict progression of mammary cancer has been recently developed based on a wound-healing gene expression signature.[27] Patients displaying the wound-healing signature had a significantly increased risk of metastasis compared with those without the signature, indicating that genomic data from normal physiological conditions may help to predict

the prognosis of cancer patients. It is important to obtain additional tumor-independent signatures from multiple species that are unique for different physiological conditions, such as liver development, regeneration, hepatic stem cell activation, that can be integrated with gene expression patterns from human HCC. Although the clinical application of gene expression profiling to identify prognostic markers and therapeutic targets for HCC is still immature, the progress over the last few years suggest that prospective clinical studies are well justified and indeed needed.

It seems reasonable to predict that the genomic technologies will play an increasingly important role in clinical oncology. The immediate focus undoubtedly will be on using the current genomic technologies to improve the diagnosis and treatment of cancer. However, with the beginning of affordable whole genome sequencing and the current expansion of the cancer genome atlas,[28] one can certainly expect significant progress in the treatment of liver cancer.

References

1. Parkin DM, Bray F, Ferlay J, Pisani P. Global cancer statistics, 2002. *CA Cancer J Clin* 2005;55:74.
2. El Serag HB. Hepatocellular carcinoma: recent trends in the United States. *Gastroenterology* 2004,127: S27.
3. El-Serag HB, Hampel H, Javadi F. The association between diabetes and hepatocellular carcinoma: a systematic review of epidemiologic evidence. *Clin Gastroenterol Hepatol* 2006;4(3):369.
4. Libbrecht L, Desmet V, Roskams T. Preneoplastic lesions in human hepatocarcinogenesis. *Liver Int* 2005;25(1):16.
5. Thorgeirsson SS, Grisham JW. Molecular pathogenesis of human hepatocellular carcinoma. *Nat Genet* 2002;31:339.
6. Bruix J, Boix L, Sala M, Llovet JM. Focus on hepatocellular carcinoma. *Cancer Cell* 2004;5:215.
7. Quackenbush J. Microarray analysis and tumor classification. *N Engl J Med* 2006;354(23):2463.
8. Hood L, Heath JR, Phelps ME, Lin B. Systems biology and new technologies enable predictive and preventative medicine. *Science* 2004;306:640.
9. Pinkel D, Albertson DG. Array comparative genomic hybridization and its applications in cancer. *Nat Genet* 2005;37(Suppl):S11.
10. Moinzadeh P, Breuhahn K, Stutzer H, Schrmacher P. Chromosome alterations in human hepatocellular carcinomas correlate with aetiology and histological grade—results of an explorative CGH meta-analysis. *Br J Cancer* 2005;14:92:935.
11. Poon TCW, Wong N, Lai PBS, et al. A tumor progression model for hepatocellular carcinoma: bioinformatics analysis of genomic data. *Gastroenterology* 2006;131:1262.
12. Davies JJ, Wilson IM, Lam WL. Array CGH technologies and their applications to cancer genomes. *Chromosome Res* 2005;13: 237.
13. Woo HG, Park ES, Lee JS, et al. Identification of potential driver genes in human liver carcinoma by genomewide screening. *Cancer Res* 2009; 69(9):4059
14. Kim CK, Lim JH, Lee WJ. Detection of hepatocellular carcinomas and dysplastic nodules in cirrhotic liver: accuracy of ultrasonography in transplant patients. *J Ultrasound Med* 2001;20:99.
15. Kojiro M, Roskams T. Early hepatocellular carcinoma and dysplastic nodules. *Semin Liver Dis* 2005;25:133.
16. Kaposi-Novak P, Libbrecht L, Woo HG, et al. Central role of c-Myc during malignant conversion in human hepatocarcinogenesis. *Cancer Res* 2009;69 (7):2775.
17. Thorgeirsson SS, Lee JS, Grisham JW. Molecular prognostication of liver cancer: end of the beginning. *J Hepatol* 2006;44(4):2006.
18. Lee JS, Chu IS, Heo J, et al. Classification and prediction of survival in hepatocellular carcinoma by gene expression profiling. *Hepatology* 2004;40:667.
19. Boyault S, Rickman DS, de Reynies A, et al. Transcriptome classification of HCC is related to gene alterations and to new therapeutic targets. *Hepatology* 2007;45(1):42.
20. Hoshida Y, Nijman SM, Kobayashi M, et al. Integrative transcriptome analysis reveals common molecular subclasses of human hepatocellular carcinoma. *Cancer Res* 2009;69(18):7385.
21. Woo HG, Lee JH, Yoon JH, et al. Identification of a cholangiocarcinoma-like gene expression trait in hepatocellular carcinoma. *Cancer Res* 2010;70(8):3034.
22. Lee JS, Thorgeirsson SS. Comparative and integrative functional genomics of HCC. *Oncogene* 2006;25(27):3801.
23. Lee JS, Chu IS, Mikaelyan A, et al. Application of comparative functional genomics to identify best-fit mouse models to study human cancer. *Nat Genet* 2004;36(12):1306.
24. Ellwood-Yen K, Graeber TG, Wongvipat J, et al. Myc-driven murine prostate cancer shares molecular features with human prostate tumors. *Cancer Cell* 2003;4:223.
25. Sweet-Cordero A, Mukherjee S, Subramanian A, et al. An oncogenic KRAS2 expression signature identified by cross-species gene-expression analysis. *Nat Genet* 2005; 37:48.
26. Lee JS, Heo J, Libbrecht L, et al. A novel prognostic subtype of human hepatocellular carcinoma derived from hepatic progenitor cells. *Nat Med* 2006;12(4):410.
27. Chang HY, Nuyten DS, Sneddon JB, et al. Robustness, scalability, and integration of a wound-response gene expression signature in predicting breast cancer survival. *Proc Natl Acad Sci U S A* 2005;102:3738.
28. International Cancer Genome Consortium. International network of cancer genome projects. *Nature* 2010;464(7291): 993.

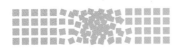

CHAPTER 19 COLORECTAL CANCER

RAMESH A. SHIVDASANI

The cumulative lifetime risk of developing colorectal cancer (CRC) in the United States is about 6%, and this increases about fourfold in persons with a history of CRC in first- or second-degree relatives. Although fewer than 5% of cases occur in patients with uncommon inherited predisposition syndromes and most CRCs are accordingly considered to be sporadic, 20% to 30% of cases might have a familial basis despite absence of a known germline defect. Characteristic somatic mutations, epigenetic alterations, and defects in DNA repair or chromosomal stability promote disease progression and malignant behaviors. Well-characterized predisposing conditions and somatic mutations profoundly inform the molecular understanding of CRC and serve as a paradigm for the genetic basis of cancer.

THE ADENOMA–CARCINOMA SEQUENCE AND MULTISTEP MODELS OF COLORECTAL TUMORIGENESIS

The genetic basis of CRC is best appreciated in light of the adenoma–carcinoma sequence and the premise that CRCs arise from benign precursor polyps. Most hyperplastic polyps harbor little potential for invasive cancer, although those of the sessile serrated variety may represent precursors of cancers with microsatellite instability.[1,2] By contrast, adenomatous polyps are known to be the important precursor lesions, with those larger than 1 cm carrying an estimated 15% risk of progression to adenocarcinoma over 10 years; endoscopic removal of such adenomas reduces CRC incidence and mortality.[3] Adenomas are marked by epithelial overgrowth, dysplasia, and abnormal differentiation, sometimes with small foci of invasive cells; residual areas of benign adenomatous tissue are frequently identified in surgical CRC specimens.

The prevalence of adenomas in the United States, estimated at 25% by age 50 and up to 50% by age 70,[4] dwarfs the 6% cumulative lifetime risk of CRC. This is because few adenomas progresses to invasive cancer, in a process that unfolds over one to three decades.[5] Alterations in three classes of genes drive tumors: oncogenes, tumor suppressor genes, and genes that prevent DNA damage. Although oncogenic events may have a genetic (mutational) or epigenetic basis, at present more is known about the somatic mutations that fuel step-wise increases in malignant potential.[6] The order of mutations can vary and most tumors do not carry every known genetic alteration. Nevertheless, certain mutations appear at appreciable frequency in different tumor stages, allowing assignment of a typical sequence (Fig. 19.1). Considered in light of the adenoma–carcinoma sequence, these mutations support the idea of cancer as a multifaceted disease that breaches natural checks on cell survival, growth, and invasion.[7] Individual mutations rarely correlate precisely with a particular feature, such as survival or angiogenesis, and common mutations often impinge on multiple cell functions. Nevertheless, the combination of somatic mutations defines cancer subtypes, their unique properties, and sensitivity to certain therapies. Specific mutations illuminate the normal controls on colonic epithelium, reveal key cellular pathways as rational targets for therapy, and may guide future prevention strategies. Furthermore, knowledge of the mutations classifies CRC into subgroups with distinctive features. For example, *KRAS* or *BRAF* gene mutations (together accounting for nearly half of all U.S. cases) predict for lack of response to epidermal growth factor receptor (EGFR) antibodies.[8,9] *KRAS* mutation status is now used to dictate EGFR antibody therapy in CRC, a practice likely to expand as the prognostic and predictive value of additional molecular features becomes apparent.

Global Events in Colorectal Cancer

In light of the central importance of somatic mutations, cellular conditions that elevate mutation rates might enable or accelerate tumor progression. Over 80% of CRCs display widespread

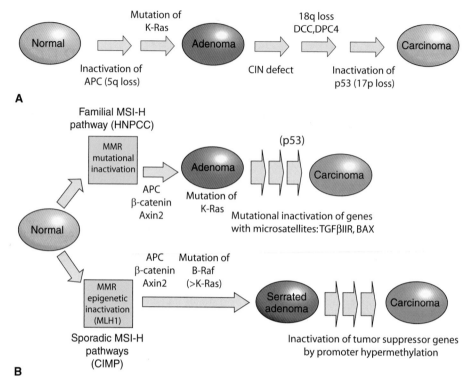

FIGURE 19.1 Genetic pathways to colorectal carcinoma. All colorectal cancers (CRCs) arise within benign adenomatous precursors, fueled by mutations that serially enhance malignant behavior. Mutations that activate the Wnt signaling pathway seem to be necessary initiating events, following which two possible courses contribute to accumulation of additional mutations. A: Chromosomal instability is a feature of up to 80% of CRCs and is commonly associated with activating *KRAS* point mutations and loss of regions that encompass *P53* and other tumor suppressors on 18q and 17p, often but not necessarily in that order. B: About 20% of CRCs are euploid but defective in DNA mismatch repair (MMR), resulting in high microsatellite instability (MSI-Hi). MMR defects may develop sporadically, associated with CpG island methylation (CIMP), or as a result of familial predisposition in hereditary nonpolyposis colorectal cancer (HNPCC). Mutations accumulate in the *KRAS* or *BRAF* oncogenes, *p53* tumor suppressor, and in microsatellite-containing genes vulnerable to MMR defects, such as *TGFβIIR*. Epigenetic inactivation of the MMR gene *MLH1* and activating *BRAF* point mutations are especially common in serrated adenomas, which progress in part through silencing of tumor suppressor genes by promoter hypermethylation. Progression from adenoma to CRC takes years to decades, a process that accelerates in the presence of MMR defects.

chromosomal gains and losses, phenomena that favor amplification of oncogenes and loss of tumor suppressors.[10] Chromosomal segregation defects may account for this background of chromosomal instability (CIN), as illustrated by the segregation factor Bub1 in mice,[11] but few specific gene defects are implicated with confidence. The remaining fraction of CRCs appears euploid at the level of whole chromosomes but may carry thousands of point mutations, small deletions, and insertions near nucleotide repeat tracts, a defect known as microsatellite instability (MSI).[12] Molecular determinants of progression in MSI+ adenomas differ from those associated with CIN; for example, *BRAF V600E* mutations occur more commonly in MSI+ serrated adenomas than in other subtypes.[13] Hypermutability with CIN or MSI results in many inconsequential or detrimental "passenger" mutations, an important consideration that focuses attention on "driver" changes. Such changes are distinguished by their appearance in a significant proportion of tumor specimens and, ideally, by laboratory demonstration of their contribution toward malignancy.

Epigenetic mechanisms are probably as significant as mutations in cancer but also less well understood. Various covalent histone modifications and methylation of cytosine residues in DNA represent the principal means for gene regulation, the latter far better characterized in CRC than the former. The 5'-CpG-3' dinucleotide pairs are particular targets for methylation in localized areas of high CpG content in promoters, where abundant methylation silences adjacent genes. Compared to normal tissue, CRCs show 8% to 15% lower total DNA methylation,[14] even in colorectal adenomas.[15] Reduced pericentromeric methylation might decrease the fidelity of chromosomal segregation, and altered methylation and loss of imprinting at the *IGF2* locus are associated with increased CRC risk,[16] suggesting broad effects of global hypomethylation on cell growth. However, because some animal models show increased tumor susceptibility with global hypomethylation,[17] whereas *Apc^Min* mice that lack or overexpress the *de novo* DNA methyltransferase DNMT3B show reduced or increased progression of small adenomas, respectively,[18,19] its precise significance is unclear. Against the background of genomewide hypomethylation, a subset of CRCs show coordinate hypermethylation of characteristic CpG-rich promoter islands, conferring the CpG island methylator phenotype (CIMP), with transcriptional attenuation of associated genes, including tumor suppressors such as *HIC1* and the secreted Wnt-inhibiting secreted Frizzled-related proteins (sFRPs).[20,21] Adenomatous precursors of CIMP cancers show the distinctive histology of sessile serrated adenomas, with dysplasia within an architectural pattern typical of hyperplastic polyps.

There are few variations to the adenoma–carcinoma sequence. A tenfold elevated risk of CRC in patients with long-standing inflammatory bowel disease, especially ulcerative colitis (UC),[22] probably reflects heightened mutation and tumorigenesis with repeated cycles of mucosal injury and repair. Such cancers arise not only from typical polyps but also within flat adenomatous plaques and nonadenomatous areas of dysplasia. A *p53* gene mutation tends to occur earlier in the cancer sequence,[23] and *APC* gene inactivation is less common than in sporadic CRC. Conversely, even in the absence of CIMP, methylation of the *p16^INK4a* tumor suppressor gene, which is rare in sporadic CRC, is common in UC-associated cancers.[24]

EARLY EVENTS AND CRITICAL PATHWAYS IN COLORECTAL TUMORIGENESIS HIGHLIGHTED BY INHERITED SYNDROMES OF INCREASED CANCER RISK

Two uncommon but highly penetrant inherited syndromes, familial adenomatous polyposis (FAP) and hereditary nonpolyposis colorectal cancer (HNPCC), together account for about 5% of all CRC cases. Other rare syndromes, familial juvenile polyposis (FJP), Peutz-Jeghers syndrome (PJS), and Cowden disease, each occurring in fewer than 1 in 200,000 births, also elevate the risk of CRC, and some genes responsible for these autosomal dominant disorders have been identified (Table 19.1). Elucidation of the corresponding molecular defects serves not only in accurate molecular diagnosis, risk assessment, and disease prevention in affected families but also informs understanding of the considerably larger proportion of sporadic cases.

Familial Adenomatous Polyposis and the Central Importance of Wnt Signaling

In FAP, an autosomal dominant monogenic disorder that underlies about 0.5% of all CRCs, individuals develop hundreds to thousands of colonic polyps by their teens or early 20s, and the lifetime risk of progression to invasive cancer approaches 100%, with cancer diagnosed at a median age of 39. Extraintestinal manifestations include duodenal and gastric adenomas; congenital hypertrophy of the retinal pigmented epithelium; osteomas and mesenteric desmoid tumors in the Gardner syndrome variant[25]; and less commonly, brain tumors in the Turcot syndrome variant,[26] cutaneous cysts, thyroid tumors, and adrenal adenomas. Although most features are benign, rare patients develop hepatoblastoma or thyroid cancer. Reflecting the similar regulation of small bowel and colonic epithelia, patients have a 5% to 10% risk of developing duodenal or ampullary adenocarcinoma, mandating close endoscopic monitoring of the upper intestine after prophylactic colectomy.[27]

The gene affected by mutations in this disorder, adenomatous polyposis coli (*APC*) on chromosome 5q21, encodes a 2842-residue protein. Germline mutations occur throughout the locus but cluster in the 5′ half and exon 15,[28] mostly introducing stop codons or frame shifts that truncate the protein. Although a few mutations correlate with phenotypic severity or specific extraintestinal manifestations, identical mutations can produce different clinical features. In the attenuated APC (AAPC) variant, disease onset is delayed, individuals develop fewer colonic polyps or cancers, and mutations cluster in the extreme 5′ or 3′ ends of *APC* exons.[29] The *I1307K* allele, present in the Ashkenazi Jewish population, barely doubles the lifetime risk of CRC and does not affect APC protein function but replaces an $(A)_3T(A)_4$ coding sequence with an extended $(A)_8$ tract that is occasionally targeted for nearby truncating mutations.[30] Identification of an *APC* mutation in a proband allows reliable testing of family members. Carriers should have screening colonoscopy annually after age 10, gastroduodenoscopy after age 25, and treatment with nonsteroidal anti-inflammatory drugs to reduce the risk of progression to cancer.[31] Prophylactic colectomy is highly recommended, with subsequent monitoring of the rectal stump and other at-risk tissues.

TABLE 19.1

GENETICS OF INHERITED COLORECTAL TUMOR SYNDROMES

Syndrome	Features Commonly Seen in Affected Individuals	Gene Defect
Syndromes with adenomatous polyps		
Familial adenomatous polyposis (FAP)	Multiple adenomas (>100) and colorectal carcinomas; duodenal polyps and carcinomas; gastric fundus polyps; congenital hypertrophy of retinal epithelium	*APC* (>90%)
Gardner syndrome	Same as FAP, with desmoid tumors and mandibular osteomas	*APC*
Turcot syndrome	Polyposis and CRC with brain tumors (medulloblastoma, glioblastoma)	*APC, MLH1*
Attenuated adenomatous polyposis (AAPC)	Less than 100 polyps, although marked variation in polyp number (from ~5 to >1,000 polyps) seen in mutation carriers within a single family	*APC* (5′ mutations)
Hereditary nonpolyposis colorectal cancer (HNPCC)	Colorectal cancer with modest polyposis; high risk of endometrial cancer; some risk of ovarian, gastric, urothelial, hepatobiliary, and brain cancers	*MSH2, MLH1, MSH6* (together >90%), may be *PMS2*
MYH-associated polyposis (MAP)	Multiple gastrointestinal polyps, autosomal recessive	*MYH*
Syndromes with hamartomatous polyps		
Peutz-Jeghers syndrome	Hamartomatous polyps throughout the gastrointestinal (GI) tract; mucocutaneous pigmentation; estimated 9- to 13-fold increased risk of GI and non-GI cancers	*STK11* (30%–70%)
Cowden disease	Multiple hamartomas involving breast, thyroid, skin, brain, and GI tract; increased risk of breast, uterus, thyroid, and some GI cancers	*PTEN* (85%)
Juvenile polyposis syndrome	Multiple hamartomas in youth, predominantly in colon and stomach; variable increase in colorectal and stomach cancer risk; facial changes	*BMPR1A* (25%), *SMAD4* (15%), *ENG*

The larger significance of the *APC* gene derives from its somatic inactivation in about 80% of sporadic CRCs and early colorectal adenomas.[32] Indeed, somatic *APC* mutations are found in tiny adenomas, containing few dysplastic glands. Attesting to the tumor suppressor function, tumors arising sporadically or in FAP patients show biallelic *APC* gene inactivation and loss of heterozygosity, with one copy usually lost by deletion. Except for the small bowel, *APC* mutations are rare in other cancers, including those in other digestive organs. *APC* gene inactivation is a rate-limiting step for development of adenomas, and its designation as a gatekeeper gene in CRC is now well supported by knowledge of its cellular functions. *APC* encodes several functional domains and proteins truncated by mutation that could in principle interfere with a wide range of cellular activities. Disruption of its known role in chromosome segregation might, for example, contribute to CIN.[33] However, attention on *APC* centers rightfully on its control of the Wnt signaling pathway. About half the sporadic CRCs with intact *APC* function carry activating point mutations in the *CTNNB1* gene,[34,35] which encodes β-catenin, a transcriptional effector of Wnt signaling. Moreover, acute loss of APC function in mice produces intestinal defects identical to those observed upon Wnt pathway activation.[36]

The Wnt glycoproteins are secreted morphogens with diverse functions in development and homeostasis. In the absence of Wnt signaling, cells use a complex containing APC, Axin2, and other cytoplasmic proteins to promote phosphorylation, by casein kinase I and glycogen synthase kinase (GSK)-3β, of several conserved serine and threonine residues in the β-catenin N-terminus, thereby targeting β-catenin for ubiquitin-mediated proteasomal degradation.[37] When Wnt ligands bind a surface protein complex that contains a member of the Frizzled protein family and the obligate coreceptor LRP5/6, they antagonize APC/Axin2 activity and thereby stabilize β-catenin. *CTNNB1* mutations in CRC alter consensus residues for N-terminal phosphorylation and render the mutant protein resistant to

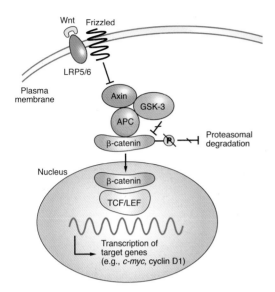

FIGURE 19.2 Outline of Wnt signaling, the key driver pathway in colorectal cancer. Members of the Wnt family of glycoprotein morphogens bind the cell surface coreceptors Frizzled and LRP5/6. In the absence of Wnt binding, normal cells use a complex containing adenomatous polyposis coli (APC), Axin, and other cytoplasmic proteins to promote glycogen synthase kinase (GSK)-3β-mediated phosphorylation of the β-catenin N-terminus, which targets β-catenin for proteasomal degradation (from ref. 37.). Binding of a Wnt ligand to Frizzled and its obligate coreceptor LRP5/6 antagonizes the APC/Axin destruction complex, stabilizing β-catenin (CTNNB1), which moves into the nucleus and coactivates genes through T-cell factor/lymphoid enhancer factor (TCF/LEF) transcription factors. Either of the two principal gatekeeper events in colorectal cancer, inactivating *APC* or activating *CTNNB1* mutations, results in constitutive, Wnt-independent stabilization of β-catenin and unregulated activation of the cognate transcriptional program. Wnt signaling in the intestine is normally confined to crypt progenitors, and its aberrant activation by *APC* or *CTNNB1* mutations confers a permanent cryptlike state that favors cell replication.

degradation. Thus, inactivating *APC* or activating *CTNNB1* mutations, two alternative lesions in CRC, have the same effect: constitutive, Wnt-independent stabilization of β-catenin (Fig. 19.2). Accumulated β-catenin translocates to the cell nucleus, where it acts as a transcriptional coactivator for the T-cell factor/lymphoid enhancer factor (TCF/LEF) family of transcription factors. Nuclear β-catenin provides TCF/LEF proteins with an activating partner, resulting in transcription of target genes.[38] Of the four known TCF/LEF proteins, TCF4 is the most important in normal bowel epithelium and CRC.[34,39] Among the many components of the Wnt signaling cascade, rare *AXIN2* mutations of uncertain significance are reported in MSI+ cases,[40] but mutations in CRC are otherwise found only in *APC* and *CTNNB1*.

Although Wnt ligands signal in many tissues, intestinal homeostasis is particularly dependent on this pathway. Wnt signaling in the intestine is confined to proliferative crypt stem and progenitor cells. In mice, cycling crypt cells that express the surface marker LGR5 are far more susceptible to Wnt-induced transformation than their differentiated progeny, implying that CRC arises in a primitive stem or progenitor cell and not in mature descendants.[41] Moreover, the Wnt-dependent transcriptional program in CRC cell lines overlaps materially with that in intestinal crypts.[42] Wnt signaling is hence necessary for intestinal epithelial self-renewal, and constitutive, ligand-independent activation imposed by *APC* or *CTNNB1* mutations induces and sustains adenomas. Among the diverse transcriptional targets of the TCF-β-catenin complex identified to date, *CMYC* seems especially important because its absence in mice abrogates the effects of acute APC loss in the intestine.[43,44] Mice that lack CD44, another prominent Wnt-pathway target, develop fewer adenomas in an APC-deficient background.[45] Gene expression profiling offers an expanded list of over 100 candidate transcriptional targets,[42,46] but the individual significance of each will take many years to investigate.

Hereditary Nonpolyposis Colorectal Cancer and the Role of DNA Mismatch Repair

HNPCC, an autosomal dominant disorder that confers a nearly 80% lifetime risk of developing CRC, usually before age 50, is estimated to account for 2% to 4% of all CRC cases in the United States.[47] Affected individuals do not lack intestinal polyps (nearly all CRCs, syndromic or sporadic, arise within adenomatous precursors) but develop many fewer colonic polyps than patients with FAP, a condition that must be excluded to satisfy criteria for diagnosis of HNPCC (Table 19.2).[48] Cancers tend to develop in the ascending colon, and patients are further predisposed to develop tumors of the endometrium, small intestine, stomach, upper urothelium, ovary, biliary tract, and brain, a spectrum reflected in the revised Amsterdam II criteria (Table 19.2). The lifetime risk of endometrial cancer, in particular, is 35% to 50% and that of urologic and ovarian cancers is 7% to 8%.[49] Cancers in HNPCC show pronounced variation in the lengths of microsatellite DNA sequences in tumors compared with unaffected tissues. Cancers showing such MSI at two or more among a panel of five mono- and dinucleotide tracts (BAT26, BAT25, D5S346, D2S123, and D17S250) carry the MSI-Hi designation. Most other CRCs harbor CIN and show microsatellite stability (MSS) or, in a small fraction, instability at only one of the five test tracts (MSI-Lo), a finding of uncertain significance.

TABLE 19.2

CRITERIA FOR CLINICAL DIAGNOSIS OF HEREDITARY NONPOLYPOSIS COLORECTAL CANCER

A. *Revised Amsterdam criteria (clinical diagnosis)*
   1. Three or more family members with histologically verified hereditary nonpolyposis colorectal cancer (HNPCC)-related cancers, one of whom is a first degree relative of the other two.
   2. Two successive affected generations.
   3. One or more of the HNPCC-related cancers diagnosed before age 50.
   4. Exclusion of Familial adenomatous polyposis (FAP).
B. *Revised Bethesda guidelines (criteria to prompt MSI testing of tumors)*
   1. Diagnosis of colorectal cancer before age 50.
   2. Synchronous or metachronous presence of CRC or other HNPCC-associated cancer.
   3. CRC diagnosed before age 60 with histopathologic features associated with MSI-Hi.
   4. CRC in at least one first-degree relative with an HNPCC-related tumor, with one of the cancers diagnosed before age 50.
   5. CRC in 2 or more first-degree relatives with HNPCC-related tumors, regardless of age.
C. *Spectrum of sites for HNPCC-related cancers*

Colon and rectum, endometrium, stomach, ovary, pancreas, ureter and renal pelvis, biliary tract, small intestine, brain, sebaceous gland adenomas, and keratoacanthomas.

HNPCC results from germline mutations in any of several genes that enable DNA mismatch repair (MMR), a proofreading process that corrects base-pair mismatches and short insertions and deletions in the normal course of DNA replication. MMR in mammalian cells is mediated by homologs of bacterial and yeast repair proteins: MutS homologs (MSH) 1-6, MutL homologs (MLH) 1-3, and PMS1 and PMS2. MLH1 and PMS2 are recruited to sites of DNA mismatch as a MutLα complex and in turn recruit MSH2-MSH6 (MutSα) or MSH2-MSH3 (MutSβ) heterodimers to sites of 1-bp or 2- to 4-bp errors, respectively. These proteins excise the strand that carries the mismatch, and they resynthesize and ligate the repaired DNA. Germline mutations in *MSH2*, *MLH1*, and *MSH6* together explain more than 90% of kindreds[50,51]; the significance of mutations in other canonical MMR pathway genes, *PMS1* and *PMS2*, is less certain.[52]

MSI-Hi colorectal cancers commonly show lymphocytic infiltrates, mucinous signet-ring differentiation, and a medullary growth pattern; Bethesda guidelines (Table 19.2) combine clinical and phenotypic features to facilitate diagnosis of HNPCC.[53] When these criteria are met, tumor DNA should either be tested for MSI in a simple, PCR-based assay or by immunohistochemistry for absence of the commonly implicated MLH1, MSH2, and MSH6 proteins.[54] A positive result should prompt genetic testing for *MLH1*, *MSH2*, or *MSH6* mutations; the personal and family history can predict the probability of identifying mutations.[55] Genetic testing identifies the mutant allele and carriers, allowing targeting of a recommendation for biannual colonoscopic screening between the ages of 20 and 40, with annual screening thereafter. Women should undergo

annual endometrial evaluation soon after age 25, and carriers should consider prophylactic subtotal colectomy, hysterectomy, and oophorectomy.

In incipient cancers, random events first disrupt function of the wild type allele of a mutant MMR gene, and the resulting "mutator phenotype" induces brisk accumulation of DNA replication errors.[50] Consequently, adenomas progress into carcinomas over 3 to 5 years instead of two or more decades.[56] Paradoxically, the prognosis for patients with MSI-Hi colorectal cancers is better than for those with MSS disease, perhaps because many resulting somatic mutations are disadvantageous. Cancer develops, of course, because some mutations activate oncogenes or inactivate tumor suppressor genes. One frequently inactivated tumor suppressor gene in MSI-Hi colorectal cancers, *TGFβRII*, encodes the type II transforming growth factor-beta (TGF-β) receptor and contains a vulnerable mononucleotide tract in the coding sequence.[57] TGF-β inhibits proliferation of many normal epithelial cells, including intestinal cells, and biallelic *TGFβRII* inactivation is detected in over 90% of MSI-Hi and 15% of MSS, sporadic CRCs.[58] Other genes mutated in MSI-Hi colorectal cancers encode proapoptotic molecules, such as CASP5 and BAX,[59] transcription factors, including TCF4,[60] and the epidermal growth factor receptor.[61] Notably, all CRCs, regardless of MMR status, seem to require mutational deregulation of the gatekeeper APC-β-catenin pathway.[62]

Another recessively inherited syndrome of multiple adenomas and CRC, MUTYH-associated polyposis (MAP), is caused by germline mutations in *MYH*, the human homolog of *Escherichia coli MutY*, another base excision-repair gene.[63] Disease begins later in life than in FAP, polyp numbers vary widely, and extracolonic tumors are less frequent than in HNPCC. Because *MYH* encodes a DNA glycosylase that mediates oxidative DNA damage, tumors are not associated with MSI but with somatic G:C to T:A mutations, including in the *APC* gene. Two alleles, *Y165C* and *G382D*, account for most cases, and cancers develop in homozygotes or compound heterozygotes; monoallelic carriers show no increased risk.[64] Surveillance recommendations are similar to those in HNPCC.

The cancer spectrum in HNPCC and the particular predilection for CRC remain unexplained. Colonic, endometrial, and selected other epithelial cells may be especially sensitive to the class of mutations that occur in the MMR setting; loss of the wild type MMR allele may occur more readily in these tissues; or they may lack repair safeguards that protect other cell types. MSI-Hi is observed in 12% to 15% of sporadic cases of CRC.[65] Most such tumors are believed to arise from serrated adenomas in the ascending colon and do not reflect unrecognized germline mutation or somatic disruption of a known MMR gene.[66] Rather, most sporadic MSI-Hi cases reflect epigenetic inactivation of the *MLH1* gene by promoter hypermethylation, often in association with the CIMP phenotype and with activating *BRAF* mutations.[67–69]

Familial Juvenile Polyposis (FJP)

Patients with FJP develop three to ten or more premalignant hamartomatous polyps in the stomach or small or large intestine in childhood or adolescence.[70,71] Although affected individuals often have the appropriate family history, a significant minority represents the first case in their families. Germline mutations in genes that encode the bone morphogenetic protein (BMP) receptor *BMPR1A*, the accessory TGF-β receptor endoglin, *ENG*, or the *SMAD4* signal transducer point to the TGF-β signaling pathway in disease pathogenesis.[72,73] Indeed, sporadic CRCs are frequently insensitive to the growth inhibitory effects of TGF-β, and loss of BMP function in mice expands stem and progenitor cells, leading to polyposis or ectopic crypts.[74–76] Not all patients carry these mutations, indicating that additional genes remain undiscovered. Notably, conditional loss of *Smad4* in mouse intestinal cells does not affect growth, whereas selective loss in T lymphocytes causes intestinal mucosal thickening and polyposis.[77] These results complicate interpretation of TGF-β functions and implicate stromal inflammation in intestinal tumorigenesis.

Peutz-Jeghers Syndrome

Patients with PJS develop hamartomatous polyps, benign tumors containing differentiated but disorganized cells, mainly in the small intestine but also in the colon or stomach; these grow to variable size, often leading to hemorrhage or intussusception. PJS shows autosomal dominant inheritance and is associated with macular lesions on the skin and buccal mucosa; bladder and bronchial polyps; and a propensity to develop a range of cancers, including those of the lung, breast, and female reproductive organs. The lifetime risk for all cancers exceeds 90% and the incidence of digestive tract cancers, especially in the small intestine, stomach, and pancreas, is elevated 50- to 500-fold over the general population; CRC risk is nearly 100 times greater.[78]

Serine–threonine kinase 11 (*STK11*) or *LKB1* is a recessive oncogene that shows loss of heterozygosity in PJS tumors and somatic mutations in sporadic pulmonary, pancreatic and biliary carcinomas, and melanoma.[79] Its product is a complex protein that functions at the intersection of several cellular pathways and points to the central importance of cell polarity and metabolism in cancer. Although LKB1 is implicated in diverse functions, its principal activity, exerted through the adenosine monophosphate (AMP)-activated protein kinase AMPK, seems to be in linking nutrient and energy utilization to controls over cellular structure and, in particular, polarity.[80] LKB1 also modulates the Rheb-GDP:Rheb-GTP cycle and downstream activity of the tuberous sclerosis gene *TSC2* and the mammalian target of rapamycin (mTOR),[81] key regulators of protein synthesis and cell growth. Determining how LKB1's roles in cell polarity and metabolism contribute to tumor suppression is an intense and exciting area of cancer biology, likely to hold many surprises and useful clues for rational therapy.

Cowden Syndrome

In Cowden syndrome, the lifetime risk of developing colon or thyroid cancer approaches 10%, whereas the risk of breast cancer is nearly 50%. A diverse array of oral and gastrointestinal mucosal lesions, including lipomas, fibromas, ganglioneuromas, and hamartomas, occur together with specific cutaneous lesions (facial trichilemmomas and acral verrucous papules) and benign breast fibroadenomas, neurofibromas, lipomas, uterine leiomyomas, and meningiomas.[82] Cowden syndrome results from germline mutations in *PTEN*, the tumor suppressor gene encoding the phosphatase and tensin homolog deleted on chromosome 10.[83] PTEN is a lipid phosphatase that dephosphorylates key phosphoinositide signaling molecules[84] and is accordingly a negative regulator of intracellular growth signaling through PI-3 kinase and its downstream effectors AKT and mTOR. *PTEN* is the second most frequently mutated gene in cancers, after *TP53*. Although mutations are rarely seen in sporadic CRC, PTEN immunostaining is lost in about 40% of cases, often as a result of promoter hypermethylation in the MSI-Hi setting,[85] emphasizing its tumor suppressor function in this disease.

Significance of Inherited Syndromes of Elevated Colorectal Cancer Risk

Following a clinical diagnosis of the above syndromes, known germline mutations should be tested and patients provided with genetic counseling and advice on cancer prevention and screening. Elucidation of the corresponding molecular defects profoundly informs understanding of sporadic CRC, revealing in particular that *APC* gene inactivation or *CTNNB1* activation are early, rate-limiting events and the seminal role of the Wnt signaling pathway. Likewise, *LKB1* and *PTEN* loss in inherited and sporadic CRCs shed light on vital molecular pathways, and HNPCC helps in classifying the disease and appreciating the significance of MSI, a feature seen in 12% to 15% of sporadic cases. Even in the absence of a well-recognized predisposition syndrome, individuals with a history of CRC in a first-degree relative are up to four times more likely to develop CRC than those without a family history.

Specific environmental factors that compound the risk of developing CRC are complex and insufficiently characterized but might include obesity, excessive consumption of red meat, lack of exercise, and vitamin D deficiency.[86] As many of these factors converge on insulin signaling, some experts propose that insulin and insulinlike growth factors play a seminal role in CRC.[87] However, three of every four CRCs arise in individuals lacking a well-defined risk factor, and it is unknown to what extent particular genotypes confer sensitivity to environmental variables.

Insights from Genomewide Association Studies

The quarter or more of sporadic CRC cases with a familial component[88,89] probably have diverse molecular etiologies, with low risk conferred by some common genetic variants and interaction of individual risk alleles with other genes and with environmental factors. One early study linked colon cancer to chromosomal segment 9q22-31,[90] which reinforced the idea that single risk loci might contribute to susceptibility in nonsyndromic forms of familial disease; the authors recently narrowed the interval to a 7.7-cM distance covering five genes.[91] Genomewide association studies (GWAS) have interrogated thousands of genomes to uncover statistical association of CRC risk with at least seven distinct loci, including those linked to single nucleotide polymorphisms (SNPs) rs6983267 at 8q24.21, rs4939827 on 18q21, and rs3802842 at 11q23 (Table 19.3). Risk alleles typically elevate the rate of CRC 10% to 25% above the background in persons with the nonrisk allele.[92,93] Homozygosity for some risk alleles and combinations of risk alleles at different loci compound the risk, to 50% to 250% over the background.

The causal significance of most of these DNA sequence variants is unclear, and many localize in gene deserts or poorly characterized regions of the

TABLE 19.3

SINGLE NUCLEOTIDE POLYMORPHISMS (SNPs) CONFERRING INCREASED RISK OF COLORECTAL CANCER

Chromosomal Location	SNP-Risk Allele	Nearest Gene	Risk Allele Frequency in Controls	Odds Ratio [95% CI]	P Value
8q24.21	rs10505477-A	*MYC*	0.50	1.17 [1.12–1.23]	3×10^{-11}
	rs6983267-G		0.49	1.27 [1.16–1.39]	1×10^{-14}
	rs10795668-A		0.48	1.12 [1.10–1.16]	3×10^{-13}
	rs7014346-A	*POU5FIP1, DQ515897*	0.18	1.19 [1.15–1.23]	9×10^{-26}
18q21.1	rs4939827-T	*SMAD7*	0.53	1.2 [1.16–1.24]	8×10^{-28}
15q13.3	rs4779584		0.19	1.23 [1.14–1.34]	5×10^{-7}
10p14	rs10795668-A		0.48	1.12 [1.10–1.16]	3×10^{-13}
8q23.3	rs16892766-A	*EIF3H*	0.07	1.27 [1.20–1.34]	3×10^{-18}
11q23.1	rs3802842-C		0.43	1.11 [1.08–1.15]	6×10^{-10}
16q22.1	rs9929218-A	*CDH1*	0.29	1.1 [1.06–1.12]	1×10^{-8}
19q13.11	rs10411210-C	*RHPN2*	0.90	1.15 [1.10–1.20]	5×10^{-9}
14q22.2	rs4444235-C	*BMP4*	0.46	1.11 [1.08–1.15]	8×10^{-10}
20p12.3	rs961253-A		0.36	1.12 [1.08–1.16]	2×10^{-10}

TABLE 19.4

SOMATIC MUTATIONS IN ONCOGENES AND TUMOR SUPPRESSOR GENES

Gene	Type of Mutation	Frequency of Alterations (%)
Oncogenes		
KRAS	Point mutation (codons 12, 13, 61)	40% (majority at codon 12)
PIK3CA	Point mutations activating kinase activity	14%–35%
BRAF	Point mutation (V600E)	5%–8%
CTNNB1	Point mutation and in-frame deletions (amino-terminus)	~5%
HER-2/ERBB2	Amplification	<5%
Tumor suppressor genes		
p53	Point mutation, LOH	>60% (most are missense mutations)
APC	Small insertion or deletion, point mutation, LOH	>80% (most result in a truncated protein)
SMAD4	LOH, point mutation	60% LOH; 10%–15% missense, nonsense mutations
SMAD2	LOH, point mutation, small deletion,	60% LOH; <5% missense mutations, small deletions
TGF-βRII	Small insertion or deletion	10%–15%; higher (>90%) in MSI-Hi disease
DCC	LOH, insertion, deletion	~60% LOH; 10%–15% microsatellite insertions in intron

LOH, loss of heterozygosity; MSI-Hi, high microsatellite instability.

genome. Addressing the role of TGF-β in CRC, one group of risk polymorphisms on chromosome 18q21 is linked to the *SMAD7* locus.[94] Particularly strong association occurs with the SNP rs6983267 at 8q24.21, which lies in a gene desert near low-risk susceptibility alleles for breast and prostate cancers. Molecular studies indicate that each of the culpable regions acts as a tissue-specific enhancer, controlling expression of the nearest neighboring structural gene, *CMYC*,[95] a highly plausible factor in disease susceptibility. In summary, common predisposition alleles confer some risk of CRC with low penetrance. Their pathophysiologic functions should be studied in greater detail to inform prevention and screening strategies and to determine how risk alleles interact with particular habits or environmental factors.

ONCOGENE AND TUMOR SUPPRESSOR GENE MUTATIONS IN COLORECTAL CANCER PROGRESSION

Building on the foundation established upon loss of the *APC* gatekeeper function, somatic mutations in cellular protooncogenes and tumor suppressor genes contribute cumulatively to the acquisition of malignant properties. The limited spectrum of recurring mutations in CRC provides a context for refined appreciation of the adenoma–carcinoma sequence and points to rational targets for therapy. The most frequent genetic events (Table 19.4) are discussed below, with reference to clinical associations and their impact on cell growth and differentiation.

KRAS, *BRAF*, and *PIK3CA* Oncogene Mutations

The Ras family of small G-proteins transduces growth factor signals and is aberrantly activated in a wide variety of cancers. *KRAS* gene mutations are detected in about 40% of colorectal carcinomas,[96] mostly clustered in codons 12 and 13, with fewer than 10% occurring at codon 61. These mutations can be present in small polyps, and their frequency increases with lesion size.[97] The significance of the same mutations in lesions of low malignant potential, such as hyperplastic polyps or aberrant crypt foci lacking dysplasia, is uncertain.[98] *KRAS* mutation is not required to initiate adenomas but almost certainly contributes to their progression, and disruption of mutant *KRAS* alleles in colon cancer cells impedes growth.[99,100]

Oncogenic *KRAS* mutations have the potential to deregulate several effector pathways for cell

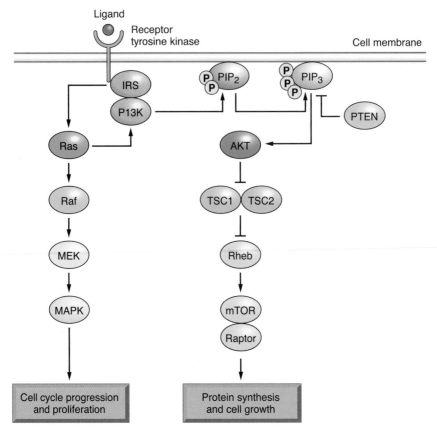

FIGURE 19.3 Signaling pathways, oncogenic mutations, and therapeutic opportunities in colorectal cancer (CRC). It is instructive to consider common genetic alterations in CRC in light of a common canonical outline of signaling through receptor tyrosine kinases, among which the epidermal growth factor receptor is a prime example. *KRAS*, the oncogene mutated in up to 40% of CRCs, signals receptor activation through RAF proteins (including BRAF, which is mutated in 5% to 8% of CRCs) and phosphatidylinositol 3-kinase (PI3K), whose catalytic PIK3CA subunit is mutated in 15% to 20% of CRCs. These transducers in turn activate the intracellular mitogen-activated protein kinase and AKT or mammalian target of rapamycin (mTOR) pathways, respectively. Common mutations hence confer growth factor independence on cells, resulting in dysregulated proliferation, protein synthesis, and metabolism. They also represent promising targets for therapeutic interference with aberrantly activated signaling cascades.

proliferation, survival, and metastasis (Fig. 19.3). Constitutive phosphorylation of extracellular signal-regulated kinases, ERK-1 and ERK2, frequently accompanies *KRAS* mutation, reflecting activation of the mitogen-activated protein kinase (MAPK) pathway. This KRAS-mediated growth factor signaling cascade recruits RAF kinases to the plasma membrane and triggers ERK kinases MEK1 and MEK2 to activate ERK1 and ERK2, which phosphorylate factors that control the G_1-S cell cycle transition, among other substrates.[101] Although other, non-KRAS-mediated growth factor pathways also activate the MAPK cascade, signaling in cancer is most often deregulated through activating mutations in *KRAS* or *BRAF*. *BRAF* is mutated in 5% to 8% of CRCs, especially those associated with MSI-Hi or CIMP.[102,103] The most common

BRAF mutation in colorectal and other cancers such as melanoma, *V599E*, affects a residue within the activation loop of the kinase domain and constitutively activates the kinase function, perhaps as a phosphomimetic.[104] Like mutant KRAS, activated BRAF also phosphorylates MEKs and ERKs, leading to dysregulated growth. Notably, KRAS and BRAF mutations are mutually exclusive in CRC,[102] reinforcing the role of the two oncogenes in a common cellular pathway and possibly reflecting alternative routes to the same end. However, patients with BRAF-mutant CRCs have a worse prognosis than those with KRAS-mutant tumors,[9] indicating the presence of distinctive features.

Besides the MAPK cascade, KRAS signals through the phosphatidylinositol 3-kinase (PI3K) pathway,[105] which phosphorylates the intracellular signaling lipid phosphatidylinositol-4,5-bisphosphate at the 3 position, triggering a cascade that promotes cell growth and survival.[106] Between 15% and 35% of CRCs carry activating mutations in *PIK3CA*, the gene encoding the catalytic p110 subunit of PI3K; most mutations cluster in exons 9 and 20 and seem to arise late in the adenoma–carcinoma sequence, perhaps coincident with invasion.[107] Curiously, although both PI3K and BRAF act downstream of KRAS, only the *BRAF-KRAS* mutant pair is mutually exclusive; *PIK3CA* mutations appear in nearly 10% of KRAS-mutant CRCs, implying that activation of both oncogenes may not be redundant. One reason could be that mutant KRAS activates PI3K signaling inefficiently[108]; more likely, oncogenic signaling pathways are less strictly linear than is convenient to depict. Indeed, the overtly parallel streams of KRAS signaling through RAF-MEK and PI3K (Fig. 19.3) interact extensively with one another and, in particular, both streams modulate mTOR, which coordinates cell growth with nutrient responses.[109] Such considerations notwithstanding, the recurrence of *KRAS*, *BRAF*, and *PIK3CA* mutations in CRC, at a collective frequency that rivals growth factor pathway aberrations in any carcinoma, appropriately places these oncogenes and their effectors at the center of research and drug development efforts.

The *p53* Tumor Suppressor

Allelic loss of chromosome 17p is observed in three of four colorectal carcinomas but fewer than 10% of adenomatous polyps.[97] The remaining *p53* allele is inactivated in most tumors with 17p loss of heterozygosity (LOH), most often at codons 175, 245, 248, 273, or 282.[110] LOH of 17p and mutations in *p53* thus appear to arise during the transition from adenoma to carcinoma, perhaps facilitating progression. When faced with stress from DNA damage, hypoxia, reduced nutrient access, and aneuploidy, cells with intact *p53* function undergo cell cycle arrest and apoptosis. The loss of *p53* may allow cells to overcome such barriers to tumor survival and progression.

Chromosome 18q Loss of Heterozygosity

LOH of chromosome 18q is rare in adenomas, except for large villous adenomas, observed in over 60% of primary CRCs, and present in nearly all liver metastases from colorectal primary tumors lacking MSI.[111] This sequence implicates loss of one or more genes on chromosome 18q in disease progression. Recent studies[112] challenge early ideas that 18q LOH conferred a poor prognosis.[113] The minimal common region of LOH on 18q21 contains two candidate tumor suppressor genes.[114] One of these genes, *SMAD4 (DPC4)*, is deleted in about one-third of cases and the remainder show loss of the other candidate gene, *DCC* (deleted in colorectal cancer), which encodes a cell surface receptor for the netrin family of axonal guidance proteins. *SMAD4/DPC4* and *SMAD2* are implicated as positive and negative regulators of TGF-β signaling, respectively, and lie close together on chromosome 18q. Somatic *SMAD4* deletions or localized mutations are present in 10% to 15% of CRCs, with 18q LOH and germline mutations noted in some FJP kindreds[115]; but *SMAD2* is somatically inactivated in fewer than 5% of CRCs.[116] Although *DCC* messenger RNA and protein are lost in more than 50% of CRCs,[117] few specific *DCC* coding mutations are known. Together with the low frequency of *SMAD4* or *SMAD2* mutations in 18q-deficient tumors, these findings suggest a complex, multifactorial basis for selection of 18q LOH in CRC.

INFREQUENT CHANGES AND CURRENT VIEWS OF THE MUTATIONAL LANDSCAPE OF COLORECTAL CANCER

Few cellular oncogenes besides *KRAS*, *BRAF*, and *PIK3CA* are common targets of point mutations in CRC (Table 19.4). Sequencing of the kinase domains in 133 tyrosine kinase (TK) and TK-like genes and 340 serine-threonine kinase (STK) genes revealed few recurrent nonsynonymous somatic mutations, including a handful in the *NTRK2*, *NTRK3*, and *FES* receptor TK genes[118] and the STK genes *MAPK24* and *MYLK2*.[119] Analysis of tyrosine phosphatases similarly identified scattered mutations of uncertain pathogenic significance in up to a quarter of CRCs.[120] In principle, increased expression by epigenetic mechanisms or gene amplification can have the same effect as activating point mutations, but oncogenes such as *HER-2* (*ErbB2*), *MYC*, *MYB*, and *CCND1* are amplified in fewer than 5% of cases in aggregate.

Most studies summarized in this chapter suffer from biased or opportunistic testing of genes, gene families, and pathways. To avoid such bias, groups have assessed copy number alterations (CNAs) by array hybridization and begun to sequence all exons and full genomes. Analysis of more than 13,000 genes in 11 CRCs revealed a substantially larger number of mutations than expected, with a conservative average estimate of 81 per tumor, but few of these mutations recur frequently and most make small, if any, contribution to the neoplastic process.[121] The results are nevertheless informative because they reveal, for example, substantive differences in the nature of mutations in different tumor types, with CRCs showing a genomewide bias toward C:G to T:A transitions at 5′-CpG-3′ sites and a lower frequency of mutations in 5′-TpC-3′ dinucleotides than observed in breast cancer.[121] Such findings may find value in linking specific environmental contributors to the mutational spectrum in initiation and progression of disease. For nearly half of the 50 CNAs—28 amplifications and 22 deletions—identified in one study, 15 of them were recurrent and encompassed fewer than 12 genes[122] and were also detected in other cancers, presumably reflecting selection for common genetic events. A subsequent study found that CRCs carry an average of 17 genes that are deleted or amplified to 12 or more copies per cell.[123] Pathways controlling cell adhesion, signaling, DNA topology, and cell cycle were most commonly affected by these changes or by point mutations, confirming that CRCs reflect disturbances in selected pathways for replicative and tissue homeostasis. Although affected cellular processes may be common to most cancers, the specific molecular defects in CRC identify the best targets for rational, directed therapy.

Prognostic and Predictive Value of Molecular Properties and Tumor Genotypes

Phenotypes and specific genetic alterations in a cancer can hold useful clues about clinical behavior, prognosis, and response to therapy. Aneuploidy and tetraploidy confer a poor prognosis and MSI-Hi imparts a relatively favorable outcome in early stage CRC.[124] Benefit from adjuvant 5-fluorouracil monotherapy may be confined to patients with MSS tumors.[125,126] As nearly all CRCs have constitutive Wnt pathway activity, this factor alone has limited prognostic value, and outcomes seem unaffected by whether Wnt activity was stimulated by APC or CTNNB1 mutations. The presence of KRAS or BRAF mutations and possibly also PIK3CA mutation or loss of PTEN expression predicts a lack of response to EGFR monoclonal antibodies.[8,127] These observations are important because they direct treatment decisions and because, unlike acute leukemia or breast cancer, CRC had previously resisted subgrouping on the basis of specific genetic alterations. For example, mutations in the two most frequently affected oncogenes, KRAS or PIK3CA, seem not to impact survival in stage III or IV disease treated with current drug regimens.[9,128] Patients with metastatic BRAF-mutant disease have especially low survival and respond poorly to current chemotherapy regimens.[9]

Mouse Models of Colorectal Cancer

The laboratory mouse has immense value in genetic analysis of CRC. The most informative mouse line, *multiple intestinal neoplasia (Min)*, carries a mutagen-induced nonsense mutation in the murine homolog of APC and phenocopies human FAP with respect to intestinal adenomatosis,[129] although species' differences place the burden mainly in the small intestine instead of the colon. APC^Min mice serve as a cornerstone for genetic analysis of intestinal tumors and deregulated Wnt signaling. Modifications of the murine APC locus influence disease phenotypes, as detailed in other reviews[130]; the D716 allele increases the number of adenomas, all showing LOH of the wild type copy,[131] whereas the APC^1638N mutation results in fewer adenomas, more of which appear in the colon.[132] Apc^Pirc rats carry a stop codon at position 1137 and develop more than half the tumors in the colon, similar to humans.[133] Deletion of the N-terminal degradation domain of β-catenin also stabilizes the protein and produces widespread intestinal polyposis in mice.[134] Expression of Kras^G12D or Kras^G12V in the intestinal epithelium of otherwise intact mice has subtle consequences on cell signaling and proliferation, whereas expression in mutant Apc backgrounds expands progenitor cell numbers and hastens adenoma progression,[135] modeling the sequence of mutations in human colon cancer. Finally, the *in vivo* requirements of each MMR gene have been analyzed by introducing inactivating mutations in all murine *mutS* and *mutL* homologs.[136] These mice generally develop lymphomas more often than intestinal tumors, and some mutants show neither MSI nor intestinal tumors, highlighting species differences. Nevertheless, the defects point to an essential role for some MMR genes in meiosis and underscore the importance of MMR in protecting cells from mutation and malignancy.

Selected References

The full list of references for this chapter appears in the online version.

1. Noffsinger AE. Serrated polyps and colorectal cancer: new pathway to malignancy. *Annu Rev Pathol* 2009;4:343.
3. Levin B, Lieberman DA, McFarland B, et al. Screening and surveillance for the early detection of colorectal cancer and adenomatous polyps, 2008: a joint guideline from the American Cancer Society, the US Multi-Society Task Force on Colorectal Cancer, and the American College of Radiology. *Gastroenterology* 2008;134:1570.
5. Jones S, Chen WD, Parmigiani G, et al. Comparative lesion sequencing provides insights into tumor evolution. *Proc Natl Acad Sci U S A* 2008;105:4283.

6. Vogelstein B, Kinzler KW. Cancer genes and the pathways they control. *Nat Med* 2004;10:789.

8. Van Cutsem E, Kohne CH, Hitre E, et al. Cetuximab and chemotherapy as initial treatment for metastatic colorectal cancer. *N Engl J Med* 2009;360:1408.

9. Souglakos J, Philips J, Wang R, et al. Prognostic and predictive value of common mutations for treatment response and survival in patients with metastatic colorectal cancer. *Br J Cancer* 2009;101:465.

12. Ionov Y, Peinado MA, Malkhosyan S, Shibata D, Perucho M. Ubiquitous somatic mutations in simple repeated sequences reveal a new mechanism for colonic carcinogenesis. *Nature* 1993;363:558.

14. Goelz SE, Vogelstein B, Hamilton SR, Feinberg AP. Hypomethylation of DNA from benign and malignant human colon neoplasms. *Science* 1985;228:187.

17. Eden A, Gaudet F, Waghmare A, Jaenisch R. Chromosomal instability and tumors promoted by DNA hypomethylation. *Science* 2003;300:455.

20. Toyota M, Ahuja N, Ohe-Toyota M, et al. CpG island methylator phenotype in colorectal cancer. *Proc Natl Acad Sci U S A* 1999;96:8681.

22. Jess T, Loftus EV Jr, Velayos FS, et al. Risk of intestinal cancer in inflammatory bowel disease: a population-based study from Olmsted county, Minnesota. *Gastroenterology* 2006;130:1039.

34. Morin PJ, Sparks AB, Korinek V, et al. Activation of beta-catenin-Tcf signaling in colon cancer by mutations in beta-catenin or APC. *Science* 1997;275:1787.

36. Sansom OJ, Reed KR, Hayes AJ, et al. Loss of Apc in vivo immediately perturbs Wnt signaling, differentiation, and migration. *Genes Dev* 2004;18:1385.

37. Clevers H. Wnt/beta-catenin signaling in development and disease. *Cell* 2006;127:469.

41. Barker N, Ridgway RA, van Es JH, et al. Crypt stem cells as the cells-of-origin of intestinal cancer. *Nature* 2009;457:608.

42. van de Wetering M, Sancho E, Verweij C, et al. The beta-catenin/TCF-4 complex imposes a crypt progenitor phenotype on colorectal cancer cells. *Cell* 2002;111:241.

43. He TC, Sparks AB, Rago C, et al. Identification of c-MYC as a target of the APC pathway. *Science* 1998;281:1509.

44. Sansom OJ, Meniel VS, Muncan V, et al. Myc deletion rescues Apc deficiency in the small intestine. *Nature* 2007;446:676.

48. Vasen HF, Watson P, Mecklin JP, Lynch HT. New clinical criteria for hereditary nonpolyposis colorectal cancer (HNPCC, Lynch syndrome) proposed by the International Collaborative group on HNPCC. *Gastroenterology* 1999;116:1453.

50. Fishel R, Kolodner RD. Identification of mismatch repair genes and their role in the development of cancer. *Curr Opin Genet Dev* 1995;5:382.

53. Umar A, Boland CR, Terdiman JP, et al. Revised Bethesda guidelines for hereditary nonpolyposis colorectal cancer (Lynch syndrome) and microsatellite instability. *J Natl Cancer Inst* 2004;96:261.

57. Markowitz S, Wang J, Myeroff L, et al. Inactivation of the type II TGF-beta receptor in colon cancer cells with microsatellite instability. *Science* 1995;268:1336.

62. Huang J, Papadopoulos N, McKinley AJ, et al. APC mutations in colorectal tumors with mismatch repair deficiency. *Proc Natl Acad Sci U S A* 1996;93:9049.

63. Sieber OM, Lipton L, Crabtree M, et al. Multiple colorectal adenomas, classic adenomatous polyposis, and germline mutations in MYH. *N Engl J Med* 2003;348:791.

65. Thibodeau SN, French AJ, Cunningham JM, et al. Microsatellite instability in colorectal cancer: different mutator phenotypes and the principal involvement of hMLH1. *Cancer Res* 1998;58:1713.

66. Liu B, Nicolaides NC, Markowitz S, et al. Mismatch repair gene defects in sporadic colorectal cancers with microsatellite instability. *Nat Genet* 1995;9:48.

69. Weisenberger DJ, Siegmund KD, Campan M, et al. CpG island methylator phenotype underlies sporadic microsat-

ellite instability and is tightly associated with BRAF mutation in colorectal cancer. *Nat Genet* 2006;38:787.

73. Sweet K, Willis J, Zhou XP, et al. Molecular classification of patients with unexplained hamartomatous and hyperplastic polyposis. *J Am Med Assoc* 2005;294:2465.

79. Hemminki A, Markie D, Tomlinson I, et al. A serine/threonine kinase gene defective in Peutz-Jeghers syndrome. *Nature* 1998;391:184.

81. Shaw RJ, Bardeesy N, Manning BD, et al. The LKB1 tumor suppressor negatively regulates mTOR signaling. *Cancer Cell* 2004;6:91.

82. Rustgi AK. The genetics of hereditary colon cancer. *Genes Dev* 2007;21:2525.

83. Liaw D, Marsh DJ, Li J, et al. Germline mutations of the PTEN gene in Cowden disease, an inherited breast and thyroid cancer syndrome. *Nat Genet* 1997;16:64.

85. Goel A, Arnold CN, Niedzwiecki D, et al. Frequent inactivation of PTEN by promoter hypermethylation in microsatellite instability–high sporadic colorectal cancers. *Cancer Res* 2004;64:3014.

87. Slattery ML, Fitzpatrick FA. Convergence of hormones, inflammation, and energy-related factors: a novel pathway of cancer etiology. *Cancer Prev Res* 2009;2:922.

90. Wiesner GL, Daley D, Lewis S, et al. A subset of familial colorectal neoplasia kindreds linked to chromosome 9q22.2-31.2. *Proc Natl Acad Sci U S A* 2003;100:12961.

92. Tomlinson I, Webb E, Carvajal-Carmona L, et al. A genome-wide association scan of tag SNPs identifies a susceptibility variant for colorectal cancer at 8q24.21. *Nat Genet* 2007;39:984.

95. Ahmadiyeh N, Pomerantz MM, Grisanzio C, et al. 8q24 prostate, breast, and colon cancer risk loci show tissue-specific long-range interaction with MYC. *Proc Natl Acad Sci U S A* 2010;107:9742.

96. Bos JL, Fearon ER, Hamilton SR, et al. Prevalence of ras gene mutations in human colorectal cancers. *Nature* 1987;327:293.

97. Vogelstein B, Fearon ER, Hamilton SR, et al. Genetic alterations during colorectal-tumor development. *N Engl J Med* 1988;319:525.

101. Downward J. Targeting RAS signalling pathways in cancer therapy. *Nat Rev Cancer* 2003;3:11.

102. Rajagopalan H, Bardelli A, Lengauer C, et al. Tumorigenesis: RAF/RAS oncogenes and mismatch-repair status. *Nature* 2002;418:934.

104. Davies H, Bignell GR, Cox C, et al. Mutations of the BRAF gene in human cancer. *Nature* 2002;417:949.

107. Samuels Y, Wang Z, Bardelli A, et al. High frequency of mutations of the PIK3CA gene in human cancers. *Science* 2004;304:554.

110. Baker SJ, Fearon ER, Nigro JM, et al. Chromosome 17 deletions and p53 gene mutations in colorectal carcinomas. *Science* 1989;244:217.

115. Howe JR, Roth S, Ringold JC, et al. Mutations in the SMAD4/DPC4 gene in juvenile polyposis. *Science* 1998;280:1086.

121. Sjoblom T, Jones S, Wood LD, et al. The consensus coding sequences of human breast and colorectal cancers. *Science* 2006;314:268.

123. Leary RJ, Lin JC, Cummins J, et al. Integrated analysis of homozygous deletions, focal amplifications, and sequence alterations in breast and colorectal cancers. *Proc Natl Acad Sci U S A* 2008;105:16224.

127. Sartore-Bianchi A, Di Nicolantonio F, Nichelatti M, et al. Multi-determinants analysis of molecular alterations for predicting clinical benefit to EGFR-targeted monoclonal antibodies in colorectal cancer. *PLoS One* 2009;4:e7287.

129. Moser AR, Pitot HC, Dove WF. A dominant mutation that predisposes to multiple intestinal neoplasia in the mouse. *Science* 1990;247:322.

134. Harada N, Tamai Y, Ishikawa T, et al. Intestinal polyposis in mice with a dominant stable mutation of the beta-catenin gene. *EMBO J* 1999;18:5931.

MOLECULAR BIOLOGY OF INDIVIDUAL CANCERS

CHAPTER 20 KIDNEY CANCER

W. MARSTON LINEHAN AND LAURA S. SCHMIDT

Kidney cancer or renal cell carcinoma (RCC) affects more than 209,000 people annually worldwide, resulting in 102,000 deaths each year.[1] A variety of risk factors, including obesity, hypertension, tobacco smoking, and certain occupational exposures, have been shown to increase one's risk for developing RCC. Our current understanding of the molecular genetics of kidney cancer has come from studies of families with an inherited predisposition to develop renal tumors. Individuals with a family history of RCC have a 2.5-fold greater chance for developing renal cancer during their lifetimes[2] and comprise about 4% of all RCC.

Kidney cancer is not a single disease but is classified into tumor subtypes based on histology.[3] Over the past two decades, studies of families with inherited renal carcinoma enabled the identification of five inherited renal cancer syndromes, and their predisposing genes (Table 20.1), which implicate diverse biological pathways in renal cancer tumorigenesis.[4] The von Hippel-Lindau (*VHL*) tumor suppressor gene was discovered in 1993.[5] Subsequently, activating mutations were identified in the *MET* protooncogene in patients with hereditary papillary renal carcinoma (HPRC).[6] More recently, the gene for Krebs cycle enzyme fumarate hydratase (FH), responsible for hereditary leiomyomatosis and renal cell carcinoma (HLRCC),[7] and *FLCN*, the gene for Birt-Hogg-Dubé (BHD) syndrome, were identified.[8] Germline mutations in the gene encoding another Krebs cycle enzyme, succinate dehydrogenase subunit B (SDHB), have been found in patients with familial renal cancer.[9] Discovery of the genes for the inherited forms of renal cancer has enabled the development of diagnostic genetic tests for presymptomatic diagnosis and improved prognosis for at-risk individuals.

VON HIPPEL-LINDAU

VHL is an autosomal dominantly inherited multisystem neoplastic disorder that is characterized by clear cell renal tumors, retinal angiomas, central nervous system hemangioblastomas, tumors of the adrenal gland (pheochromocytoma), endolymphatic sac and pancreatic islet cell, and cysts in the pancreas and kidney. VHL occurs in about 1 in 36,000 and develops during the second to fourth decades of life with nearly 70% penetrance by age 60. Bilateral, multifocal renal tumors with clear cell histology develop in 25% to 45% of VHL patients[10] that can have metastatic potential when they reach 3.0 cm.

Genetics of Von Hippel-Lindau

Loss of heterozygosity (LOH) on chromosome 3p in clear cell renal tumors suggested the location of a predisposing gene for RCC.[11] Positional cloning in VHL kindreds defined the disease locus to chromosome 3p25-26, leading to the cloning of the *VHL* gene in 1993.[5] *VHL* is a tumor suppressor gene in which both copies of *VHL* must be inactivated for tumor initiation. Germline *VHL* mutations that predispose to VHL encompass the entire mutation spectrum, including large deletions, protein-truncating mutations, and missense mutations that exchange the amino acid in the VHL protein. Over 1,000 different *VHL* mutations have been identified in more than 945 VHL families worldwide. Mutations are located throughout the entire gene with the exception of the first 35 residues in the acidic domain.[10] With the development of new methods for detection of deletions, *VHL* mutation detection rates are approaching 100%.[12,13] VHL subclasses based on the predisposition to develop pheochromocytomas, and high or low risk of RCC are established with interesting genotype-phenotype associations.[14]

Gene Mutated in Renal Cancer Families with Chromosome 3p Translocations

In 1979 Cohen et al.[15] described a family with a constitutional t(3;8)(p14;q24) balanced translocation that cosegregated with bilateral multifocal clear cell renal tumors. Loss of the derivative chromosome carrying the 3p segment and differ-

TABLE 20.1

HEREDITARY RENAL CANCER SYNDROMES

Syndrome	Chromosome Location	Predisposing Gene	Histology	Frequency of Gene Mutations	
				Germline (Ref.)	Sporadic RCC (Ref.)
Von Hippel-Lindau (VHL)	3p25	VHL	Clear cell	100% (12)	92% (20)
Hereditary papillary renal carcinoma type 1 (HPRC)	7q31	MET	Type 1 papillary	100% (6,25,26)	13% (29)
Birt-Hogg-Dubé syndrome (BHD)	17p11.2	FLCN	Chromophobe, hybrid	90% (47)	11% (56)
Hereditary leiomyomatosis and renal cell carcinoma (HLRCC)	1q42–43	FH	Type 2 papillary	93% (71)	TBD
Succinate dehydrogenase (SDH)-associated familial renal cancer	1p35–36 11q23	SDHB SDHD	Clear cell, chromophobe	TBD	TBD

ent somatic mutations in the remaining copy of VHL were identified in the tumors from this translocation family. Based on these data Schmidt et al.[16] proposed a three-step tumorigenesis model in 3p translocation families: (1) inheritance of the constitutional translocation, (2) loss of the derivative chromosome bearing 3p25, and (3) mutation of the remaining copy of VHL, resulting in inactivation of both copies of VHL and predisposing to clear cell RCC. A number of chromosome 3 translocation families have been described.[17,18] Loss of the derivative chromosome concomitant with somatic mutation of the remaining copy of VHL in these families provides strong evidence for the three-step tumorigenesis model and implicates VHL loss in clear cell RCC that develops in chromosome 3 translocation kindreds.

Gene for Clear Cell Kidney Cancer

Mutation of the VHL gene is found in a high percentage of tumors from patients with clear cell kidney cancer.[19] Nickerson et al.[20] recently identified mutation or methylation of the VHL gene in 92% of clear cell kidney cancers. VHL gene mutation is not found in papillary, chromophobe, collecting duct, medullary, or other types of kidney cancer.

Function of the VHL Protein

The most well-understood function of the VHL protein pVHL is the substrate recognition site for the hypoxia-inducible factor (HIF)-α family of transcription factors targeting them for ubiquitin-mediated proteasomal degradation (Fig. 20.1).[14] pVHL binds through its α domain to elongin C and forms an E3 ubiquitin ligase complex with elongin B, cullin-2, and Rbx-1. Under normal oxygen conditions, HIF-α becomes hydroxylated on critical prolines by a family of HIF prolyl hydroxylases (PHD) that require 2-oxoglutarate, molecular oxygen, ascorbic acid, and iron as cofactors. pVHL then binds to hydroxylated HIF-α through its β domain, targeting HIF-α for ubiquitylation by the E3 ligase complex. Under hypoxic conditions when PHDs are unable to function or when pVHL is mutated, altering its binding to HIF-α or elongin C binding, HIF-α cannot be recognized by pVHL. HIF-α accumulates and transcriptionally up-regulates a number of genes important in blood vessel development (EPO, VEGF), cell proliferation (PDGFβ, TGFα), and glucose metabolism (GLUT-1).[14] HIF-α dependent up-regulation of target genes involved in neovascularization provides an explanation for the increased vascularity of central nervous system (CNS) hemangioblastomas and clear cell renal tumors in VHL. Germline VHL mutations frequently occur in the pVHL binding domains for HIF-α and elongin C.[21] HIF-2α, rather than HIF-1α, stabilization appears to be critical for renal tumor development.[22,23] Additional HIF-dependent and HIF-independent functions for pVHL have been reported.[10,14]

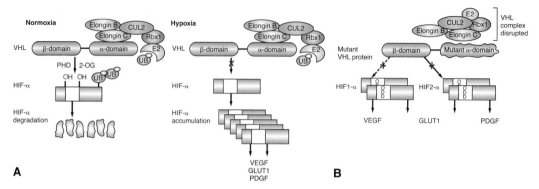

FIGURE 20.1 The von Hippel-Lindau (VHL) E3 ubiquitin ligase complex targets hypoxia-inducible factor (HIF)-α for ubiquitin-mediated degradation. **A:** Under normal oxygen conditions, HIF-α is hydroxylated on critical prolines by HIF prolyl hydroxylase (PHD), requiring molecular oxygen, 2-oxoglutarate, and iron as cosubstrates. The VHL protein (pVHL) can then recognize and bind hydroxylated HIF-α, enabling its ubiquitylation by the VHL E3 ligase complex and degradation by the proteasome. Under hypoxic conditions, PHD is unable to function properly, pVHL cannot recognize HIF-α, and HIF-α accumulates, leading to up-regulation of HIF-target genes (*VEGF*, *GLUT1*, *PDGF*) that support tumor growth and neovascularization. **B:** When *VHL* is mutated and pVHL is unable to bind HIF-α, HIF-α stabilization leads to transcriptional up-regulation of HIF target genes. (From ref. 4, with permission.)

HEREDITARY PAPILLARY RENAL CARCINOMA TYPE 1

HPRC is an autosomal dominant hereditary cancer syndrome in which affected individuals are at risk for the development of multifocal, bilateral papillary type 1 kidney cancer.[24] HPRC develops in the fifth and sixth decades with age-dependent penetrance estimated at 67% by 60 years of age[25]; however, early onset HPRC has been described.[26] This rare disorder has been reported in less than 40 kindreds worldwide.[24]

Genetics of Hereditary Papillary Renal Carcinoma: *MET* Protooncogene

In 1995 Zbar et al.[27] described ten families in which multifocal, bilateral papillary renal tumors were inherited in an autosomal dominant fashion and suggested that these families might represent a hereditary counterpart to sporadic papillary tumors. Schmidt et al.[6] localized the HPRC disease locus to chromosome 7q31.1-34 by linkage analysis. Since trisomy of chromosome 7 was described as a hallmark feature of papillary renal tumors,[28] a gain-of-function oncogene seemed a likely candidate disease gene; in fact, germline missense mutations were identified in the tyrosine kinase domain of the *MET* protooncogene located at 7q31 in affected HPRC family members.[6] Mutations of the *MET* gene have been detected in 13% of sporadic papillary renal tumors.[6,29] Further studies to determine the role of *MET* and related genes in papillary type 1 kidney cancer are currently under way.

Hereditary Papillary Renal Carcinoma: Functional Consequences of *MET* Mutations

The *MET* protooncogene encodes the hepatocyte growth factor/scatter factor (HGF/SF) receptor tyrosine kinase. Binding of ligand HGF to MET triggers autophosphorylation of critical tyrosines in the intracellular tyrosine kinase domain, subsequent phosphorylation of tyrosines in the multifunctional docking site, and recruitment of a variety of transducers of downstream signaling cascades that regulate cellular programs, leading to cell growth, branching morphogenesis, differentiation, and "invasive growth."[30] Although MET overexpression has been demonstrated in a number of epithelial cancers,[31] HPRC was the first cancer syndrome for which germline *MET* mutations were identified. The missense *MET* mutations in HPRC are constitutively activating without ligand stimulation, display oncogenic potential *in vitro*,[32,33] and are predicted by molecular modeling to stabilize active MET kinase.[34] Nonrandom duplication of the chromosome 7 bearing the mutant *MET* allele was demonstrated in papillary renal tumors from HPRC patients[35] and may represent the second step in HPRC tumor pathogenesis. The presence of two copies of mutant *MET* may give kidney cells a proliferative growth advantage and lead to tumor progression.

XP11.2 TRANSLOCATION RENAL CELL CANCER

Xp11.2 translocation renal cell carcinomas, typically presenting with papillary architecture and clear or eosinophilic cytoplasm, are uncommon tumors often detected in young children and adolescents. Translocations involving Xp11.2 and 1q 21.2 associated with sporadic papillary renal carcinoma, and first described in a 2-year-old child,[36] generate a fusion between a novel gene, PRCC, and the basic helix-loop-helix family transcription factor gene, TFE3.[37] The encoded fusion protein, PRCC-TFE3, acts as a stronger transcriptional activator than native TFE3, and loss of the majority of native TFE3 transcripts is observed in these tumors. This deregulation of normal TFE3 transcriptional control caused by the chromosomal translocation may be important to the development of sporadic papillary renal cell carcinoma.[38,39] Xp11.2 translocation renal cell carcinomas involving at least five different TFE3 gene fusions and resulting in deregulation of TFE3 transcription activity have been described, including the identical ASPL-TFE3 fusion associated with alveolar soft part sarcoma.[40] Tsuda et al.[41] have shown that these TFE3 fusion proteins are strong transcriptional activators of the MET gene, resulting in inappropriate MET-directed cell proliferation and invasive growth. Given the physiologic consequences of TFE3 fusion protein expression, therapeutic targeting of MET may be an effective treatment for Xp11.2 translocation renal tumors.

BIRT-HOGG-DUBÉ SYNDROME

BHD syndrome is a rare autosomal-dominant inherited cancer syndrome characterized by benign tumors of the hair follicle (fibrofolliculoma), pulmonary cysts and spontaneous pneumothorax, and a sevenfold increased risk for renal cancers.[42–45] Fibrofolliculomas and lung cysts are the most common manifestations (>85% of BHD patients).[46–48] Renal tumors with variable histologies develop in about 30% of BHD-affected individuals (median age 48 to 50 years), most frequently chromophobe renal carcinoma and hybrid oncocytic tumors.[46,49] Metastases may develop from BHD renal tumors, but they are uncommon.

Genetics of Birt-Hogg-Dubé: Folliculin Gene

Linkage analysis performed in BHD kindreds led to localization of the disease locus to the short arm of chromosome 17[50,51] and the identification of the BHD gene, FLCN.[8] Almost all BHD-associated

FLCN mutations are predicted to truncate the BHD protein, folliculin, including insertion or deletion, nonsense, and splice-site mutations,[8,46,47,52] but recently several missense mutations located in conserved amino acid residues have been described.[47,53] The mutation detection rate in several large BHD cohorts approached 90%, and germline mutations were distributed throughout the entire length of the FLCN gene with no clear genotype-phenotype correlations.[46,47,54] Vocke et al.[55] identified second "hit" somatic mutations or LOH in 70% of renal tumors from BHD patients, supporting a role for FLCN as a tumor suppressor gene that predisposes to renal tumors when both copies are inactivated. Gad et al.[56] detected FLCN mutations in 11% of chromophobe renal cell carcinomas; others found infrequent FLCN mutations in other histologic variants of RCC.[57–59] Further studies are currently in progress to evaluate the role of FLCN and related genes in chromophobe kidney cancer.

Function of the Birt-Hogg-Dubé Protein, Folliculin

The function of the BHD protein, FLCN, is currently under investigation. Baba et al.[60] identified a novel folliculin interacting protein, FNIP1, and showed that FNIP1 interacts with the γ subunit of 5' adenosine monophosphate (AMP)-activated protein kinase (AMPK), an energy sensor in cells that negatively regulates mammalian target of rapamycin (mTOR), the master switch for protein translation and cell proliferation, through TSC1/2.[61,62] A second folliculin interacting protein, FNIP2, was subsequently identified that displayed similar biochemical properties to FNIP1.[63,64] FLCN, through FNIP1/2, may play a role in regulation of the AMPK-TSC1/2-mTOR signaling pathway (Fig. 20.2). Published data supporting mTOR activation[65,66] as well as mTOR inhibition[67–69] as a consequence of FLCN inactivation in in vivo models and BHD renal tumors has led to the hypothesis that the mechanism by which FLCN interacts with and modulates mTOR is context dependent.[68]

HEREDITARY LEIOMYOMATOSIS AND RENAL CELL CARCINOMA

HLRCC is an autosomal dominantly inherited disorder that predisposes to the development of skin and uterine leiomyomas and an aggressive type 2 papillary renal carcinoma. Fewer than 150 HLRCC families have been reported worldwide.[70,71] Renal tumors, which are often unilateral and solitary,[70,72] may develop with early age of onset in 15% to 62% of affected individuals[70,71] and can be aggressive, metastasize, and cause death within 5 years of diagnosis.

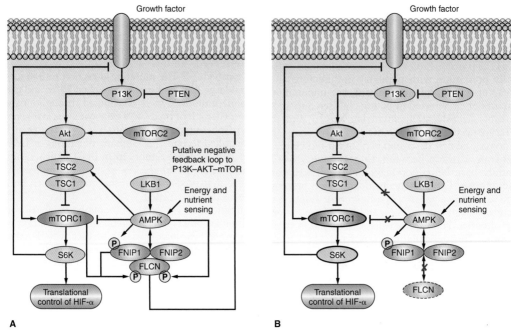

FIGURE 20.2 The putative Birt-Hogg-Dubé gene (*FLCN*) pathway. **A:** *FLCN* binds through FNIP1/2 to adenosine monophosphate (AMP)-activated protein kinase (AMPK) and may become phosphorylated by AMPK or by a rapamycin-sensitive kinase (i.e., mammalian target of rapamycin [mTOR]). **B:** When *FLCN* is inactivated and, presumably, FLCN protein is absent, mTOR is dysregulated, potentially driving kidney tumor formation in BHD patients. (From ref. 4, with permission.)

Genetics of Hereditary Leiomyomatosis and Renal Cell Carcinoma: Fumarate Hydratase Gene

Linkage localized the HLRCC disease locus to chromosome 1q42-43,[73] but an association with renal cancer was not appreciated until Launonen et al.[74] demonstrated linkage to chromosome 1q in two Finnish MCUL kindreds with solitary, highly aggressive papillary type 2 renal tumors. The disorder was renamed *hereditary leiomyomatosis and renal cell carcinoma* and the locus was subsequently mapped to a 1.6Mb region of 1q42. Germline mutations were identified in the fumarate hydratase (*FH*) gene, a Krebs cycle enzyme that converts fumarate to malate in HLRCC-affected family members.[7] *FH* mutations in HLRCC include missense, frameshift, nonsense, and splice-site mutations as well as partial and complete gene deletions.[70,72,75,76] Missense mutations are most common (57%) and occur mainly at evolutionarily conserved residues.[72,75,76] Mutations are found throughout the entire length of the *FH* gene excluding exon 1, which encodes a mitochondrial signal peptide, and no clear genotype–phenotype associations have been reported.[70] *FH* acts as a classic tumor suppressor gene with loss or somatic mutation of the wild type *FH* allele at high frequency in renal tumors and skin and uterine leiomyomata.[7] *FH* mutations are rarely detected in sporadic uterine and skin leiomyomata or sporadic RCC.[77]

Functional Consequences of Fumarate Hydratase Mutations

FH mutations reduce FH activity by 20% to 80%[7,75,78] in lymphoblastoid cell lines from HLRCC patients. HLRCC-associated missense mutations significantly lowered FH activity compared with truncating mutations,[75] suggesting that mutant FH monomers might act in a dominant negative manner to alter proper conformation of FH tetramers. Loss of FH activity in HLRCC leads to accumulation of fumarate and, to a lesser extent, succinate, due to a block in the Krebs cycle.[79,80] Pollard et al.[79] have confirmed that the accumulation of fumarate and succinate resulted in elevation of HIF-1α and HIF-target genes (*VEGF, BNIP*), and increased microvessel density[81] in HLRCC-associated uterine fibroids. Isaacs et al.[80] showed that stabilization of HIF-1α resulted from competitive inhibition of the HIF PHD cosubstrate,

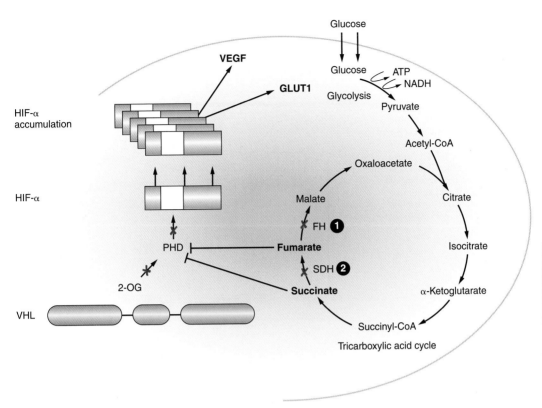

FIGURE 20.3 Fumarate hydratase (FH) and succinate dehydrogenase (SDH) deficient kidney cancer. *FH* and *SDH* subunit *B* and *D* mutations reduce FH and SDH enzyme activity, leading to the accumulation of fumarate and succinate, which inhibits hypoxia-inducible factor (HIF) prolyl hydroxylase (PHD) by competitive inhibition of 2-oxoglutarate (2-OG). Consequently, HIF-α is not hydroxylated, not recognized by pVHL, and accumulates. This pseudohypoxia is associated with the development of aggressive tumors that develop in hereditary leiomyomatosis and renal cell carcinoma (HLRCC) and SDH-familial renal cancer. (From ref. 4, with permission.)

2-oxoglutarate, by fumarate accumulation, leading to abrogation of PHD function and release of HIF-1α from proteasomal degradation. This pseudohypoxic drive, resulting from loss of FH activity, HIF-1α stabilization, and up-regulation of HIF-inducible genes explains the aggressive nature of HLRCC-associated renal tumors (Fig. 20.3). Recently Sudarshan et al.[82] demonstrated that *FH* mutations in an HLRCC-derived cell line led to glucose-mediated generation of reactive oxygen species (ROS) and ROS-dependent HIF-1α stabilization, supporting an alternate mechanism by which pseudohypoxic drive could support renal tumorigenesis in HLRCC.

FAMILIAL RENAL CANCER: SUCCINATE DEHYDROGENASE GENE

Bilateral multifocal renal tumors with early onset (<40 years of age) have been reported in the set-

ting of hereditary head and neck paragangliomas (HPGL) and adrenal or extra-adrenal pheochromocytomas.[9] Most frequently, clear cell RCC develops; however, chromophobe RCC, papillary type 2 RCC, and renal oncocytoma have been described.[83–85]

Genetics of Familial Renal Cancer: Succinate Dehydrogenase Subunit B and D Mutations

Germline mutations in the gene encoding succinate dehydrogenase subunit D (SDHD) were initially associated with HPGL and later with familial and sporadic pheochromocytomas.[86,87] Subsequently, inactivating mutations in *SDHB* were found in kindreds with familial pheochromocytoma only and with HPGL and one case of sporadic pheochromocytoma.[88] Later early onset clear cell RCC was diagnosed in two individuals with HPGL and germline *SDHB* mutations.[9] Renal carcinomas with various histologies were reported in patients with

FIGURE 20.4 The genetic basis of kidney cancer. The seven renal cancer predisposing genes—*VHL, MET, FLCN, FH, SDH, TSC1,* and *TSC2*—have been identified through studies of the inherited kidney cancer syndromes. These genes interact through common nutrient and energy sensing pathways. Our understanding of the molecular mechanisms by which these genes interact in these pathways has enabled the development of targeted therapeutic agents to benefit kidney cancer patients. (From ref. 4, with permission.)

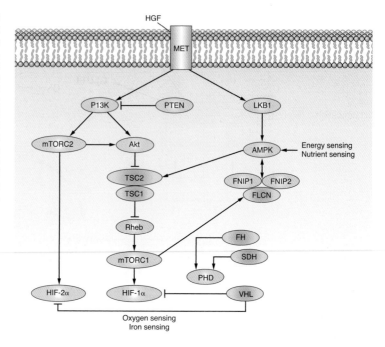

germline missense, frameshift, and nonsense mutations in *SDHB* and *D*.[83–85,89]

Functional Consequences of Succinate Dehydrogenase Subunit B and D Mutations

Mutational inactivation of the *SDH* gene results in reduced SDH enzyme activity and accumulation of succinate in renal tumors. In a mechanism similar to *FH* mutations in HLRCC (Fig. 20.3), accumulation of succinate serves to competitively inhibit 2-oxoglutarate and block PHD activity.[79,80] In the absence of PHD, HIF-α accumulates and drives transcriptional activation of HIF-α target genes that support tumor neovascularization, growth and invasion.

TUBEROUS SCLEROSIS COMPLEX

The tuberous sclerosis complex (TSC) is a multisystem, autosomal dominant disorder affecting both children and adults and is characterized by facial angiofibromas, renal angiomyolipomas, lymphangiomyomatosis of the lung, and disabling neurologic manifestations. The disease is phenotypically heterogeneous, and many patients have only minimal symptoms of disease.[90]

The predominant renal manifestations in TSC are bilateral multifocal angiomyolipomas (AML),

benign tumors composed of abnormal vessels, immature smooth muscle cells, and fat cells. The lifetime risk of renal cancer in TSC patients is 2% to 3%, which is similar to the general population.[90] The most common histologic type of renal tumor is clear cell; however, there are rare reports of papillary RCC, chromophobe RCC, and oncocytoma in TSC patients.[90] TSC is caused by mutations in one of two genes—*TSC1* that encodes hamartin[91] or *TSC2* that encodes tuberin[92]—leading to loss of TSC1/2 negative regulation of mTOR signaling.[61,62,93] Drug therapy targeting the mTOR pathway may be most effective for treating TSC-associated AMLs and renal tumors.[94]

CONCLUSION

Seven renal cancer predisposing genes—*VHL, MET, FLCN, FH, SDH, TSC1,* and *TSC2*—have been identified through studies of the inherited renal cancer syndromes, VHL, HPRC, BHD, HLRCC, SDH-related familial renal cancer and TSC (Fig. 20.4). These studies have provided valuable insight into the genetic events that lead to the development of renal tumors and the biochemical mechanisms that contribute to their progression and, ultimately, in some cases, metastasis. These findings have enabled the development of diagnostic genetic testing and provided the foundation for the development of targeted therapeutic agents for patients with the common form of sporadic kidney cancer.

Selected References

The full list of references for this chapter appears in the online version.

4. Linehan WM, Srinivasan R, Schmidt LS. The genetic basis of kidney cancer: a metabolic disease. *Nat Rev Urol* 2010;7:277.

5. Latif F, Tory K, Gnarra J, et al. Identification of the von Hippel-Lindau disease tumor suppressor gene. *Science* 1993;260:1317.

6. Schmidt L, Duh FM, Chen F, et al. Germline and somatic mutations in the tyrosine kinase domain of the MET protooncogene in papillary renal carcinomas. *Nat Genet* 1997;16:68.

7. Tomlinson IP, Alam NA, Rowan AJ, et al. Germline mutations in FH predispose to dominantly inherited uterine fibroids, skin leiomyomata and papillary renal cell cancer. *Nat Genet* 2002;30:406.

8. Nickerson ML, Warren MB, Toro JR, et al. Mutations in a novel gene lead to kidney tumors, lung wall defects, and benign tumors of the hair follicle in patients with the Birt-Hogg-Dubé syndrome. *Cancer Cell* 2002;2:157.

9. Vanharanta S, Buchta M, McWhinney SR, et al. Early-onset renal cell carcinoma as a novel extraparaganglial component of SDHB-associated heritable paraganglioma. *Am J Hum Genet* 2004;74:153.

10. Nordstrom-O'Brien M, van der Luijt RB, van Rooijen E, et al. Genetic analysis of von Hippel-Lindau disease. *Hum Mutat* 2010;31(5):521.

14. Kaelin WG. The von Hippel-Lindau tumor suppressor protein: O2 sensing and cancer. *Nat Rev Cancer* 2008;8:865.

15. Cohen AJ, Li FP, Berg S, et al. Hereditary renal-cell carcinoma associated with a chromosomal translocation. *N Engl J Med* 1979;301:592.

21. Stebbins CE, Kaelin WG Jr, Pavletich NP. Structure of the VHL-ElonginC-ElonginB complex: implications for VHL tumor suppressor function. *Science* 1999;284:455.

22. Kondo K, Kico J, Nakamura E, Lechpammer M, Kaelin W. Inhibition of HIF is necessary for tumor suppression by the von Hippel-Lindau protein. *Cancer Cell* 2002;1:237.

23. Maranchie JK, Vasselli JR, Riss J, et al. The contribution of VHL substrate binding and HIF1-alpha to the phenotype of VHL loss in renal cell carcinoma. *Cancer Cell* 2002;1:247.

24. Dharmawardana PG, Giubellino A, Bottaro DP. Hereditary papillary renal carcinoma type I. *Curr Mol Med* 2004;4:855.

27. Zbar B, Glenn G, Lubensky I, et al. Hereditary papillary renal cell carcinoma: clinical studies in 10 families. *J Urol* 1995;153:907.

29. Schmidt L, Junker K, Nakaigawa N, et al. Novel mutations of the MET proto-oncogene in papillary renal carcinomas. *Oncogene* 1999;18:2343.

30. Gentile A, Trusolino L, Comoglio PM. The Met tyrosine kinase receptor in development and cancer. *Cancer Metastasis Rev* 2008;27:85.

31. Birchmeier C, Birchmeier W, Gherardi E, Vande Woude GF. Met, metastasis, motility and more. *Nat Rev Mol Cell Biol* 2003;4:915.

34. Miller M, Ginalski K, Lesyng B, et al. Structural basis of oncogenic activation caused by point mutations in the kinase domain of the MET proto-oncogene: modeling studies. *Proteins* 2001;44:32.

35. Zhuang Z, Park WS, Pack S, et al. Trisomy 7: harboring non-random duplication of the mutant MET allele in hereditary papillary renal carcinomas. *Nat Genet* 1998;20:66.

37. Sidhar SK, Clark J, Gill S, et al. The t(X;1)(p11.2;q21.2) translocation in papillary renal cell carcinoma fuses a novel gene PRCC to the TFE3 transcription factor gene. *Hum Mol Genet* 1996;5:1333.

39. Weterman MA, van Groningen JJ, den Hartog A, Geurts van Kessel A. Transformation capacities of the papillary renal cell carcinoma-associated PRCCTFE3 and TFE3PRCC fusion genes. *Oncogene*. 2001;20:1414.

41. Tsuda M, Davis IJ, Argani P, et al. TFE3 fusions activate MET signaling by transcriptional up-regulation, defining another class of tumors as candidates for therapeutic MET inhibition. *Cancer Res* 2007;67:919.

42. Birt AR, Hogg GR, Dubé WJ. Hereditary multiple fibrofolliculomas with trichodiscomas and acrochordons. *Arch Dermatol* 1977;113:1674.

43. Toro JR, Glenn GM, Duray PH, et al. Birt-Hogg-Dubé syndrome: a novel marker of kidney neoplasia. *Arch Dermatol* 1999;135:1195.

44. Zbar B, Alvord WG, Glenn GM, et al. Risk of renal and colonic neoplasms and spontaneous pneumothorax in the Birt-Hogg-Dubé syndrome. *Cancer Epidemiol Biomarkers Prev* 2002;11:393.

46. Schmidt LS, Nickerson ML, Warren MB, et al. Germline BHD-mutation spectrum and phenotype analysis of a large cohort of families with Birt-Hogg-Dubé syndrome. *Am J Hum Genet* 2005;76:1023.

47. Toro JR, Wei MH, Glenn GM, et al. BHD mutations, clinical and molecular genetic investigations of Birt-Hogg-Dubé syndrome: a new series of 50 families and a review of published reports. *J Med Genet* 2008;45:321.

49. Pavlovich CP, Walther MM, Eyler RA, et al. Renal tumors in the Birt-Hogg-Dubé syndrome. *Am J Surg Pathol* 2002;26:1542.

50. Schmidt LS, Warren MB, Nickerson ML, et al. Birt-Hogg-Dubé syndrome, a genodermatosis associated with spontaneous pneumothorax and kidney neoplasia, maps to chromosome 17p11.2. *Am J Hum Genet* 2001;69:876.

55. Vocke CD, Yang Y, Pavlovich CP, et al. High frequency of somatic frameshift BHD gene mutations in Birt-Hogg-Dubé-associated renal tumors. *J Natl Cancer Inst* 2005; 97:931.

60. Baba M, Hong SB, Sharma N, et al. Folliculin encoded by the BHD gene interacts with a binding protein, FNIP1, and AMPK, and is involved in AMPK and mTOR signaling. *Proc Natl Acad Sci U S A* 2006;103:15552.

61. Inoki K, Corradetti MN, Guan KL. Dysregulation of the TSC-mTOR pathway in human disease. *Nat Genet* 2005; 37:19.

63. Hasumi H, Baba M, Hong SB, et al. Identification and characterization of a novel folliculin-interacting protein FNIP2. *Gene* 2008;415:60.

65. Baba M, Furihata M, Hong SB, et al. Kidney-targeted Birt-Hogg-Dubé gene inactivation in a mouse model: Erk1/2 and Akt-mTOR activation, cell hyperproliferation, and polycystic kidneys. *J Natl Cancer Inst* 2008;100:140.

66. Hasumi Y, Baba M, Ajima R, et al. Homozygous loss of BHD causes early embryonic lethality and kidney tumor development with activation of mTORC1 and mTORC2. *Proc Natl Acad Sci U S A* 2009;106:18722.

67. van Slegtenhorst M, Khabibullin D, Hartman TR, et al. The Birt-Hogg-Dubé and tuberous sclerosis complex homologs have opposing roles in amino acid homeostasis in Schizosaccharomyces pombe. *J Biol Chem* 2007;282:24583.

68. Hudon V, Sabourin S, Dydensborg AB, et al. Renal tumor suppressor function of the Birt-Hogg-Dubé syndrome gene product folliculin. *J Med Genet* 2010;47(3):182.

69. Hartman TR, Nicolas E, Klein-Szanto A, et al. The role of the Birt-Hogg-Dubé protein in mTOR activation and renal tumorigenesis. *Oncogene* 2009;28:1594.

70. Kiuru M, Launonen V. Hereditary leiomyomatosis and renal cell cancer (HLRCC). *Curr Mol Med* 2004;4:869.

71. Wei MH, Toure O, Glenn GM, et al. Novel mutations in FH and expansion of the spectrum of phenotypes expressed in families with hereditary leiomyomatosis and renal cell cancer. *J Med Genet* 2006;43:18.

73. Alam NA, Bevan S, Churchman M, et al. Localization of a gene (MCUL1) for multiple cutaneous leiomyomata and uterine fibroids to chromosome 1q42.3-q43. *Am J Hum Genet* 2001;68:1264.

74. Launonen V, Vierimaa O, Kiuru M, et al. Inherited susceptibility to uterine leiomyomas and renal cell cancer. *Proc Natl Acad Sci U S A* 2001;98:3387.

75. Alam NA, Rowan AJ, Wortham NC, et al. Genetic and functional analyses of FH mutations in multiple cutaneous and uterine leiomyomatosis, hereditary leiomyomatosis and renal cancer, and fumarate hydratase deficiency. *Hum Mol Genet* 2003;12:1241.

79. Pollard PJ, Briere JJ, Alam NA, et al Accumulation of Krebs cycle intermediates and over-expression of HIF1alpha in tumours which result from germline FH and SDH mutations. *Hum Mol Genet* 2005;14:2231.

80. Isaacs JS, Jung YJ, Mole DR, et al. HIF overexpression correlates with biallelic loss of fumarate hydratase in renal cancer: novel role of fumarate in regulation of HIF stability. *Cancer Cell* 2005;8:143–53.

82. Sudarshan S, Sourbier C, Kong HS, et al. Fumarate hydratase deficiency in renal cancer induces glycolytic addiction and hypoxia-inducible transcription factor 1alpha stabilization by glucose-dependent generation of reactive oxygen species. *Mol Cell Biol* 2009;29:4080.

85. Ricketts C, Woodward ER, Killick P, et al. Germline SDHB mutations and familial renal cell carcinoma. *J Natl Cancer Inst* 2008;100:1260.

90. Crino PB, Nathanson KL, Henske EP. The tuberous sclerosis complex. *N Engl J Med* 2006;355:1345.

91. van Slegtenhorst M, de Hoogt R, Hermans C, et al. Identification of the tuberous sclerosis gene TSC1 on chromosome 9q34. *Science* 1997;277:805.

92. The European Chromosome 16 Tuberous Sclerosis Consortium. Identification and characterization of the tuberous sclerosis gene on chromosome 16. *Cell* 1993;75:1305.

93. Shaw RJ, Bardeesy N, Manning BD, et al. The LKB1 tumor suppressor negatively regulates mTOR signaling. *Cancer Cell* 2004;6:91.

CHAPTER 21 BLADDER CANCER

MARGARET A. KNOWLES

MOLECULAR BIOLOGY OF INDIVIDUAL CANCERS

Understanding of the molecular changes that underlie bladder cancer development has progressed rapidly.[1-4] Most studies have focused on urothelial carcinomas (UCs), which comprise the majority (>90%) of tumors diagnosed in the Western world. Where the parasite *Schistosoma haematobium* is endemic, squamous tumors predominate, and there is evidence that these differ at the molecular level.[5,6] This chapter will focus on somatic alterations identified in UC by genomic and RNA profiling. There is also much information about germline polymorphisms that confer increased risk of UC development and the reader is referred to recent reviews on this topic.[7-9]

At diagnosis more than 70% of UCs are non-invasive (Ta) or superficially invasive (T1) papillary lesions. These commonly recur, but progression to muscle invasion is infrequent (10% to 20%) and prognosis is good. In contrast, tumors that are muscle invasive at diagnosis (≥T2) have poor prognosis (<50% survival at 5 years). Carcinoma *in situ* (CIS) is a high-grade lesion, that is "superficial" in the strict sense, but has poor prognosis. It is not yet clear whether, or how often, papillary low-grade tumors become invasive. This has led to an ongoing debate, which is as yet unresolved.[1] The divergent behavior of these tumor groups is reflected in striking differences in their molecular profiles.[1-4]

MOLECULAR ALTERATIONS IN SUPERFICIAL UROTHELIAL CARCINOMA

Low-grade Ta papillary UCs are genetically stable and commonly contain point mutations or loss of entire chromosomes of chromosome arms rather than complex chromosomal rearrangements. Recent findings also indicate significant alteration or microRNA (miRNA) expression. Common alterations are deletions of chromosome 9 (>50%), mutations of FGF receptor 3 (*FGFR3*), and mutations of the p110α catalytic subunit of phosphatidylinositol-3-kinase (PI3K) (*PIK3CA*)

(Table 21.1). These tumors are often near diploid. Loss of heterozygosity (LOH) of 11p is found in approximately 40% of UCs, including some Ta tumors, but is more common in tumors of higher grade and stage. Gains of 1q, 17, and 20q, amplifications of 11q, and loss of 10q have been identified but are not common (Table 21.1). Amplifications of 11q include the cyclin D1 gene (*CCND1*), which is involved in cell-cycle progression from G1 to S phase (Fig. 21.1).

Promoter hypermethylation of *APC*, *CDKN2A* (p14ARF), and *RASSF1A* has been found in DNA from urine of bladder cancer patients including those with low-grade/stage tumors.[10] However, this is more common in tumors of high tumor grade and stage.[11] Some hypermethylation in Ta/T1 tumors is associated with increased risk of progression.[12] A study that related regional gene expression to DNA copy number, identified genomic regions with altered expression that were copy number-independent, most showing downregulation. Genes known to show promoter methylation in UC were not located in these regions, indicating other mechanisms of gene silencing.[13]

Low-grade Ta tumors are genetically stable. Thus, synchronous or metachronous tumors from the same patient show great genetic similarity, although some clonal evolution can be detected over time. LOH of chromosome 9 and mutation of *FGFR3* are the least divergent events, and widely believed to represent early genetic changes.[14,15] Flat urothelial hyperplasia, a predicted tumor precursor, shows more frequent chromosome 9 loss than *FGFR3* mutation, suggesting that this occurs earlier.[16]

Chromosome 9

More than 50% of UCs of all of grades and stages show chromosome 9 LOH, many with loss of an entire homologue.[17-19] A critical region on 9p21 and at least three regions on 9q (9q22, 9q32–q33, and 9q34) have been identified. Candidate genes within these regions are *CDKN2A* (p16/p14ARF) and *CDKN2B* (p15) at 9p21,[20-24] *PTCH* (Gorlin syndrome gene) at 9q22,[25,26] *DBC1* at 9q32–q33,[27-29]

TABLE 21.1

GENETIC CHANGES IDENTIFIED IN Ta BLADDER TUMORS

Gene (Cytogenetic Location)	Alteration	Frequency (%) (Ref.)
ONCOGENES		
HRAS (11p15)/NRAS (1p13)/ KRAS2 (12p12)	Activating mutations	15 (60, 199–201)
FGFR3 (4p16)	Activating mutations	60–80 (40, 42, 43)
CCND1 (11q13)	Amplification/ overexpression	10–20 (72, 202)
PIK3CA (3q26)	Activating mutations	27 PUNLMP; 16–30 Ta (39, 69)
MDM2 (12q13)	Overexpression	~30 overexpression (103, 203)
TUMOUR SUPPRESSOR GENES		
CDKN2A (9p21)	Homozygous deletion/ methylation/mutation	HD 20–30 (21, 23, 24) LOH ~60 (17)
PTCH (9q22)	Deletion/mutation	LOH ~60; mutation frequency low (25, 26)
DBC1 (9q32–33)	Deletion/methylation	LOH ~60 (38, 204)
TSC1 (9q34)	Deletion/mutation	LOH ~60; mutation ~12 (31, 33, 39)
DNA COPY NUMBER CHANGES[a]		
2q, 8p, 10p, 10q, 11p, 13q, 17p, 18q, Y	Deletion	~10 (186, 205, 206)
9p, 9q	Deletion	36–47 (186, 205, 206)
1q, 17q, 20q	Gain	11–17 (186, 205, 206)
8p12, 11q13 (including CCND1)	Amplification	Occasional (205, 206)

HD, homozygous deletion; LOH, loss of heterozygosity.
[a]Comparative genomic hybridization analyses.

and *TSC1* (tuberous sclerosis syndrome gene 1) at 9q34[30–33] (Table 21.1).

CDKN2A (9p21) encodes the two cell-cycle regulators, p16 and p14ARF, which share coding region in exons 2 and 3 but have distinct exons 1. The protein products are translated in different reading frames to generate two entirely different proteins. p16 is a negative regulator of the Rb pathway and p14ARF, a negative regulator of the p53 pathway (Fig. 21.1). Inactivation of this locus in UC is commonly by homozygous deletion (HD). There are conflicting reports on association of 9p21 deletion with clinical parameters but HD appears to be associated with high tumor grade and stage.[34] Reduced copy number of 9p21 is present in approximately 45% of UC, indicating that, as suggested by knockout mice and *in vitro* experiments.[35,36] p16 and/or p14ARF may be haploinsufficient.[34]

On 9q, three genes are implicated. *PTCH*, the Gorlin syndrome gene (9q22) shows infrequent mutation,[26] but many tumors have reduced mRNA expression.[25] *DBC1* (9q33) shows HD in a few tumors[29,37] and no mutations, but is commonly silenced by hypermethylation.[27,38] LOH of 9q34 and mutation of the retained copy of *TSC1* is found in approximately 13% of UC.[39] The protein acts in complex with the TSC2 protein to negatively regulate mTOR, a central molecule in the control of protein synthesis and cell growth (Fig. 21.2).

FGFR3

Since the initial identification of *FGFR3* mutations in UC,[40] 11 different mutations have been identified.[41–54] These are in hot-spot codons in exons 7, 10, and 15 (Fig. 21.3A) and are all predicted to constitutively activate the receptor.[55] Mutation is associated with low tumor grade and stage, with up to 80% of low-grade Ta tumors showing mutation.[42] Mutations are also found in urothelial papilloma, a likely precursor of superficial UC.[50] Mutation is not associated with tumor recurrence or progression in Ta tumors overall,[43,54,56] but there is evidence that mutant Ta grade 1 tumors show a higher risk of recurrence.[43] Tumors with *FGFR3* mutation show increased FGFR3 protein expression, as do a significant number of tumors without mutation.[57]

Mutant FGFR3 proteins are oncogenic in rodent mesenchymal cells.[58,59] In cultured normal urothelial cells, mutant FGFR3 activates

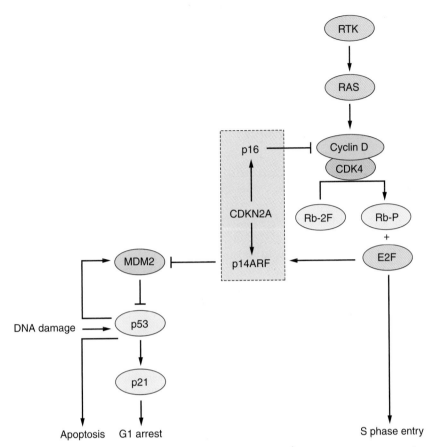

FIGURE 21.1 Key interactions in the Rb and p53 pathways. The *CDKN2A* locus encodes p16 and p14ARF that act as negative regulators of the Rb and p53 pathways, respectively. This interrelated signaling network is central to tumor suppression via the mechanisms of cell-cycle arrest and apoptosis. Stimulation by mitogens induces cyclin D1 expression. Phosphorylation of Rb by CDK4-cyclin D1 complexes releases E2F family members to induce expression of genes required for progression into S phase. The cyclin D-CDK4 complexes also sequester p27 and p21 (not shown). This allows formation of cyclin E-CDK2, which reinforces the inactivation of Rb. p16 negatively regulates this process by interacting with CDK4. The p53 pathway responds to stress signals (e.g., DNA damage). p21 expression is induced and this leads to cell-cycle arrest. MDM2 is a ubiquitin ligase responsible for inactivation of p53. In turn p53 regulates MDM2 expression providing a negative feedback loop. The p53 and Rb pathways are connected by p14ARF, which sequesters (inactivates) MDM2 in the nucleus and is up-regulated by E2Fs and in response to mitogenic signaling. Overexpression of E2Fs and oncogenes such as *MYC* can both result in p53-triggered cell-cycle arrest via p14ARF.

the RAS-MAPK pathway, induces increased cell survival and stimulates continued proliferation to high cell density at confluence.[59] This *in vitro* phenotype suggests that *FGFR3* mutation could contribute to clonal expansion or the development of hyperplasia within the urothelium *in vivo*. RAS gene and *FGFR3* mutations are mutually exclusive events. Mutation of either a RAS gene or *FGFR3* was found in 82% of low-grade tumors, indicating that virtually all superficial UCs may share activation of the RAS-MAPK pathway.[60] Mutations of *FGFR3* and *TP53* are also some-what mutually exclusive.[41,61] However, as *TP53* mutation is found predominantly in high-grade/stage UCs, which are thought to represent a distinct pathogenic pathway (see following discussion), it is predicted that these events are not biologically equivalent.

FGFR3 is considered a good therapeutic target in superficial UC.[62] Several studies indicate that inhibition of mutant *FGFR3* by knockdown or inhibition using small molecules or antibodies has a profound effect of UC cell phenotype including inhibition of xenograft growth *in vivo*.[58,63–68]

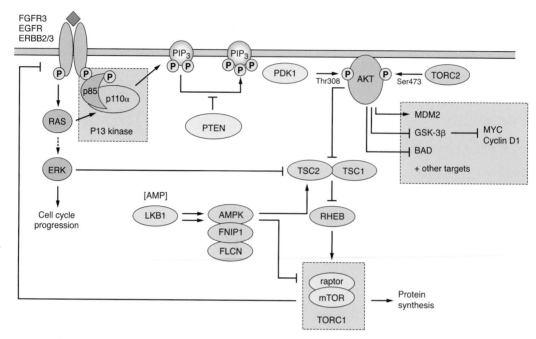

FIGURE 21.2 Oncogenic signaling via the RAS-MAPK and PI3K pathways. Growth factor-mediated signaling or mutational activation of Ras oncogenes can activate both of these pathways. Signaling via the RAS/RAF/MEK/ERK cascade leads to phosphorylation of many substrates that can have multiple cellular effects depending on the intensity and duration of signaling. In many situations proliferation is induced. Activated receptor tyrosine kinases bind p85, the regulatory subunit of PI3K, and recruit the enzyme to the membrane where it phosphorylates phosphatidyinositol-4, 5-bisphosphate (PIP2) to generate PIP3, which in turn recruits PDK1 and AKT to the membrane where AKT is activated by phosphorylation to regulate a wide range of target proteins (not all shown). Among these are cyclin D1 and MDM2, which are up-regulated either directly or indirectly, resulting in a positive stimulus via the Rb or p53 pathways, respectively. AKT also phosphorylates and inactivates tuberin the *TSC2* gene product, leading to activation of mTOR complex 1 (TORC1), which controls protein synthesis. The *TSC1* product hamartin forms an active complex with tuberin, and loss of function of either protein leads to dysregulated mTOR signaling. MYC expression is induced as a consequence of both by ERK and AKT signaling.

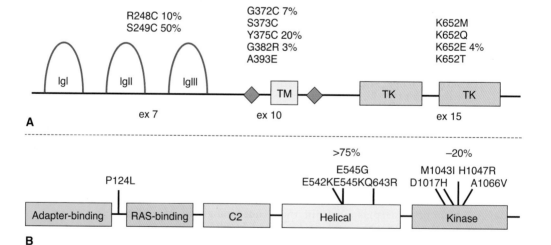

FIGURE 21.3 A: *FGFR3* mutations identified in bladder cancer. Positions of hot-spot mutations in exons 7, 10, and 15 that are found in bladder cancer are shown in relation to protein structure. The relative frequency of the more common mutations is given as a percentage. IgI, IgII, IgIII, immunoglobulinlike domains; TM, transmembrane domain; TK, tyrosine kinase domain. **B:** *PIK3CA* mutations identified in bladder cancer in relation to protein structure.

PIK3CA

PI3K plays a pivotal role in signaling from receptor tyrosine kinases (Fig. 21.2). Activating mutations of the p110α catalytic subunit (*PIK3CA*) are found in UC. One study identified mutations in 13%, with a significant association with low tumor grade and stage[69] and a second reported a frequency of 27%.[39] The development of a low-cost, high-throughput assay to detect the common variants should facilitate studies to clarify the exact frequency and clinical associations of these mutations.[70] The *PIK3CA* mutation spectrum (Fig. 21.3B) differs significantly from that in other cancers. Mutations E542K and E545K in the helical domain are most common (24% and 52%, respectively) and the kinase domain mutation H1047R, which is the most common mutation in other cancers, is less frequent (13% compared with 46% reported for other cancers in COSMIC, Catalogue of Somatic Mutations in Cancer [www.sanger.ac.uk/genetics/CGP/cosmic/]). The selective pressure for helical domain mutation in UC is not yet understood, although recent studies of the structure of p110α and the effect of the common activating mutations reveal different mechanisms of activation by helical domain and kinase domain mutations.[71]

Cyclin D1

CCND1 (11q13) is amplified in some superficial and invasive UCs[72] and the protein is overexpressed in an even larger number.[73–76] Overexpression in many cases may be the consequence of other alterations, such as activation of the MAPK or PI3K pathways (Fig. 21.2). There is no consensus on the clinical significance of overexpression, but up-regulation is more common in Ta tumors.[75,76]

MicroRNA Expression

There are several reports of altered miRNA expression in UC. Changes in apparently "normal" urothelium from UC patients indicate that such alterations may occur early in disease development.[77] Comparison of superficial and advanced UC indicates significant differences in profile.[77] Predominantly down-regulation of miRNAs was found in Ta tumors compared with normal urothelium. Interestingly, two of the down-regulated miRNAs, miR-99a and miR-100, were found to regulate FGFR3.[77] Low levels of miR-7 have also been reported to be associated with *FGFR3* mutation.[78]

CARCINOMA IN SITU

CIS is the predicted precursor of muscle-invasive UC.[79] It is usually recognized only retrospectively in paraffin-embedded samples, and few studies have assessed genetic changes. Alterations include *TP53* mutation, chromosome 9 loss, up-regulated ERBB2 expression, and a range of alterations similar to those found in muscle-invasive UC.[80–83] Array-based studies have revealed significant genomic instability. Gains of 5p, 6p22.3, 10p15.1, and losses of 5q and 13q13-q14 were common. The genomic profile was similar to that of high-risk Ta and T1 tumors with associated CIS and lacking *FGFR3* mutation.[84] *FGFR3* mutation has not been found in CIS. One study reported that chromosome 9 loss was infrequent in primary CIS but common in CIS associated with synchronous carcinoma,[84] indicating two forms of CIS with different developmental pathways.

MOLECULAR ALTERATIONS IN INVASIVE UROTHELIAL CARCINOMA

Many genetic alterations are found in muscle-invasive UC, including alterations to known genes and genomic alterations for which the target genes are currently unknown (Table 21.2).

Oncogenes

ERBB2 (17q23), a receptor tyrosine kinase of the *EGFR* gene family, is amplified in 10% to 20% and overexpressed in 10% to 50% of invasive UC.[85–89] The prognostic significance of these alterations is controversial.[90–94] As this receptor cannot bind ligand and relies on heterodimerization with ERBB3, it is likely that ERBB3 status and/or ligand expression may have significant influence.[95,96] Up to 70% of invasive tumors overexpress EGFR, and this is associated with poor prognosis.[97,98] Both ERBB2 and EGFR represent potential therapeutic targets in advanced UC.[99] These changes may activate the RAS-MAPK and/or the PI3K pathways (Fig. 21.2).

RAS gene mutation is not associated with either invasive or superficial disease.[60] *In vitro* experiments in tumor cells indicate that HRAS can induce an invasive phenotype.[100] In mice expressing mutant H-ras in the urothelium, superficial papillary tumors develop rather than muscle-invasive tumors.[101] Thus, RAS mutation may contribute to development of both forms of UC. *FGFR3* is mutated less frequently than in superficial UC. Approximately 15% of T2 tumors show mutation.[42,57,61] However, protein expression is up-regulated in 40% to 50% of nonmutant-invasive UC.[57,67] FGFR1 is also overexpressed in many of these cancers,[102] indicating that FGFR-targeted therapies may be applicable to both noninvasive and invasive UC.

Some UCs (4% to 6%) show amplification of *MDM2* (12q14).[103,104] MDM2 regulates p53 levels, and overexpression provides an alternative

TABLE 21.2

GENETIC CHANGES FOUND IN INVASIVE (≥T2) BLADDER TUMORS

Gene (Cytogenetic Location)	Alteration	Frequency (%) (Ref.)
ONCOGENES		
HRAS (11p15)/NRAS (1p13)/ KRAS2 (12p12)	Activating mutations	10–15 (60, 199–201)
FGFR3 (4p16)	Activating mutations	0–34 (40, 42, 49, 54)
ERBB2 (17q)	Amplification/overexpression	10–14 amplification (87, 89, 207)
CCND1 (11q13)	Amplification/overexpression	10–20 amplification (72, 202, 208)
MDM2 (12q13)	Amplification/overexpression	4 amplification (103, 203)
E2F3 (6p22)	Amplification/overexpression	9–11 amplification in ≥T1 (108, 111)
TUMOR SUPPRESSOR GENES		
CDKN2A (9p21)	Homozygous deletion/ methylation/mutation	HD 20–30 (21, 23, 24) LOH ~60 (17)
PTCH (9q22)	Deletion/mutation	LOH ~60 (25, 26) Mutation frequency low
DBC1 (9q32–33)	Deletion/methylation	LOH ~60 (38, 204)
TSC1 (9q34)	Deletion/mutation	LOH ~60 (31, 33, 39) Mutation ~12
PTEN (10q23)	Homozygous deletion/ mutation	LOH 30–35 (129–131, 133, 134); mutation 17 (132)
RB1 (13q14)	Deletion	37% (117–119)
TP53 (17p13)	Deletion/mutation	70% (209–211)
DNA COPY NUMBER CHANGES[a]		
2q, 5q, 6q, 8p, 9p, 9q, 10q, 11p, 11q, 13q, 15q, 16q, 17p, 18q, Y	Deletion in >12%	(186, 212)
1q, 3q, 5p, 7p, 8q, 10p, 17q, 20p, 20q	Gain in >12%	(186, 212)
1q22, 3p24, 6p22, 8p12, 8q21–22 and q24, 10p13–14, 12q15, 17q21, 20q13	Amplification <5% (5%–10% for 6p22)	(111, 186, 212)

HD, homozygous deletion; LOH, loss of heterozygosity.
[a]Comparative genomic hybridization analyses.

mechanism to inactivate p53 function (Fig. 21.1). There is no consensus on the relationship of up-regulated MDM2 to tumor grade, stage, or prognosis. MYC is up-regulated in many bladder tumors, although the mechanism for this is unclear.[105] Although amplifications of 8q are found in some invasive UC, MYC is not the major target. However, additional copies of the whole of 8q are common and may lead to overexpression.[106,107] MYC may also be up-regulated in response to other molecular events (e.g., MAPK pathway stimulation). An amplicon on 6p in 14% of muscle-invasive UC and cell lines[108–110] contains E2F3, and functional studies indicate that E3F3 can drive urothelial cell proliferation (Fig. 21.1).[111,112] E2F transcription factors interact with and are regulated by Rb

and tumors with E2F3 amplification have Rb inactivated.

Tumor Suppressor Genes

As in other aggressive cancers, the tumor suppressor genes TP53, RB1, CDKN2A, and PTEN are implicated in invasive UC. The pathways controlled by p53 and Rb regulate cell-cycle progression and responses to stress (Fig. 21.1). TP53 mutation is common in invasive UC (mutations are listed in the International Agency for Research on Cancer TP53 database).[113] Although immunohistochemical detection of p53 protein with increased half-life identifies many mutant p53 proteins and is commonly used as a surrogate marker for mutation, many *TP53* mutations (~20%) yield unstable or truncated proteins that cannot be detected in this way. Thus, p53 protein accumulation is not a useful prognostic marker. Two meta-analyses indicate only a small association between p53 positivity and poor prognosis.[114,115] A recent study that examined both protein expression and mutation of *TP53* confirmed limited concordance of these measurements but found that the combined measurements provided useful prognostic information.[116]

The Rb pathway regulates cell-cycle progression from G1 to S phase (Fig. 21.1). *RB1* has not been screened for mutations in UC but homozygous deletions, LOH of 13q14, and loss of Rb protein expression are detected in tumors of high grade and stage.[117–120] Altered Rb protein expression including both loss of expression, and the up-regulation which is associated with loss of p16 expression,[121] has been found in about 54% of cystectomy tumor samples.[122] *CDKN2A* (encoding p16 and p14ARF) is hemizygously deleted in more than 50% of UCs of all grades and stages, and homozygous deletion is associated with invasion.[34] These proteins link the Rb and p53 pathways (Fig. 21.1), and due to multiple regulatory feedback mechanisms, inactivation of both pathways together is predicted to have greater impact than inactivation of either pathway alone.[123] Assessment of Rb, p53, and p21 bear this out.[124] More recent studies indicate that broad analysis of changes that deregulate the G1 checkpoint achieves greater predictive power.[122,125–127] It is also reported that alterations of p53 and loss of p16 expression predict progression in Ta tumors.[128]

PTEN (phosphatase and tensin homologue deleted on chromosome 10) (10q23), a negative regulator of the PI3K pathway by virtue of its lipid phosphatase activity toward PtIns(3,4,5)P3 (Fig. 21.2), is deleted in 24% to 58% of invasive UCs.[129–131] Mutations of the retained copy are infrequent but HD has been detected in tumor cell lines.[39,132–134] Reduced expression is common[39,135] and is associated with p53 alteration. Many tumors (41%) with altered p53 show down-regulation of *PTEN*, and this combined alteration is associated with poor outcome.[136] As *PTEN* is haploinsufficient in mouse models,[137] loss of function of one allele in UC may lead to altered phenotype. In mice, conditional deletion of *Pten* in the urothelium led to early urothelial hyperplasia[135,138] and late development of tumors resembling human papillary superficial tumors. A study that induced stochastic deletion of *p53* and/or *Pten* in mice showed that deletion of either gene alone did not lead to tumor formation but dual deletion led to early development of aggressive UC, with frequent metastases.[136] PTEN loss may affect proliferation, apoptosis, and migration. Re-expression in PTEN-null UC cells has revealed effects on cell chemotaxis,

anchorage independent growth, and tumor growth *in vivo*.[139–141] UC cell invasion can be inhibited by the protein phosphatase activity of PTEN alone.[141] Thus, loss of both lipid and protein phosphatase activities of PTEN may contribute in different ways to urothelial tumorigenesis. The *TSC1* product hamartin acts in the PI3K pathway downstream of PTEN (Fig. 21.2), providing an alternative mechanism of pathway activation in 13% of invasive UC.[31,39]

The Rho family GDP dissociation inhibitor RhoGDI2 has been implicated as a tumor suppressor in UC. Expression is reduced in an isogenic cell line model of metastasis[142] and low expression is associated with reduced survival in UC patients.[143] Phosphorylation by SRC appears to enhance the suppressive action of RhoGDI2 and down-regulation of SRC and RHOGDI2 are mutually exclusive in UC,[144] suggesting that SRC may play an important role in some cases.[145]

Other Genomic Changes in Invasive Urothelial Carcinoma

Large numbers of genomic changes have been detected in invasive UC. These include numerous losses and gains in DNA copy number and several regions of high-level amplification that may contain novel oncogenes (Table 21.2). To date the target genes within most of these regions have not been identified.

Invasive UC displays genetic instability with rapid genetic divergence of related tumors from the same patient. This is commonly chromosomal instability rather than microsatellite instability. No significant differences have yet been found between minimally invasive (T1) and deeply invasive tumors (T2 or greater), suggesting that T1 tumors with the ability to break through the basement membrane are aggressive lesions. Although T1 tumors often have good outcome, this may reflect complete resection rather than lack of tumor aggression. Some alterations, including gains of 3p22–25 and 5p and losses of 4p11–15, 5q15–23, 6q22–23, and 10q24–26, are associated with T1 tumor progression.[146] In one comparative genomic hybridization (CGH) study, muscle-invasive tumor samples and paired metastatic samples were compared, but no significant metastasis-associated markers were identified.[147]

MicroRNA Expression

Many miRNAs show altered expression in invasive UC.[78] In comparison with normal urothelium, invasive tumors are reported to show predominantly up-regulation of miRNAs rather than down-regulation.[77] Two studies have directly compared invasive and noninvasive samples[77] and several have shown association of specific changes with either poor outcome or the invasive phenotype.[78,148,149] Functional studies indicate potential roles for miR-145 and miR-221 in regulating urothelial cell survival,[150,151] miR-200 in regulating epithelial-mesenchymal transition,[152] miR-145 and miR-133a in regulating the cytoskeletal gene FSCN1,[153] and miR-101 in modulation of expression of the Polycomb Repressive Complex 2 gene EZH1.[154]

INFORMATION FROM EXPRESSION AND GENOMIC MICROARRAY PROFILING

Microarray analysis provides extensive information that is contributing to improved tumor classification and understanding of UC pathogenesis.[155] Molecular signatures for the known histopathologic subtypes (grade and stage), for CIS, the presence of metastases, and treatment response have been reported and some have been validated or are being validated in multicenter studies with the aim of introduction into clinical practice. Several reports have generated expression signatures for diagnostic classification.[156–161] Profiles of superficial tumors showed that the presence of FGFR3 mutation has a major impact on expression profile.[162] One study[163] examined differences between normal urothelium, PUNLMP or low-grade Ta and high-grade Ta tumors.[164] Cytoskeletal genes differed most between normal urothelium and low-grade tumors, and changes in high-grade tumors were related to the cell cycle.

Signatures for prediction of recurrence in Ta grade 2 tumors and the presence of CIS in patients with Ta tumors have been generated.[165–168] Interestingly "normal" mucosa from cystectomy specimens with adjacent CIS contained the CIS signature, indicating that in such bladders there may be widespread urothelial alteration.[167] This CIS signature has been validated in a large multicenter study.[165] In another study a "no CIS" classification was correlated with FGFR3 mutation.[54] Progression of superficial tumors has been predicted with relatively high sensitivity and specificity[159,169] and one of the signatures[169] validated in a multicenter study.[165] A recent study using large training and validation sets identified signatures for recurrence and progression in superficial and muscle-invasive tumors.[170] Real-time polymerase chain reaction confirmed an eight-gene predictor of progression in noninvasive disease. The other signatures were not confirmed, emphasizing the need for validation using an independent technique in a large sample set. The application of two forms of artificial intelligence to expression data from the study of Wild et al.[159] has also resulted in

the identification of 11 genes associated with progression of noninvasive UC.[171] A panel of antibodies to six of these genes was predictive of outcome.

Muscle-invasive UC with known outcome have not been studied in large numbers, but in one study, tumors with good (survival ≥18 months) or bad (survival <18 months) prognosis were classified with 78% success.[158] Two other studies showed less ability to identify poor survival,[161,172] but one protein identified (synuclein) showed significant association with outcome.[172] Signatures for the presence of lymph node metastases have been presented[161,172] but robust predictors have not emerged.

Profiles of muscle-invasive UC reveal enrichment for markers of an epithelial-mesenchymal transition,[173] indicating that this may be an important feature of CIS->invasive UC progression. Immunohistochemistry results support this.[174,175] UC cell lines with epithelial-mesenchymal transition show resistance to EGFR inhibitors.[176,177] Tumor molecular profile may have profound effects not only on response to targeted therapies but to radiotherapy and conventional chemotherapy. Two studies have examined response to neoadjuvant M-VAC (methotrexate, vinblastine, doxorubicin, and cisplatin) chemotherapy. Profiles from responders and nonresponders were used to generate a gene signature that correctly predicted response in eight of nine test cases.[178] In a second study, expression profiles from 30 patients yielded 55 genes that correlated with postchemotherapy survival, 2 of which (emmprin and survivin) were validated by immunohistochemistry and had significant correlation with therapeutic response and overall outcome in patients with no metastases.[179] Prediction models for response to both chemotherapy and targeted agents have also been developed using profiles of UC cell lines.[180,181] The same group developed a bioinformatics approach to predict drug sensitivity (COXEN), using expression profiles and known response of the NCI-60 panel of cell lines to predict response of cell lines based on expression profile. This predicted sensitivity of UC cell lines to several agents that was confirmed by in vitro testing[182] and has been shown to predict patients' response to chemotherapy.[183]

Genomic profiling has used array-based CGH (aCGH) and single nucleotide polymorphism (SNP) array analysis. aCGH provides high-resolution copy number profiles and has precisely defined regions of high-level amplification.[109,184–187] Used in concert with expression analysis, candidate "drivers" of these amplicons have been identified.[187] SNP array analysis has allowed novel chromosomal regions of allelic imbalance to be identified.[83,188] More regions of both copy number alteration and allelic imbalance have been found with increasing tumor stage. Despite a large body of data, no robust genetic markers to predict Ta tumor recurrence or progression of high-risk Ta tumors have been identified to date.

SIGNALING PATHWAYS IN UROTHELIAL CARCINOMA

There is overwhelming evidence for activation of the RAS-MAPK and PI3K pathways. In superficial UC, *FGFR3* and RAS mutation in almost all cases suggests dependence on RAS-MAPK pathway activation. As *FGFR3* activation does not activate the PI3K pathway in cultured normal urothelial cells,[59] the presence of *PIK3CA* mutations in superficial UC, including those with *FGFR3* mutation, implies that additional activation of the PI3K pathway is required. RAS mutation may activate both pathways. Inactivation of *TSC1* and activating mutations of *AKT1* in superficial and invasive UC, and *PTEN* inactivation in invasive UC, may also activate the PI3K pathway. Upstream activators of the pathway, including ERBB receptors, may also contribute. It is noteworthy that alterations in three of the key genes in the pathway (*PIK3CA*, *TSC1*, and *PTEN)* are not mutually exclusive,[39] implying that combined mutations have additive or synergistic effects and that noncanonical effects may be critical. This may be particularly important for *TSC1*. The widely studied functions of *TSC1* and *TSC2* are attributed to the *TSC1/TSC2* complex that regulates mTOR activity. Although independent functions have been ascribed to *TSC2*, independent function of *TSC1* is not clear. The finding of *TSC1* mutations in bladder but not other cancers and the lack of mutual exclusivity with *PIK3CA* and *PTEN* alterations may indicate an independent *TSC1* function in the urothelium. The known cross-talk between the MAPK and PI3K pathways via RAS and ERK (Fig. 21.2) could place the PI3K pathway at center stage and indicate utility of inhibitors of this pathway in treatment of both groups of UC. As targeted agents for inhibition of these pathways are now available or in development, it will be important to confirm these predictions by direct measurement of pathway activation in tumor samples.

UROTHELIAL TUMOR-INITIATING CELLS

There is evidence for the existence within heterogeneous urothelial tumor cell populations of a highly tumorigenic subpopulation with stem cell–like characteristics. As cancer stem cells in other tumor types show resistance to chemotherapy agents and are predicted to be the cause of posttreatment disease relapse, there is great interest in characterizing these stem cells and identifying markers that may allow specific targeting. Two recent studies provide clear evidence for such a population within urothelial cancers.[189,190] He et al.[190] identified a population of tumor cells with urothelial basal cell-like characteristics that reside at the tumor-stromal interface in tumors and xenografts and possess most of the tumor-forming ability of the parental tumor. A second study identified a CD44+ population of cells in primary tumors that expressed the basal cell marker CK5 and was enriched for tumor-initiating cells.[189] Expression profiling in both studies provides the basis for future attempts to identify tumor-initiating cells and examine relationships to therapeutic response and outcome.[191]

MOLECULAR PATHOGENESIS AND TUMOR CLONALITY

UC are commonly multifocal and show frequent recurrence. In many cases, the macroscopically "normal" urothelium shows areas of microscopic dysplasia or CIS, and it is easy to envisage how new lesions may develop following resection of a primary tumor. The issue of clonality of UC has received much attention, and most studies have found only monoclonal tumors with shared genetic changes in multiple tumors resected from the same patient. However, there are some examples of more than one unrelated monoclonal tumor in the same bladder (oligoclonality) (reviewed in ref 192).

Macroscopically normal urothelium from tumor-bearing bladders has shown LOH in several genomic regions. Detailed mapping identified candidate genes whose involvement is predicted to be at a very early stage in tumor development. These have been termed "forerunner" genes and functional studies suggest that some regulate key cellular functions.[193,194]

Based on molecular and histopathological observations, a model for the molecular pathogenesis of UC has been developed (Fig. 21.4). *FGFR3* and *TP53* mutation are predominantly confined to one of the two major subgroups of UC and currently are the best molecular markers for these groups. It is not yet clear how often T1 tumors develop directly from flat dysplasia or from papillary Ta tumors. Similarly, the pathogenesis of high-grade papillary tumors and their relationship to flat dysplastic lesions is not well understood and is therefore represented as a potential third pathway in Figure 21.4. Further work is required to examine T1 tumors in more detail, to determine whether these are invasive tumors caught in their journey toward muscle, whether any develop from papillary Ta tumors or whether they represent a third

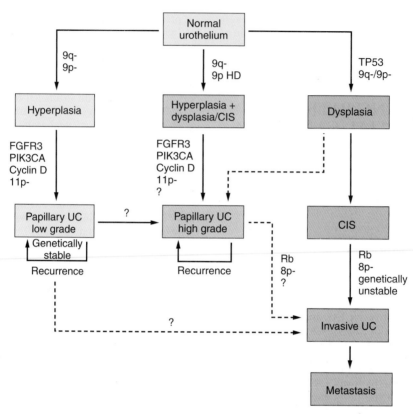

FIGURE 21.4 Potential pathways of urothelial tumorigenesis. Low-grade papillary tumors (*left*) may arise via simple hyperplasia and minimal dysplasia and are characterized at the molecular level by deletions of chromosome 9 and activating mutations of *FGFR3* and *PIK3CA*. Invasive carcinoma (*right*) is believed to arise via the flat high-grade lesion carcinoma *in situ* (CIS), and in this case *TP53* mutation occurs early, chromosome 9 deletions (9q) are less common, and *FGFR3* mutations are infrequent. These genetically unstable tumors accumulate genomic alterations, including *RB1* inactivation, 8p deletions, and many other genetic events. The finding of dysplasia in association with high-grade papillary tumors that lack *TP53* mutation but have frequent chromosome 9 losses suggests that an independent route to high-grade papillary tumors may exist (*center*).

distinct group. More detailed examination of differences between primary and UC-associated dysplasia/CIS may confirm the existence of a third pathway to urothelial neoplasia. To date, no molecular alterations can differentiate muscle invasive UC from their metastases. This may reflect early migration of cells to distant sites without requirement for additional changes, or that determinants of progression and metastasis are yet to be identified. Additional alterations may also remain to be identified in Ta tumors that show only one or two molecular events.

Attempts have been made to apply bioinformatic modeling to define possible genetic pathways of UC development. Two potential cytogenetic pathways, one initiated by −9, followed by −11p and 1q+ and a second initiated by +7 followed by 8p− and +8q were identified, the latter group containing more aggressive tumors (T1–T3) and the former, Ta–T2 tumors.[195] A Bayesian network model using LOH data for 17 chromosomes in papillary UC (all grades) showed 9p and 9q loss as the most probable primary event with 8p− and 17− as major subsequent events[196] and a subsequent analysis based on cytogenetic data confirmed several of these associations and predicted two distinct pathways that ultimately converge, one initiated by +7 and the other by −9.[197]

Undoubtedly, application of array-based genomic and expression approaches in combination with high throughput mutation scanning will answer some of the outstanding questions relating to pathogenesis. Key to this will be appropriate selection of tissues for study, and there will be great advantages if archival samples from clinical trials can be used. It will be essential to test the effects of key molecular alterations on human urothelial cell phenotype. The recent development of immortal normal human urothelial cell lines will facilitate this.[198]

Selected References

The full list of references for this chapter appears in the online version.

1. Knowles MA. Molecular subtypes of bladder cancer: Jekyll and Hyde or chalk and cheese? *Carcinogenesis* 2006;27(3):361–373.

4. Cordon-Cardo C. Molecular alterations associated with bladder cancer initiation and progression. *Scand J Urol Nephrol Suppl* 2008:154–165.

7. Kiemeney LA, Grotenhuis AJ, Vermeulen SH, et al. Genome-wide association studies in bladder cancer: first results and potential relevance. *Curr Opin Urol* 2009; 19:540–546.

9. Wu X, Hildebrandt MAT, Chang DW. Genome-wide association studies of bladder cancer risk: a field synopsis of progress and potential applications. *Cancer Metastasis Rev* 2009;28:269–280.

10. Cairns P. Gene methylation and early detection of genitourinary cancer: the road ahead. *Nat Rev Cancer* 2007;7:531–543.

14. Takahashi T, Habuchi T, Kakehi Y, et al. Clonal and chronological genetic analysis of multifocal cancers of the bladder and upper urinary tract. *Cancer Res* 1998;58: 5835–5841.

30. Pymar LS, Platt FM, Askham JM, et al. Bladder tumour-derived somatic TSC1 missense mutations cause loss of function via distinct mechanisms. *Hum Mol Genet* 2008;17:2006–2017.

34. Chapman EJ, Harnden P, Chambers P, et al. Comprehensive analysis of CDKN2A status in microdissected urothelial cell carcinoma reveals potential haploinsufficiency, a high frequency of homozygous co-deletion and associations with clinical phenotype. *Clin Cancer Res* 2005;11:5740–5747.

39. Platt FM, Hurst CD, Taylor CF, et al. Spectrum of phosphatidylinositol 3-kinase pathway gene alterations in bladder cancer. *Clin Cancer Res* 2009;15:6008–6017.

40. Cappellen D, De Oliveira C, Ricol D, et al. Frequent activating mutations of FGFR3 in human bladder and cervix carcinomas. *Nat Genet* 1999;23:18.

42. Billerey C, Chopin D, Aubriot-Lorton MH, et al. Frequent FGFR3 mutations in papillary non-invasive bladder (pTa) tumors. *Am J Pathol* 2001; 158:1955–1959.

54. Zieger K, Dyrskjot L, Wiuf C, et al. Role of activating fibroblast growth factor receptor 3 mutations in the development of bladder tumors. *Clin Cancer Res* 2005;11:7709–7719.

57. Tomlinson DC, Baldo O, Harnden P, et al. FGFR3 protein expression and its relationship to mutation status and prognostic variables in bladder cancer. *J Pathol* 2007;213: 91–98.

58. Bernard-Pierrot I, Brams A, Dunois-Larde C, et al. Oncogenic properties of the mutated forms of fibroblast growth factor receptor 3b. *Carcinogenesis* 2006;27:740–747.

59. di Martino E, L'Hôte CG, Kennedy W, et al. Mutant fibroblast growth factor receptor 3 induces intracellular signaling and cellular transformation in a cell type- and mutation-specific manner. *Oncogene* 2009;28:4306–4316.

60. Jebar AH, Hurst CD, Tomlinson DC, et al. FGFR3 and Ras gene mutations are mutually exclusive genetic events in urothelial cell carcinoma. *Oncogene* 2005; 24:5218–5225.

61. van Rhijn BW, van der Kwast TH, Vis AN, et al. FGFR3 and P53 characterize alternative genetic pathways in the pathogenesis of urothelial cell carcinoma. *Cancer Res* 2004; 64:1911–1914.

63. Tomlinson DC, Hurst CD, Knowles MA. Knockdown by shRNA identifies S249C mutant FGFR3 as a potential therapeutic target in bladder cancer. *Oncogene* 2007;26: 5889–5899.

65. Qing J, Du X, Chen Y, et al. Antibody-based targeting of FGFR3 in bladder carcinoma and t(4;14)-positive multiple myeloma in mice. *J Clin Invest* 2009;119:1216–1229.

68. Martinez-Torrecuadrada JL, Cheung LH, Lopez-Serra P, et al. Antitumor activity of fibroblast growth factor receptor 3-specific immunotoxins in a xenograft mouse model of bladder carcinoma is mediated by apoptosis. *Mol Cancer Ther* 2008;7:862–873.

69. Lopez-Knowles E, Hernandez S, Malats N, et al. PIK3CA mutations are an early genetic alteration associated with FGFR3 mutations in superficial papillary bladder tumors. *Cancer Res* 2006;66:7401–7404.

77. Catto JWF, Miah S, Owen HC, et al. Distinct microRNA alterations characterize high- and low-grade bladder cancer. *Cancer Res* 2009;69:8472–8481.

78. Veerla S, Lindgren D, Kvist A, et al. MiRNA expression in urothelial carcinomas: important roles of miR-10a, miR-222, miR-125b, miR-7 and miR-452 for tumor stage and metastasis, and frequent homozygous losses of miR-31. *Int J Cancer* 2009;124:2236–2242.

95. Memon AA, Sorensen BS, Meldgaard P, et al. The relation between survival and expression of HER1 and HER2 depends on the expression of HER3 and HER4: a study in bladder cancer patients. *Br J Cancer* 2006;94:1703–1709.

96. Amsellem-Ouazana D, Bieche I, Tozlu S, et al. Gene expression profiling of ERBB receptors and ligands in human transitional cell carcinoma of the bladder. *J Urol* 2006;175:1127–1132.

99. Dovedi SJ, Davies BR. Emerging targeted therapies for bladder cancer: a disease waiting for a drug. *Cancer Metastasis Rev* 2009;28:355–367.

102. Tomlinson DC, Lamont FR, Shnyder SD, et al. Fibroblast growth factor receptor 1 promotes proliferation and survival via activation of the mitogen-activated protein kinase pathway in bladder cancer. *Cancer Res* 2009;69:4613–4620.

108. Oeggerli M, Tomovska S, Schraml P, et al. E2F3 amplification and overexpression is associated with invasive tumor growth and rapid tumor cell proliferation in urinary bladder cancer. *Oncogene* 2004;23:5616–5623.

109. Hurst CD, Fiegler H, Carr P, et al. High-resolution analysis of genomic copy number alterations in bladder cancer by microarray-based comparative genomic hybridization. *Oncogene* 2004;23:2250–2263.

111. Hurst CD, Tomlinson DC, Williams SV, et al. Inactivation of the Rb pathway and overexpression of both isoforms of E2F3 are obligate events in bladder tumours with 6p22 amplification. *Oncogene* 2008;27:2716–2727.

112. Olsson AY, Feber A, Edwards S, et al. Role of E2F3 expression in modulating cellular proliferation rate in human bladder and prostate cancer cells. *Oncogene* 2007;26: 1028–1037.

116. George B, Datar RH, Wu L, et al. p53 gene and protein status: the role of p53 alterations in predicting outcome in patients with bladder cancer. *J Clin Oncol* 2007;25: 5352–5358.

123. Mitra AP, Birkhahn M, Cote RJ. p53 and retinoblastoma pathways in bladder cancer. *World J Urol* 2007;25:563–571.

136. Puzio-Kuter AM, Castillo-Martin M, Kinkade CW, et al. Inactivation of p53 and Pten promotes invasive bladder cancer. *Genes Dev* 2009;23:675–689.

145. Said N, Theodorescu D. Pathways of metastasis suppression in bladder cancer. *Cancer Metastasis Rev* 2009; 28:327–333.

148. Dyrskjot L, Ostenfeld MS, Bramsen JB, et al. Genomic profiling of microRNAs in bladder cancer: miR-129 is associated with poor outcome and promotes cell death in vitro. *Cancer Res* 2009;69:4851–4860.

152. Adam L, Zhong M, Choi W, et al. miR-200 expression regulates epithelial-to-mesenchymal transition in bladder cancer cells and reverses resistance to epidermal growth factor receptor therapy. *Clin Cancer Res* 2009;15:5060–5072.

155. Orntoft TF, Dyrskjot L. Gene signatures for risk-adapted treatment of bladder cancer. *Scand J Urol Nephrol Suppl* 2008;(218):166–174.

MOLECULAR BIOLOGY OF INDIVIDUAL CANCERS

162. Lindgren D, Liedberg F, Andersson A, et al. Molecular characterization of early-stage bladder carcinomas by expression profiles, FGFR3 mutation status, and loss of 9q. *Oncogene* 2006;25:2685–2696.

167. Dyrskjot L, Kruhoffer M, Thykjaer T, et al. Gene expression in the urinary bladder: a common carcinoma in situ gene expression signature exists disregarding histopathological classification. *Cancer Res* 2004;64:4040–4048.

169. Dyrskjot L, Zieger K, Kruhoffer M, et al. A molecular signature in superficial bladder carcinoma predicts clinical outcome. *Clin Cancer Res* 2005;11:4029–4036.

172. Sanchez-Carbayo M, Socci ND, Lozano J, et al. Defining molecular profiles of poor outcome in patients with invasive bladder cancer using oligonucleotide microarrays. *J Clin Oncol* 2006;24:778–789.

173. McConkey DJ, Choi W, Marquis L, et al. Role of epithelial-to-mesenchymal transition (EMT) in drug sensitivity and metastasis in bladder cancer. *Cancer Metastasis Rev* 2009;28:335–344.

179. Als AB, Dyrskjøt L, von der Maase H, et al. Emmprin and survivin predict response and survival following cisplatin-containing chemotherapy in patients with advanced bladder cancer. *Clin Cancer Res* 2007;13:4407–4414.

186. Blaveri E, Brewer JL, Roydasgupta R, et al. Bladder cancer stage and outcome by array-based comparative genomic hybridization. *Clin Cancer Res* 2005;11:7012–7022.

192. Hafner C, Knuechel R, Stoehr R, et al. Clonality of multifocal urothelial carcinomas: 10 years of molecular genetic studies. *Int J Cancer* 2002;101:1–6.

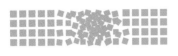

CHAPTER 22 PROSTATE CANCER

YU CHEN, VIVEK K. ARORA, AND CHARLES L. SAWYERS

Prostate cancer is the most common malignancy and the second leading cause of cancer death in Western men. It is highly heterogeneous with a disease specific mortality of one in seven. Many men survive decades without treatment, while others succumb quickly despite aggressive management. Among men who require systemic treatment, response rates to therapies are also highly variable—most notably some patients respond to androgen deprivation therapy for decades while a minority do not respond at all. Currently, the combination of clinical stage (tumor size on palpation), serum level of the prostate specific antigen (PSA), and histological grade (reported as Gleason score) is used to guide treatment decisions. Although useful for some clinical decisions, the modest predictive value of these parameters results both in overtreatment of many man and ineffective treatment for others. To achieve a "personalized medicine" approach to prostate cancer, it is important to define the repertoire of molecular lesions in prostate cancer, to identify the effect of these lesions on disease aggressiveness, and to identify therapies that have specific effectiveness against individual molecular lesions. Precedent for the ultimate success of this approach comes from other malignancies, such as the target specific kinase inhibitors erlotinib and PF-02341066 in lung cancers harboring epidermal growth factor receptor (EGFR) mutations and *EML4-ALK* fusions, respectively, the anti-HER2 antibody trastuzumab in breast cancers harboring HER2 amplification, and the kinase inhibitor PLX4032 in melanomas harboring BRAF mutations.[1-5] In prostate cancer, recent work is beginning to define disease subtypes driven by different oncogenic genetic lesions. Ongoing research is expected to result in a more personalized treatment approach in prostate cancer, including who to screen, who to treat, and what form of treatment to use.

GENETIC PREDISPOSITION

Prostate cancer has a significant genetic component. A large Nordic study of 44,788 pairs of twins con-

cluded that 42% of prostate cancers are attributable to genetic risk.[6] Men with one, two, and three first degree relatives afflicted with prostate cancer have a 2-, 5-, and 11-fold risk of developing the disease, respectively.[7] Given that large-scale screening of the general population is associated with small overall survival benefit and excess morbidity from curative surgery or radiation therapy for low risk disease,[8,9] identification of genetic predispositions—especially of aggressive disease—could guide screening decisions.

Early work identified rare mutations of several genes—*ELAC2, MSR1, RNAseL*—that confer increased risk of prostate cancer development but affect a small group of patients. Polymorphisms of genes in the androgen signaling pathway have been extensively studied with conflicting results.[10] With the technology to detect single nucleotide polymorphisms (SNP), genome-wide association studies (GWAS) of large cohorts have discovered novel genomic regions associated with prostate cancer risk. A number of independent reports showed that polymorphisms of multiple loci on chromosome 8q24 account for 10% and 30% of prostate cancer cases among European and African ancestry, respectively.[11-15] One challenge is to identify mechanisms by which these SNPs confer prostate cancer susceptibility since the 8q24 loci are located at a "gene desert." Recent work suggests that at least one loci may serve as an enhancer for *MYC*, which is approximately 300 kb away.[16] In addition, other loci have been recently discovered,[17,18] but none have shown a significant enough increase in the odds ratio of developing cancer to warrant screening of the general population. There is some evidence that simultaneous presence of multiple risk-associated SNPs in the same individual is associated with a significantly higher risk of prostate cancer.[19]

GENETIC LANDSCAPE OF PROSTATE CANCER

Like other epithelial tumors, many prostate cancers have a large number of genetic and epigenetic lesions associated with hallmark properties of

MOLECULAR BIOLOGY OF INDIVIDUAL CANCERS

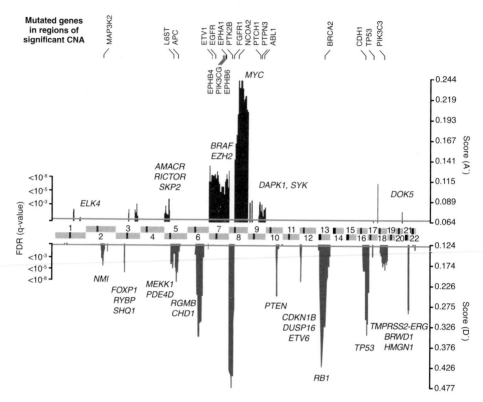

FIGURE 22.1 Genomic aberrations in prostate cancer. Regions of amplification (*red*) or deletion (*blue*) with false discovery rate (FDR) 10% or less are plotted, with chromosomes indicated at the center and centromeres in red. Genes with somatic nonsynonymous mutations are listed on top (*black*). Additional genes of interest targeted by copy-number alterations alone are also indicated (*gray*) (From ref. 21 with permission).

malignancies.[20] Types of lesions include overexpression of oncogenes and underexpression of tumor suppressor genes, genomic amplifications and deletions, translocations, and, more rarely, point mutations. One recent large-scale study that combines gene expression profiling, comparative genomic hybridization (array CGH) to characterize amplifications and deletions, and targeted resequencing for somatic mutations has shed light onto the genetic landscape of prostate cancer.[21] On average, prostate cancer is characterized by a relatively low mutation rate of genes commonly mutated in other malignancies, such as *KRAS*, *BRAF*, or *p53*, but a relatively large number of genomic alterations (Fig. 22.1). Recurrent amplifications and deletions, some focal, covering single to a handful of genes, and others spanning entire arms covering thousands of genes, are present in many tumors at diagnosis. On average, higher grade and stage tumors contain a greater number of genomic alterations. The most common genomic alteration is loss in the chromosomal arm 8p followed by a gain of chromosomal 8q. Some focal genomic alterations, such as deletion of *PTEN* or deletion of the interstitial region between *TMPRSS2* and *ERG* that creates the TMPRSS2-

ERG fusion gene, results in a clearly established oncogenic driver lesion. But for most genomic alterations, the specific genes responsible for oncogenesis are a subject of speculation.

Although many individual genes are rarely affected in prostate cancer, several key oncogenic and tumor suppressor pathways are commonly involved when the individual genes in each pathway are considered collectively. Four pathways—the phosphatidylinositol 3-phosphate kinase (PI3K)/AKT pathway, the RAS/MAP kinase pathway, the retinoblastoma pathway, and the androgen receptor (AR) pathway—are altered in one-third of primary cancers and almost all of metastatic lesions. This suggests that in prostate cancer, different individual genes in the pathway may be targeted to activate or suppress a common pathway lesion (Fig. 22.2). The sections below focus on those pathways where prostate cancer is most validated.

Androgen Receptor Pathway

It has been 70 years since Higgins and Hodges made the seminal observation that prostate cancers

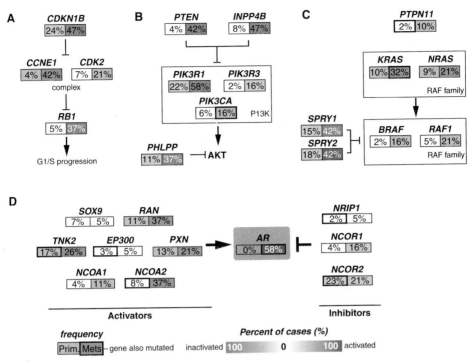

FIGURE 22.2 Alterations in the retinoblastoma (**A**), phosphatidylinositol 3-kinase (PI3K) (**B**), RAS/MAP kinase (**C**), and androgen receptor (AR) (**D**) pathways in prostate cancer. Alteration frequencies are shown for individual genes and for the entire pathway in primary and metastatic tumors. Alterations are defined as those having significant up- or down-regulation compared with normal prostate samples, or by somatic mutations, and are interpreted as activation (*red*) or inactivation (*blue*) of protein function. (From ref. 21 with permission.)

regress after surgical orchiectomy or suppression of androgen production by administration of exogenous estrogens.[22] These observations proved that prostate cancer is an androgen-dependent malignancy, and androgen deprivation therapy became the first targeted therapy in oncology—leading to a Nobel Prize for Charles Huggins in 1966.

Androgens exert their cellular actions through the AR, a 110 kb steroid receptor transcription factor, located on Xq12.[23,24] Upon binding androgen, AR mediates transcription of a number of genes involved in survival and differentiation of prostate epithelial cells. AR activity is required for development of both normal and malignant prostate tissue as men with germline AR inactivating mutations or men orchiectomized at a young age do not develop a prostate gland. AR plays a critical role in early pathogenesis as well as progression to advanced disease, and drugs that inhibit AR function remain the primary treatment for advanced prostate cancer.

Early Pathogenesis

Several lines of evidence suggest that enhanced AR signaling may play a causative role in prostate cancer initiation. Polymorphisms of three genes in the AR pathway, *AR* itself, *CYP17*, and *SRD5A2*,

are low penetrant risk factors for prostate cancer development in some but not all studies.[6] Overexpression of AR in both mouse and human primary prostate cells confers tumor forming ability when injected orthotopically into mice.[25,26] In rat models of carcinogen-induced prostate cancer, implantation of testosterone pellets results in an increased number of tumors.[27] Transgenic mice that overexpress AR in the prostate develop prostatic intraepithelial neoplasia (PIN).[28]

Pathway analysis from a recent large-scale prostate cancer genomic project found AR pathway alterations in 60% of primary tumors. The most commonly altered AR pathway member was *NCOA2* (also called *SRC2*), an AR coactivator that potentiates AR transcriptional output. Copy gains or somatic mutations of the *NCOA2* gene were found in approximately 20% of primary tumors. In addition, several other AR coactivators showed increased expression, while AR corepressors were down-regulated (Fig. 22.2D).

Cancer Progression and Castration-Resistant Growth

Because of the dependence of the prostate lineage on AR function, chemical castration through suppression of testicular function has become the mainstay in systemic treatment of prostate cancer. In normal prostate tissue, castration results in atrophy and cessation of PSA production indefinitely until restoration of testosterone levels. However, prostate cancers progress to the lethal castration-resistant prostate cancer (CRPC) after a variable duration of response. Cancer progression is usually accompanied by restoration of PSA secretion, indicating reactivation of AR activity. Thus, instead of bypassing the requirement for AR function, most castrate-resistant tumors have reactivation of the AR pathway, likely through multiple mechanisms.[23]

Alterations of AR itself represent the best characterized mechanism of castration resistance. Mutations of AR are detected in up to 10% of CRPCs and result in activation by other hormone ligands such as corticosteroids or, paradoxically, by antiandrogens.[29] Overexpression of AR is seen in the majority of CRPCs, and the AR gene is amplified in approximately 30% of cases.[30-32] AR overexpression is sufficient to activate AR in the milieu of castrate levels of androgens and to convert the antiandrogen, bicalutamide, into a weak agonist.[33] Alternative splicing of AR mRNA can lead to a truncated protein containing the N-terminal transcriptional activation and DNA binding domains but missing the ligand binding domain. Some of these variants have constitutive transcriptional activity in the absence of androgens and can be detected in CRPC samples. Overexpression of at least two variants can confer castration resistance in preclinical models.[34-36]

Alterations in AR pathway genes are found in 100% of metastases and may enhance AR activity in the presence of castrate androgen levels. NCOA2, for example, increases the magnitude of AR signaling across a broad range of androgen concentrations. Several other androgen receptor coactivators, including NCOA1, TNK2, and EP300, are up-regulated in metastatic disease, while AR corepressors, including NRIP1, NCOR1, and NCOR2, are down-regulated (Fig. 22.2D).

Intratumoral androgens are not completely eliminated by castration and may be increased in CRPC.[37] Direct measurements of intratumoral androgens by mass spectrometry showed that castration-resistant metastatic tumors in men treated with gonadotropin-releasing hormone (GnRH) agonists such as leuprolide have higher levels of testosterone than primary tumors in untreated men.[38] There is some evidence that CRPC may synthesize androgens to activate AR in an autocrine loop. Two expression profiling studies that compared metastatic CRPC with primary tumors have shown that enzymes involved in androgen synthesis are up-regulated in CRPC. Holzbeierlein et al.[32] found overexpression of enzymes involved in synthesis of cholesterol, the common steroid precursor, from acetyl-CoA, and Stanbrough

et al.[39] found overexpression of enzymes involved in synthesis of testosterone and the more potent androgen dihydrotestosterone (DHT) from cholesterol. A third study of patient samples at all stages of disease found an abundance of the enzymes AKR1C3 and SRD5A1 necessary for conversion of androstenedione to DHT. However, the samples lacked high expression of enzymes necessary for de novo steroidogenesis.[40] These data suggest that autocrine androgen synthesis may allow tumors to grow despite low serum androgen levels, but that this process may in part be dependent on adrenal precursors (Fig. 22.3).

Multiple kinase signaling pathways have been implicated in CRPC—most notably the HER2 and AKT pathways—with evidence that they exert their effects, in part, through modulation of AR activity. The HER2 receptor tyrosine kinase is progressively overexpressed in more advanced CRPC, though it is seldom amplified as seen in breast cancer. In experimental systems, forced overexpression of HER2 results in castration resistance, while pharmacologic inhibition or protein knockdown results in growth suppression.[41] Loss of PTEN and activation of the AKT pathway, commonly seen in CRPC (Fig. 22.2B), can contribute to castration resistance. Primary tumors with loss of PTEN have lower response rates to neoadjuvant bicalutamide.[42] Prostate cancer in mice with genetically engineered loss of PTEN rapidly develop castration resistance, and PTEN knockdown in murine hormone-sensitive prostate cancer cells confers castration-resistant growth.[43,44]

Androgen Receptor Targeting

Androgen deprivation therapy (ADT), most commonly delivered by administration of GnRH such as leuprolide, remains the cornerstone of prostate cancer systemic therapy. With the discovery that CRPC is associated with reactivation of AR and remains AR dependent, there have been many recent efforts to develop alternative AR targeting strategies (Fig. 22.3).

Antiandrogens

Antiandrogens compete with endogenous androgens for the ligand binding pocket of AR. Similar to androgens, antiandrogens promote translocation of AR from the cytoplasm into the nucleus and DNA binding but induce conformational changes that prevent optimal transcriptional activity. In the United States, there are three nonsteroidal antiandrogens currently in use—flutamide, bicalutamide, and nilutamide. Although generally active upon treatment initiation, each compound has been associated with the antiandrogen withdrawal response, whereby treated patients with progressive disease derive clinical benefit when the antiandrogen is stopped,[45] indicating that they

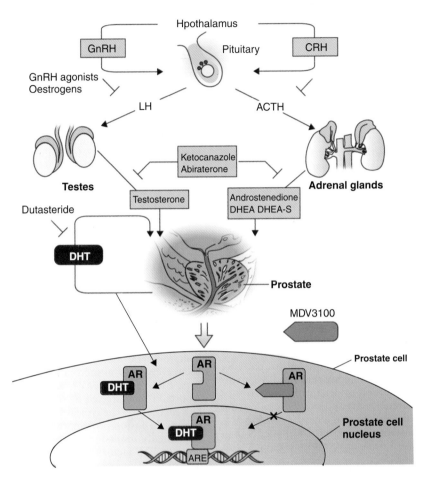

FIGURE 22.3 The androgen-signaling axis and its inhibitors. Testicular androgen synthesis is regulated by the gonadotropin-releasing hormone–luteinizing hormone (GnRH–LH) axis, whereas adrenal androgen synthesis is regulated by the corticotrophin-releasing hormone (CRH)-adrenocorticotropic hormone (ACTH) axis. GnRH agonists and corticosteroids inhibit stimulation of the testes and adrenals, respectively. Abiraterone inhibits CYP17, a critical enzyme in androgen synthesis. MDV3100 competitively inhibits the binding of androgens to androgen receptors. DHEA, dehydroepiandrosterone; DHEA-S, dehydroepiandrosterone sulphate; DHT, dihydrotestosterone; AR, androgen receptor; ARE, androgen-response element. (From ref. 98 with permission.)

have potential to act as AR agonists despite their intended role as antagonists. Indeed, overexpression of AR can convert bicalutamide from an antagonist into an agonist.[33]

Novel antiandrogens that have no agonistic properties would likely be clinically superior, and several efforts to identify such compounds are ongoing. Currently, the most promising compound, MDV3100, binds to AR with high affinity and prevents AR binding to DNA. MDV3100 is highly active in preclinical models of castration resistance where bicalutamide functions as an agonist.[46] In a phase 1/2 trial of MDV3100 in 140 CRPC patients previously treated with bicalutamide, the clinical response rate was greater than 50% as measured by a sustained, greater than 50% decline in serum PSA and radiographic evidence of partial response or

stable disease. Among those who where chemotherapy naive, PSA response rate was 62% and time to progression was 41 weeks—both compare favorably to docetaxel chemotherapy. Among the more advanced patients refractory to docetaxel, PSA response rate was 51% and time to progression was 21 weeks.[47] A phase 3 trial of MDV3100 in men with chemotherapy-refractory CRPC is ongoing.

Androgen Lowering Therapies

The most commonly used form of ADT, leuprolide, inhibits testicular androgen synthesis but does not impact other sources of androgen sources such as the adrenal glands and the purported autocrine androgen synthesis by tumor cells. Second-line ADT agents such as aminoglutethimide and ketoconazole inhibit adrenal androgen synthesis and have modest activity in CRPC, but their clinical utility is limited by side effects due to off target activities that preclude dose escalation.

CYP17 is a key P450 enzyme in the androgen biosynthesis pathway that functions in the testes and adrenal glands to catalyze the conversion of pregnenolone and progesterone into the weak androgens dehydroepiandrosterone (DHEA) and androstenedione, respectively. These weak androgens are further converted into testosterone and DHT, which may occur in peripheral tissues and in prostate tumor cells. Therefore, specific inhibition of CYP17 should decrease androgen synthesis without affecting the production of other essential steroids. The experimental drug abiraterone acetate is a pregnenolone derivative that is a selective, high affinity (half maximal inhibitory concentration [IC50] = 2 nM), irreversible inhibitor of CYP17. In phase 2 studies, two-thirds of chemotherapy-naive and half of postdocetaxel patients had PSA responses.[48–50] One potentially undesirable consequence of abiraterone treatment is increased production of adrenal progestins (generated by enzymes upstream of the CPY17 block). These progestins may have agonist activity in CRPC patients whose tumors have a highly sensitized AR pathway. Indeed, addition of dexamethasone to suppress this adrenal activity (and to rescue from potential adrenal insufficiency) reversed abiraterone resistance in one-third of patients (Fig. 22.3).[48] Phase 3 trials of abiraterone in men with CRPC are ongoing.

Indirect Approaches

AR activity requires the cooperation of numerous other proteins, some of which can be pharmacologically targeted. AR is stabilized by binding to the molecular chaperone, heat shock protein 90 (HSP90). Indeed, HSP90 inhibitors emerged as hits in a broad screen for chemical compounds that inhibit AR signaling. The clinical HSP90 inhibitor 17-AAG destabilizes AR and causes regression of prostate cancer in preclinical models.[51,52] To activate transcription, AR requires coordinated activity of chromatin remodeling enzymes, including histone deacetylases (HDAC). HDAC inhibitors suppress AR activity and prostate cancer growth in preclinical models.[53,54] Despite these promising preclinical results, clinical trials of HSP90 and HDAC inhibitors in CRPC have been disappointing, but this may be due to limitations in dose and schedule of these early generation inhibitors.[55]

ETS TRANSCRIPTION FACTORS

In 2005, using bioinformatic analysis of prostate cancer gene expression data, Tomlins et al.[56] made the seminal discovery that one of several members of the E26 transformation-specific (ETS) transcription factors are translocated in over half of all prostate cancers. This discovery also led to the recognition that recurrent genomic translocations, which had previously been observed only in hematopoietic malignancies and sarcomas, can occur commonly in solid tumors. Four ETS members, *ERG*, *ETV1*, *ETV4*, and *ETV5*, have been reported to be targeted by translocations in prostate cancer.[56–58] The typical translocation does not result in a fusion protein. Instead, the translocation usually results in aberrant expression of the targeted ETS factor in the prostate by juxtaposition to the promoter of highly expressed prostate gene—similar to the translocations of *MYC* and *BCL2* to *IgG* locus in Burkitt and follicular lymphomas (Fig. 22.4). The most prevalent translocation is between the androgen-regulated *TMPRSS2* gene and *ERG*, occurring in approximately 50% of all prostate cancers. Both genes are located on 21q22, and the fusion frequently occurs due to an interstitial deletion, which can be detected by high-density CGH approaches.[21]

FIGURE 22.4 Schematic of *TMPRSS2-ERG* and *ETV1* fusions. A: *TMPRSS2* and *ERG* are separated by 3Mb on 21q22. *TMPRSS2-ERG* fusion is usually formed by interstitial deletion resulting in exon 2 of TMPRSS2 juxtaposed to exon 4 of ERG. Fusion results in slightly truncated protein starting from exon 4. B: *ETV1* located on 7p21, can be fused to a number of genomic loci, some of which are shown. Many fusions result in a truncated protein starting in exon 6 but full length protein is also observed. Arrow indicates ATG translation initiation sites.

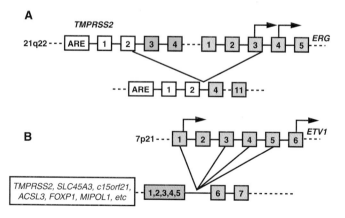

ETS Fusions as Prognostic and Predictive Factors

The discovery of the ETS translocations immediately raised questions about their prognostic value, which are still under debate. Just prior to the discovery of the translocation, one study noted *ERG* mRNA overexpression in a large subset of prostate cancers (almost certainly a consequence of the TMPRSS2-ERG translocation) reported a favorable prognosis.[59] Yet, presence of the *TMPRSS2-ERG* fusion (detected by fluorescence *in situ* hybridization [FISH]) strongly predicted for increased disease-specific mortality in a watchful waiting cohort from Sweden.[60] Larger studies (of U.S. populations) have found no prognostic role of *ERG* translocation.[61,62] It has been more difficult to assess the effect of the other, non-ERG ETS factors on prognosis due to the much smaller number of affected patients, although several reports consistently report that *ETV1* overexpression is associated with poor prognostic features.[61,63,64]

Given that the most common ETS fusions are expressed under the control of the androgen-regulated *TMPRSS2* promoter, their presence may be predictive of response to androgen deprivation therapy. In one small study, *ERG* rearrangement was associated with improved response to abiraterone acetate, but larger confirmatory studies are needed.[65]

ETS Fusions Occur Early in the Pathogenic Process

Analysis of primary and metastatic human tumors indicates that the TMPRSS2-ERG fusion (and most likely the rarer ETV fusions) are early events in prostate oncogenesis. Interestingly, independent prostate cancer loci in the prostatectomy sample from a single patient may harbor different types of ETS fusions, raising the possibility of multiple, concurrent primaries. However, studies of metastatic lesions uniformly contain the same type of ETS fusion, suggesting that the fusion is a premetastatic event and that not all fusion-positive tumors progress.[66–68] This pattern contrasts with genomic *PTEN* loss or *AR* amplification where the prevalence increases in castration-resistant metastatic lesions, suggesting these may represent later events. The role of ETS fusions in prostate cancer initiation is more controversial, particularly since mice engineered to express ETS fusions in the prostate do not develop cancers. Using FISH, early studies suggests that ETS fusions are rare in PIN. However, immunohistochemistry studies with a highly specific ERG antibody reveal that PIN lesions associated with ERG-positive carcinoma are generally positive for ERG.[69]

Oncogenic Role of ETS Factors

ETS factors are atypical oncogenes in that they can be highly expressed in some normal tissues (e.g., *ERG* in endothelial cells and *ETV1* in neurons). Furthermore, forced ETS overexpression in cells in culture is usually not transforming. Like many transcription factors, aberrant expression under specific contexts is likely required for oncogenesis. In the prostate, activation of the PTEN/AKT pathway provides one context for ETS-mediated tumorigenesis. In mouse models, overexpression of *ERG* or *ETV1* alone in the prostate has only modest effects.[56,70,71] Yet, in the context of PTEN loss or AKT activation, *ERG* overexpression is oncogenic. Indeed, in human prostate cancers, there is a strong correlation between *ERG* overexpression and loss of PTEN.[72–74]

The transcriptional program governed by aberrantly overexpressed ETS in prostate cancer is currently not well understood. To address this question, the genomic binding sites of ERG have recently been mapped in prostate cancer. Surprisingly, there is an extraordinarily high overlap between ERG and AR binding sites—suggesting that ERG can modulate AR activity.[75] Since AR can promote both cellular growth and differentiation, one hypothesis is that ERG expression modulates AR function away from differentiation and toward proliferation.

The PTEN/AKT Pathway

The PTEN (*p*hosphatase and *ten*sin homolog deleted on chromosome 10) tumor suppressor gene, originally identified through studies in breast cancer and glioblastoma, is lost in a significant fraction of prostate cancers through deletion, mutation, or epigenetic silencing.[76] Studies using high-density SNP arrays show that *PTEN* is the only gene in the overlapping chromosomal regions lost in a large set of prostate cancers displaying deletion of 10q23.[77] Examination of nine prostate cancer xenografts with neither *PTEN* loss of heterozygosity (LOH) nor mutations showed that five had epigenetic silencing.[78] Three independently generated mouse models with prostate-specific homozygous deletions of *Pten* all developed prostate cancer with progression from PIN to adenocarcinoma to metastasis similar to human disease.[79–81] These data unambiguously implicate *PTEN* as a critical lesion in prostate cancer pathogenesis. Whether *PTEN* loss occurs early or late in prostate tumorigenesis is not clear. Complete genomic loss of *PTEN* is seen in greater than 50% of metastatic lesions but in only approximately 20% of localized lesions. Within the same patient, *PTEN* loss can be observed in metastatic but not primary lesions,[68] suggesting that genomic *PTEN* loss is involved in disease progression but not initiation. However, heterozygous

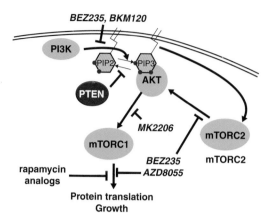

FIGURE 22.5 Schematic of the phosphatidylinositol 3-kinase (PK3K) pathway and inhibitors. PI3K phosphorylates PIP2 into PIP3, while the PTEN phosphatase catalyzes the opposite reaction. PIP3 activates AKT by recruitment to the membrane, activation of mammalian target of rapamycin complex 2 (mTORC2) and pyruvate dehydrogenase kinase (PDK) kinases. AKT activates many growth pathways include mTORC1. BEZ235 is a dual-specificity kinase inhibitor that inhibits both PI3K and mTOR, the common kinase component of mTROC1 and mTORC2 complexes. BKM120 and AZD8055 are kinase inhibitors that inhibit PI3K and mTOR, respectively. Rapamycin analogues (e.g., sirolimus, temsirolimus, everolimus) specifically inhibit assembly of the mTORC1 complex. MK2206 is a new generation allosteric inhibitor of AKT.

PTEN loss or decreased PTEN protein expression by immunohistochemistry has been reported in approximately 25% of PIN and greater than 50% of primary cancers, suggesting that PTEN may be a haploinsufficient tumor suppressor. Partial loss could be important for early tumorigenesis, with progression to complete loss at metastasis.[82] Mouse models have confirmed a dosage effect of Pten in prostate cancer progression.

PTEN is the major negative regulator of the PI3K/AKT pathway (Fig. 22.5). PI3K, which can be activated by many growth factors, phosphorylates PIP2 into PIP3 at the plasma membrane and PIP3 recruits pleckstrin homology (PH) domain–containing proteins, including AKT. As a lipid phosphatase, PTEN converts PIP3 back to PIP2 thereby limiting normal activity of the pathway. PI3K also activates mammalian target of rapamycin (mTOR) C2 complex (which contains the kinase mTOR complexed with distinct regulatory factors), which directly phosphorylates and activates AKT. Activated AKT phosphorylates a number of crucial substrates implicated in cell growth and survival, including downstream activation of the other mTOR complex, mTORC1 (Fig. 22.5).

The PTEN→AKT→mTOR pathway has garnered special attention due to the large number of mutations in the genes in this pathway, including PTEN, PI3K, AKT, as well as upstream kinases.

Mouse models of prostate cancer suggest that both AKT and mTORC2 are essential mediators of PTEN-loss–mediated tumorigenesis—prostate-specific deletions of either gene abolish the tumor phenotype of Pten loss prostate.[83,84] This pathway is also amenable to pharmaceutical inhibition using approved drugs such as rapamycin, and its analogues, which inhibit mTORC1; investigational kinase inhibitors targeting PI3K, mTORC1 and mTORC2, and AKT are in clinical development (Fig. 22.5). Preclinical data provide strong rationale for their trials in prostate cancer. In addition to AKT, PTEN loss likely has other crucial targets, evidenced by the observation that overexpression of active AKT in mice causes PIN that does not progress into cancer while $Pten^{(-/-)}$ mice develop invasive cancer. One candidate pathway involves CDC42 and JNK.[85]

Chromosome 8p Loss and 8q Gain

NKX3.1

Heterozygous loss of 8p21 is the most frequent chromosomal aberration in prostate cancer, affecting 60% of PIN and 85% of prostate cancers.[86] The most studied candidate tumor suppressor gene mapping to this region is the AR regulated, prostate specific homeobox transcription factor NKX3.1. However, unlike classic tumor suppressor genes, the remaining NKX3.1 allele is not mutated or deleted, leading to the hypothesis that NKX3.1 haploinsufficiency is sufficient for oncogenesis. Prostate development in mice with targeted deletion of Nkx3.1 proceeds normally, albeit with subtle defects in prostate morphogenesis.[86] Mechanistic studies suggest NKX3.1 facilitates terminal differentiation. In castrated mice, introduction of testosterone results in an early intense proliferative response to reconstitute the gland followed by differentiation and quiescence. In $Nkx3.1^{(+/-)}$ and $Nkx3.1^{(-/-)}$ mice, there is a delay in differentiation, resulting in hypertrophy.[87,88] When crossed into $Pten^{(+/-)}$ mice, loss of Nkx3.1 is reported to accelerate prostate neoplasia. Furthermore, prostate tumors that develop in two genetically engineered mouse models caused by distinct initiating lesions (transgenic expression of Myc and conditional Pten deletion) both show reduced Nkx3.1 expression.[79,89] In the case of Pten loss, the decline in Nkx3.1 expression is most likely explained by crosstalk between Pten and Nkx3.1 rather than selection for Nkx3.1 loss as a progression event.[90]

Other evidence argues against NKX3.1 as the 8p tumor suppressor. Despite monoallelic loss, mRNA expression is still quite high in prostate tumors. In fact, tumors that harbor single copy loss of NKX3.1 do not have lower levels of NKX3.1 transcript. Furthermore, the minimal common deleted region on 8p does not always span NKX3.1.

Thus, there may be other tumors suppressors in 8p21 whose loss mediate prostate tumorigenesis.

MYC

Gain of 8q is the second most common chromosomal abnormality in prostate cancer with peaks of amplification located at both *MYC* and *NCOA2*. Metastatic lesions often have further amplicons at the *MYC* locus on 8q24. MYC is a transcription factor that heterodimerizes with Max to regulate the expression of a large number of genes (up to 15% of the genome) and serves as an integrator of numerous growth signals. Physiologically, *MYC* expression correlates with proliferation, and levels are tightly controlled at multiple levels—by transcription, mRNA stability, and protein stability. There is strong experimental evidence implicating *MYC* dysregulation in prostate cancer. *MYC* overexpression in primary prostate epithelial cells leads to transformation,[25] and transgenic mice expressing *MYC* in the prostate develop PIN followed by adenocarcinoma,[89] which histologically represents the closest mimic of human prostate cancer among current mouse models.[91]

Epigenetic Changes

In addition to genetic alternations, a number of epigenetic changes have been implicated in prostate cancer progression, such as altered DNA methylation and histone modifications, that lead to changes in gene expression.[92] One early change in prostate cancer is silencing of the π-class glutathione *S*-transferase (*GSTP*) gene through DNA methylation at CpG islands in transcriptional regulatory regions. *GSTP* is frequently overexpressed in many cancers, perhaps due to oncogenic and chemotherapy stress. Unexpectedly, GSTπ expression is silenced in the vast majority of prostate cancers and PIN lesions through methylation of the GSTπ promoter.[93]

DNA is packaged around the core histone proteins H2A, H2B, H3, and H4 to form chromatin. The amino termini of histones, particularly H3 and H4, are subject to posttranslational modification through lysine acetylation or methylation and arginine methylation, all of which influence gene expression. Altered histone modifications, such as H3K4 methylation and H4R3 methylation, have been reported to correlate with reduced risk of recurrence in surgically resected prostate cancer.[94] Changes in expression of the proteins responsible for these histone modifications have been implicated in prostate cancer. For example, EZH2 (enhancer of Zeste homolog 2) is a polycomb group protein overexpressed in high-grade localized as well as castrate-resistant metastatic prostate cancer.[95] EZH2 is part of a larger suppressive complex that recruits DNA methyltransferases to CpG islands. EZH2 methylates lysine 27 of histone H3 and forms a bridge between suppressive histone and DNA methylation.[96] High levels of EZH2 may be oncogenic through suppression of gene expression due to H3K27 methylation of critical target genes such as the RasGAP family member DAB2IP.[97]

MOLECULAR BIOLOGY OF INDIVIDUAL CANCERS

Selected References

The full list of references for this chapter appears in the online version.

6. Nelson WG, De Marzo AM, Isaacs WB. Prostate cancer. *N Engl J Med* 2003;349:366.
7. De Marzo AM, Platz EA, Sutcliffe S, et al. Inflammation in prostate carcinogenesis. *Nat Rev Cancer* 2007;7:256.
8. Schroder FH, Hugosson J, Roobol MJ, et al. Screening and prostate-cancer mortality in a randomized European study. *N Engl J Med* 2009;360:1320.
9. Andriole GL, Crawford ED, Grubb RL 3rd, et al. Mortality results from a randomized prostate-cancer screening trial. *N Engl J Med* 2009;360:1310.
11. Amundadottir LT, Sulem P, Gudmundsson J, et al. A common variant associated with prostate cancer in European and African populations. *Nat Genet* 2006;38:652.
12. Gudmundsson J, Sulem P, Manolescu A, et al. Genome-wide association study identifies a second prostate cancer susceptibility variant at 8q24. *Nat Genet* 2007; 39:631.
13. Haiman CA, Patterson N, Freedman ML, et al. Multiple regions within 8q24 independently affect risk for prostate cancer. *Nat Genet* 2007;39:638.
14. Yeager M, Orr N, Hayes RB, et al. Genome-wide association study of prostate cancer identifies a second risk locus at 8q24. *Nat Genet* 2007;39:645.

15. Al Olama AA, Kote-Jarai Z, Giles GG, et al. Multiple loci on 8q24 associated with prostate cancer susceptibility. *Nat Genet* 2009;41:1058.
16. Ahmadiyeh N, Pomerantz MM, Grisanzio C, et al. 8q24 prostate, breast, and colon cancer risk loci show tissue-specific long-range interaction with MYC. *Proc Natl Acad Sci U S A* 2010;107:9742.
17. Eeles RA, Kote-Jarai Z, Giles GG, et al. Multiple newly identified loci associated with prostate cancer susceptibility. *Nat Genet* 2008;40:316.
18. Thomas G, Jacobs KB, Yeager M, et al. Multiple loci identified in a genome-wide association study of prostate cancer. *Nat Genet* 2008;40:310.
19. Zheng SL, Sun J, Wiklund F, et al. Cumulative association of five genetic variants with prostate cancer. *N Engl J Med* 2008;358:910.
21. Taylor BS, Schultz N, Hieronymus H, et al. Integrative genomic profiling of human prostate cancer. *Cancer Cell* 2010;18:11.
22. Huggins C, Hodges CV. Studies on prostatic cancer. I. The effect of castration, of estrogen and of androgen injection on serum phosphatases in metastatic carcinoma of the prostate. *Cancer Res* 1941;1:293.
24. Chen Y, Sawyers CL, Scher HI. Targeting the androgen receptor pathway in prostate cancer. *Curr Opin Pharmacol* 2008;8:440.

25. Berger R, Febbo PG, Majumder PK, et al. Androgen-induced differentiation and tumorigenicity of human prostate epithelial cells. *Cancer Res* 2004;64:8867.

30. Visakorpi T, Hyytinen E, Koivisto P, et al. In vivo amplification of the androgen receptor gene and progression of human prostate cancer. *Nat Genet* 1995;9:401.

32. Holzbeierlein J, Lal P, LaTulippe E, et al. Gene expression analysis of human prostate carcinoma during hormonal therapy identifies androgen-responsive genes and mechanisms of therapy resistance. *Am J Pathol* 2004;164:217.

33. Chen CD, Welsbie DS, Tran C, et al. Molecular determinants of resistance to antiandrogen therapy. *Nat Med* 2004;10:33.

36. Sun S, Sprenger CC, Vessella RL, et al. Castration resistance in human prostate cancer is conferred by a frequently occurring androgen receptor splice variant. *J Clin Invest* 2010;120:2715.

38. Montgomery RB, Mostaghel EA, Vessella R, et al. Maintenance of intratumoral androgens in metastatic prostate cancer: a mechanism for castration-resistant tumor growth. *Cancer Res* 2008;68:4447.

39. Stanbrough M, Bubley GJ, Ross K, et al. Increased expression of genes converting adrenal androgens to testosterone in androgen-independent prostate cancer. *Cancer Res* 2006;66:2815.

41. Mellinghoff IK, Vivanco I, Kwon A, et al. HER2/neu kinase-dependent modulation of androgen receptor function through effects on DNA binding and stability. *Cancer Cell* 2004;6:517.

45. Kelly WK, Scher HI. Prostate specific antigen decline after antiandrogen withdrawal: the flutamide withdrawal syndrome. *J Urol* 1993;149:607.

46. Tran C, Ouk S, Clegg NJ, et al. Development of a second-generation antiandrogen for treatment of advanced prostate cancer. *Science* 2009;324:787.

47. Scher HI, Beer TM, Higano CS, et al. Antitumour activity of MDV3100 in castration-resistant prostate cancer: a phase 1-2 study. *Lancet* 2010;375:1437.

49. Danila DC, Morris MJ, de Bono JS, et al. Phase II multicenter study of abiraterone acetate plus prednisone therapy in patients with docetaxel-treated castration-resistant prostate cancer. *J Clin Oncol* 2010;28:1496.

52. Hieronymus H, Lamb J, Ross KN, et al. Gene expression signature-based chemical genomic prediction identifies a novel class of HSP90 pathway modulators. *Cancer Cell* 2006;10:321.

54. Welsbie DS, Xu J, Chen Y, et al. Histone deacetylases are required for androgen receptor function in hormone-sensitive and castrate-resistant prostate cancer. *Cancer Res* 2009;69:958.

56. Tomlins SA, Laxman B, Dhanasekaran SM, et al. Distinct classes of chromosomal rearrangements create oncogenic ETS gene fusions in prostate cancer. *Nature* 2007;448:595.

58. Tomlins SA, Rhodes DR, Perner S, et al. Recurrent fusion of TMPRSS2 and ETS transcription factor genes in prostate cancer. *Science* 2005;310:644.

60. Demichelis F, Fall K, Perner S, et al. TMPRSS2:ERG gene fusion associated with lethal prostate cancer in a watchful waiting cohort. *Oncogene* 2007;26:4596.

62. Gopalan A, Leversha MA, Satagopan JM, et al. TMPRSS2-ERG gene fusion is not associated with outcome in patients treated by prostatectomy. *Cancer Res* 2009;69:1400.

72. Carver BS, Tran J, Gopalan A, et al. Aberrant ERG expression cooperates with loss of PTEN to promote cancer progression in the prostate. *Nat Genet* 2009;41:619.

73. King JC, Xu J, Wongvipat J, et al. Cooperativity of TMPRSS2-ERG with PI3-kinase pathway activation in prostate oncogenesis. *Nat Genet* 2009;41:524.

74. Zong Y, Xin L, Goldstein AS, et al. ETS family transcription factors collaborate with alternative signaling pathways to induce carcinoma from adult murine prostate cells. *Proc Natl Acad Sci U S A* 2009;106:12465.

75. Yu J, Mani RS, Cao Q, et al. An integrated network of androgen receptor, polycomb, and TMPRSS2-ERG gene fusions in prostate cancer progression. *Cancer Cell* 2010;17:443.

78. Whang YE, Wu X, Suzuki H, et al. Inactivation of the tumor suppressor PTEN/MMAC1 in advanced human prostate cancer through loss of expression. *Proc Natl Acad Sci U S A* 1998;95:5246.

79. Wang S, Gao J, Lei Q, et al. Prostate-specific deletion of the murine Pten tumor suppressor gene leads to metastatic prostate cancer. *Cancer Cell* 2003;4:209.

83. Chen ML, Xu PZ, Peng XD, et al. The deficiency of Akt1 is sufficient to suppress tumor development in Pten+/− mice. *Genes Dev* 2006;20:1569.

84. Guertin DA, Stevens DM, Saitoh M, et al. mTOR complex 2 is required for the development of prostate cancer induced by Pten loss in mice. *Cancer Cell* 2009;15:148.

85. Vivanco I, Palaskas N, Tran C, et al. Identification of the JNK signaling pathway as a functional target of the tumor suppressor PTEN. *Cancer Cell* 2007;11:555.

87. Kim MJ, Bhatia-Gaur R, Banach-Petrosky WA, et al. Nkx3.1 mutant mice recapitulate early stages of prostate carcinogenesis. *Cancer Res* 2002;62:2999.

88. Magee JA, Abdulkadir SA, Milbrandt J. Haploinsufficiency at the Nkx3.1 locus. A paradigm for stochastic, dosage-sensitive gene regulation during tumor initiation. *Cancer Cell* 2003;3:273.

89. Ellwood-Yen K, Graeber TG, Wongvipat J, et al. Myc-driven murine prostate cancer shares molecular features with human prostate tumors. *Cancer Cell* 2003;4:223.

90. Lei Q, Jiao J, Xin L, et al. NKX3.1 stabilizes p53, inhibits AKT activation, and blocks prostate cancer initiation caused by PTEN loss. *Cancer Cell* 2006;9:367.

94. Seligson DB, Horvath S, Shi T, et al. Global histone modification patterns predict risk of prostate cancer recurrence. *Nature* 2005;435:1262.

95. Varambally S, Dhanasekaran SM, Zhou M, et al. The polycomb group protein EZH2 is involved in progression of prostate cancer. *Nature* 2002;419:624.

98. Chen Y, Clegg NJ, Scher HI. Anti-androgens and androgen-depleting therapies in prostate cancer: new agents for an established target. *Lancet Oncol* 2009;10:981.

CHAPTER 23 GYNECOLOGIC CANCERS

KUNLE ODUNSI, TANJA PEJOVIC, AND MATTHEW L. ANDERSON

MOLECULAR BIOLOGY OF INDIVIDUAL CANCERS

Gynecologic cancer research has mirrored all cancer research programs in that it has focused largely on molecular defects in oncogenes, tumor-suppressor genes, and DNA repair mechanisms. Several research groups have also channeled their resources into various carcinogenic phenomena such as apoptotic pathway defects, growth signaling, angiogenesis, tissue invasion, or metastasis. These efforts have led to a broad understanding of the chromosomal and molecular abnormalities that underlie malignancies of the female genital tract (vulva, vagina, cervix, uterus, ovaries, and fallopian tubes). It is clear that an improvement in outcome of these malignancies can only be achieved if (1) early diagnosis is achieved, (2) there is accurate prediction of progression and response, and (3) new treatment options reflecting the molecular pathogenesis and progression are developed. This requires detailed disease-specific understanding of the diverse molecular changes in gynecologic malignancies that ultimately lead cells to develop the following hallmarks of cancer: abnormalities in self-sufficiency of growth signals, evasion of apoptosis, insensitivity to antigrowth signals, limitless replicative potential, sustained angiogenesis, and tissue invasion and metastases. Moreover, there is growing evidence for the concept of cancer immunosurveillance and immunoediting based on (1) protection against development of spontaneous and chemically induced tumors in animal systems and (2) identification of targets for immune recognition of human cancer.[1] This concept is supported by several studies in gynecologic cancers and has opened new avenues for the development of novel biomarkers and therapeutic targets. It is the purpose of this chapter to highlight and summarize some of the recent basic findings in gynecologic malignancies, with an emphasis on clinically applicable developments.

OVARIAN CANCER

Origins of Epithelial Ovarian Cancer

Epithelial ovarian cancer (EOC) arises primarily from the ovarian surface epithelium (OSE), with a subset possibly originating in the adjacent fimbria.[2,3] The OSE forms a monolayer surrounding the ovary, but is composed of relatively few cuboidal cells (107 cells per ovary, or 0.05% of the entire organ). Developmentally it derives from the celomic epithelium, which also gives rise to the peritoneal mesothelium and oviductal epithelium.[4] The OSE appears generally stable, uniform, and quiescent, though it can undergo proliferation *in vivo*.[5] Despite the small number of cells within the OSE and their apparent inactivity, the risk for EOC is nearly 2%, suggesting a high malignant potential. The basis for such a high potential is poorly understood. No physiological role for the primate OSE has been established,[6] and the lack of any obvious function could contribute to the asymptomatic nature of early stage EOC.

In other organs, such as colon, distinct premalignant lesions have been identified and found to accumulate genetic defects that ultimately result in malignancy. However, the search to identify similar epithelial precursors in the human ovary has proven only partially fruitful, in large part because normal ovaries are only rarely biopsied or examined. Histologic findings consistent with a preinvasive lesion for ovarian cancer have been described by a number of studies where ovaries were removed from women who eventually developed peritoneal carcinomas, ovaries from high-risk women who were undergoing prophylactic oophorectomy, and in areas of ovarian epithelium adjacent to early-stage ovarian cancers that demonstrate a transition from normal to malignant cells.[7] The hypothesis that these lesions are premalignant is strengthened by observations that regions of epithelial irregularity express levels of p53 and Ki-67 intermediate between those found in normal ovarian epithelium and ovarian cancers.

Each of these observations is consistent with the hypothesis that, similar to cancers originating in other organs, ovarian cancer evolves from an intraepithelial precursor. If so, improved means to detect and/or eradicate these lesions may prove fruitful for preventing ovarian cancer.

Molecular Pathways to Ovarian Cancer

Inherited Syndromes of Ovarian Cancers

Linkage analysis of familial breast and ovarian cancers provided some of the first insights into the molecular basis of ovarian cancer. These efforts ultimately identified two gene products, *BRCA1* and *BRCA2*, each clearly associated with an increased incidence of ovarian cancer. Although only a minority (8% to 10%) of diagnosed ovarian cancers are familial, most (76% to 92%) familial ovarian cancers are associated with mutations at the *BRCA1* locus, located on 17q21. Hundreds of mutations in *BRCA1* have now been identified, most commonly loss of function nonsense or frameshift mutations. Two specific mutations, 185delAG and 5382insC, are found in 1% and 0.1% of Ashkenazi Jewish women.

Functionally, *BRCA1* regulates *p53*, an oncogene frequently implicated in ovarian cancer. Thus, loss of *BRCA1* allows DNA damage to accumulate via a loss of its activation of *p53*. However, mutations in *BRCA1* also likely contribute to ovarian cancer by mechanisms other than its interactions with *p53*. These include its ability to specifically regulate X chromosome gene expression mediated by an association of Xist with the inactive X chromosome.[8] Consistent with this observation, site-specific dysregulation of X-linked gene expression in *BRCA1*-associated epithelial ovarian malignancies have been described.

Although mutations in *BRCA1* or *BRCA2* are only rarely observed in sporadic, nonfamilial ovarian cancers, it is possible that the mutations in pathways by which *BRCA1* regulates X-chromosome gene expression do, in fact, contribute to this disease. Characterization of genome-wide patterns of gene expression in sporadic breast cancers has allowed investigators to classify these tumors as either BRCA1-like or BRCA2-like in the patterns of their gene expression. This observation implicates the contribution of alterations in other components of the BRCA1 or BRCA2 regulated pathways to sporadic breast cancers and, possibly, ovarian cancer. Any understanding of the role of *BRCA1* in ovarian cancer is further complicated by reports of women with high-risk mutations in *BRCA1* who fail to develop ovarian cancer. These observations speak clearly to the role of genetic modifiers in determining whether *BRCA1* or *BRCA2* mutations ultimately lead to malignancy. For example, CAG repeat polymorphism in the androgen receptor has been shown to modify the subsequent risk of ovarian cancer in women with known mutations in *BRCA1*.

Genomic Instability

Genomic instability, manifested as a cell's ability to tolerate DNA damage, is a hallmark of all cancer, including epithelial ovarian cancers. Tolerance to DNA damage can be achieved by alterations in any of the six major DNA repair pathways: base excision repair, mismatch repair, nucleotide excision repair, homologous recombination, nonhomologous recombination, and translesion DNA synthesis. The specific DNA pathway affected often predicts the specific type of mutations observed in particular cancers, its sensitivity to drugs, as well as clinical outcome of affected patients.

Fanconi Anemia DNA Repair Pathway

Studies on the pathogenesis of rare inherited DNA repair disorders, such as Fanconi anemia (FA), have helped define the molecular basis of defective DNA damage responses linked to cancer risk. FA is a rare genetic disorder characterized by skeletal anomalies, progressive bone marrow failure, cancer susceptibility, and cellular hypersensitivity to DNA cross-linking agents. To date, 13 FA genes have been cloned: *FANCA, -B, -C, -D1, -D2, -E, -F, -G, -J, -L, -M, -N,* and *-I*. Of these, *FANCA, FANCB, FANCC, FANCE, FANCF, FANCG, FANCL,* and *FANCM* form a nuclear core complex. Although the functional scope of this complex has not been fully defined, it is clear that it must be completely intact to facilitate monoubiquitination of the downstream FANCD2 and FANCI proteins, a change that allows FANCD2 and FANCI to colocalize with *BRCA1, BRCA2* (and presumably FANCJ and FANCN), and *RAD51* in damage-induced nuclear foci.[9]

Four lines of evidence link the FA pathway with ovarian carcinogenesis. first, *BRCA2* has been identified as the FA gene *FANCD1*. As a result, heterozygotes for *BRCA2* mutations have a high risk of tissue-specific epithelial cancers, while homozygotes develop FA. Second, an increased prevalence of epithelial cancers, including ovarian malignancies, has been observed in FANCD2 nullizygous mice. Functionally significant silencing of *FANCF* in ovarian cancer through promoter hypermethylation has also been described. Lastly, low levels of FANCD2 protein are found in ovarian surface epithelia from women at risk for ovarian cancer. Taken together, these data suggest that the FA pathway is important in defining predisposition to ovarian (and breast) cancer, and that aberrations of FA genes may account for some familial ovarian cancer cases not accounted for by *BRCA1* and *BRCA2* mutations.

In sporadic ovarian cancers, the epigenetic silencing of FA pathway through methylation of the FA gene promoter region is one of the frequent mechanisms of inactivation. One study found that 4 of 19 primary ovarian carcinomas had *FANCF* methylation, although a larger study of 106 ovarian tumors did not identify loss of FANCF expression. Loss of *BRCA2* mRNA and protein has been reported in 13% of ovarian carcinomas, and in contrast to other FA genes, methylation is not a cause of the protein loss. Epigenetic silencing of

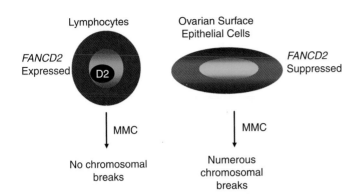

Lymphocytes

Ovarian Surface
Epithelial Cells

FANCD2
Expressed

D2

FANCD2
Suppressed

MMC

MMC

No chromosomal
breaks

Numerous
chromosomal
breaks

FIGURE 23.1 Tissue-restricted genetic instability in ovarian epithelial cells from women at risk for ovarian cancer with no BRCA mutations. Mitomycin C–induced chromosomal breakage is high and FANCD2 levels are low in ovarian epithelial cells but normal in peripheral blood lymphocytes and may antedate the onset of overt carcinoma. (We thank Dr. Grover Bagby for helping to create this figure.)

BRCA1 through methylation was found in 23% of advanced ovarian carcinomas (Fig. 23.1).

Interestingly, tumors with inactivated BRCA2 are responsive to cisplatin. However, due to their low accuracy of DNA repair, these cells accumulate secondary genetic modifications that can lead to reversal of BRCA2 mutation, allowing these cells to acquire resistance to crosslinking agents.[10]

Other DNA Repair Pathways

Similar to the FA/BRCA pathway, disruptions of other DNA repair pathways have been observed in ovarian cancer. These disruptions account, at least in part, for the specific drug sensitivity of the tumors. Recent studies indicate translesion DNA synthesis defect in ovarian cancer is a consequence of elevation in activity of POLB, an error-prone polymerase. Inhibition of POLB in these cells results in resensitization to cisplatin.[11] Overall it is believed that although inactivation of one DNA repair pathway may confer advantage to tumors, cancer cells may rely more on other repair pathways. Therefore, inactivation of the second pathway would be deleterious for these cells, causing synthetic lethality. An RNA interference screen identified the ataxia-telangiectasia mutated (ATM) pathway to be synthetically lethal with FA.[12] Similarly a strategy for synthetic lethality is under investigation, using base excision repair poly(adenosine diphosphate-ribose) polymerase 1 (PARP1) inhibitors in the treatment of homologous recombination deficient ovarian cancer.[13,14] PARP inhibition has been shown to be up to 1,000 times selectively more toxic to cancer cells than to wild type cells. PARP inhibitors act by exploiting a tumor cell's defect in homologous recombination, a type of DNA repair. This is because following PARP inhibition, cells require homologous recombination to repair common types of DNA damage. Although normal cells can use homologous recombination for repair of this damage and survive, certain types of tumors (e.g., those with BRCA1 or BRCA2 defects) have lost the ability to repair by homologous recombination and will die.

Genome Wide Association Studies. The identification of common ovarian cancer susceptibility variants may have clinical implications in the future for identifying patients at greatest risk of the disease. In this regard, several genome wide association study (GWAS) have been performed in ovarian cancer. The most striking of these was a recent study by the Ovarian Cancer Association Consortium to identify common ovarian cancer susceptibility alleles.[15] A total of 507,094 single nucleotide polymorphisms (SNPs) were genotyped in 1,817 cases and 2,353 controls from the United Kingdom; and 22,790 top ranked SNPs were also genotyped in 4,274 cases and 4,809 controls of European ancestry from Europe, the United States, and Australia. Twelve SNPs were identified at 9p22 associated with disease risk ($P < 10^{-8}$). The most significant SNP (rs3814113; $P = 2.5 \times 10^{-17}$) was genotyped in a further 2,670 ovarian cancer cases and 4,668 controls, confirming its association (combined data odds ratio [OR] = 0.82 95% confidence interval [CI], 0.79 to 0.86; $P_{trend} = 5.1 \times 10^{-19}$). The association was strongest for serous ovarian cancers (OR 0.77; 95% CI, 0.73 to 0.81; $P_{trend} = 4.1 \times 10^{-21}$).

Transcriptional Profiling of Ovarian Cancer Histologic Subtypes

Several gene expression studies using cDNA microarrays have been performed in ovarian cancer. Additionally, several studies have focused on the alterations demonstrated in the DNA copy number.[16–18] Array-based technology has shown that the different histological subtypes of ovarian carcinoma are distinguishable based on their overall genetic expression profiles. A common finding among several studies is the ability to distinguish low-grade serous ovarian carcinoma from high-grade carcinoma based on their gene expression profiles.[17,19–23] A number of genes shown to be differentially expressed in EOC are known to be involved in many important cellular mechanisms, including cell cycle regulation, apoptosis, tumor invasion, and control of local immunity.[20,24,25]

Increased mutagenic signaling by receptor tyrosine kinases plays a major role in ovarian carcinogenesis (Table 23.1). Overexpression of

TABLE 23.1

GENETIC ALTERATIONS IN OVARIAN CANCER

Gene	Alteration	Frequency (%)
DNA REPAIR GENES		
BRCA1	Nonsense	5
BRCA2	Frame-shift mutation	3
MLH1	Mutation	1
ONCOGENES		
EGFR	Amplification/overexpression	20
ERBB2	Amplification/overexpression	30
(Her2/neu)		
FMS	Coexpression with CSF-1	50
PI3K3	Mutation/amplification	12–20
AKT2	Mutation/amplification	20
TGF-β	Mutation/overexpression	12
TβR I	Mutation	33
TβR II	Mutation	25
TUMOR SUPPRESSOR GENES		
p53	Mutation/overexpression	20–50
km23	Mutation	42

epidermal growth factor receptor (EGFR) (ERBB1), ERBB2/HER2/neu, and c-FMS has been reported repeatedly in ovarian cancer. One of the major downstream mediators of signaling initiated by these receptors is the phosphatidylinositol 3-kinase (PI3K)–AKT pathway. Aberrations in this pathway including increased AKT1 kinase activity, AKT2 and PI3K amplification, and PI3KR1 mutations may provide opportunities for therapeutic intervention.

It has been reported that more than 75% of ovarian carcinomas are resistant to transforming growth factor-beta (TGF-β),[26] and the loss of TGF-β responsiveness may play an important role in the pathogenesis or progression of ovarian cancer. In addition, it has been shown that TGF-β1, the TGF-β receptors (TβR-II and TβR-I), and the TGF-β signaling component Smad2 are altered in ovarian cancer. Alterations in TβR-II have been identified in 25% of ovarian carcinomas, whereas mutations in TβR-I were reported in 33% of such cancers.[27] Protooncogene transformation might lead either to an overexpression of mitogenic molecules or an inactivation of those with inhibitory action, thus contributing to neoplastic transformation and development. The most important protooncogenes of the first group are undoubtedly constituted by FMS and HER2/neu. The first one encodes a transmembrane tyrosine kinase receptor, which binds MCSF. It is possible that FMS-MCSF both stimulates epithelial cell proliferation and induces a chemical attraction for macrophages that, in turn, can produce mitogenic stimulating factor. Elevated plasma concentrations of MCSF

are present in the sera of 70% of patients with ovarian cancer.[28] The second protooncogene, HER2/neu, encodes another tyrosine kinase, which is similar to EGFR. Its action may consist of amplification of mitogenic action in target cells; this oncogene is overexpressed in 30% to 35% of ovarian cancer and is associated with a poor prognosis.[29]

Metastasis of Ovarian Cancers

Metastasis is the functional hallmark of all cancer. In general, metastasis involves the invasion of transformed epithelial cells across their basement membrane, through the underlying stroma, and into blood vessels and lymphatic channels, which subsequent disseminate them to distant sites. Only a tiny fraction of cells released into circulation by a tumor ever results in metastasis; understanding the mechanisms by which those cells can land and grow is a priority for cancer researchers. Given the unique need to accommodate the survival of exfoliated cells as well as their subsequent attachment and growth, it seems reasonable to assume that expression and functional organization of molecular pathways important for promoting the metastasis of ovarian cancers will differ from breast and other cancers that depend on hematogenous or lymphatic dissemination. Nonetheless, a wide variety of gene products implicated in the metastasis of other cancers have also been implicated in the metastasis of ovarian cancer. These include growth factor receptors such as EGFR, insulinlike growth factor receptors (IGFRs), and kinases, such as *jak/stat*, focal adhesion kinase, PI3K, and c-met. Comparisons of primary and metastatic ovarian cancers by transcriptional profiling have failed to reveal significant differences in the expression of gene products likely related to the metastatic process.

Particular attention has recently focused on the role of lysophosphatidic acid (LPA) in promoting the metastasis of ovarian cancers. LPA is constitutively produced by mesothelial cells lining the peritoneal cavity; its levels are increased in the ascites of women with both early- and late-stage ovarian cancers.[30] When applied to ovarian cancer cell lines *in vitro*, LPA promotes both the migration of these cells in a manner dependent on Ras MEK kinase-1 as well as their invasion across artificial barriers analogous to a basement membrane. At a molecular level, exogenous LPA enhances ovarian cancer invasiveness both by activating matrix metalloproteinase-2 via membrane-type-1-matrix metalloproteinase (MT1-MMP) and down-regulating the expression of specific tissue inhibitors of metalloproteinases (TIMP-2 and -3).[31] Its application to cultured ovarian cancer cells has also been shown to promote disassembly of intracellular stress fibers and focal adhesions,[32] observations consistent with the idea that LPA promotes dissemination of ovarian cancer by loss of cell adhesion. However, LPA has also been shown to promote the invasiveness of ovarian cancers by additional mechanisms dependent on interleukin-8. The G12/13-RhoA and cyclooxygenase pathways have also been implicated in the LPA-induced migration of ovarian cancers. These mechanisms appear to be independent of the ability of LPA to induce changes in *MMP2* expression. Lastly, it should be noted that LPA appears to promote ovarian cancer metastasis by stimulating *fas*-ligand expression and the shedding of *fas*-ligand–containing microvesicles, potentially leading to an evasion of tumor immunity.

Until recently, the metastasis of ovarian cancer has been almost exclusively studied as a process involving individual cells. However, multicellular clusters of self-adherent cells, known as *spheroids*, can be isolated from the ascitic fluid of women with ovarian cancer. Spheroids readily adhere to both extracellular matrix proteins, such as collagen IV, and mesothelial cells in monolayer culture using beta-1 integrins. Once adherent, the cells contained in spheroids disaggregate, allowing them to invade underlying mesothelial cells and create invasive foci.[33] These observations are consistent with the hypothesis that ovarian cancer spheroids play an important role in the metastatic potential of ovarian cancer. Recent evidence has shown that a loss of circulating gonadotropins results in a dose-dependent decrease in the expression of vascular endothelial growth factor (VEGF) in the outer, proliferating cells of ovarian cancer

spheroids,[34] indicating that these cell clusters remain responsive to signals in their microenvironment that may promote metastasis.

The presence of spheroids in ascites may also help to explain the frequent persistence and frequent recurrence of ovarian cancer after treatment. Spheroids express high levels of p27 and P-glycoprotein that contribute, at least in part, to their relative resistance to the cytotoxic effects of paclitaxel when compared with ovarian cancer cells in monolayer culture. Ovarian cancer spheroids have also been shown to be relatively resistant to the cytotoxic effects of radiation.[35] These observations are consistent with *in vitro* studies that demonstrate that the signals generated by adhesion to specific components of the extracellular matrix, such as collagen IV, can modify the sensitivity of ovarian cancers to chemotherapy. However, the mechanisms by which the aggregation of malignant cells promote or enhance cell survival remain unclear. It is also unclear how the aggregation of these malignant cells might promote or enhance the migration, attachment, or invasion of ovarian cancer cells. Insight into these questions is likely to come from genetic models, such as the migration of the border cell cluster in *Drosophila*. Analyses of border cell migration indicate that specific shifts in epithelial polarity, known as the *epithelial-mesenchymal transition* (EMT), and changes in the patterns of signals arising at junctional complexes are necessary for the invasion and migration of epithelial clusters.[36] Signals arising from these junctional proteins appear to be integrated by a specific steroid receptor coactivator, known as AIB1 (Amplified in Breast Cancer 1; SRC3). Ironically, overexpression of AIB1 is a frequent feature of ovarian cancers, suggesting that the pathways regulated by this transcriptional coactivator may also play a critical role in promoting ovarian cancer metastasis. Other proteins first identified in *Drosophila*, such as *Snail*, also appear to play an important role in regulating the EMT of transformed ovarian epithelia, further lending credence to the utility of this genetic model.

Angiogenesis

Growth of both primary ovarian cancers and their metastases requires the formation of new blood vessels to support adequate perfusion. This process, known as *angiogenesis*, mechanistically involves both the branching of new capillaries as well as the remodeling of larger vessels. Other processes, such as vasculogenic mimicry, have also been implicated in tumor angiogenesis.

Angiogenesis is tightly regulated by a balance of pro- and antiangiogenic factors. These include growth factors, such as TGF-β, VEGF, and platelet-derived growth factor; prostaglandins, such as prostaglandin E2; cytokines, such as interleukin 8;

and other factors, such as the angiopoietins (Ang-1, Ang-2), and hypoxia-inducible factor-1α (HIF-1α). Many of these angiogenic factors have been implicated in ovarian cancer. For example, VEGF is a family of secreted polypeptides with critical roles in both normal development and human disease. Many cancers, including ovarian carcinomas, release VEGF in response to the hypoxic or acidic conditions typical in solid tumors. Near universal, albeit variable, levels of VEGF expression have been reported in ovarian cancers, in which higher levels correlate with advanced disease and poor clinical prognosis.[37] Circulating levels of VEGF have also been reported to be higher in the serum of women with ovarian cancers when compared with those with benign tumors. Expression of HIF-1 correlates well with microvessel density in ovarian cancers and has been proposed to up-regulate VEGF expression.[38] Culturing ovarian cancer cell lines under hypoxic conditions stimulates the expression of both HIF-1α and VEGF expression in ovarian cancer cell lines; addition of prostaglandin E2 potentiates the ability of hypoxia to induce the expression of both proangiogenic factors.[39]

Ironically, many of the molecules implicated in regulating angiogenesis in cancer, such as c-met, also regulate other processes critical for cancer metastasis, such as cell migration and invasiveness. Inhibition of PI3K decreases transcription of VEGF in ovarian cancer cells, an effect that is reversed by the forced expression of AKT. Such observations are consistent with reports that hypoxia not only induces angiogenesis, but also increases the invasiveness of ovarian cancer cells.[40] Likewise, an acidic environment induces increased interleukin-8 expression in ovarian cancer in a manner dependent on transcription factors AP-1 and nuclear factor-κB–like factor, suggesting that feedback between these pathways may also determine how tumors interact with their external environment. Undoubtedly, better insight into these interactions will help to define the suitability of these molecules as therapeutic targets.

Epigenetics

It has become increasingly apparent that epigenetic events can lead to cancer as frequently as loss of gene function due to mutations or loss of heterozygosity. The overall level of genomic methylation is reduced in cancer (global hypomethylation), but hypermethylation of promoter regions of specific genes is a common event that is often associated with transcriptional inactivation of specific genes.[41] This is critical because the silenced genes are often tumor suppressor genes, and their loss of function can be evident in early stages of cancer but can also drive neoplastic progression and metastasis. Epigenetic gene silencing is a complex series of events that includes DNA hypermethylation of CpG islands within gene-promoter regions, histone deacetylation, methylation or phosphorylation, or histone demethylation. Global hypermethylation of CpG islands appears to be prevalent but highly variable in ovarian cancer tissue.[42] Multiple genes are abnormally methylated in ovarian cancer compared with normal ovarian tissue, including p16, RAR-β, H-cadherin, GSTP1, MGMT, RASSF1A, leukotriene B4 receptor, MTHFR, progesterone receptor, CDH1, IGSF4, BRCA1, TMS1, estrogen receptor-α, the putative tumor suppressor km23 (TGFB component), and others.[43] The degree of DNA methylation and the demethylation activity of chemotherapeutic drugs and the sensitive relations of histone acetylation and the specificity of demethylation of select genes are important to ensure the success of treatment and prevent disease recurrence.

Role of Specific Immune Responses

The novel observation by William Coley in the 1890s that severe bacterial infections could induce an antitumor response in patients with partially resected tumors has evolved into an understanding that the immune system can recognize tumor-associated antigens and direct a targeted response. The concept of "cancer immunoediting" suggests that the immune system not only protects the host against the development of primary cancers but also dynamically sculpts tumor immunogenicity.[44] In epithelial ovarian cancer, support for the role of immune surveillance of tumors comes from recent observations that the presence of infiltrating T lymphocytes (TILS) in tumors is associated with improved survival of patients with the disease.[45,46] In one study, there was improved survival of patients with higher frequencies of intraepithelial CD8+ TIL (55 months vs. 26 months; hazard ratio [HR] 0.33; 95% CI, 0.18 to 0.60; P = .0003).[46] In addition, the subgroups with a high versus low intraepithelial CD8+/CD4+ TIL ratio had a median survival of 74 versus 25 months (HR 0.30; 95% CI, 0.16 to 0.55; P = .0001). This unfavorable effect of CD4+ T cells on prognosis was found to be due to CD25+ Forkhead box P3+ regulatory cells (T$_{reg}$, suppressor T cells), as indicated by survival in patients with high versus low CD8+/T$_{reg}$ ratios (median, 58 months vs. 23 months; HR 0.31; 95% CI, 0.17 to 0.58; P = .0002).[46]

Finally, advanced-stage ovarian cancer patients can have detectable tumor-specific cytotoxic T cell and antibody immunity. This was illustrated in a recent study that indicated that immunity to p53 predicted improved overall survival in patients with advanced-stage disease.[47] All of these observations support clinical trials of immunotherapy for epithelial ovarian cancer in an effort to elicit effective antitumor responses. Major obstacles include the identification of tumor-restricted immunogenic targets, generation of a sufficient immune response to cause tumor rejection, and approaches to overcome tumor evasion of immune attack.

Ovarian Cancer-Specific Antigens

The development of approaches for analyzing humoral and cellular immune reactivity to cancer in the context of the autologous host has led to the molecular characterization of tumor antigens recognized by autologous CD8+ T cells or antibodies. As a consequence of these advances, human tumor antigens defined to date can be classified into one or more of the following categories: (1) differentiation antigens, such as tyrosinase, Melan-A/MART-1, and gp 100; (2) mutational antigens, such as CDK4, β-catenin, caspase-8, and P53; (3) amplification antigens, such as Her2/neu and p53; (4) splice variant antigens, such as NY-CO-37/PDZ-45 and ING1; (5) viral antigens, such as human papillomavirus (HPV) and Epstein-Barr virus; and (6) cancer-testis antigens, such as MAGE, NY-ESO-1, and LAGE-1. Thus, it is clear that some antigens may play a crucial role in progression of tumor cells (e.g., Her2/neu) and could be useful as biomarkers of disease progression and targets of therapy. On the other hand, in considering an antigenic target for ovarian cancer immunotherapy, an ideal candidate antigen should not only demonstrate high-frequency expression in the tumor tissues and restricted expression in normal tissues, but also provide evidence for inherent immunogenicity. In this regard, the cancer-testis antigens are a distinct and unique class of differentiation antigens with high levels of expression in adult male germ cells, but generally not in other normal adult tissues, and aberrant expression in a variable proportion of a wide range of different cancer types. Among cancer-testis antigens, NY-ESO-1, initially defined by serologic analysis of recombinant cDNA expression (SEREX) libraries in esophageal cancer, is particularly immunogenic, eliciting both cellular and humoral immune responses in a high proportion of patients with advanced NY-ESO-1 expressing ovarian cancer.[48]

The reasons for the aberrant expression of cancer-testis antigens in cancer are currently unknown. Nevertheless, the fact that the expression of these antigens is restricted to cancers, gametes, and trophoblast suggests a link between cancer and gametogenesis. Although possible mechanisms include global demethylation and histone deacetylation, the induction of a "gametogenic" program in cancer has also been proposed.[49] Although several lines of evidence have shown that spontaneous or vaccine-induced tumor-antigen–specific T cells can recognize ovarian cancer targets, prolongation of survival in patients treated with immunization has only rarely been observed. This is probably a reflection of several *in vivo* immunosuppressive mechanisms in tumor-bearing hosts. A recently described mechanism in ovarian cancer is the expression of inhibitory molecules such as programmed death-1 (PD-1) and lymphocyte activation gene-3 (LAG-3).[50] Together, these molecules render ovarian tumor infiltrating CD8+ T cells "hyporesponsive," wherein effector function is most impaired in antigen-specific LAG-3+PD-1+CD8+ TILs.

ENDOMETRIAL CANCER

The current concept of endometrial cancer integrates histopathology with molecular genetic mechanisms of cancer development. Two major pathogenetic variants of endometrial carcinoma, type I (endometrioid) and type II (serous), evolve via divergent pathways and different precursor lesions, different genetic abnormalities, and ultimately different clinical outcomes parallel their distinct histology.

Type I Cancers

More than 90% of uterine cancers arise in the self-renewing glandular epithelium that lines the uterine cavity. The endometrium epithelium responds to steroid hormones with well-characterized patterns of growth and maturation critical for its role in normal reproduction. Estrogen is a well-recognized growth factor for the endometrium, promoting glandular proliferation. Subsequent exposure to the progestin-rich environment that follows ovulation results in an arrest of endometrial proliferation accompanied by glandular luteinization. Several decades of epidemiologic evidence has convincingly demonstrated that continued, unopposed exposure to estrogen is associated with an increased risk of developing endometrial cancer. These risks are particularly notable among postmenopausal women treated with estrogen-only hormone replacement. Following the introduction of hormone replacement therapy, the incidence of endometrial cancer among women in the United States rose steadily. An association between the growth-promoting effects of estrogen and endometrial carcinomas is thought to underlie the epidemiologic associations found for endometrial cancers, medical conditions such as anovulation, obesity, and other epidemiologically defined risk factors, including early age at menarche and nulliparity.

The estrogen-related endometrioid adenocarcinomas account for 80% of endometrial cancer, demonstrate large number of genetic changes, and appear to arise via a progression pathway. Common genetic changes in this type of endometrial carcinoma include microsatellite instability (MSI), or specific mutations of *PTEN*, *K-ra*s, and *βB*-catenin genes.

Microsatellite Instability

Microsatellites are short segments of repetitive DNA found predominantly in noncoding DNA and scattered through the genome. The MSI phenotype is expressed in the cells with changes in the number of repeat elements as compared with normal tissue because of DNA repair error during replication. Approximately 20% of type I endometrial cancers demonstrate MSI phenotype, while MSI in type II cancers is very rare, present in less than 5% of the cases.[51] MSI is due to inactivation of any of the mismatch repair genes and proteins: *MLH1*, *MSH2*, *MSH3*, and *MSH6*. The most common mechanism of MSI in the endometrium is inactivation of *MLH1* by epigenetic silencing of its promoter through hypermethylation of CpG islands, followed by *MSH6* mutation and *MSH3* frame shift mutations. In contrast, the MSI present in colon cancer is predominantly due to mutations in *MSH2*, followed by *MLH1* and *MSH6* mutations. MSI is an early event in type I cancers and it has been described in precancerous lesions. Once established, MSI may specifically target or inactivate genes with susceptible repeat elements, such as TGF-β1 receptors and IGFIIR, resulting in new subclones with altered capacity to invade and metastasize.

PTEN

Inactivation of *PTEN* (phosphatase and tensin homolog) tumor suppressor gene located at 10q23 is the most common genetic defect in type I endometrial cancers, and it is present in more than 80% of tumors that are preceded by histologically distinct premalignant phase.[52] The predominant *PTEN* activity is a lipid phosphatase that converts inositol triphosphates into inositol biphosphate, thus inhibiting survival and proliferative pathways that are activated by inositol triphosphatase. PTEN protein functions in maintaining G_1 arrest and enabling apoptosis via an AKT-dependent mechanism. *PTEN* inactivation is caused by various mechanisms. The most common *PTEN* defect in endometrial cancer is its complete loss of function through inactivation of both alleles. Mutations or deletions that result in loss of heterozygosity at *PTEN* locus are also observed with high frequency. The *PTEN* mutations pattern is different in microsatellite stable and MSI cancers. MSI tumors have a higher frequency of deletions, involving three or more base pairs, as compared with the microsatellite-stable tumors. In addition, the mutations in MSI tumors only rarely involve the polyadenine repeat of exon 8, which is the expected target.

KRAS

KRAS mutations have been found in up to 30% of type I endometrial cancers. The frequency of KRAS mutations is particularly high in MSI-positive tumors.[53]

β-catenin

β-catenin (3p21) is a component of the E-cadherin–catenin complex essential for cell dif-ferentiation and maintenance of normal tissue architecture, and it also plays a role in signal transduction. The APC protein down-regulates β-catenin levels, inducing phosphorylation of serine-threonine residues coded in exon 3 of the β-catenin and its degradation via ubiquitin-proteosome pathway. Gain of function mutations in β-catenin exon 3 are seen in 25% to 38% of type I cancers.[54] These mutations result in protein stabilization, accumulation, and transcriptional activation. β-catenin mutations have been found also in premalignant endometrial lesions. β-catenin changes may characterize pathways of endometrial cancer separate from PTEN mutations and are characterized by squamous differentiation. Several genes may be targets of dysregulated β-catenin pathway. Although in colon cancer elevated β-catenin levels trigger cyclin D1 expression and uncontrolled progression of tumor cells into the cell cycle, in type I endometrial cancers, β-catenin may regulate expression of MMP-7, which has a role in the establishment of microenvironment necessary for maintenance of tumor growth.

Type II Endometrial Cancer

The more aggressive, non–estrogen-related, non-endometrioid cancers (predominantly serous and clear cell carcinomas) are characterized by p53 mutations and Her2/neu amplification and bcl-2 changes. These high-grade tumors are known to be associated in some cases with an identifiable intraepithelial neoplasia component. The same pattern of genetic changes is seen in the preneoplastic atrophic endometrium, suggesting that these are early events in type II tumors carcinogenesis[55] (Table 23.2).

CERVIX, VAGINAL, AND VULVAR CANCERS

Role of Human Papillomavirus

Persistent infections with specific high-risk HPV genotypes (e.g., HPV-16, HPV-18, HPV-31, HPV-33, and HPV-45) have been identified as an essential, although not sufficient, factor in the pathogenesis of majority of cancers of the cervix, vagina, and vulva.[56] The existence of papilloma viruses was first demonstrated by Shope in the 1930s using an ultrafiltrate of warts from rabbits.[57] Since then, papilloma viruses with an epithelial tropism have been demonstrated in nearly every mammalian species, including humans. The HPVs are encapsulated DNA viruses containing a double-stranded DNA genome of approximately 7,800 base pairs. After infecting a suitable epithelium, viral DNA replication takes place in the

TABLE 23.2

GENETIC ALTERATIONS IN ENDOMETRIAL CANCER

Gene	Class	Alteration	Frequency (%)	Type
MSI				
MLH1	DNA repair	Promoter hypermethylation	20 (all repair gene	I
MSH6	DNA repair	Frame-shift mutation	alterations	
MSH3	DNA repair	Frame-shift mutation	together)	
ONCOGENES				
KRAS	G protein	Mutation	20	II
β-catenin	Transcription factor	Mutation	25–38	I
Her2/neu	Tyrosine kinase	Amplification/overexpression	10	I
BCL2	Antioxidant, prevents apoptosis	Amplification/overexpression		II
TUMOR SUPPRESSOR GENES				
p53	Transcription factor	Mutation/overexpression	20	II
PTEN	Tyrosine phosphatase	Mutation, biallelic loss of function	80	I

MSI, microsatellite instability.

basal cells of the epidermis, where the HPV genome is stably retained in multiple copies, guaranteeing its persistence in the epithelium's proliferative cells. This occurs early in preneoplastic lesions, when the viral genome still persists in an episomal state. In most invasive cancers and also in a few high-grade dysplastic lesions, however, integration of high-risk HPV genomes into the host genome is observed. Integration seems to be a direct consequence of chromosomal instability and an important molecular event in the progression of preneoplastic lesions. In a review of more than 190 reported integration loci, HPV integration sites are found to be randomly distributed over the whole genome with a clear predilection for genomic fragile sites. No evidence for targeted disruption or functional alteration of critical cellular genes by the integrated viral sequences could be found.[58]

The ability of high-risk HPVs to transform human epithelia relates to the transcription of specific viral gene products. Transcription from the HPV genome occurs in two waves: an early phase with seven to eight gene products and a late phase with two gene products (L1, L2). Early-phase gene products play a critical role in viral DNA replication (E1, E8) and regulation of transcription (E2, E8). In contrast, the L1 and L2 genes code for the capsid's primary and secondary proteins, respectively. The ability of different high-risk HPVs to transform human epithelia has been primarily associated with the expression of two specific viral gene products, E6 and E7. Transformation of human genital tract epithelium likely requires the expression of both E6 and E7; transfection of human keratinocytes in vitro with either is insufficient to accomplish this phenomenon.

At a molecular level, E6 and E7 interfere with important control mechanisms of the cell cycle, apoptosis, and maintenance of chromosomal stability by directly interacting with p53 and pRB, respectively. Moreover, recent studies demonstrated that the two viral oncoproteins cooperatively disturb the mechanisms of chromosome duplication and segregation during mitosis and thereby induce severe chromosomal instability associated with centrosome aberrations, anaphase bridges, chromosome lagging, and breaking.[59] They have also been shown to interact with a number of other cellular proteins whose role in epithelial transformation remains unclear, including transcriptional coactivators, such as p300, and components of junctional complexes, such as hDlg1. Altered expression of hDlg1 has been observed in high-grade cervical dysplasias, consistent with the hypothesis that these gene products play an early role in the HPV-induced progression to cervical cancer. Specific sequence differences have been associated with different levels of risk for ultimately developing cervical cancers. For example, recent evidence demonstrates that the sequence of E6 found in Ashkenazi populations confers a protective advantage against developing cervical cancer, previously attributed to the practice of circumcision. Although much less understood, other early genes, such as E2, have also been implicated in the transformation.

Immune Evasion by Human Papillomavirus

HPV infection has a transitory pattern, whereby most individuals (70% to 90%) eliminate the virus 12 to 24 months after initial diagnosis.[60] HPV has evolved several strategies to evade immune attack. Most obviously, papillomaviruses do not infect and replicate in antigen-presenting cells that are located in the epithelium, nor do they lyse keratinocytes, so there is no opportunity for antigen-presenting cells to engulf virions and present virion-derived antigens to the immune system. Furthermore, there is no blood-borne phase of infection, so the immune system outside the epithelium has little opportunity to detect the virus. Additionally, HPVs have exploited the redundancy of the genetic code to keep the levels of "late" proteins low.[61] Papillomavirus capsid protein production in mammalian cells is markedly up-regulated if the "viral" codons are replaced by the ones that are used by mammals, thereby limiting opportunities for the host to mount an effective immune attack. Following viral integration and subsequent malignant change, the local tumor environment at the cervical lesion is immunosuppressive. Thus, antigen-loaded dendritic cells (DCs) fail to mature, and immature DCs transmit a tolerogenic, rather than an immunogenic, signal to T cells bearing antigen-directed T-cell receptors in draining lymph nodes.

Human Papillomavirus Vaccines

The aim of prophylactic vaccination is to generate neutralizing antibodies against the HPV L1 and L2 capsid proteins. Prophylactic vaccine development against HPV has focused on the ability of the L1 and L2 virion structural proteins to assemble into viruslike particles (VLPs). VLPs mimic the natural structure of the virion and generate a potent immune response. Because the VLPs are devoid of DNA, they are not infectious or harmful. HPV VLPs can be generated by expressing the HPV capsid protein L1 in baculovirus or yeast. They consist of five L1 subunits that multimerize into immunogenic pentamers. Seventy-one L1 pentamers, in turn, multimerize into an HPV VLP. Initial studies have shown that VLPs are capable of inducing high titers of neutralizing antibodies to L1 and L2 epitopes.[62] Furthermore, VLPs have proven effective in generating HPV type-specific protection from viral challenge in animal papillomavirus models.

With the approval of preventive HPV vaccines that encompass HPV-16, -18, -6, and -11, large prevention clinical trials targeting the most prevalent HPV types in different regions of the world are warranted. Questions such as the necessity of repeat vaccinations and longevity of protection from HPV infection remain to be determined. It is estimated that if women were vaccinated against all high-risk types of HPV before they become sexually active, there should be a reduction of at least 85% in the risk of cervical cancer, and a decline of 44% to 70% in the frequency of abnormal Papanicolaou (Pap) smears attributable to HPV.[63] Unfortunately, even after vaccination is implemented, a reduction in the incidence of cervical cancer could not be expected to become apparent for at least a decade.[64] Therefore, therapeutic vaccines are still very much needed to reduce the morbidity and mortality associated with cervical cancer.

The therapeutic approach to patients with pre-invasive and invasive cervical cancers is to develop vaccine strategies that induce specific CD8+ cytotoxic T lymphocyte (CTL) responses aimed at eliminating virus-infected or transformed cells. The majority of cervical cancers express the HPV-16-derived E6 and E7 oncoproteins, which are thus attractive targets for T-cell–mediated immunotherapy. Several HPV vaccine strategies have successfully elicited immune responses against HPV E6 and E7 epitopes and have prevented tumor growth on challenge with HPV-16-positive tumor cells in mice. Early-phase human trials using therapeutic vaccines have shown that they are safe, as no serious adverse effects have been reported. Other approaches currently undergoing preclinical development include the use of recombinant alpha viruses such as Venezuelan equine encephalitis virus, Semliki Forest virus, and naked DNA vaccination.

GESTATIONAL TROPHOBLASTIC DISEASE

Gestational trophoblastic disease (GTD) encompasses a diverse group of diseases with unique cytogenetic and molecular pathogenesis. The current concept implies that the abnormal trophoblastic tissue in GTD recapitulates the trophoblast present in the early developing placenta and the implantation site. Complete mole is diploid, usually 46, XX is androgenetic in origin, resulting from duplication of a haploid paternal genome (23X). More than 90% of complete moles contain this DNA content, and the remaining group are also androgenetic except 46, XY, and formed by dispermy. Partial moles are triploid, and diandric, usually XXY (58%), XXX (40%), and XYY (2%). Predominance of paternal chromosomes is therefore characteristics of molar pregnancy. Synergistic up-regulation of *CMYC*, *ERBB2*, *CFMS*, and *BCL2* has been suggested in pathogenesis of complete mole,[65] and similar findings have been confirmed in choriocarcinoma, while mutational analysis of *p53* and *KRAS* failed to show mutations in either complete mole or choriocarcinoma. The other genes involved in the development of choriocarcinoma include *DOC-2*, a candidate tumor-suppressor gene and a putative tumor suppressor at 7p12-7q11.23,[66] and the RAS guanosine triphosphate hydrolase (GTPase) activating protein. It has been postulated that GTD develops by a mechanism of monoallelic contribution, when the gene susceptible to inactivation would be affected by one-hit kinetics. Alternatively, uniparental transmission of genes that are parentally imprinted would impair their regulation.

Placental-site trophoblastic tumor (PSTT) represents neoplastic transformation of implantation site intermediate trophoblast. Placental-site trophoblastic tumor is characterized by aberrant expression of cyclins and p53. Further efforts are needed for better understanding of persistent trophoblastic disease.

Selected References

The full list of references for this chapter appears in the online version.

1. Dunn GP, Old LJ, Schreiber RD. The immunobiology of cancer immunosurveillance and immunoediting. *Immunity* 2004;21(2):137.
3. Levanon K, Crum C, Drapkin R. New insights into the pathogenesis of serous ovarian cancer and its clinical impact. *J Clin Oncol* 2008;26:5284.
5. Wright JW, Pejovic T, Fanton J, Stouffer RL. Induction of proliferation in the primate ovarian surface epithelium in vivo. *Hum Reprod* 2008;23:129.
6. Wright JW, Pejovic T, Lawson M, et al. Ovulation in the absence of the ovarian surface epithelium in the primate. *Biol Reprod* 2010;82:599.
8. Ganesan S, Richardson AL, Wang ZC, et al. Abnormalities of the inactive X chromosome are a common feature of BRCA1 mutant and sporadic basal-like breast cancer. *Cold Spring Harb Symp Quant Biol* 2005;70:93.
9. Garcia-Higuera I, Taniguchi T, Ganesan S, et al. Interaction of the Fanconi anemia proteins and BRCA1 in a common pathway. *Mol Cell* 2001;7(2):249.
10. Sakai W, Swisher EM, Karlan BY, et al. Secondary mutations as a mechanism of cisplatin resistance in BRCA2-mutated cancers. *Nature* 2008;451:1116.
11. Boudsocq F, Benaim P, Canitrot Y, et al. Modulation of cellular response to cisplatin by a novel inhibitor of DNA polymerase beta. *Mol Pharmacol* 2005;67(5):1485.
12. Kennedy RD, Chen CC, Stuckert P, et al. Fanconi anemia pathway-deficient tumor cells are hypersensitive to inhibition of ataxia telangiectasia mutated. *J Clin Invest* 2007;117:1440.
13. Bryant HE, Schultz N, Thomas HD, et al. Specific killing of BRCA2-deficient tumours with inhibitors of poly(ADP-ribose) polymerase. *Nature* 2005;434:913.
14. Farmer H, McCabe N, Lord CJ, et al. Targeting the DNA repair defect in BRCA mutant cells as a therapeutic strategy. *Nature* 2005;434:917.
15. Song H, Ramus SJ, Tyrer J, et al. A genome-wide association study identifies a new ovarian cancer susceptibility locus on 9p22.2. *Nat Genet* 2009;41:996.
17. Meinhold-Heerlein I, Bauerschlag D, Hilpert F, et al. Molecular and prognostic distinction between serous ovarian carcinomas of varying grade and malignant potential. *Oncogene* 2005;24:1053.
24. Landen CN Jr, Birrer MJ, Sood AK. Early events in the pathogenesis of epithelial ovarian cancer. *J Clin Oncol* 2008;26:995.
25. Berchuck A, Iversen ES, Lancaster JM, et al. Prediction of optimal versus suboptimal cytoreduction of advanced-stage serous ovarian cancer with the use of microarrays. *Am J Obstet Gynecol* 2004;190:910.
26. Hu W, Wu W, Nash MA, et al. Anomalies of the TGF-beta postreceptor signaling pathway in ovarian cancer cell lines. *Anticancer Res* 2000;20(2A):729.
28. van Haaften-Day C, Shen Y, Xu F, et al. OVX1, macrophage-colony stimulating factor, and CA-125-II as tumor markers for epithelial ovarian carcinoma: a critical appraisal. *Cancer* 2001;92(11):2837.
30. Ren J, Xiao YJ, Singh LS, et al. Lysophosphatidic acid is constitutively produced by human peritoneal mesothelial cells and enhances adhesion, migration, and invasion of ovarian cancer cells. *Cancer Res* 2006;66(6):3006.
31. Sengupta S, Kim KS, Berk MP, et al. Lysophosphatidic acid down-regulates tissue inhibitor of metalloproteinases, which are negatively involved in lysophosphatidic acid-induced cell invasion. *Oncogene* 2007;26:2894.
32. Do TV, Symowicz JC, Berman DM, et al. Lysophosphatidic acid down-regulates stress fibers and up-regulates pro-matrix metalloproteinase-2 activation in ovarian cancer cells. *Mol Cancer Res* 2007;5(2):121.
33. Burleson KM, Hansen LK, Skubitz AP. Ovarian carcinoma spheroids disaggregate on type I collagen and invade live human mesothelial cell monolayers. *Clin Exp Metastasis* 2004;21(8):685.
34. Schiffenbauer YS, Abramovitch R, Meir G, et al. Loss of ovarian function promotes angiogenesis in human ovarian carcinoma. *Proc Natl Acad Sci U S A* 1997;94(24):13203.
36. Szafranski P, Goode S. A Fasciclin 2 morphogenetic switch organizes epithelial cell cluster polarity and motility. *Development* 2004;131(9):2023.
37. Kassim SK, El-Salahy EM, Fayed ST, et al. Vascular endothelial growth factor and interleukin-8 are associated with poor prognosis in epithelial ovarian cancer patients. *Clin Biochem* 2004;37(5):363.
41. Baylin SB, Ohm JE. Epigenetic gene silencing in cancer—a mechanism for early oncogenic pathway addiction? *Nat Rev Cancer* 2006;6(2):107.
42. Wei SH, Chen CM, Strathdee G, et al. Methylation microarray analysis of late-stage ovarian carcinomas distinguishes progression-free survival in patients and identifies candidate epigenetic markers. *Clin Cancer Res* 2002;8(7):2246.
44. Smyth MJ, Dunn GP, Schreiber RD. Cancer immunosurveillance and immunoediting: the roles of immunity in suppressing tumor development and shaping tumor immunogenicity. *Adv Immunol* 2006;90:1.
45. Zhang L, Conejo-Garcia JR, Katsaros D, et al. Intratumoral T cells, recurrence, and survival in epithelial ovarian cancer. *N Engl J Med* 2003;348(3):203.
46. Sato E, Olson SH, Ahn J, et al. Intraepithelial CD8+ tumor-infiltrating lymphocytes and a high CD8+/regulatory T cell ratio are associated with favorable prognosis in ovarian cancer. *Proc Natl Acad Sci U S A* 2005;102(51):18538.
47. Goodell V, Salazar LG, Urban N, et al. Antibody immunity to the p53 oncogenic protein is a prognostic indicator in ovarian cancer. *J Clin Oncol* 2006;24(5):762.
48. Odunsi K, Jungbluth AA, Stockert E, et al. NY-ESO-1 and LAGE-1 cancer-testis antigens are potential targets for immunotherapy in epithelial ovarian cancer. *Cancer Res* 2003;63(18):6076.
49. Old LJ. Cancer/testis (CT) antigens—a new link between gametogenesis and cancer. *Cancer Immunity* 2001;1:1.
50. Matsuzaki J, Gnjatic S, Mhawech-Fauceglia P, et al. Tumor-infiltrating NY-ESO-1-specific CD8+ T cells are negatively regulated by LAG-3 and PD-1 in human ovarian cancer. *Proc Natl Acad Sci U S A* 2010;107:7875.
51. Mutter GL, Boynton KA, Faquin WC, Ruiz RE, Jovanovic AS. Allelotype mapping of unstable microsatellites establishes

direct lineage continuity between endometrial precancers and cancer. *Cancer Res* 1996;56(19):4483.

52. Mutter GL, Lin MC, Fitzgerald JT, et al. Altered PTEN expression as a diagnostic marker for the earliest endometrial precancers. *J Natl Cancer Inst* 2000;92(11):924.

54. Mirabelli-Primdahl L, Gryfe R, Kim H, et al. Beta-catenin mutations are specific for colorectal carcinomas with microsatellite instability but occur in endometrial carcinomas irrespective of mutator pathway. *Cancer Res* 1999;59(14):3346.

56. zur Hausen H. Papillomaviruses causing cancer: evasion from host-cell control in early events in carcinogenesis. *J Natl Cancer Inst* 2000;92(9):690.

58. Wentzensen N, Vinokurova S, von Knebel Doeberitz M. Systematic review of genomic integration sites of human papillomavirus genomes in epithelial dysplasia and invasive cancer of the female lower genital tract. *Cancer Res* 2004;64(11):3878.

60. Ho GY, Bierman R, Beardsley L, Chang CJ, Burk RD. Natural history of cervicovaginal papillomavirus infection in young women. *N Engl J Med* 1998;338(7):423.

62. Koutsky LA, Ault KA, Wheeler CM, et al. A controlled trial of a human papillomavirus type 16 vaccine. *N Engl J Med* 2002;347(21):1645.

63. Walboomers JM, Jacobs MV, Manos MM, et al. Human papillomavirus is a necessary cause of invasive cervical cancer worldwide. *J Pathol* 1999;189(1):12.

66. Matsuda T, Sasaki M, Kato H, et al. Human chromosome 7 carries a putative tumor suppressor gene(s) involved in choriocarcinoma. *Oncogene* 1997;15(23):2773.

CHAPTER 24 BREAST CANCER

ERIN WYSONG HOFSTATTER, GINA G. CHUNG, AND LYNDSAY N. HARRIS

It has been said that cancer is a genetic disease and can be best understood by studying the DNA alterations that lead to the development of cancer. However, a deeper understanding of carcinogenesis requires insight into how these genetic changes alter cellular programs that lead to growth, invasion, and metastasis. This chapter is presented following the logical progression of DNA to RNA to protein, and it describes, at each step, the lesions that contribute to breast cancer carcinogenesis. The chapter also introduces new concepts in epigenetics, microRNAs, and gene expression analyses that illustrate how new biologic discoveries, and novel technologies, have profoundly affected our understanding of breast cancer pathogenesis within the past decade.

GENETICS OF BREAST CANCER

Breast cancer is a heterogeneous disease fundamentally caused by progressive accumulation of genetic aberrations, including point mutations, chromosomal amplifications, deletions, rearrangements, translocations, and duplications.[1,2] Germline mutations account for only about 10% of all breast cancers, while the vast majority of breast cancers appear to occur sporadically and are attributed to somatic genetic alterations (Fig. 24.1).[3]

HEREDITARY BREAST CANCER

One of the most important risk factors for breast cancer is family history. Though familial forms comprise nearly 20% of all breast cancers, most of the genes responsible for familial breast cancer have yet to be identified. Breast cancer susceptibility genes can be categorized into three classes according to their frequency and level of risk they confer: rare high-penetrance genes, rare intermediate-penetrance genes, and common low-penetrance genes and loci[4] (Table 24.1).

High-Penetrance, Low-Frequency Breast Cancer Predisposition Genes

BRCA1 and BRCA2

BRCA1 and *BRCA2* mutations account for approximately half of all dominantly inherited hereditary breast cancers. These mutations confer a relative risk of breast cancer 10 to 30 times that of women in the general population, resulting in a nearly 85% lifetime risk of breast cancer development.[5] *BRCA1* and *BRCA2* mutation carriers are quite rare among the general population, however, the prevalence is substantially higher in certain founder populations, most notably in the Ashkenazi Jewish population, where the carrier frequency is 1 in 40.

More than a thousand germline mutations have been identified in *BRCA1* and *BRCA2*. Pathogenic mutations most often result in truncated protein products, although mutations that interfere with protein function also exist.[4,5] Interestingly, penetrance of pathogenic *BRCA1* and *BRCA2* mutations and age of cancer onset appear to vary both within and among family members. Specific BRCA mutations as well as gene–gene and gene–environment interactions as potential modifiers of *BRCA*-related cancer risk are areas of active investigation.[6,7]

BRCA1-related breast cancers are characterized by features that distinguish them from both *BRCA2*-related and sporadic breast cancers.[4] *BRCA1*-related tumors typically occur in younger women and have more aggressive features, with high histologic grade, high proliferative rate, aneuploidy, and absence of estrogen and progesterone receptors and human epidermal growth factor receptor 2 (HER2). This "triple-negative" phenotype of *BRCA1*-related breast cancers is further characterized by a "basal-like" gene expression profile of cytokeratins 5/6, 14, and 17, epidermal growth factor and P-cadherin.[8]

Though *BRCA1* and *BRCA2* genes encode large proteins with multiple functions, they primarily act as classic tumor suppressor genes that function to maintain genomic stability by facilitating double-strand DNA repair through homologous

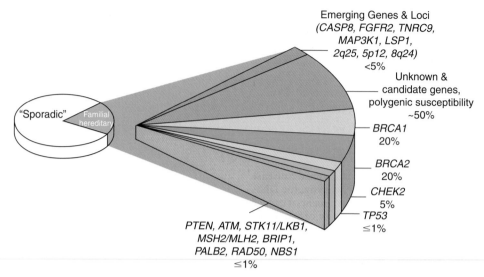

FIGURE 24.1 Genetic susceptibility to breast cancer. Familial breast cancer comprises approximately 20% to 30% of all breast cancers. *BRCA1* and *BRCA2* are two major high-penetrance genes associated with hereditary breast and ovarian cancer syndrome, which together account for nearly half of inherited breast cancers. Other rare breast cancer susceptibility genes have been identified, such as *CHEK2, TP53, PTEN,* and *STK11.* Several emerging low-penetrance genes and loci recently discovered by genomewide association studies account for a small proportion of familial breast cancers (<5%). To date, about half of familial breast cancers remain unexplained but are likely attributable to as yet unknown genes and/or polygenic susceptibility. (From Olopade O, et al. Advances in breast cancer: pathways to personalized medicine. *Clin Cancer Res* 2008;14(24): Fig 1.)

recombination.[8,9] When loss of heterozygosity (LOH) occurs via loss, mutation, or silencing of the wild type *BRCA1* or *BRCA2* allele, the resultant defective DNA repair leads to rapid acquisition of additional mutations, particularly during DNA replication, and ultimately sets the stage for cancer development.

The integral role of BRCA1 and BRCA2 in double-strand DNA repair holds potential as a therapeutic target for *BRCA*-related breast cancers. For example, platinum agents cause interstrand crosslinks, thereby blocking DNA replication and leading to stalled replication forks. Poly(adenosine diphosphate-ribose) polymerase-1 (PARP1) inhibitors additionally show promise as specific therapy for *BRCA*-related tumors. PARP1 is a cellular enzyme that functions in single-strand DNA repair through base excision and represents a major alternative DNA repair pathway in the cell.[10,11] When PARP inhibition is applied to a background deficient in double-strand DNA repair, as is the case in *BRCA*-related tumor cells, the cells are left without adequate DNA repair mechanisms and ultimately undergo cell cycle arrest, chromosome instability, and cell death.[4] Given their phenotypic similarities to *BRCA1*-related breast cancers, sporadic basal-like breast tumors may display sensitivity to PARP inhibition as well.[11] Phase 2 studies are currently under way to explore the use of PARP inhibitors in both *BRCA*- and basallike, non-*BRCA*-related breast tumors.

Other High-Penetrance Genes

A small number of other high-risk, low frequency breast cancer susceptibility genes exist, and they include *TP53, PTEN, STK11/LKB1,* and *CDH1.*[4–6] These high-penetrance genes confer an eight- to tenfold increase in risk of breast cancer as compared to noncarriers, but they collectively account for less than 1% of cases of breast cancer. Like *BRCA1* and *BRCA2,* these genes are inherited in an autosomal dominant fashion and function as tumor suppressors.[12] The hereditary cancer syndromes associated with each gene are usually characterized by multiple cancers in addition to breast cancer, as summarized in Table 24.1.

Moderate-Penetrance, Low Frequency Breast Cancer Predisposition Genes

Four genes have been identified that confer an elevated but moderate risk of developing breast cancer, namely *CHEK2, ATM, BRIP1,* and *PALB2* (Table 24.1). Each of these genes confers approximately a two- to threefold relative risk of breast cancer in mutation carriers, though this risk may be higher in select clinical settings.[5] Mutation frequencies in the general population are rare, on the order of 0.1% to 1%, though some founder

TABLE 24.1

BREAST CANCER SUSCEPTIBILITY GENES AND LOCI

Gene/Locus	Associated Syndrome/Clinical Features	Breast Cancer Risk	Mutation/Minor Allele Frequency
HIGH PENETRANCE GENES			
BRCA1 (17q21)	**Hereditary breast/ovarian cancer:** bilateral/multifocal breast tumor, prostate, colon, liver, bone cancers	60%–85% (lifetime); 15%–40% risk of ovarian cancer	1/400
BRCA2 (13q12.3)	**Hereditary breast/ovarian cancer:** male breast cancer, pancreas, gall bladder, pharynx, stomach, melanoma, prostate cancer. Also causes D1 Fanconi anemia (biallelic mutations)	60%–85% (lifetime); 15%–40% risk of ovarian cancer	1/400
TP53 (17p13.1)	**Li-Fraumeni syndrome:** breast cancer, soft tissue sarcoma, central nervous system tumors, adrenocortical cancer, leukemia, prostate cancer	50%–89% (by age 50); 90% in Li-Fraumeni survivors	<1/10,000
PTEN (10q23.3)	**Cowden syndrome:** breast cancer, hamartoma, thyroid, oral mucosa, endometrial, brain tumor	25%–50% (lifetime)	<1/10,000
CDH1 (16q22.1)	**Familial diffuse gastric cancer:** lobular breast cancer, gastric cancer	RR 6.6	<1/10,000
STK11/LKB1 (19p13.3)	**Peutz-Jeghers syndrome:** breast, ovary, testis, pancreas, cervix, uterine, colon cancers; melanocytic macules of lips/digits; gastrointestinal hamartomatous polyps	30%–50% (by age 70)	<1/10,000
MODERATE PENETRANCE GENES			
CHEK2(22q12.1)	**Li-Fraumeni 2 syndrome(?):** breast, prostate, colorectal, and brain tumors, sarcomas	OR 2.6 (for 1100delC mutation)	1/100–200 (in certain populations)
BRIP1 (17q22)	**Breast cancer:** also causes FA-J Fanconi anemia(biallelic mutations)	RR 2.0	<1/1000
ATM (11q22.3)	**Ataxia-telangiectasia:** breast, ovarian, leukemia, lymphoma, possible stomach/pancreas/bladder cancers; immunodeficiency	RR 2.37	1/33–333
PALB2 (16p12)	**Breast, pancreatic, prostate cancers:** also causes FA-N Fanconi anemia(biallelic mutations)	RR 2.3	<1/1000
LOW PENETRANCE GENES AND LOCI			
FGFR2 (10q26)	Breast cancer	OR 1.26	0.38
TOX3 (16q12.1)	Breast cancer	OR 1.14	0.46
LSP1 (11p15.5)	Breast cancer	OR 1.06	0.3
TGFB1 (19q13.1)	Breast cancer	OR 1.07	0.68
MAP3K1 (5q11.2)	Breast cancer	OR 1.13	0.28
CASP8 (2q33-34)	Breast cancer (protective)	OR 0.89	0.13
6q22.33	Breast cancer	OR 1.41	0.21 (in Ashkenazi Jewish)
2q35	Breast cancer	OR 1.11	0.11–0.52
8q24	Breast cancer	OR 1.06	0.4
5p12	Breast cancer	OR 1.19	0.2–0.31

OR, overall risk; RR, relative risk.

mutations have been identified. Together, these genes account for approximately 2.3% of inherited breast cancer. The moderate relative risk of breast cancer of these genes in conjunction with the low population frequency renders this class of genes very difficult to detect with typical association studies. However, these genes were specifically selected for study as candidate breast cancer genes based on their known roles in signal transduction and DNA repair in close association with BRCA1 and BRCA2.[6]

Low-Penetrance, High Frequency Breast Cancer Predisposition Genes and Loci

Both candidate gene and genome-wide association studies (GWAS) have identified a low-risk panel of approximately ten different alleles and loci in 15% to 40% of women with breast cancer[5] (Table 24.1). Despite their frequency, the relative risk of breast cancer conferred by any one of these genetic variants alone is minimal, on the order of less than 1.5.[4] Nevertheless, these alleles and loci may become clinically relevant in their suggestion of interactions with other high-, moderate-, and low-risk genes; these additive or multiplicative relationships could account for a measurable fraction of population risk. For example, association studies of FGFR2 and MAP3K1 within *BRCA* families showed that these single nucleotide polymorphisms (SNPs) conferred an increased risk in the presence of *BRCA2* mutations.

Recent studies suggest that microRNA (miRNA) SNPs may also contribute to breast cancer susceptibility, and miRNAs appear to regulate many tumor suppressor genes (TSGs) and oncogenes via degradation of target mRNAs or repression of their translation. Thus, genetic variations in miRNA genes or miRNA binding sites could affect expression of TSGs or oncogenes and, thereby, cancer risk. For example, specific SNPs located within pre-miR-27a and miR-196a-2 genes have been associated with reduced breast cancer risk.[13]

SOMATIC CHANGES IN BREAST CANCER

The vast majority of breast cancers are sporadic in origin, ultimately caused by accumulation of numerous somatic genetic alterations.[1] Recent data suggest that a typical individual breast cancer harbors anywhere from 50 to 80 different somatic mutations.[2] Many of these mutations occur as a result of erroneous DNA replication; others may occur through exposure to exogenous and endogenous mutagens. To date, hundreds of candidate somatic breast cancer genes have been identified

through GWAS.[14,15] Yet the full range of somatic mutations will not be clear until hundreds more breast tumor samples are sequenced. To this end, international efforts are currently underway to produce a comprehensive catalog of these genetic alterations.

Determining the role of each identified mutation in the development of breast cancer remains a substantial challenge. Data suggest that the vast majority of identified somatic DNA mutations in a given tumor are "passenger" mutations, representing harmless, biologically neutral changes that do not contribute to oncogenesis.[1,2] Conversely, "driver" mutations confer a growth advantage on the cell in which they occur and appear to be implicated in cancer development. By definition, driver mutations are found in candidate cancer genes (CAN).[15]

Although the catalog of somatic mutations and CAN genes is still incomplete, it is comprehensive enough that various structural features are starting to emerge. When specific driver mutations are cataloged among several different breast tumors, a bimodal cancer "genomic landscape" appears, comprising a small number of commonly mutated gene "mountains" among hundreds of infrequently mutated gene "hills."[1,2] Gene mountains correspond to the most frequently mutated genes found within breast tumors, such as TP53, CDH1, phosphatidylinositol 3-kinase (PI3K), cyclin D, PTEN, and AKT.[6] Each individual gene hill, on the other hand, is typically found in less than 5% of breast tumors.[1,16] This substantial heterogeneity of DNA mutations among breast tumors may explain the wide variations in phenotypes, both in terms of tumor behavior as well as responsiveness to therapy.

Historically, the focus of genetic research has been on the gene mountains, in part because they were the only mutations that available technology could identify. However emerging data suggest that it is actually the gene hills that play a much more pivotal role in breast cancer, consistent with the idea that having a large number of mutations, each associated with a small survival advantage, drives tumor progression. Recent studies have shown that a substantial number of these infrequent somatic mutations sort out among a much smaller number of biologic groups and cell signaling pathways that are known to be pathogenic in breast cancer, thereby vastly reducing the complexity of the genomic landscape. Examples of such pathways include interferon signaling, cell cycle checkpoint, BRCA1/2-related DNA repair, p53, AKT, transforming growth factor-β (TGF-β) signaling, Notch, epidermal growth factor receptor (EGFR), FGF, ERBB2, RAS, and PI3K. In short, it appears that common pathways, rather than individual gene mutations, govern the course of breast cancer development.[16]

Although recurrent point mutations are less common in breast cancer than other solid tumors,

TABLE 24.2

RECURRENT AMPLIFICATIONS IN BREAST CANCER CELL LINES AND HUMAN TUMORS

Cell Line	8q24	11q13	17q12	17q22	20q13
BT-474		11q13-q14	17q12	17q22-24 (avg 49 copies)	20q13 (avg 37 copies)
SKBR-3	8q23.2-q24.21		17q12	17q24	20q13
MCF-7		11q13		17q21-q22, 17q23	20q13.1, 20q13.2-q13.31
MCF-10A			No amplification		
UACC-893		11q13-q14	17q12-q21.2	17q22-24	
UACC-812			17q12	17q23	20q13
MDA-MB361		11q13.4-q14.1	17q12-q21.1	17q23.2-q24.1	
SUM-190		11q13.4-q14.1			
ZR-75-1		11q13.2-q13.4			
ZR-75-30	8q24.22, 8q24.3		17q12-q21.2	17q23.2-q24.2	

emerging data show that particular regions of the genome are commonly amplified and these regions contain genes that drive cancer progression (Table 24.2). The best example of an important amplified region is the 17q12 amplicon that harbors the *HER2* oncogene. This amplicon leads to a more aggressive tumor phenotype, now the target of a highly successful antibody therapy, trastuzumab (Herceptin). It has been observed that RNAi knockdown of coamplified genes within the 17q12 amplicon results in decreased cell proliferation and increased apoptosis.[17] Thus, the 17q12 amplicon appears to encode a concerted genetic program that contributes to the oncogenesis.

There are several other amplicons, in addition to 17q12 (*HER2*), that seem to drive the cancer phenotype and have prognostic significance in breast cancers, for example, 11q13 (*CCDN1*) and 8q24 (*MYC*), 20q13.[18] These regions contain gene sets that are important in DNA metabolism and maintenance of chromosomal integrity, suggesting that response to DNA damaging agents used as anticancer therapy might be modulated by the presence of particular amplicons. Indeed, these coamplicons are frequent in *HER2* amplified tumors and may modify tumor behavior and patient outcome.[19,20] The contribution of these genomic alterations to functional consequences, may lie not in the overexpression of individual genes, but of gene cassettes on the amplicon.

Direct clinical translation of the growing catalog of somatic alterations in breast cancer has yet to evolve. However, with advancing technology and further identification and categorization of genetic mutations, new opportunities for individualized diagnosis and treatment options are likely to emerge.

GENE EXPRESSION PATTERNS IN BREAST CANCER

The cellular programs that are encoded by DNA are enacted by transcription into messenger RNA (mRNA) and translated into protein. Not surprisingly, the DNA alterations described above lead to either under- or overexpression of their associated mRNAs; consequently abnormal gene expression patterns are a common finding in breast tumors. Gene expression profiling has been introduced into the clinical literature during the past decade as research suggests that assessing the expression of multiple genes in a tumor sample may reflect programs turned on by DNA alternations and predict tumor behavior. So-called molecular signatures hold promise for improving diagnosis, prediction of recurrence, and selection of therapies for individual patients.

Several technologies have been developed to generate molecular signatures, including cDNA and oligonucleotide arrays and multiplex polymerase chain reaction (PCR) technologies. These technologies and newly developed statistical methodologies now allow evaluation of hundreds and even thousands of mRNAs simultaneously with grouping of samples based on coexpressed genes.

Molecular Classification of Breast Cancer

The seminal work by Perou et al.[21] and Sorlie et al.[22] suggests a classification of breast cancer subtypes based on gene expression patterns they termed "molecular portraits" of breast cancer.

Among the categories they defined were the luminal A and B tumor types (typically estrogen receptor [ER] or progesterone receptor [PR] positive), *HER2* gene-amplified tumors, and a newly recognized class termed "basal-like" due to the expression of basal keratins. Basal tumors typically lack ER, PR, and *HER2*, and are often referred to as triple negative, although not all basal-like tumors are triple negative and the reverse. Although the exact definition of molecular subtypes is an area of active debate, it is clear that these subtypes are reproducible in multiple, unrelated data sets, and their prognostic impact has been validated in these settings.[21,23,24] As a result, clinical trials are now being designed to subdivide patients by ER/PR and *HER2* status to validate claims that therapeutic approaches should address these groups rather than the population of breast cancer patients as a whole.

Prognostic Signatures

Around the same time period, van't Veer et al.[24] and van de Vijver et al.[25] were the first to apply gene expression analysis to define a subgroup of breast cancer patients with increased likelihood of metastasis. The estimated hazard ratio for distant metastases in the group with a poor prognosis signature, as compared with the group with the good prognosis signature, was 5.1 (95% confidence interval, 2.9 to 9.0; P <.001). The European Organisation for Research and Treatment of Cancer (EORTC) and the Breast International Group (BIG) are currently conducting a prospective clinical trial to validate the utility of this assay for sparing patients from systemic chemotherapy (the MINDACT study).[26] In a preliminary analysis, the 70-gene profile signature was strongly prognostic, outperforming classic prognostic criteria such as those used by the St. Gallen consensus panel[27]; however, the magnitude of effect was much less than previously reported with hazard ratios for time to distant metastases of 1.85 (1.14 to 3.0) and for overall survival of 2.5 (1.4 to 4.5). The 70-gene signature is now commercialized as the MammaPrint and has received clearance by the U.S. Food and Drug Administration (FDA) as a class 2, 510(k) product.

Other groups have developed prognostic gene expression signatures, including the 76-gene Rotterdam signature, which identifies a high-risk group of node-negative patients, and the Genomic Grade Index (GGI), which distinguishes poor and good prognosis groups in breast tumors of intermediate histologic grade.[28] The potential value of these signatures has yet to be clearly defined, but it emphasizes the role of gene expression profiling at distinguishing prognostic groups not otherwise recognizable by standard histologic or clinical parameters.

Predictive Signatures

Endocrine Therapy

Several groups have applied gene expression profiling analysis to better define the likelihood of benefit from therapy. Such predictive signatures may have particular value as they help oncologists counsel patients about appropriate choices for treatment. Genomics Health Inc (Redwood City, California) developed the Oncotype DX® assay as a predictor of benefit from antiestrogen therapy using multiple real-time reverse transcriptase polymerase chain reaction (RT-PCR) assays in formalin fixed paraffin-embedded tissue. The assay was developed from 250 candidate genes selected from published literature, genomic databases, and in-house experiments performed on frozen tissue. From these data, a panel of 16 cancer-related genes and 5 reference genes were used to develop an algorithm to compute a recurrence score, ranging from 0 to 100, that can be used to estimate the odds of recurrence over 10 years from diagnosis.[29] Paik et al.[29] reported an analysis of two randomized controlled trials: National Surgical Adjuvant Breast and Bowel Project NSABP-B14, in which node-negative patients with ER-positive tumors were randomly assigned to tamoxifen or nil; and NSABP-B20, in which node-negative patients with ER-positive tumors were randomly assigned to tamoxifen alone or with cyclophosphamide, methotrexate, and fluorouracil (CMF) chemotherapy. Using the tissue samples from NSABP-B20, patients were categorized into three recurrence score groups: low risk (recurrence score less than 18), intermediate risk (recurrence score 18 to 30), and high risk (recurrence score 31 to 100). Samples from NSABP-B14 were then analyzed and found to be 6.8% (4.0% to 9.6%), 14.3% (8.3% to 20.3%) and 30.5% (23.6% to 37.4%). Paik et al. further analyzed the performance of the Oncotype DX assay to include patients in the other arms of NSABP-B14 and NSABP-B20 and found that the Oncotype DX assay was a strong predictor of benefit from CMF in NSABP-B20, with little or no benefit from chemotherapy for patients with low or intermediate recurrence scores but substantial benefit for those with high recurrence scores. Conversely, in NSABP-B14, the benefit from tamoxifen versus observation was confined to the low and intermediate risk categories (P value for interaction of .001). These data suggest that in patients who have an apparent favorable prognosis based on clinical features (negative nodes, positive ER), the Oncotype DX assay helps determine those most likely to benefit from tamoxifen only (low recurrence scores) versus those most likely not to benefit from tamoxifen but likely to benefit from chemotherapy (high recurrence scores). The benefits of chemotherapy in the 25% of patients who have intermediate recurrence scores remains uncertain and are the basis of an ongoing prospective randomized trial (Tailor Rx) where those with high recurrence scores will receive endocrine therapy and chemotherapy, those with low recurrence scores will receive endocrine therapy alone, and intermediate recurrence scores are randomly assigned to endocrine therapy versus endocrine and chemotherapy. A recent study by Albain et al.[30] suggests that a low recurrence score predicts a lack of benefit of fluorouracil (5-FU), Adriamycin (doxorubicin), and cyclophosphamide (FAC) chemotherapy in node-positive breast cancer patients treated on Southwest Oncology Group SWOG-8814. Although these provocative data suggest a similar utility for Oncotype DX in node-positive patients, they do not include the use of taxanes and require additional validation with modern-day regimens. The value of the Oncotype DX assay in predicting benefit from hormonal therapy in patients treated with aromatase inhibitor therapy has recently been published, demonstrating that the assay performs equally similarly with both tamoxifen and anastrazole but does not distinguish benefit of one over the other.[31]

Additional predictors for ER-positive breast cancer include the Breast Cancer 2-Gene Expression Ratio (AvariaDx Inc, Carlsbad, California), a quantitative RT-PCR–based assay that measures the ratio of the *HOXB6* and *IL17BR* genes, and is marketed as a marker of recurrence risk in untreated ER-positive/node-negative patients.[32,33] The Breast Cancer Gene Expression Ratio is significantly and independently associated with poorer disease-free survival in two studies of lymph node–negative, ER-positive, tamoxifen-treated patients with breast cancer. In these two studies, patients who were low risk by the two-gene expression ratio had average 10-year recurrence rates of approximately 17% to 25%. Further validation is awaited.

Chemotherapy

Defining predictors of response to chemotherapy and targeted therapies has been more challenging. Ayers et al.[34] from the M. D. Anderson Cancer Center were the first to report that multigene analysis of fine needle aspiration specimens predicts response to neoadjuvant T-FAC chemotherapy. These results require validation and are the subject of a prospective trial of chemotherapy with randomization based on the predictor (F. Symmans, personal communication). Another approach to the development of predictive signatures was pioneered by the group at Duke Center for Health Policy and Informatics where gene signatures were defined in model systems and applied to human data sets. While initially tested in lung cancer, these signatures are now the subject of several prospective randomized trials in breast cancer, and other tumor types.[35] Validation of gene signatures is of utmost importance in the future to determine the value of these expression profiles at predicting treatment response, and clinical outcome, in breast cancer patients. National organizations such as the American Society of Clinical Oncology, National Comprehensive Cancer Network, and College of American Pathologists have ongoing efforts to interpret the data from the burgeoning field of multigene biomarker tests to help the practicing clinician interpret their clinical utility.[36]

EPIGENETICS OF BREAST CANCER

Cells maintain their stable identity and phenotype over many generations without external stimuli or signaling events. This cellular memory is encoded in the epigenome, a collection of heritable information that exists alongside the genomic sequence. DNA methylation and chromatin modification are major epigenetic mechanisms in higher eukaryotes and are tightly coupled to basic genetic processes, such as DNA replication, transcription, and repair. DNA methylation at the promoter proximal CpG sequences is associated with gene silencing. Similarly, specific histone modifications control transcriptional status or capacity of the underlying sequence by regulating the activity of chromatin domains in an active or inactive state. Euchromatin or active chromatin is enriched with acetylated histones H3, H4, and H2A and histone H3 methylated at lysine residues K4, K40, and K36.[37] In contrast, heterochromatin or silent chromatin is depleted of histone acetylation while enriched in histone H3 methylated at lysine resides K9, K27, and K79. It is well documented that cancers, including breast cancer, have altered patterns of DNA methylation and histone acetylation, leading to alterations in transcription that appear to be oncogenic.[37,38] Hence, epigenetic therapies have received intense interest from a large number of clinical and basic cancer studies.

Major epigenetic cancer drugs include DNA methyltransferase (DNMT) and histone deacetylase (HDAC) inhibitors. Preclinical studies show promise that HDAC inhibitors may have activity in breast cancer cells, and many clinical phase 1 and 2 studies are in progress.[39,40]

MicroRNAs: A Newly Discovered Class of Molecules that Regulate Gene Expression

miRNAs are small noncoding RNAs that belong to a novel class of regulatory molecules that control expression of hundreds of target mRNA transcripts. miRNAs are generated from large RNA precursors (termed pre-miRNAs) that are processed in the nucleus into approximately 70 nucleotide pre-miRNAs, which fold into imperfect stem-loop structures.[41] The pre-miRNAs undergo an additional processing step within the cytoplasm, and mature miRNAs of 18 to 25 nucleotides in length are excised from one side of the pre-miRNA hairpin by Dicer. miRNAs regulate gene expression in two ways. First, miRNAs that bind to protein-coding mRNA sequences that are exactly complementary to the miRNA induce the RNA-mediated interference (RNAi) pathway. Messenger RNA targets are then cleaved by ribonucleases in the RNA-induced silencing complex (RISC). Second, miRNAs bind to imperfect complementary sites within the 3′-untranslated regions (3′UTRs) of their target protein-coding mRNAs and repress the expression of these genes at the level of translation.[42]

miRNAs are known to be associated with breast cancer in both cell lines and clinical samples. For example, *miR-21*, *miR-155*, *miR-7*, and *miR-210* are overexpressed in aggressive human breast cancers,[43,44] while *let-7* and *miR-125a* have been shown to be down-regulated in breast cancers.[45] It has also been shown that *miR-125a* may function as a tumor suppressor by inhibiting ERBB2 and ERBB3.

MicroRNAs Predict Response to Cancer Treatment

Soon after they were discovered to be misregulated in cancer, miRNA misexpression patterns were found to be associated with cancer outcome and response to treatment, including radiation and chemotherapy. Certain miRNAs associated with hypoxia, such as *miR-210*, have been shown to be biomarkers of poor outcome in breast cancer.[43] Furthermore, *in vitro* data show that certain miRNAs are associated with resistance to doxorubicin[46] or tamoxifen.[47] In patient samples, an association of miRNA's tumor subtypes have specific miRNA patterns and this is associated with poor outcome. Defining the role of miRNAs as biomarkers for prognosis and prediction, as well as their potential as targeted therapies, is an active area of research in breast cancer.

PROTEIN/PATHWAY ALTERATIONS

The molecular mechanisms that lead to cancer have been characterized as the hallmarks of cancer, as proposed by Hanahan and Weinberg.[48] They include self-sufficiency in growth signals, insensitivity to antigrowth factor signals, evasion of apoptosis, infinite replicative potential, invasion and metastasis, and sustained angiogenesis. The effectors of genetic and epigenetic abnormalities are in most cases reflected in the abnormal levels, functions, and interactions of proteins and signaling pathways. Undoubtedly, numerous alterations coordinate to result in the malignant phenotype; however, a number of key proteins and their pathways have emerged as critical drivers of breast cancer development and growth as well as potential therapeutic targets.

Therapeutic Targets in Breast Cancer

Estrogen Signaling

Most breast cancers are intimately linked with exposure to estrogen and alterations in the estrogen receptor signaling pathway. Estrogen is a steroid hormone that exerts its actions by binding to the nuclear ER. Upon activation by its ligand, ER binds in a coordinated fashion with a number of coregulatory proteins to estrogen response elements in the promoter region of estrogen-responsive genes. This in turn directs the transcription of numerous growth-promoting genes, including PR. Although ER is overexpressed in as many as 70% of invasive breast cancers, the precise mechanism by which this occurs is unclear. Amplification of the gene appears to be one mechanism; however, it was present in only approximately 50% of cases with ER overexpression in one study, suggesting that transcriptional deregulation and posttranscriptional modifications (such as alteration of mRNA levels by miRNAs) may also play a role. The level of ER expression is not only of biologic interest, but it is a highly effective predictor for response to antiestrogens, which is a recommended treatment for all ER-expressing tumors.

Estrogen exerts its actions through both genomic (described above) and nongenomic mechanisms. In contrast to the genomic actions of ER, nongenomic actions of ER are extremely rapid (within seconds to minutes of estrogen exposure) and are believed to result from the hormone-dependent activation of membrane-bound or cytosolic ERs. These nonnuclear ER actions result in rapid phosphorylation and activation of important growth regulatory kinases including EGFRs, insulinlike growth factor-1R (IGF-1R), c-Src, Shc, and the p85α regulatory subunit of PI3K.[5] This "crosstalk" between ER and growth factor receptors is bidirectional: constitutive HER2, for example, can increase ER signaling to the point where it is unresponsive to antiestrogen treatments. These findings suggest a role for HER2/IGF-1R/EGFR activation in both acquired and *de novo* resistance to treatment with antiestrogens.[49]

The ER pathway has proven to be an invaluable target for therapeutic treatments in breast cancer. A number of agents have been developed over the prior decades that can inhibit this pathway by either binding to the receptor itself (e.g., selective ER modulators such as tamoxifen) or by decreasing the production of endogenous estrogen (e.g., aromatase inhibitors and ovarian ablation). Although these agents are highly effective and have made a significant impact on breast cancer morbidity and mortality, unfortunately, *de novo* and acquired resistance is also quite common.

As described above, the Oncotype DX assay adds additional insight into the behavior of ER-positive tumors and provides useful information for treatment decision making.

Growth Factor Receptor Pathways

Growth factor receptor pathways, and in particular tyrosine kinase receptors, play an essential role in initiating both proliferative and cell survival pathways in tissue and are normally tightly regulated. In breast cancer biology, the ErbB family has been studied most extensively, but an expanding number of other growth factors, such as insulin-like growth factor receptors, have also been the subject of intense scrutiny in hopes of identifying effective therapeutic targets.[50] These receptors have an extracellular ligand-binding region, a transmembrane region, and a cytoplasmic tyrosine kinase–containing domain that can activate downstream signaling cascades. These growth factor receptor pathways can be constitutively activated by a number of mechanisms, including excessive ligand levels, gain-of-function mutations, overexpression with or without gene amplification, and gene rearrangements and resultant fusion proteins with oncogenic potential. This can ultimately lead to inappropriate kinase activity and growth promoting second messenger activation (Fig. 24.2).

Human Epidermal Growth Factor Receptor 2

HER2 (EGFR2 or ErbB2) is a member of a family of receptor tyrosine kinases that also includes EGFR (HER1, ErbB1), ErbB3, and ErbB4. Ligand binding to the extracellular domains of the ErbB1, ErbB3, or ErbB4 receptors induces homo- and heterodimerization and kinase activation. The HER2 protein exists in a closed conformation and has no ligand, but it is the preferred partner for dimerization with HER1, -3, and -4. At a molecular level, *HER2* amplification is associated with deregulation of G_1/S phase cell cycle control via up-regulation of cyclins D1, E, and cdk6, as well as p27 degradation. HER2 also interacts with important second messengers including SH2 domain-containing proteins (e.g., Src kinases).

More important, HER2 amplification or protein overexpression (found in 20% to 30% of invasive breast cancers) is clearly associated with accelerated cell growth and proliferation, poor clinical outcome, and response to the monoclonal anti-HER2 antibody, trastuzumab. In the adjuvant setting, several independent randomized studies have shown that the addition of trastuzumab to chemotherapy reduced the rate of recurrence by over 50% among women with HER2-positive early stage breast cancer.[51] Based on these results, trastuzumab in combination with standard chemotherapy was approved by the FDA in 2006 for use in the adjuvant setting.

The precise mechanism of action of trastuzumab (and therefore mechanism of resistance as well) remains controversial. Trastuzumab appears to inhibit several major pathways that regulate tumor growth. First, trastuzumab may disrupt heterodimeric interaction of HER2 (and also block cleavage of HER2 at the juxtamembrane region). Second, trastuzumab modulates host immunity, activating natural killer cells involved in antibody-dependent cellular cytotoxicity (ADCC). In both animal models and more recently in clinical studies, the FcγR genotype required for ADCC was associated with trastuzumab effectiveness in HER2 overexpressed breast cancer. Third, trastuzumab also appears to affect angiogenesis at multiple levels, including a decrease in tumor-associated microvessel density, reduction in proangiogenic factors, and "normalization" of neovascularization. Finally, trastuzumab partially inhibits numerous downstream signaling pathways, most notably the ras/raf/MEK/MAPK and the PI3K/AKT pathways, and studies suggest that activation of these pathways by alternate receptors (e.g., IGF-1R, c-met) or deregulation through loss of PTEN or P13K mutation may lead to resistance to trastuzumab[52] (Fig. 24.2).

Human Epidermal Growth Factor Receptor 2/Epidermal Growth Factor Receptor

As HER2 signaling is effected through heterodimer formation with other EGFRs, targeting HER2 and EGFR simultaneously, for example, may provide therapeutic synergy. The tyrosine kinase inhibitor lapatinib competes with adenosine triphosphate to bind to the activation loop of target kinases, thereby inhibiting their activity. Lapatinib inhibits the tyrosine phosphorylation of both EGFR and HER2 and in turn inhibits activation of the proproliferative kinases ERK1/2 and AKT. Lapatinib has now been FDA approved in combination with capecitabine in advanced HER2-positive breast cancer previously progressed on trastuzumab, based on a phase 3 trial showing a significant benefit for the combination over capecitabine alone.

Insulinlike Growth Factor-1R

In addition to activation of the EGFR pathway, signaling via insulinlike growth factor (IGF-1 and IGF-2) and their receptor (IGF-1R) can result in phosphorylation and activation of a variety of oncogenic kinases. IGF-1R is the primary response mediator of IGF and is expressed in all epithelial cell types. However, elevated IGF-1 levels and IGF-1R signaling have been implicated in increased

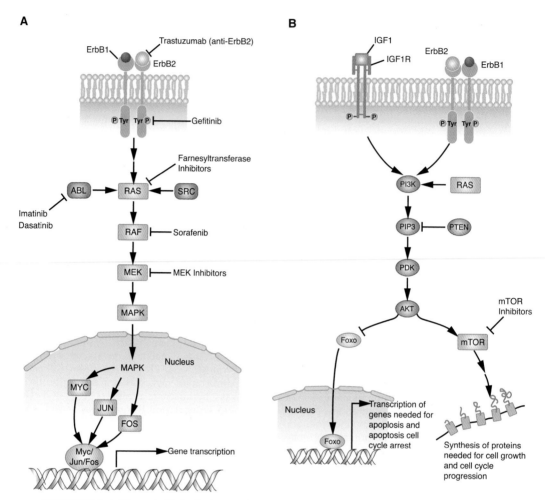

FIGURE 24.2 A: The ras/raf/MEK/MAPK pathway is activated by multiple growth factor receptors (here exemplified by ErbB1 and ErbB2) as well as several intracellular tyrosine kinases such as SRC and ABL. Activated RAS stimulates a sequence of phosphorylation events mediated by RAF, MEK, and ERK (MAP) kinases. Activated MAP kinase (MAPK) translocates to the nucleus and activates proteins such as MYC, JUN, and FOS that promote the transcription of numerous genes involved in tumor growth. **B:** The phosphatidylinositol 3-kinase (PI3K)pathway is activated by RAS and by a number of growth factor receptors (here exemplified IGF1R and the ErbB1/ErbB2 heterodimer). Activated PI3K generates phosphatidylinositol-3,4,5-triphosphate (PIP3), which activates phosphoinositide-dependent kinase-1 (PDK). In turn, PDK phosphorylates AKT. PTEN is an endogenous inhibitor of AKT activation. Phosphorylated AKT transduces multiple downstream signals, including activation of the mammalian target of rapamycin (mTOR) and inhibition of the FOXO family of transcription factors. mTOR activation promotes the synthesis of proteins required for cell growth and cell cycle progression. (Redrawn from Golan DE, Tashjian AH, Armstrong EJ. *Principles of pharmacology: the pathophysiologic basis of drug therapy.* 2nd ed. Baltimore: Wolters Kluwer Health, 2008.)

risk of breast and other cancers. The IGF-1R has in particular been shown to be an effective target in preclinical studies. Similar to ErbB receptor inhibition, IGF-1R inhibitors have focused primarily on neutralizing antibodies and tyrosine kinase inhibitors. Currently more than eight monoclonal antibodies directed against IGF-1R are in various stages of clinical development in a variety of cancers. Notably, extensive cross-talk of IGF-1R downstream signaling pathways with other impor-

tant signaling pathways in breast cancer suggests that combining IGF-1R inhibitors with other targeted agents may be an effective therapeutic strategy. For example, IGF-1R up-regulation has been suggested as a mechanism of resistance to HER2 and EGFR inhibitors through sustained activation of the PI3K/AKT pathway. Similarly, IGF-1R up-regulation has also been seen in breast cancer cells that have developed resistance to antiestrogen and HER2 treatments.

Ras and Phosphatidylinositol 3-Kinase Pathways

Redundancies and cross-talk of numerous different signaling pathways are a common theme. Several downstream messengers, however, bear special consideration due to their functional importance and therapeutic implications. PI3K/AKT is a central signaling pathway downstream of many receptor tyrosine kinases and regulates cell growth and proliferation (Fig. 24.2B). Activating mutations in the gene encoding the p110α catalytic subunit of PI3K (PI3CKA) may be an important contributing factor to mammary tumor progression. Activating mutations of the AKT gene family are rare.

PTEN dephosphorylates, and therefore inactivates, the p110 catalytic domain of PI3K and is either mutated or underexpressed (e.g., via methylation) in many breast cancers. Activation of the PI3K pathway, in turn, results in the 3-phosphoinositide-dependent kinase-mediated activation of several known kinases including AKT1, AKT2, and AKT3. Interestingly, activated AKT1 appears to be antiapoptotic but also plays an antiinvasive role in tumor formation. In addition to the AKTs, downstream proliferative effectors of the PI3K pathway also include the mammalian target of rapamycin (mTOR) complex 1 (TORC1), which consists of mTOR, raptor, and mLst8. It is currently believed that TORC1 mediates its progrowth effects through the activation of S6-kinase1 and suppression of 4E-BP1, an inhibitor of cap-dependent translation. These observations all point to mTOR-raptor as a critical target in cancer therapy, and indeed, several mTOR inhibitors known as rapamycin analogues (e.g., CCI-779, RAD-001, AP-23576) are undergoing clinical trials for the treatment of breast cancer.

The ras/raf/MEK/MAPK pathway is also a critical signaling pathway for numerous growth factor receptors (Fig. 24.2A). Thus far in breast cancer, agents that target the MEK pathway (e.g., raf inhibitor sorafenib) have had modest success as single agents, but studies in combination with other treatments hold more promise.

Angiogenesis

Angiogenesis is normally a tightly regulated process of vessel formation during physiologic events such as wound healing and pregnancy. It has also been shown to be an important part of tumor growth and spread. In contrast to physiologic angiogenesis, tumor-associated angiogenesis is highly dysregulated with disorganized and distorted vasculature and increased vascular permeability. Thus, in recent years, angiogenesis has become a frequent target for the treatment of many cancers.

Central to this process is the proangiogenic factor, vascular endothelial growth factor (VEGF), which together with its receptors, regulate endothelial cell growth and new vessel formation.[53] VEGFRs, like EGFRs, are also tyrosine kinase receptors. VEGF-A binds to both VEGFR1 (Flt-1) and VEGFR2 (KDR/Flk1). VEGFR2 appears to mediate most of the known cellular responses to VEGFs, while the function of VEGFR1 is less well defined. Bevacizumab, a humanized monoclonal antibody directed against VEGF-A, has been the most extensively studied thus far. To date, three large randomized trials have shown a statistically significant benefit in progression-free survival when bevacizumab was added to a variety of different chemotherapies in the first-line metastatic setting. Multitargeted VEGFR tyrosine kinase inhibitors such as sunitinib (VEGFR, PDGFR, and c-kit blockade) and sorafenib (VEGFR and RAF kinase blockade) have also been studied extensively in breast and other cancers. Despite the success of some of these agents, identification of predictive factors for antiangiogenic response have thus far proven to be elusive and is not recommended as a selection criteria for treatment or for entry into clinical trials.

Selected References

The full list of references for this chapter appears in the online version.

1. Bell DW. Our changing view of the genomic landscape of cancer. *J Pathol* 2010;220(2):231.
2. Wood LD, Parsons DW, Jones S, et al. The genomic landscapes of human breast and colorectal cancers. *Science* 2007;318(5853):1108.
4. Turnbull C, Rahman N. Genetic predisposition to breast cancer: past, present, and future. *Annu Rev Genomics Hum Genet* 2008;9:321.
5. Foulkes WD. Inherited susceptibility to common cancers. *N Engl J Med* 2008;359(20):2143.
6. Hirshfield KM, Rebbeck TR, Levine AJ. Germline mutations and polymorphisms in the origins of cancers in women. *J Oncol* 2010;2010:297671.
7. Narod SA. Modifiers of risk of hereditary breast cancer. *Oncogene* 2006;25(43):5832.
8. Turner NC, Reis-Filho JS. Basal-like breast cancer and the BRCA1 phenotype. *Oncogene* 2006;25(43):5846.
9. Venkitaraman AR. Cancer susceptibility and the functions of BRCA1 and BRCA2. *Cell* 2002;108(2):171.
10. Fong PC, Boss DS, Yap TA, et al. Inhibition of poly(ADP-ribose) polymerase in tumors from BRCA mutation carriers. *N Engl J Med* 2009;361(2):123.
11. Iglehart JD, Silver DP. Synthetic lethality—a new direction in cancer-drug development. *N Engl J Med* 2009;361(2):189.
12. Stratton MR, Rahman N. The emerging landscape of breast cancer susceptibility. *Nat Genet* 2008;40(1):17.
13. Hoffman AE, Zheng T, Yi C, et al. microRNA miR-196a-2 and breast cancer: a genetic and epigenetic association

study and functional analysis. *Cancer Res* 2009;69(14):5970.

14. Forbes SA, Bhamra G, Bamford S, et al. The catalogue of somatic mutations in cancer (COSMIC). *Curr Protoc Hum Genet* 2008;chapter 10:unit 10.11.

15. Stratton MR, Campbell PJ, Futreal PA. The cancer genome. *Nature* 2009;458(7239):719.

16. Copeland NG, Jenkins NA. Deciphering the genetic landscape of cancer—from genes to pathways. *Trends Genet* 2009;25(10):455.

17. Kao J, Pollack JR. RNA interference-based functional dissection of the 17q12 amplicon in breast cancer reveals contribution of coamplified genes. *Genes Chromosomes Cancer* 2006;45(8):761.

18. Chin K, DeVries S, Fridlyand J, et al. Genomic and transcriptional aberrations linked to breast cancer pathophysiologies. *Cancer Cell* 2006;10(6):529.

19. Bentires-Alj M, Gil SG , Chan R, et al. A role for the scaffolding adapter GAB2 in breast cancer. *Nature Med* 2005;12(1):114.

21. Perou CM, Sørlie T, Eisen MB, et al. Molecular portraits of human breast tumours. *Nature* 2000;406(6797):747.

22. Sorlie T, Perou CM, Tibshirani R, et al. Gene expression patterns of breast carcinomas distinguish tumor subclasses with clinical implications. *Proc Natl Acad Sci U S A* 2001;98 (19):10869.

23. Gruvberger S, Ringnér M, Chen Y, et al. Estrogen receptor status in breast cancer is associated with remarkably distinct gene expression patterns. *Cancer Res* 2001;61(16):5979.

24. van't Veer LJ, Dai H, van de Vijver MJ, et al. Gene expression profiling predicts clinical outcome of breast cancer. *Nature* 2002;415(6871):530.

25. van de Vijver MJ, He YD, van't Veer LJ, et al. A gene-expression signature as a predictor of survival in breast cancer. *N Engl J Med* 2002;347(25):1999.

26. Piccart MJ, Loi S, Van'tVeer L, et al. Multi-center external validation study of the Amsterdam 70-gene prognostic signature in node negative untreated breast cancer: are the results still outperfoming the clinical-pathological criteria? *Breast Cancer Res Treat* 2004;88(S17): (abst 38).

27. Goldhirsch A, Wood WC, Gelber RD, et al. Meeting highlights: updated international expert consensus on the primary therapy of early breast cancer. *J Clin Oncol* 2003;21 (17):3357.

28. Sotiriou C, Wirapati P, Loi S, et al. Gene expression profiling in breast cancer: understanding the molecular basis of histologic grade to improve prognosis. *J Natl Cancer Inst* 2006;98(4):262.

29. Paik S, Shak S, Tang G, et al. A multigene assay to predict recurrence of tamoxifen-treated, node-negative breast cancer. *N Engl J Med* 2004;351(27):2817.

30. Albain KS, Barlow WE, Shak S, et al. Prognostic and predictive value of the 21-gene recurrence score assay in postmenopausal women with node-positive, oestrogen-receptor-positive breast cancer on chemotherapy: a retrospective analysis of a randomised trial. *Lancet Oncol* 2010;11 (1):55.

31. Mamounas E, Tang G, Fisher B, et al. Association between the 21-gene recurrence score assay and risk of locoregional recurrence in node-negative, estrogen receptor-positive breast cancer: results from NSABP B-14 and NSABP B-20. *J Clin Oncol* 2010;28(10):1677.

32. Ma XJ, Hilsenbeck SG, Wang W, et al. The HOXB13:IL17BR expression index is a prognostic factor in early-stage breast cancer. *J Clin Oncol* 2006;24(28):4611.

33. Ma XJ, Wang Z, Ryan PD, et al. A two-gene expression ratio predicts clinical outcome in breast cancer patients treated with tamoxifen. *Cancer Cell* 2004;5(6):607.

34. Ayers M, Symmans WF, Stec J, et al. Gene expression profiles predict complete pathologic response to neoadjuvant paclitaxel and fluorouracil, doxorubicin, and cyclophosphamide chemotherapy in breast cancer. *J Clin Oncol* 2004;22(12):2284.

35. Acharya CR, Hsu DS, Anders CK, et al. Gene expression signatures, clinicopathological features, and individualized therapy in breast cancer. *JAMA* 2008;299(13):1574.

36. Harris L, Fritsche H, Mennel R, et al. American Society of Clinical Oncology 2007 update of recommendations for the use of tumor markers in breast cancer. *J Clin Oncol* 2007; 25(33):5287.

37. Barski A, Cuddapah S, Cui K, et al. High-resolution profiling of histone methylations in the human genome. *Cell* 2007;129(4):823.

38. Veeck J, Esteller M. Breast cancer epigenetics: from DNA methylation to microRNAs. *J Mammary Gland Biol Neoplasia* 2010;15(1):5.

39. Fiskus W, Ren Y, Mohapatra A, et al. Hydroxamic acid analogue histone deacetylase inhibitors attenuate estrogen receptor-alpha levels and transcriptional activity: a result of hyperacetylation and inhibition of chaperone function of heat shock protein 90. *Clin Cancer Res* 2007;13(16):4882.

40. Zhou Q, Shaw PG, Davidson NE. Inhibition of histone deacetylase suppresses EGF signaling pathways by destabilizing EGFR mRNA in ER-negative human breast cancer cells. *Breast Cancer Res Treat* 2009;117(2):443.

42. Reinhart B, Slack FJ, Basson M, et al. The 21 nucleotide let-7 RNA regulates *C. elegans* developmental timing. *Nature* 2000;403:901.

43. Camps C, Buffa FM, Colella S, et al. hsa-miR-210 is induced by hypoxia and is an independent prognostic factor in breast cancer. *Clin Cancer Res* 2008;14(5):1340.

44. Foekens JA, Sieuwerts AM, Smid M, et al. Four miRNAs associated with aggressiveness of lymph node-negative, estrogen receptor-positive human breast cancer. *Proc Natl Acad Sci U S A* 2008;105(35):13021.

45. Iorio MV, Casalini P, Tagliabue E, et al. microRNA profiling as a tool to understand prognosis, therapy response and resistance in breast cancer. *Eur J Cancer* 2008;44(18):2753.

48. Hanahan D, Weinberg RA. The hallmarks of cancer. *Cell* 2000;100(1):57.

50. Yarden Y, Sliwkowski MX. Untangling the ErbB signalling network. *Nat Rev Mol Cell Biol* 2001;2(2):127.

51. Hudis CA. Trastuzumab—mechanism of action and use in clinical practice. *N Engl J Med* 2007;357(1):39.

52. Hynes NE, Dey JH. PI3K inhibition overcomes trastuzumab resistance: blockade of ErbB2/ErbB3 is not always enough. *Cancer Cell* 2009;15(5):353.

53. Ellis LM, Hicklin DJ. VEGF-targeted therapy: mechanisms of anti-tumour activity. *Nat Rev Cancer* 2008;8(8):579.

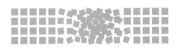

CHAPTER 25 ENDOCRINE TUMORS

SAMUEL A. WELLS, Jr.

MOLECULAR BIOLOGY OF INDIVIDUAL CANCERS

Over the past two decades, the remarkable advances in endocrine oncology have been enhanced by powerful and sophisticated molecular technology. In this regard studies of hereditary endocrine tumors have been especially fruitful, not only in defining the molecular genetic basis of these complex diseases, but in understanding the pathogenesis of the individual component tumor of the syndromes as well as their sporadic counterparts.

THE MULTIPLE ENDOCRINE NEOPLASIA SYNDROMES

Most endocrine tumors involve a single endocrine gland, are usually benign, and occur sporadically. Rarely, endocrine tumors occur in a familial pattern where they are multiple, involving more than one endocrine gland. Over the past 50 years at least six multiple endocrine neoplasia (MEN) syndromes have been described, including MEN-1, MEN-2, von Hippel-Lindau (VHL) disease, neurofibromatosis type 1, Carney complex (CNC), and the McCune-Albright syndrome (MAS). The genetic mutation causing each of these six MEN syndromes has been identified, in many cases leading to improved diagnosis and treatment of patients with a specific syndrome. It is not possible to address each of these syndromes in detail in this chapter, accordingly, the most common ones will be addressed.

Multiple Endocrine Neoplasia Type 1

Clinical Features

In 1954 Wermer[1] described a family with hyperparathyroidism and tumors of the pancreatic islet cells and the pituitary gland. This hereditary syndrome has since been named multiple endocrine neoplasia (MEN) type 1 (MEN-1) (Mendelian Inheritance in Man [MIM] 13001) and over 20 separate endocrine or nonendocrine tumors may occur in patients with this disease. The prevalence of MEN-1 is 2 to 3 per 100,000, and males and females are equally affected. MEN-1 is characterized by high penetrance but variable expressivity. Virtually all patients develop parathyroid hyperplasia by age 40, 50% develop malignant pancreatic islet cell tumors (usually gastrinomas, less often insulinomas, and rarely glucagonomas, or vasoactive intestinal polypeptide secreting tumors [VIPomas]), and 25% develop pituitary tumors (usually prolactinomas). The diagnosis of MEN-1 is established either when a previously unaffected member of a family with MEN-1 develops a single characteristic endocrine tumor, or when a patient with hyperparathyroidism develops a pituitary tumor or a pancreatic islet cell tumor.

Molecular Genetics

Chandrasekharappa et al.[2] discovered the genetic mutation for MEN-1. The *MEN1* gene spans a 9.8 kb segment of chromosome 11q13 and consists of 10 exons with a 1,830 base pair region that encodes transcripts of 2.7 and 3.1 kb. The transcripts, expressed in almost all tissues, encode a novel, highly conserved 610 amino acid, 67 kDa protein, menin.[3] *MEN1*, a putative tumor suppressor gene, mainly resides in the nucleus but is also found in the cytoplasm. The amino acid sequence of menin does not have homologies in the genome, thus clues to its mechanism of action have primarily come from identification of menin partnering to proteins or chromatin. Approximately 25 protein partners for menin have been identified, the first of which was junD, followed by others, such as MLL-containing complex, SMAD3, PEM, NM23, and nuclear factor B; however, at present no one menin partner has been shown convincingly to be critical to MEN-1 tumogenesis. The crystal structure of menin is unknown, and there is no direct evidence that menin binds directly to DNA; however, the protein appears to play a critical role in the regulation of gene transcription, apoptosis, and genome stability. Homozygous mice null for *Men1* die during embryogenesis, while heterologous mice, *Men1*[+/], develop a pattern of endocrine tumors very similar to that of patients with MEN-1.

The first "hit" in the *MEN1* gene that leads to tumorigenesis involves small mutations in one or several bases, broadly distributed across the *MEN1* open reading frame, such that half of newly diagnosed index cases are found to have novel mutations.[4,5] The second "hit" is a chromosomal mutation in somatic tissue that causes frameshift (deletions, insertions, or splice site defects) and nonsense mutations, including a portion or all of the *MEN1* gene. Approximately 75% of kindreds with MEN-1 will be found to have *MEN1* mutations, however, in patients who demonstrate hyperparathyroidism and pituitary tumors, the incidence of *MEN1* mutations is approximately 10%, suggesting another genetic cause of this MEN-1 variant. To date approximately 400 unique germline or somatic mutations of *MEN1* have been described (Fig. 25.1).[6] There is little correlation between genotype and phenotype, and presymptomatic diagnosis by direct DNA testing is useful only in identifying family members and then monitoring them for the development of specific endocrine tumors associated with MEN-1. There is no rationale for prophylactic removal of the parathyroid glands, the pancreas, or the pituitary gland in asymptomatic patients who have inherited a mutated *MEN1* allele.

The endocrine tumors characteristic of MEN-1 occur more commonly in a sporadic setting, where 25% of gastrinomas, 10% to 20% of insulinomas, 50% of VIPomas, 25% to 35% of bronchial carcinoids, and 20% of parathyroid adenomas express somatic *MEN1* mutations. Conversely, somatic *MEN1* mutations rarely if ever occur in sporadic adrenocortical tumors, pituitary tumors, or thyroid tumors.[6]

Other Hereditary Endocrinopathies Involving the Parathyroid and Pituitary Glands

The Parathyroid Gland

While familial hyperparathyroidism is most commonly a component of MEN-1, it can occur in

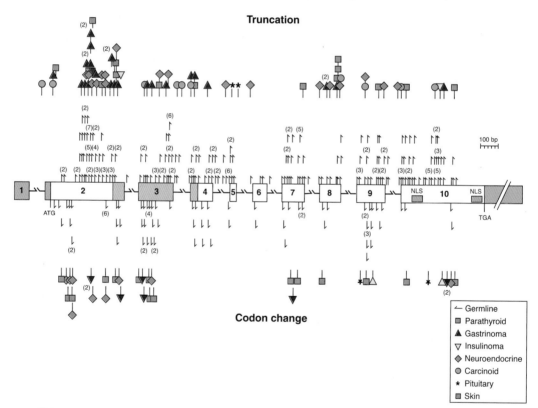

FIGURE 25.1 A schematic diagram of the genomic organization of the gene responsible for multiple endocrine neoplasia type 1 (MEN-1), including MEN-1 germline and somatic mutations. The gene contains ten exons (the first of which remains untranslated) and extends across 9 kb. It encodes a 610 amino acid protein, menin. Mutations shown above the exons cause menin truncation; those shown below the exons cause an amino acid or codon change. All unique mutations are represented; numbers in parentheses represent multiple reports of the same mutation in apparently unrelated individuals. The green-shaded areas indicate the untranslated regions. The location of the two nuclear localization signals (NLS), at codons 479–497 and 588–608, are indicated. Missense mutations in a region of menin (amino acids 139–242, identified by blue shading) prevented interaction with the AP1 transcription factor JunD. (From ref. 6, with permission.)

other settings, the most notable being familial (benign) hypocalciuric hypercalcemia (FHH), the hyperparathyroidism jaw-tumor (HPT-JT) syndrome, familial isolated hyperparathyroidism (FIHP), and MEN-2A.

Familial Hypocalciuric Hypercalcemia (FHH, MIM 145980). The calcium-sensing receptor (CASR), a critical regulator of extracellular calcium homeostasis, is a seven-transmembrane-spanning G-protein–coupled receptor, which is expressed in cells of the parathyroid gland and the kidney tubule. The discovery of the CASR was a surprise, since previously no small cation had been shown capable of acting as a ligand for a G-protein–coupled receptor.[7] The human CASR, encoded by six exons of the gene located on chromosome 3q113.3-q21, is sensitive to changes in the ambient calcium concentration and when activated it inhibits parathyroid hormone (PTH) secretion and the renal reabsorption of calcium. With heterogenous inactivating mutations of the *CASR* gene the parathyroid cell fails to sense properly an increased serum calcium concentration, and the resulting increase in PTH secretion causes FHH, an autosomal dominant disease characterized by hypocalciuria, hypercalcemia, and parathyroid hyperplasia. It is important for clinicians to recognize this relatively mild form of familial hyperparathyroidism; although parathyroidectomy reduces the serum calcium level, it is only temporary. With inactivating mutations in both alleles of the *CASR* gene, neonatal severe hyperparathyroidism ([NSHPT] MIM 239200) develops with serum calcium levels in the range of 15 to 20 mg/dL. This disease represents a life-threatening emergency and urgent parathyroidectomy is indicated.[8] Conversely, activating mutations of the *CASR* gene cause the parathyroid cells to sense that serum calcium is "elevated" when it is actually normal. There is a resulting decrease in the blood calcium level expressed as the syndrome of autosomal dominant hypoparathyroidism ([ADH] MIM 168468).[9] To date approximately 115 mutations (60% inactivating and 40% activating) have been described in the *CASR* gene, and most are missense mutations clustered in exons 3, 4, and 7.

Hyperparathyroidism-Jaw Tumor Syndrome (HPT-JT, MIM 145001). HPT-JT is characterized by the autosomal dominant occurrence of hyperparathyroidism, ossifying fibromas of the mandible or maxilla, renal cysts or solid tumors, and uterine fibromas.[10] Approximately 50 families with HPT-JT have been reported and 80% of patients have hyperparathyroidism, and in 15% of cases the parathyroid tumors are malignant. It is noteworthy that the age-related penetrance of HPT-JT is approximately 40% by age 40 in contrast to MEN-1 where the age-related penetrance is 98% by age 40.[11] Members of kindreds with this disease need lifelong surveillance by physical examination and biochemical evaluation. It has even been suggested that serial ultrasound examination of the neck should be performed as parathyroid carcinoma has been reported in normocalcemic kindred members.[12]

The cause of HPT-JT appears to be a tumor suppressor gene, *HRPT2*, which is located on chromosome 1q25-q31. The *HPRT2* gene consists of 17 exons and the mutations are scattered throughout the 1593 coding region, with the majority resulting in functional loss through premature truncation.[13] Approximately 16 activating mutations of *HRPT2*, most of which are frameshift, have been identified. The *HPRT2* gene encodes a 531 amino acid protein, parafibromin (named for parathyroid tumors and jaw fibromas).[14] The function of parafibromin is unknown but it is thought to regulate posttranscriptional events and histone modification. There is recent evidence that parafibromin has pro-apoptotic activity, important as a tumor suppressor function.[15] Germline mutations in *HPRT2* have been identified in approximately half of HPT-JT families, and even in some families with MEN-2A.

Besides the evidence of germline mutations in patients with the HPT-JT somatic *HRPT2* mutations have been detected in the majority of patients with sporadic parathyroid carcinoma.[16,17] It is important to note that mutations in *HRPT2* are rarely if ever seen in sporadic parathyroid adenomas, an important diagnostic finding distinguishing benign from malignant parathyroid tumors.[15,18]

Familial Isolated Hyperparathyroidism (FIHP, MIM 145000). The syndrome of FIHP is a heterogenous condition, and some kindreds thought to have this disease have been shown to have germline mutations of *MEN1*, *CASR*, or *HRP-JT*, suggesting that the disease represents incompletely expressed forms of MEN1, FHH, or HPT-JT.[19] Over 100 families with FIHP have been reported and in most cases the causative genetic mutation is unknown, although there are convincing data that it resides on chromosome 2p13.3-14.[20]

The Pituitary Gland

There is no relationship between genotype and phenotype in patients with MEN-1, thus there is no way to predict the presence or behavior of pancreatic islet cell tumors or pituitary tumors. There are, however, important genetic mutations associated with other hereditary and sporadic pituitary tumors.

Carney Complex (CNC, MIM 160980). Pituitary adenomas can occur as a component of CNC, a familial disease characterized by hypersomatotropenemia, cardiac or cutaneous myxomas, spotty skin pigmentation, primary pigmented nodular adrenal disease, and testicular tumors.[21] About

75% of patients exhibit subclinical increases in growth hormone (GH), insulinlike growth factor-1 (IGF-1), and prolactin. Acromegaly occurs in about 10% of patients. Genetic linkage analysis has shown two loci for CNC, one on chromosome 2p16 (CNC2), and the other on chromosome 17q22-24 (CNC1). Neither locus is associated with a specific phenotype. In more than 50% of cases the CNC has been linked to an inactivating mutation in the gene coding for the protein kinase A (PKA) type 1α subunit, PRKAR1A, at 17q24. The 2p16 locus is uncharacterized.

Familial Isolated Pituitary Adenomas (FIPA, MIM 102200). Pituitary adenomas can also occur as FIPA. Daly et al.[22] evaluated 64 families with FIPA, residing in Belgium, France, Italy, and the Netherlands. Of the 138 affected family members, 55 had prolactinomas, 47 had somatotropinomas, 28 had nonsecreting adenomas, and 8 had adrenocorticotropic hormone–secreting tumors. The incidences of a homogenous (single tumor) phenotype and a heterogeneous tumors phenotype were approximately equal. Affected patients were found to have no mutations in either the MEN1 or PRKRA1A genes.

Recently, Vierimaa et al.,[23] in a study of cases of low penetrance familial pituitary adenoma in Northern Finland identified loss of mutation functions in the aryl hydrocarbon receptor interacting protein (AIP) gene. AIP forms a complex with the aryl hydrocarbon receptor (AHR) and two 90-kD heat-shock proteins (HSP90). AHR is a ligand-activated transcription factor and also participates in cellular signaling pathways.

Expression profiling in two families resulted in the identification of AIP as one of the candidate genes, and a nonsense mutation (Gln14X) was also identified and found to segregate with the GH-secreting adenomas.[23] Daly et al.[24] studied 73 FIPA families with 156 individuals and found that 11 of them harbored 10 AIP germline mutations. Kindred members with AIP mutations, compared to those without mutations, were younger and had larger tumors. Growth hormone producing tumors predominated among family members with AIP mutations.

Multiple Endocrine Neoplasia Type 2

Clinical Features

In 1968 Steiner et al.[25] described a large family with medullary thyroid carcinoma (MTC), pheochromocytoma, hyperparathyroidism, and Cushing's syndrome. The disease was named multiple endocrine neoplasia type 2, and it is now recognized that there are three related syndromes characterized by hereditary MTC: MEN-2A (MIM 171400), MEN-2B (MIM 162300), and familial medullary thyroid carcinoma (FMTC) (MIM 155240). There is near complete penetrance but variable expressivity, as virtually all patients with MEN-2A develop MTC, approximately half develop pheochromocytomas, and 30% develop hyperparathyroidism. Less often MEN-2A is associated with cutaneous lichen amyloidosis (CLA), which develops on the upper back and serves as a precocious marker of the disorder, or Hirschsprung's disease (HD), which is characterized by loss of ganglion cells in variable segments of the large bowel. Patients with MEN-2B develop MTC and pheochromocytomas with the same frequency as patients with MEN-2A, but rather than hyperparathyroidism, they express a generalized gastrointestinal neuromatosis and a characteristic physical appearance. Patients with FMTC develop only MTC. Of patients with hereditary MTC, 80% have MEN-2A, 15% have FMTC, and 5% have MEN-2B.

Medullary thyroid carcinoma originates from C cells, which are derived from the neural crest. The C cells have great biosynthetic capability and secrete the polypeptide hormone calcitonin (CTN) and the glycoprotein carcinoembryonic antigen (CEA). Plasma CTN serves as an excellent marker for MTC, and presently its main use is in detecting persistent or residual MTC following thyroidectomy.

The MTC is the most common cause of death in patients with MEN-2A, MEN-2B, and FMTC, and the only effective therapy is timely thyroidectomy as standard chemotherapy and external beam radiotherapy are not useful.

Molecular Genetics

In 1985 Takahashi et al.[26] discovered the RET (REarranged during Transfection) protooncogene. The gene is located in the pericentromeric region of chromosome 10q11.2 and includes 21 exons. RET encodes a receptor tyrosine kinase, which is expressed in neuroendocrine cells (including thyroid C cells and adrenal medullary cells), neural cells (including parasympathetic and sympathetic ganglion cells), urogenital tract cells, and the branchial arch cells.

The RET gene has an extracellular portion, which contains four cadherin-like repeats, a calcium binding site and a cysteine-rich region, a transmembrane portion, and an intracellular portion, which contains two tyrosine kinase domains. Alternate splicing of RET produces three isoforms with either 9, 43, or 51 amino acids at the C terminus, referred to as RET9, RET43, and RET51.[27,28] Mice lacking RET51 are normal, however, mice lacking RET9 have renal malformation and defects in innervation of the gut.[29]

RET is essential for the development, survival, and regeneration of many neuronal cells in the gut, the kidney, and the nervous system. A tripartite complex is necessary for RET signaling. One of four glial-derived neurotrophic factors (GDNF) family ligands (GFLs)—GDNF, neurturin, persephin, or artemin–binds *RET* in conjunction with one of four glycosylphosphatidylinositol-anchored coreceptors, designated GDNF family receptors (GFR): GFR-α1, GFR-α2, GFR-α3, or GFR-α4.[30–32] The GFL-GFR complex causes dimerization of two *RET* molecules with activation of autophosphorylation and intracellular signaling. The C-terminal of *RET* contains 16 tyrosine residues, among which Y905 is a binding site for Grb7/10 adaptors, Y1015 a binding site for phospholipase Cγ, Y981 a binding site for c-Src, and Y1096 a binding site for Grb2. Tyrosine 1072 is a multidocking binding site for such proteins as SHC, SHCC, IRS1/2, FRS2, DOK1/4/5/, and Enigma. The *RET* receptor may activate various signaling pathways through Y1072, which thereby serves as a prerequisite for initiating transformation of *RET*-derived oncogenes in cell cultures and transgenic animals.[33] The structure of the RET receptor complex and the molecular pathways activated when there is ligand binding or constitutive activation are shown in Figure 25.2.[34]

Recently, the biochemical characterization and structure of the human *RET* tyrosine kinase domain was reported showing that both the phosphorylated and nonphosphorylated forms adopt the same active kinase conformation necessary to bind adenosine triphosphate and substrate and have a preorganized activation loop conformation.[35]

In 1993 and 1994 it was shown that point mutations in the *RET* protooncogene cause MEN-2A, MEN-2B, and FMTC.[36,37] The *RET* mutations are generally of two types and affect either the extracellular ligand binding site or the tyrosine kinase domain.

MEN-2A is associated with mutations involving the extracellular cysteine codons 609, 611, 618, 620 (exon 10) 630, or 634 (exon 11). The mutations associated with FMTC involve a broad range of codons, including those associated with MEN-2A, particularly 609, 618, and 620, as well as others: 768, 790, and 791 (exon 13), 804 and 844 (exon 14), or 891 (exon 15). One must be careful in making a diagnosis of FMTC, especially in small families, which span only one or two generations.

Ninety-five percent of patients with MEN-2B have a point mutation, codon M918T (exon 16), within the intracellular domain of *RET*. A few patients with MEN-2B have a mutation in codon A883F (exon 15). Rarely, compound heterozygous mutations in V804M with either Y806C or S904C occur in patients with a phenotype resembling MEN-2B.[38] In a study of 25 patients with *de novo* MEN-2B, Carlson et al.[39] found that the new mutation was of paternal origin in all cases. The investigators also observed a distortion of the sex ratio in both *de novo* MEN-2B patients and the affected offspring of MEN-2B transmitting males, suggesting a possible role for imprinting.

In patients with MEN-2A there is a clear correlation between genotype and phenotype, concerning both the pattern of clinical expression and the severity of disease.[28,37,40] Over 85% of patients with MEN-2A have a 634 codon mutation, and a C634R substitution is most often associated with hyperparathyroidism.[41,42] Patients with MEN-2A and CLA also have mutations at codon 634. Pheochromocytomas are associated with several codon mutations, most frequently 634, 618, 620, and 791.[43] Patients with the relatively rare association of MEN-2A and Hirschsprung's disease have mutations in exon 10, particularly codons 609, 618, and 620. Recently, the American Thyroid Association published guidelines for the diagnosis and treatment of MTC, including a list of the *RET* mutations so far described in patients with MEN-2A, MEN-2B, and FMTC.[44]

The medullary thyroid carcinoma has an early onset and a very aggressive clinical course in patients with MEN-2B, and it is moderately aggressive in patients with MEN-2A, particularly in patients with *RET* mutations in codons 634, 611, 618, and 620. The MTC is least aggressive in patients with FMTC. A schematic structure of the *RET* protooncogene with the most common codon mutations is shown in Figure 25.3.

It is important to note that approximately half of the patients with sporadic MTC have somatic M918T mutations in the MTC cells, and it has been suggested that the genotype is associated with a more aggressive phenotype, although this is controversial.[45]

The molecular basis for the genotype–phenotype correlations remains poorly understood; however, Iwashita et al.[46] introduced specific *RET* codon mutations into the short and long isoforms of *RET* cDNA and transfected the mutants into NIH3T3 cells. High levels of transforming activity of the mutant *RET* genes M918T and A833F correlated with the aggressive clinical phenotypes, MEN-2B, while low levels of transforming activity of the mutant *RET* genes E768D, V804L, and S891A correlated with the less aggressive FMTC phenotype. A similar study evaluating not only transforming ability of *RET* mutants but apoptosis, anchorage-independent growth, and signaling confirmed the findings of Iwashita et al. and also demonstrated that M918T and A883F mutants significantly enhanced the suppression of apoptosis.[47] It is of interest that mutations at codons 609, 618, and 620 markedly decrease the cell surface expression of *RET*, compared to codon 634 mutants, indicating that the former mutations impair transport of *RET* to the plasma membrane. One would expect this relationship considering the centrality of these *RET* mutations in association with MEN-2A and FMTC with Hirschsprung's disease.

Recently, gene expression studies relating to MEN-2A and MEN-2B have been reported by two groups. Myers and Mulligan[48] used cDNA microarray analysis of cell lines that expressed

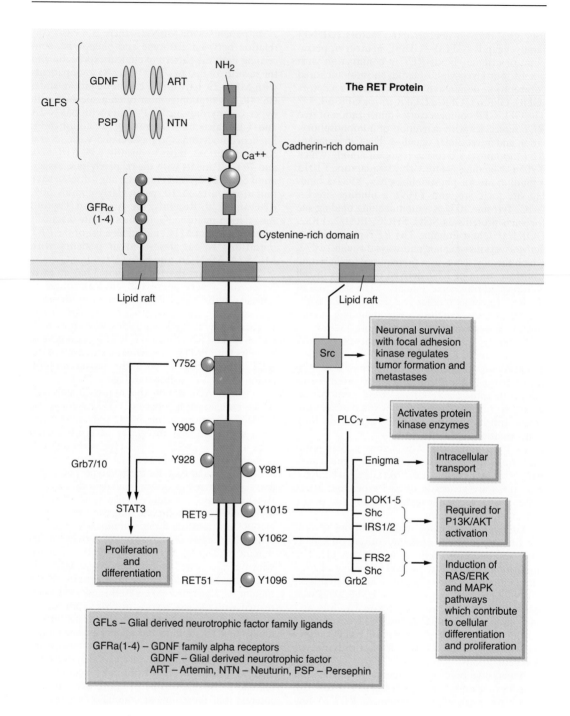

FIGURE 25.2 The RET structure and signaling network. The structure of the RET protein and the signaling network, showing docking sites and targets. RET, rearranged during transfection; GFLS, glial derived neurotrophic factor (GDNF) family ligands; ART, artemin; NTN, neurturin; PSP, persephin; GFRα, GDNF-family α receptors; Ca++, calcium ion. (From ref. 34, with permission.)

either the RET9 or the RET51 protein isoform to study *RET*-mediated gene expression patterns. They found that cells expressing *RET* have altered intercellular interactions correlated with increased expression of a number of cell surface molecules.

The most striking expression pattern observed, however, was the up-regulation of stress response genes, specifically heat shock protein's (HSP) 70 family members: HSPA1A, HSPA1B, and HSPA1L. Additionally, other members of several

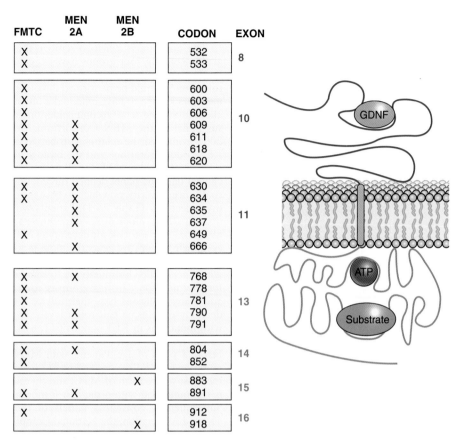

FMTC	MEN 2A	MEN 2B	CODON	EXON
X			532	8
X			533	
X			600	10
X			603	
X			606	
X	X		609	
X	X		611	
X	X		618	
X	X		620	
X	X		630	11
X	X		634	
	X		635	
	X		637	
X			649	
	X		666	
X	X		768	13
X			778	
X			781	
X	X		790	
X	X		791	
X	X		804	14
X			852	
		X	883	15
X	X		891	
X			912	16
		X	918	

FIGURE 25.3 A schematic diagram showing the RET tyrosine kinase receptor and ligand complex as well as genotype-phenotype correlations for patients with type 2 multiple endocrine neoplasia syndromes, including MEN-2A, MEN-2B, and familial medullary thyroid carcinoma (FMTC). The RET gene product is divided into intracellular (*purple*), transmembrane (*orange*), and intracellular domains containing tyrosine kinase activity (*blue*). The exons coding for each domain are shown with corresponding colors. Known *RET* codon mutations are listed and grouped according to the exons in which they occur. Phenotypically expressed clinical syndromes corresponding to each codon mutation are listed. (From You YNY, Lankhani V, Wells SA. The multiple endocrine neoplasia syndromes. In: Willard H, Ginsburg LS. *Genomic and Personalized Medicine.* 1st ed. San Diego: Academic Press; 2009:936.)

HSP families associated with stress response were up-regulated. The increased expression of HSPs, particularly of the HSP70 and HSP90 families, has been documented in breast cancer, gastrointestinal cancer, and endometrial cancer and is associated with a poor prognosis. Conversely, the expression of HSP70 levels in osteosarcomas and renal cell carcinomas is associated with an improved prognosis and a positive response to chemotherapy.[49]

Jain et al.[50] performed microarray expression analysis from pheochromocytomas and MTCs in 34 patients with MEN-2A, MEN-2B, and sporadic MTC. They found 118 probe sets that were differentially regulated in MEN-2B tumors compared to MEN-2A tumors (20 were up-regulated in MTCs from patients with MEN-2A and 98 were up-regulated in MTCs from patients with MEN-2B). Five genes were most discriminating by significance

analysis microarray and correctly classified all of the cases of MTC associated with either MEN-2A or MEN-2B. The investigators found that genes involved in the process of epithelial to mesenchymal transition, many associated with the tumor growth factor β pathway, were up-regulated in MEN-2B MTCs. Also chondromodulin-1 mRNA and protein expression were localized to the malignant C cells, and its high expression correlated with the presence of skeletal deformities in MEN-2B patients.

Several groups have studied copy number imbalance in patients with MTC. One study of 37 patients with MTC, 29 with sporadic tumors, detected altered amplifications or deletions in chromosomal regions that housed genes likely to influence tumor pathogenesis.[51] Additional studies showed copy number changes in 50% to 60% of MTC cases studied, most commonly in chromosomes 19p, 19q, 13q, and 11.[52,53]

APPLICATION OF MOLECULAR GENETICS TO CLINICAL MEDICINE

The discovery that mutations in the *RET* protooncogene cause MEN-2A, MEN-2B, and FMTC changed the management of patients with both sporadic and hereditary MTC and represents a paradigm for personalized genomic medicine.

Genetic Testing

DNA analysis for *RET* germline mutations is indicated in patients with presumably sporadic MTC, as approximately 5% of them will be found to have hereditary disease. It is imperative to screen the family members of patients with newly found germline *RET* mutations, since they are at risk for MTC and approximately half of them will be affected.[54]

Prophylactic Surgery

In patients with MEN-2A, MEN-2B, and FMTC who are shown to have inherited a mutated *RET* allele it is important to remove the thyroid before MTC develops or while it is still confined to the gland.[55] Thus, considering patients with familial cancer syndromes, hereditary MTC fulfills each of the criteria necessary for prophylactic removal of the organ at risk: (1) near complete penetrance, such that virtually all patients who have inherited a mutated allele will develop the malignancy, (2) a highly reliable genetic test to detect family members who have inherited a mutated allele, (3) the organ at risk is expendable or its function can be easily replaced, (4) resection of the organ at risk can be performed with minimal risk, and (5) there is a sensitive tumor marker, or other indicator, to determine whether the malignancy has been prevented or cured following organ removal.

The question is when to remove the thyroid gland. Recently, four groups have suggested criteria for defining the age at which prophylactic thyroidectomy should be performed in young kindred members known to have inherited a mutated *RET* allele. In the first set of recommendations a consensus panel at the MEN Consortium Meeting in 2000 evaluated the relationship between specific *RET* codon mutations and the biological aggressiveness of hereditary MTC.[40] Based on combined clinical data the panel defined three levels of thyroid cancer severity, on which to base the timing of thyroidectomy (Table 25.1). Patients with mutations in *RET* codons 609, 768, 790, 791, 804, or 891 (level 1) are at risk for developing MTC; however, their tumors are generally more indolent and develop at a later age than is the case in patients with other *RET* codon mutations. Recommendation for thyroidectomy in this group is controversial, and many clinicians base their advice for thyroidectomy on plasma calcitonin levels. In patients with mutations in RET codons 611, 618, 620, or 634 (level 2) thyroidectomy is recommended at or before 5 years of age. Patients with MEN-2B and mutations in *RET* codons 883 or 918 (level 3) have the most severe form of MTC, and thyroidectomy is recommended within the first 6 months of life. Subsequently, consensus panels of the British Thyroid Association, the National Comprehensive Cancer Network, and the American Thyroid Association have addressed this topic with largely confirmatory, and in some cases expanded, recommendations.[44,56,57]

Although these recommendations seem reasonable, it is known that there are certain factors that modify the severity of the MTC, even within individual families. For example, it has been shown in some kindreds with codon 804 *RET* mutations (generally associated with a nonaggressive form of MTC) that a concomitant somatic

---

TABLE 25.1

RECOMMENDATIONS FOR PROPHYLACTIC THYROIDECTOMY BASED ON *RET* CODON MUTATION

Risk Level for MTC	1 High	2 Higher	3 Highest
Codons	609, 768, 790, 791, 804, 891	611, 618, 620, 634	883, 918, or known MEN-2B
Thyroidectomy (age)	No consensus: By 5 to 10 years; or at first abnormal stimulated calcitonin	By 5 years	By 6 months; preferably within first month of life

MTC, medullary thyroid carcinoma; MEN, multiple endocrine neoplasia.
(Modified from ref. 40, with permission.)

918 codon mutation in MTC cells confers a highly malignant phenotype.[58] Furthermore, it has been proposed that certain specific single-nucleotide polymorphisms (SNPs) influence the clinical behavior of the MTC, however, at present this relationship is unclear.

Realizing the criticalness of removing the thyroid gland while the MTC is curable, and understanding that it is impractical to establish strict guidelines for the timing of thyroidectomy based on the various *RET* codon mutations, clinicians should err on the side of advising thyroidectomy too early rather than too late. This approach is strengthened by the fact that once the MTC has spread beyond the thyroid gland it is virtually incurable, as no chemotherapy or radiotherapy regimen has proven effective.

SPORADIC THYROID CANCERS

Papillary Thyroid Carcinoma

Malignant tumors of the thyroid gland have a great range of biological behavior, ranging from the slow growing to highly aggressive. Over the past two decades the genetic mutations and chromosomal translocations that cause most histological types of thyroid cancer have been identified and have defined potential targets of small molecule thera-

peutics. The first of these observations came in 1985 with the discovery of the *RET* protooncogene.[26] In 1987 Fusco et al.[59] demonstrated in papillary thyroid carcinoma (PTC) the fusion of the C-terminal *RET* tyrosine kinase-encoding domain to the promoter and N-terminal portion of unrelated genes. The creation of these heterologous partners resulted in the illegitimate expression of a constitutively active chimeric oncogene termed *RET/PTC*. Subsequently, more than 15 molecular fusion oncogenes in PTCs have been identified, all of which differ according to the 5′-terminal region of the heterologous gene (Fig. 25.4). The most common of these chimeric oncogenes are *H4(CCDC6)-RET*, also known as *RET/PTC1* (60% to 70%), and *ELE1-RET*, also known as *RET/PTC3* (20% to 30%). The prevalence of *RET/PTC* in the thyroid cancers of children is greater than 50%, and in youngsters in Kiev and Belarus who developed PTC following exposure to radiation from the Chernobyl accident the prevalence of such rearrangements is 67% to 87%.[60–62] Analysis of components of the chimeric oncogenes showed a physical proximity of the chromatin distribution of follicular epithelial cells, supporting radiation as a cause of the induced fusion.[63] Similar *RET/PTC* rearrangements also occur in Hürthle cell carcinomas and trabecular adenomas, but they have not been described in patients with follicular carcinoma or anaplastic carcinomas.

The reported incidence of these hybrid genes in sporadic PTCs varies widely, from less than 5% to

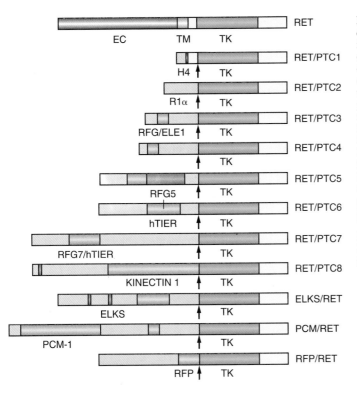

FIGURE 25.4 A schematic showing chimeric forms of the RET receptor formed by the joining of the C-terminus of RET to the promoter and N-terminus of unrelated genes. These chimeric oncogenes result in constitutive activation of RET and have been identified in patients with papillary thyroid carcinoma. EC, extracellular domain of RET; TM, transmembrane domain of RET; TK, tyrosine kinase domain of RET. H4, R1α, RFG/ELE1, RFG5, hTIF1, RFG7/hTIFR, KINECTIN1, ELKS, PCM-1, RFP represent the promoter and N-terminus of unrelated genes. (Modified from Santoro M, Melillo RM, Carlomagno F, Fusco A, Vecchio G. Molecular mechanisms of RET activation in human cancer. *Ann N Y Acad Sci* 2002;963:116, with permission.)

almost 70%, depending on tumor heterogeneity, geographic location, and the techniques used to detect *RET/PTC* rearrangements. In a study of 65 papillary thyroid carcinomas, five techniques (standard-sensitivity reverse transcription-polymerase chain reaction [RT-PCR], high-sensitivity RT-PCR, real-time LightCycler RT-PCR, Southern blot analysis, and fluorescence *in situ* hybridization) were used to detect *RET/PTC1* and *RET/PTC3* rearrangements. Three patterns of detection were evident. When a significant proportion of tumor cells (35% to 86%) contained *RET/PTC* rearrangements (clonal pattern), the translocations were detected by all five techniques. When 17% to 24% of tumor cells (subclonal), or less than 9% of tumor cells (nonclonal), contained *RET/PTC* rearrangements, less than five techniques were able to detect the translocations. Also, in contrast to clonal tumors, where neither *BRAF* nor *ras* mutations were identified, such mutations were found in 40% to 60% of subclonal or nonclonal tumors. *RET/PTC* oncogenes, found in PTC, like the *RET* mutations in the MEN-2 syndromes, potentiate the intrinsic tyrosine kinase activity of *RET* and thereby the downstream signaling events. There does not appear to be any relationship between *RET/PTC* rearrangements and the clinical behavior of PTC.

A much less frequent chromosomal rearrangement associated with PTC involves the neurotrophic receptor–tyrosine kinase *NTRK1* (also known as *TRK* and *TRKA*). Chimeric oncogenes result from the fusion of *NTRK1* and various activating genes: *TRK*, which contains sequences from the *TPM3* gene on chromosome 1q22-23; *TRK-T1* and *TRK-T2*, which contain different sequences of the *TPR* gene on chromosome 1q25; and *TRK-T3*, which combines with sequences of *TFG* on chromosome 3q11-12.[64]

The most common mutation in PTC is the *BRAF*[T17699A] mutation (V600E), which occurs in 35% to 65% of tumors.[65] There is virtually no overlap between the presence of *BRAF* mutations and *RET/PTC* gene rearrangements. Compared to the *RET/PTC* rearrangements, the *BRAF* mutations are reportedly associated with a more aggressive form of papillary carcinomas, characterized by extrathyroidal invasion, lymph node metastases, advanced tumor stage, and tumor recurrence. However, this point is controversial.

Follicular Thyroid Carcinoma

The peroxisome proliferators-activated receptor-γ (PPAR-γ), a member of the steroid-nuclear hormone receptor superfamily, is encoded by *PPARG* located on 3p25. Rearrangements involving the thyroid specific transcription factor, paired-box gene 8 (*PAX8*) with the peroxisome proliferators-activated receptor-γ (*PPAR-γ*) were first identified in follicular thyroid carcinoma (FTC) as a cytogenetically

detectable translocation t(2,3)(q13; p25).[66] The *PAX8–PPARγ* appears to be confined to atypical follicular adenomas and FTC and has not been detected in PTC or either poorly differentiated or undifferentiated (anaplastic) thyroid carcinomas. In an evaluation of 88 conventional follicular and Hürthle cell tumors analyzed for *ras* mutations and *PAX8-PPARγ* rearrangements, 49% of FTCs had *ras* mutations, 36% had *PAX8-PPARγ* rearrangements, and one had both. *Ras* mutations occurred in almost half of the follicular adenomas, and *PAX8-PPARγ* translocations were present in only 4%. Overt tumor invasiveness was associated with *PAX8-PPARγ* translocations and not *ras* mutations. *PAX8-PPARγ* rearrangements or *ras* mutations were found infrequently in Hürthle cell tumors.[67]

The *H-*, *K-*, and *N-ras* protooncogenes belong to the superfamily of membrane-associated GTP-binding proteins, which play an important role in the transduction of mitogenic signals from growth factor receptors on the cell surface. Activated *ras* phosphorylates *Raf*, which ultimately leads to activation of mitogen-activated protein kinases. Although specific patterns of *ras* mutations appear to be the rule in other tumors (*H-ras* in bladder cancer, *K-ras* in colon and pancreatic cancer, and *N-ras* in hematologic malignancies), mutations of all three *ras* genes have been reported in thyroid tumors.[68] Most often mutations of codon 61 of *H-ras* or *N-ras* are found in thyroid neoplasms, although the incidence of the mutations varies widely, perhaps due to the various techniques used by different investigators. Garcia-Rostand et al.[69] used PCR and single-strand conformational analysis to detect *H-*, *K-*, or *N-ras* mutations in 125 thyroid carcinomas. Mutations were present in 8.2% of 49 well-differentiated carcinomas (approximate equal frequencies in PTC and FTC), and in 50% to 55% of patients with poorly differentiated or anaplastic thyroid carcinomas (ATC). Furthermore, the mortality rate was two- to threefold higher in patients whose thyroid tumors had *ras* mutations, compared with those absent *ras* mutations.

Anaplastic thyroid carcinoma accounts for less than 2% of all thyroid cancers, but causes half of all thyroid cancer deaths. The tumor arises from follicular cells, and there is good evidence that it is a continuum of PTC or FTC. The tumors are relatively insensitive to standard chemotherapeutic regimens and are not responsive to external beam radiotherapy. The tumors are characterized by substantial chromosomal instability, characterized by *BRAF* or *ras* point mutations, which occur also in well-differentiated thyroid carcinomas and β-catenin (*CTNNB1*) and *p53* mutations, which occur in overt ATC but not in PTC or FTC. Mutations of *p53* have been described in over half of ATCs and represent a potential therapeutic target. The serine/threonine kinases of the *aurora* family play a central role in the regulation of the cell cycle, and the expression of Aurora B is 10- to 20-fold higher in ATC

TABLE 25.2

GENETIC MUTATIONS ASSOCIATED WITH THYROID CANCERS DERIVED FROM FOLLICULAR CELLS

| Genetic Alteration | Well-Differentiated Thyroid Carcinoma | | Poorly Differentiated Thyroid Carcinoma | Undifferentiated Thyroid Carcinoma | Post-Chernobyl Childhood Thyroid Cancer |
	Papillary Thyroid Carcinoma	Follicular Thyroid Carcinoma			
RET rearrangement	13–43%	0%	0–13%	0%	50–90%
BRAF mutation	29–69%	0%	0–13%	10–35%	0–12%
BRAF rearrangement	1%	Unknown	Unknown	Unknown	11%
NTRK1 rearrangement	5–13%	Unknown	Unknown	Unknown	3%
Ras mutation	0–21%	40–53%	18–27%	20–60%	0%
PPARG rearrangement	0%	25–63%	0%	0%	Unknown
CTNNB1 mutation	0%	0%	0–25%	66%	Unknown
TP53 mutation	0–5%	0–9%	17–38%	67–88%	Unknown

CTNNB1, *β*-catenin; NTRK1, neurotrophic tyrosine kinase receptor type 1; PPARG, peroxisome-proliferator-activated receptor-γ.
(Modified from Kondo T, Essat S, Asa SL. *Nat Rev Cancer* 2006;6:292, with permission.)

MOLECULAR BIOLOGY OF INDIVIDUAL CANCERS

compared to normal thyroid tissue and well-differentiated thyroid carcinoma.[70] A summation of the genetic mutations of thyroid cancers derived from follicular cells is shown in Table 25.2.

FUTURE DIRECTIONS

Advances in molecular genetics have elucidated the oncogenic event(s) of many solid tumors, and this is nowhere more evident than in endocrine tumors. The discovery of the mutations causing MEN-1 and MEN-2 has been important because it has led to an understanding of the pathogenesis, not only of the component hereditary tumors but their sporadic counterparts as well. These discoveries have already been of great benefit in the diagnosis and treatment of patients with endocrine tumors, as evidenced most clearly in families with hereditary MTC.

Another therapeutic benefit of the molecular research has been the identification of molecular targets for small molecule therapy. Already, clinical trials are under way to evaluate agents that have shown promise in preclinical studies, and some have shown significant activity.

Selected References

The full list of references for this chapter appears in the online version.

1. Wermer P. Genetic aspects of adenomatosis of endocrine glands. *Am J Med* 1954;16:363.
2. Chandrasekharappa SC, Guru SC, Manickam P, et al. Positional cloning of the gene for multiple endocrine neoplasia-type 1. *Science* 1997;276:404.
4. Agarwal SK, Debelenko LV, Kester MB, et al/ Analysis of recurrent germline mutations in the MEN1 gene encountered in apparently unrelated families. *Hum Mutat* 1998;12:75.
5. Owens M, Ellard S, Vaidya B. Analysis of gross deletions in the MEN1 gene in patients with multiple endocrine neoplasia type 1. *Clin Endocrinol (Oxf)* 2008;68:350.
6. Schussheim DH, Skarulis MC, Agarwal SK, et al. Multiple endocrine neoplasia type 1: new clinical and basic findings. *Trends Endocrinol Metab* 2001;12:173.

7. Brown EM, Gamba G, Riccardi D, et al. Cloning and characterization of an extracellular Ca(2+)-sensing receptor from bovine parathyroid. *Nature* 1993;366:575.
8. Pollak MR, Brown EM, Chou YH, et al. Mutations in the human Ca(2+)-sensing receptor gene cause familial hypocalciuric hypercalcemia and neonatal severe hyperparathyroidism. *Cell* 1993;75:1297.
10. Jackson CE, Norum RA, Boyd SB, et al. Hereditary hyperparathyroidism and multiple ossifying jaw fibromas: a clinically and genetically distinct syndrome. *Surgery* 1990;108:1006; discussion 1012.
12. Guarnieri V, Scillitani A, Muscarella LA, et al. Diagnosis of parathyroid tumors in familial isolated hyperparathyroidism with HRPT2 mutation: implications for cancer surveillance. *J Clin Endocrinol Metab* 2006;91:2827.
13. Bradley KJ, Cavaco BM, Bowl MR, et al. Parafibromin mutations in hereditary hyperparathyroidism syndromes

and parathyroid tumours. *Clin Endocrinol (Oxf)* 2006;64: 299.

16. Howell VM, Haven CJ, Kahnoski K, et al. HRPT2 mutations are associated with malignancy in sporadic parathyroid tumours. *J Med Genet* 2003;40:657.

17. Shattuck TM, Valimaki S, Obara T, et al. Somatic and germline mutations of the HRPT2 gene in sporadic parathyroid carcinoma. *N Engl J Med* 2003;349:1722.

19. Warner J, Epstein M, Sweet A, et al. Genetic testing in familial isolated hyperparathyroidism: unexpected results and their implications. *J Med Genet* 2004;41:155.

20. Warner JV, Nyholt DR, Busfield F, et al. Familial isolated hyperparathyroidism is linked to a 1.7 Mb region on chromosome 2p13.3-14. *J Med Genet* 2006;43:e12.

21. Carney JA, Gordon H, Carpenter PC, Shenoy BV, Go VL. The complex of myxomas, spotty pigmentation, and endocrine overactivity. *Medicine (Baltimore)* 1985;64:270.

22. Daly AF, Jaffrain-Rea ML, Ciccarelli A, et al. Clinical characterization of familial isolated pituitary adenomas. *J Clin Endocrinol Metab* 2006;91:3316.

23. Vierimaa O, Georgitsi M, Lehtonen R, et al. Pituitary adenoma predisposition caused by germline mutations in the AIP gene. *Science* 2006;312:1228.

24. Daly AF, Vanbellinghen JF, Khoo SK, et al. Aryl hydrocarbon receptor interacting protein gene mutations in familial isolated pituitary adenomas: analysis in 73 families. *J Clin Endocrinol Metab* 2007;92(5):1891.

25. Steiner AL, Goodman AD, Powers SR. Study of a kindred with pheochromocytoma, medullary thyroid carcinoma, hyperparathyroidism and Cushing's disease: multiple endocrine neoplasia, type 2. *Medicine (Baltimore)* 1968; 47:371.

26. Takahashi M, Ritz J, Cooper GM. Activation of a novel human transforming gene, ret, by DNA rearrangement. *Cell* 1985;42:581.

27. Tahira T, Ishizaka Y, Itoh F, Sugimura T, Nagao M. Characterization of ret proto-oncogene mRNAs encoding two isoforms of the protein product in a human neuroblastoma cell line. *Oncogene* 1990;5:97.

28. Myers SM, Eng C, Ponder BA, Mulligan LM. Characterization of RET proto-oncogene 3′ splicing variants and polyadenylation sites: a novel C-terminus for RET. *Oncogene* 1995;11:2039.

29. de Graaff E, Srinivas S, Kilkenny C, et al. Differential activities of the RET tyrosine kinase receptor isoforms during mammalian embryogenesis. *Genes Dev* 2001;15:2433.

33. Ichihara M, Murakumo Y, Takahashi M. RET and neuroendocrine tumors. *Cancer Lett* 2004;204:197.

34. Wells SA Jr, Santoro M. Targeting the RET pathway in thyroid cancer. *Clin Cancer Res* 2009;15:7119.

35. Knowles PP, Murray-Rust J, Kjaer S, et al. Structure and chemical inhibition of the RET tyrosine kinase domain. *J Biol Chem* 2006;281:33577.

36. Donis-Keller H, Dou S, Chi D, et al. Mutations in the RET proto-oncogene are associated with MEN2A and FMTC. *Hum Mol Genet* 1993;2:851.

37. Mulligan LM, Kwok JB, Healey CS, et al. Germ-line mutations of the RET proto-oncogene in multiple endocrine neoplasia type 2A. *Nature* 1993;363:458.

38. Miyauchi A, Futami H, Hai N, et al. Two germline missense mutations at codons 804 and 806 of the RET proto-oncogene in the same allele in a patient with multiple endocrine neoplasia type 2B without codon 918 mutation. *Jpn J Cancer Res* 1999;90:1.

39. Carlson KM, Bracamontes J, Jackson CE, et al. Parent-of-origin effects in multiple endocrine neoplasia type 2B. *Am J Hum Genet* 1994;55:1076.

40. Brandi ML, Gagel RF, Angeli A, et al. Guidelines for diagnosis and therapy of MEN type 1 and type 2. *J Clin Endocrinol Metab* 2001;86:5658.

41. Eng C, Clayton D, Schuffenecker I, et al. The relationship between specific RET proto-oncogene mutations and disease phenotype in multiple endocrine neoplasia type 2. International RET mutation consortium analysis. *JAMA* 1996;276:1575.

42. Mulligan LM, Eng C, Healey CS, et al. Specific mutations of the RET proto-oncogene are related to disease phenotype in MEN 2A and FMTC. *Nat Genet* 1994;6:70.

43. Machens A, Brauckhoff M, Holzhausen HJ, et al. Codon-specific development of pheochromocytoma in multiple endocrine neoplasia type 2. *J Clin Endocrinol Metab* 2005; 90:3999.

44. Kloos RT, Eng C, Evans DB, et al. Medullary thyroid cancer: management guidelines of the American Thyroid Association. *Thyroid* 2009;19:565.

45. Eng C, Mulligan LM, Smith DP, et al. Mutation of the RET protooncogene in sporadic medullary thyroid carcinoma. *Genes Chromosomes Cancer* 1995;12:209.

46. Iwashita T, Kato M, Murakami H, et al. Biological and biochemical properties of Ret with kinase domain mutations identified in multiple endocrine neoplasia type 2B and familial medullary thyroid carcinoma. *Oncogene* 1999;18:3919.

47. Mise N, Drosten M, Racek T, Tannapfel A, Putzer BM. Evaluation of potential mechanisms underlying genotype-phenotype correlations in multiple endocrine neoplasia type 2. *Oncogene* 2006;25:6637.

48. Myers SM, Mulligan LM. The RET receptor is linked to stress response pathways. *Cancer Res* 2004;64:4453.

49. Jaattela M. Heat shock proteins as cellular lifeguards. *Ann Med* 1999;31:261.

50. Jain S, Watson MA, DeBenedetti MK, et al. Expression profiles provide insights into early malignant potential and skeletal abnormalities in multiple endocrine neoplasia type 2B syndrome tumors. *Cancer Res* 2004;64:3907.

54. Elisei R, Romei C, Cosci B, et al. RET genetic screening in patients with medullary thyroid cancer and their relatives: experience with 807 individuals at one center. *J Clin Endocrinol Metab* 2007;92:4725.

55. Skinner MA, Moley JA, Dilley WG, et al. Prophylactic thyroidectomy in multiple endocrine neoplasia type 2A. *N Engl J Med* 2005;353:1105.

56. Sherman SI, Angelos P, Ball DW, et al. Thyroid carcinoma. *J Natl Compr Canc Netw* 2007;5:568.

57. Kendall-Taylor P. Guidelines for the management of thyroid cancer. *Clin Endocrinol (Oxf)* 2003;58:400.

59. Fusco A, Grieco M, Santoro M, et al. A new oncogene in human thyroid papillary carcinomas and their lymph-nodal metastases. *Nature* 1987;328:170.

60. Klugbauer S, Lengfelder E, Demidchik EP, Rabes HM. High prevalence of RET rearrangement in thyroid tumors of children from Belarus after the Chernobyl reactor accident. *Oncogene* 1995;11:2459.

61. Nikiforov YE, Rowland JM, Bove KE, Monforte-Munoz H, Fagin JA. Distinct pattern of ret oncogene rearrangements in morphological variants of radiation-induced and sporadic thyroid papillary carcinomas in children. *Cancer Res* 1997;57:1690.

63. Nikiforova MN, Stringer JR, Blough R, et al. Proximity of chromosomal loci that participate in radiation-induced rearrangements in human cells. *Science* 2000;290:138.

65. Kimura ET, Nikiforova MN, Zhu Z, et al. High prevalence of BRAF mutations in thyroid cancer: genetic evidence for constitutive activation of the RET/PTC-RAS-BRAF signaling pathway in papillary thyroid carcinoma. *Cancer Res* 2003;63:1454.

CHAPTER 26 SARCOMAS

SAMUEL SINGER, TORSTEN NIELSEN, AND CRISTINA R. ANTONESCU

Soft tissue sarcomas are life-threatening mesenchymal neoplasms that account for approximately 1% of all human cancer. They pose a significant therapeutic challenge because more than 50% of patients with newly diagnosed sarcoma eventually die of disease. Soft tissue sarcomas also pose significant diagnostic challenges as there are more than 50 histologic subtypes with unique molecular, pathologic, clinical, prognostic, and therapeutic features. Figure 26.1 shows the histologic appearance of the major subtypes.

The expansion in the molecular genetic and cytogenetic characterization of soft tissue sarcoma has improved classification and has divided sarcomas into two broad groups: those with simple karyotypes and those with highly complex karyotypes. Figure 26.2 shows the molecular alterations found in some of the subtypes in each group. The first group consists of sarcomas with simple genetic alterations (translocations or specific activating mutations) and with near-diploid, simple karyotypes. These alterations include translocations in myxoid/round-cell liposarcoma and synovial sarcoma, *APC* or *β*-catenin mutations in desmoid tumors, and *KIT* or *PDGFRA* activating mutations in gastrointestinal stromal tumors (GIST). Translocation-associated sarcomas typically occur in young adults, with highest incidence in the 30s and 40s. For most translocation-associated sarcomas, oncogenesis results from transcriptional deregulation induced by fusion genes. The second group consists of sarcomas with aberrant, highly complex genomes. Examples include dedifferentiated and pleomorphic liposarcoma, leiomyosarcoma, pleomorphic malignant fibrous histiocytoma, and myxofibrosarcoma. The peak incidence for these complex sarcoma types is in the 50s and 60s. Although these complex sarcoma subtypes commonly have alterations in cell-cycle genes *TP53*, *MDM2*, *RB1*, and *INK4a* and defects in specific growth-factor signaling pathways, the critical subtype-specific molecular alterations that drive sarcomagenesis largely remain to be discovered. This information will be essential for the development of therapeutics that can selectively target the driver genetic alterations required for sarcoma

survival. This idea is best illustrated by the development of imatinib, a small molecule that inhibits ABL, KIT, and PDGFRA tyrosine kinases. The discovery of activating mutations in *KIT* and *PDGFRA*, specifically in GIST, led to rapid clinical development of imatinib for GIST, in which it proved to be an effective, low toxicity therapy. This success illustrates how targeting a sarcoma-specific oncogenic mechanism can lead to dramatic responses.

Table 26.1 outlines the diagnostic histologic characteristics and molecular and cytogenetic abnormalities of the major soft tissue sarcoma subtypes.

TRANSLOCATION-ASSOCIATED SARCOMAS

Myxoid/Round Cell Liposarcoma

Myxoid liposarcoma typically presents in the thigh or other deep soft tissues in adult patients (peak age 30–50 years). The diagnosis can usually be made with confidence based on characteristic morphology: myxoid matrix, plexiform vasculature, and lipoblasts. These features may, however, be partially lost in its high-grade form, termed *round cell liposarcoma*. The great majority of myxoid/round cell liposarcomas carry a balanced translocation, t(12;16)(q13;p11),[1] fusing *FUS* (also known as *TLS*) with *DDIT3* (aka *CHOP, GADD153*).[2] In rare cases, *EWSR1* substitutes for its homologue *FUS*. At least nine *FUS-DDIT3* transcript variants have been reported,[3,4] and several are known to be capable of inducing a sarcoma phenotype in model systems.[5,6] The translocations fuse 5′ exons of *FUS* (encoding transcriptional regulatory domains that interact with the RNA polymerase II complex[7]) to the full coding sequence of *DDIT3*, a leucine-zipper transcription factor with roles in cell cycle control[8] and adipocytic differentiation.[9] The fusion oncoprotein complexes with cofactors including C/EBP*β* to deregulate gene expression, although few direct targets have been validated to date.[10,11] The net result is activation

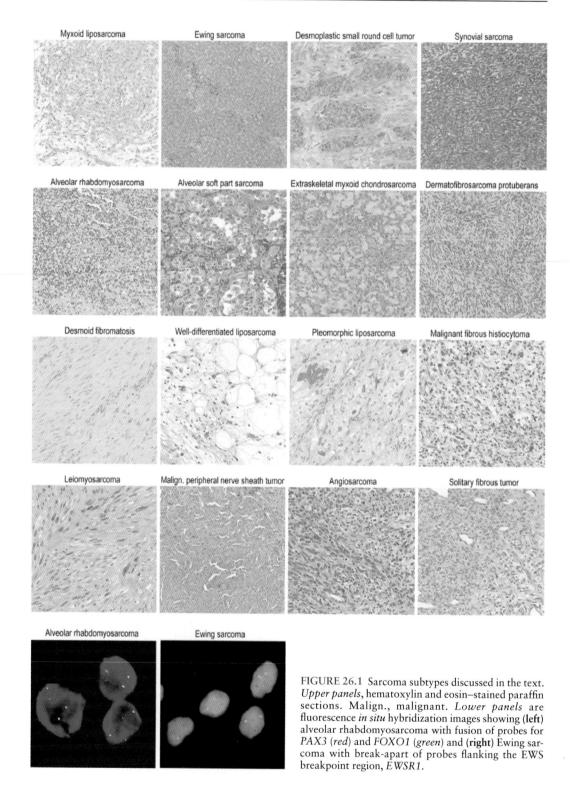

FIGURE 26.1 Sarcoma subtypes discussed in the text. *Upper panels*, hematoxylin and eosin–stained paraffin sections. Malign., malignant. *Lower panels* are fluorescence *in situ* hybridization images showing (**left**) alveolar rhabdomyosarcoma with fusion of probes for *PAX3* (*red*) and *FOXO1* (*green*) and (**right**) Ewing sarcoma with break-apart of probes flanking the EWS breakpoint region, *EWSR1*.

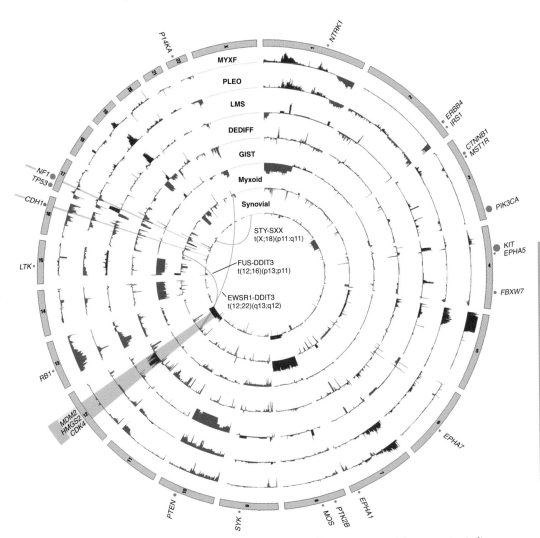

FIGURE 26.2 Nucleotide and copy number alterations in soft tissue sarcoma. The outer ring indicates chromosomal position. The second through fifth rings represent four subtypes with complex karyotypes (as labeled; MYXF, myxofibrosarcoma; PLEO, pleomorphic liposarcoma; LMS, leiomyosarcoma; DEDIFF, dedifferentiated liposarcoma). The three inner rings represent subtypes with simple karyotypes (Myxoid, myxoid/round cell liposarcoma). The plots show the statistical significance of genomic aberrations, with amplification in *red* and deletion in *blue*. *Green* curves indicate the chromosomal breakpoints of pathognomonic translocations in myxoid/round-cell liposarcoma and synovial sarcoma. Genes harboring somatic nucleotide alterations are indicated with *green circles* whose size is proportional to their frequency of occurrence. (Courtesy of Barry S. Taylor, Computational Biology Center, Memorial Sloan-Kettering Cancer. Adapted from ref. 19.)

of critical pathways including those related to the angiogenic factor interleukin (IL)-8, early adipose differentiation (PPARγ), growth factor signaling (insulinlike growth factor [IGF], the proto-oncoprotein RET), and cell-cycle control (cyclinD-CDK4).[10,12–14]

Clinically, evidence for *FUS-DDIT3* translocations from reverse transcription polymerase chain reaction (RT-PCR)[15] or fluorescence *in situ* hybridization (FISH)[16] can help confirm the diagnosis and may be useful for small biopsies dominated

by a round cell component. Fusion subtype, however, appears to have little prognostic value beyond what is known from stage and grade. In general, molecular markers in myxoid liposarcoma have been difficult to test for independent prognostic significance, given the difficulty of assembling large series with long follow-up.[17] Nevertheless, p53, IGF1R/IGF2, and RET overexpression may be adverse factors.[13,18] Such findings support IGF/Akt/mTOR and Ras-Raf-ERK/MAPK pathway inhibitors as potential targeted

TABLE 26.1

CYTOGENETIC AND MOLECULAR ABNORMALITIES IN SOFT TISSUE SARCOMAS

Disease	Diagnostic Morphology or Immunohisto-chemistry	Cytogenetic Event	Molecular Abnormality	Molecular Diagnostic[a]
Myxoid/round cell liposarcoma	Lipoblasts, plexiform vasculature, myxoid atrix	t(12;16)(q13;p11) t(12;22)(q13;q12)	FUS-DDIT3 (>90%) EWSR1-DDIT3 (<5%)	DDIT3 breaks (FISH)[16,187]
Ewing sarcoma family tumor	Small, blue, round cells; CD99 and FLI1 expression; lack of lymphoid biomarker expression	t(11;22)(q24;q12) t(21;22)(q22;q12) Alternative events: fusions of 22q12 with 7p22, 17q22, 2q33; inv 22q12; t(16;21) (p11;q22)	EWSR1-FLI1 (>80%) EWSR1-ERG (10–15%) Other ETS family partners: ETV1, ETV4, FEV, PATZ1 (~5%) FUS-ERG (<1%)	EWSR1 breaks (FISH)[36] or RT-PCR
Desmoplastic small, round cell tumor	Small, blue, round cell islands in dense stroma; positive for keratin, desmin, vimentin, and WT1	t(11;22)(p13;q12)	EWSR1-WT1 (>75%)	EWSR1 breaks (FISH)[36]
Synovial sarcoma	Biphasic histology, positive for TLE1[64]	t(X;18)(p11;q11) (>90%)	SYT-SSX1 (66%), SYT-SSX2 (33%), SYT-SSX4 (<1%)	SYT breaks (FISH)[188]
Alveolar rhabdomyosarcoma	Small, blue cells expressing desmin, myogenin, myoD1	t(2;13)(q35;q14) t(1;13)(p36;q14)	PAX3-FOXO1 (~80%) PAX7-FOXO1 (~20%) PAX3-NCOA1 (<1%) PAX3-NCOA2 (<1%)	PAX3/7 type-specific FISH or RT-PCR[189]
Alveolar soft-part sarcoma	Nested polygonal cells in vascular network; positive for TFE3[78]	t(X;17)(p11;q25)	ASPSCR1-TFE3 (>90%)	ASPSCR1-TFE3 RT-PCR[190]
Dermatofibrosarcoma protuberans	Bland spindle cells, storiform and honeycomb growth in subcutis, positive for CD34	Rings derived from t(17;22) (>75%) t(17;22)(q22; q13.1)[86,87,191] (10%)	COL1A1-PDGFB	
Embryonal rhabdomyosarcoma	Spindle cells and rhabdomyo-blasts, positive for desmin and myogenin	Trisomies 2q, 8 and 20 (>75%)	LOH at 11p15 (>75%)	

TABLE 26.1

(CONTINUED)

Disease	Diagnostic Morphology or Immunohistochemistry	Cytogenetic Event	Molecular Abnormality	Molecular Diagnostic[a]
Extraskeletal myxoid chondrosarcoma	Bland epithelioid cells arranged in reticular pattern in myxoid stroma	t(9;22)(q22;q12)	EWSR1-NR4A3 (75%)	EWSR1 breaks (FISH); RT-PCR[95–97] RT-PCR[95–97]
		t(9;17)(q22;q11)	TAF15-NR4A3 (<10%)	
		t(9;15)(q22;q21)	TCF12-NR4A3 (<10%)	
		t(3;9)(q12;q22)	TFG–NR4A3 (<5%)	
Endometrial stromal tumor	Bland spindle cells, positive for CD10 and ER	t(7;17)(p15;q21)	JAZF1-SUZ12 (30%)	
Clear cell sarcoma	Nested epithelioid cells with clear or amphophilic cytoplasm, positive for S100 and HMB-45	t(12;22)(q13;q12)	EWSR1-ATF1 (>75%)	EWSR1 breaks (FISH)[36,192]
		t(2;22)(q34;q12)	EWSR1-CREB1 (<5%)	
Infantile fibrosarcoma	Monomorphic spindle cells, herringbone pattern	t(12;15)(p13;q25)	ETV6-NTRK3 (>75%)	FISH, RT-PCR
Inflammatory myofibroblastic tumor	Myofibroblastic cells with lymphoplasmacytic infiltrate, positive for ALK	t(1;2)(q25;p23) t(2;19)(p23;p13) t(2;17)(p23;q23)	ALK-TPM34 ALK-TPM ALK-CLTC	ALK breaks (FISH)
Gastrointestinal stromal tumor	Spindle (70%), epithelioid (20%) or mixed (10%) morphology, positive for CD117 (KIT), DOG1, and CD34	Monosomies 14 and 22 (>75%) Deletion of 1p (>25)	KIT or PDGFRA mutation (>90%)[193,194]	PCR mutation analysis
Desmoid fibromatosis	Bland myofibroblastic-type cells, fascicular growth, nuclear positivity for β-catenin	Trisomies 8 and 20 (30%)	APC inactivation by mutation/ deletion (10%) CTNNB1 (β-catenin) mutations (85%)	IHC for β-catenin expression

MOLECULAR BIOLOGY OF INDIVIDUAL CANCERS

TABLE 26.1

(CONTINUED)

Disease	Diagnostic Morphology or Immunohisto-chemistry	Cytogenetic Event	Molecular Abnormality	Molecular Diagnostic[a]
Well-differentiated/dedifferentiated liposarcoma	Atypical multinucleated stromal cells, lipoblasts, positive for MDM2, CDK4	12q13-15 rings and giant markers	MDM2 and CDK4 amplification (>85%)	MDM2 amplification (FISH)
Pleomorphic liposarcoma	Pleomorphic spindle and giant cells, pleomorphic lipoblasts	Complex[b] (>90%)		None
Myxofibrosarcoma and pleomorphic MFH	Pleomorphic spindle and giant cells, storiform growth, variable myxoid stroma	Complex[b] (>90%)	SKP2 amplification	None
Leiomyosarcoma	Elongated fusiform cells with eosinophilic cytoplasm, in intersecting fascicles, positive for desmin and smooth muscle actin	Complex[b] (>50%) Deletions of 1p	RB1 point mutations/deletions	None
Malignant peripheral nerve sheath tumor	Monomorphic spindle cells, high mitotic count, geographic necrosis	Complex[b] (90%)		None
			NF1 mutation, loss or deletion (>50%)	None

FISH, fluorescence *in situ* hybridization; RT-PCR, reverse transcription polymerase chain reaction; LOH, loss of heterozygosity; IHC, immunohistochemistry; MFH, malignant fibrous histiocytoma.
[a]Refers to molecular tests that can be run on formalin-fixed paraffin-embedded material for molecular confirmation of diagnosis: quantitative RT-PCR of transcripts,[189] or FISH to interphase genomic DNA.[195]
[b]Complex karyotypes containing multiple numerical and structural chromosomal aberrations.

therapies in myxoid liposarcomas. In addition, mutations in *PIK3CA*, which were found in 18% of myxoid/round cell liposarcomas, were associated with worse outcome.[19]

The dense microvasculature and high levels of IL-8[10] and vascular endothelial growth factor (VEGF)[20] expression seen in this tumor may underlie its observed sensitivity to radiotherapy[21] and trabectedin,[22] suggesting a value for antian-

giogenic therapies. Trabectedin may also function by disrupting the binding of FUS-DDIT3 to target promoters.[11]

Ewing Sarcoma

Ewing family tumors appear most commonly in adolescents and young adults; primary sites can be either bone or soft tissues. A range of aggressive small, blue, round cell tumors with variations in clinical and morphologic features have been subsumed under the general term *Ewing sarcoma family tumor* following the recognition of common pathognomonic chromosomal translocations.[23,24] *EWSR1*, the common 5' translocation partner, is fused to one of several possible ETS family transcription factor genes (usually *FLI1*). In the fusion protein, EWSR1 provides, at minimum, its 264 amino acid N-terminal transcriptional regulatory domain, and the ETS factor provides its C-terminal DNA-binding domain. In the process, EWSR1 loses its RNA recognition domain, and the ETS factor loses its native transactivation domain. Several direct transcriptional targets for the fusion oncoprotein are supported by strong evidence. Some of these targets are upregulated (*ID2*,[25] *PTPL1*,[26] *MK-STYX*,[27] *DAX1*[28]) and some repressed (*CIP1*,[29] *TGFBR2*,[30] *IGFBP3*[31]) in Ewing sarcoma, but gene repression events, mediated by cofactors, appear to predominate overall.[32] The net result is activation of pathways driving proliferation and cell survival (including IGF signaling[33]), with concurrent repression of pathways promoting mesenchymal differentiation.[34,35]

Molecular confirmation of an *EWSR1* translocation can be critical for patient management because many of the clinical, morphologic, and immunophenotypic features of Ewing sarcoma are shared with entities such as mesenchymal chondrosarcoma and small cell osteosarcoma. Commercially available *EWSR1* split-apart FISH probes are valuable ancillary diagnostic tools (Fig. 26.1).[36] RT-PCR alternatives are complicated by the need to cover the many alternative gene and exonic fusion sites, but RT-PCR offers the advantage of identifying the specific exon fusion involved, which can have independent prognostic relevance.[37]

Several existing agents (including IGF/mTOR and histone deacetylase inhibitors[38–40]) that target recently identified, translocation-induced mechanisms and pathways are currently being tested in clinical trials for Ewing sarcoma, and novel strategies to directly inhibit the oncoprotein itself are in active development.[41]

Desmoplastic Small Round Cell Tumor

In desmoplastic small round cell tumor, the same 5' portions of *EWSR1* involved in Ewing sarcomas are fused to *WT1*,[42,43] a tumor suppressor deleted in Wilms tumor.[44] The 56-kDa EWSR1-WT1 chimeric protein includes the last three of the four WT1 DNA-binding zinc finger domains. Despite some similarities to Ewing sarcoma family tumors, desmoplastic small round cell tumors show little response to conventional chemotherapy. Prognosis is dismal, and new therapies are needed.[45] Several

transcriptional targets of the EWSR1-WT1 chimeric oncoprotein have been identified.[43] *PDGFA* expression is directly induced by EWSR1-WT1,[46] explaining the desmoplastic background and possibly the recent observation of a partial response to sunitinib.[47] *IL2RB* is also induced, and its downstream JAK/STAT signaling pathway appears active in this tumor,[43,48] representing a potential target for novel treatment approaches.

Synovial Sarcoma

Synovial sarcoma differs from most translocation-associated sarcomas in that the genes involved in its defining translocation, t(X;18)(p11;q11), encode epigenetic regulators, not transcription factors with direct DNA-binding activity.[49] The translocation fuses the widely expressed *SYT* (aka *SS18*) gene with an *SSX* gene normally expressed only in testis.[50] In the fusion oncoprotein, SYT, which interacts with components of the SWI/SNF chromatin remodeling complex,[51] retains all but the last eight amino acids from its C-terminal transcription activation domain. The SSX partner (SSX1, 2 or 4) retains only its C-terminal 78-residue repressor domain, which confers nuclear localization in association with Polycomb group proteins that mediate chromatin condensation and epigenetic gene silencing.[52] The resulting chimeric oncoprotein dysregulates transcription at the level of epigenetic modifications[53] and, when forcibly expressed in a mesenchymal stem cell background[54] or conditionally expressed in mice,[49,55] recapitulates synovial sarcoma. Direct targets of SYT-SSX include the tumor suppressors *COM1*[56] and *EGR1*[57]; both genes are repressed in synovial sarcoma, with the *EGR1* promoter undergoing SYT-SSX-dependent histone methylation.[57] Thus, transcriptional reactivation agents such as histone deacetylase inhibitors are worth investigation in this disease, as they may reactivate mesenchymal differentiation and reverse some effects of the SYT-SSX oncoprotein.[58,59]

The synovial sarcoma oncoprotein may also function by disrupting normal interactions between transcription factors and their DNA-binding sites, such as interactions between SLUG/SNAIL and the E-cadherin promoter, leading to transcriptional activation.[60] Subtle differences in such interactions may underlie the propensity of *SYT-SSX1* translocations, compared to *SYT-SSX2* translocations, to be associated with biphasic histology and poorer outcome, although prognostic differences are controversial.[61,62] The need for diagnostic molecular translocation testing, however, may be obviated by assays for TLE1, a transcriptional corepressor[63] that is highly expressed in synovial sarcoma and serves as a sensitive and specific biomarker.[64] Other oncogenic pathways that are activated, directly or indirectly, in synovial sarcoma include IGF2,[54,65,66] suggesting potential value for IGF/Akt/mTOR inhibitors in this disease.

Alveolar Rhabdomyosarcoma

In alveolar rhabdomyosarcoma, an aggressive cancer of older children and adolescents, the transcriptional activation domain of FOXO1 (aka FKHR) from 13q14 is fused to the DNA-binding domain of paired box transcription factor PAX3 (2q35) or PAX7 (1p36).[67,68] Until recently, about 20% of cases were thought to be translocation-negative, but recent work has proven that such tumors in fact represent histologic variants of embryonal rhabdomyosarcoma.[69] Furthermore, those cases with translocations involving PAX3 have a considerably worse prognosis than those involving PAX7.[70] Thus, molecular confirmation of the diagnosis by FISH (Fig. 26.1) and/or RT-PCR is required to optimize patient care.[71] Either translocation results in high-level nuclear expression of a chimeric transcription factor that abnormally activates PAX targets, many of which are genes involved in neurogenesis that are not expressed in normal skeletal muscle.[72] In addition, PAX3-FOXO1 directly induces PDGFRA; small-molecule (imatinib) and antibody inhibitors of this receptor tyrosine kinase are effective in mouse models.[73] Another probable direct target of PAX3-FOXO1, based on comparison of primary tumor and mouse model expression profiles, is the cell-cycle regulator SKP2,[74] perhaps helping explain why alveolar rhabdomyosarcoma is responsive to conventional cytotoxic chemotherapy.

Alveolar Soft-Part Sarcoma

Alveolar soft-part sarcoma has a clinical presentation and pathognomonic molecular event with many similarities to other translocation-associated sarcomas.[75] In this disease, the 5' half of the widely-expressed ASPSCR1 (aka ASPL) gene on 17q25 is fused to exon 3 or 4 of TFE3 on Xp11, the latter retaining its transcriptional activation, basic helix-loop-helix, and leucine zipper domains.[76] Interestingly, the same fusion is present in some renal cell carcinomas.[77] Although alveolar soft-part sarcoma has distinctive histology, translocation detection by RT-PCR or by immunohistochemistry for TFE3 can serve as a diagnostic adjunct.[78,79] The disease lacks validated prognostic biomarkers. Direct targets of ASPSCR1-TFE3 are not yet identified, although gene expression profiling and tissue microarray studies have highlighted prominent activation of c-Met signaling and angiogenesis pathways.[80-82] Antiangiogenic targeted therapy is effective in xenograft models[83] and has yielded partial responses in patients with metastatic disease.[84]

Dermatofibrosarcoma Protuberans

The cytogenetic hallmark of dermatofibrosarcoma protuberans (DFSP) is supernumerary ring chromosomes that contain material from chromosomes 17 and 22[85-87] or, less commonly, an unbalanced der(22)t(17;22)(q21-23;q13). The molecular consequence of both types of aberration is the overexpression of the platelet-derived growth factor-beta (PDGFB) gene on chromosome 22, through fusion with the collagen gene COL1A1 on chromosome 17.[88,89] The same fusion gene is also seen in two histologic variants: giant cell fibroblastoma and Bednar tumor (pigmented DFSP). FISH and comparative genomic hybridization (CGH) studies have indicated that increased COL1A1–PDGFB copy number is associated with fibrosarcomatous transformation of DFSP, although the copy number increase is not an invariable feature of these cases.[90,91]

The COL1A1-PDGFB fusion product signals through the PDGF receptor in an autocrine loop.[92] This signaling can be blocked using tyrosine kinase inhibitors acting at PDGFR, such as imatinib. A number of clinical studies have shown a high response rate to imatinib therapy in both locally advanced and metastatic DFSP.[85,93,94] These results support the concept that DFSP cells depend on aberrant activation of PDGF signaling for proliferation and survival.

Extraskeletal Myxoid Chondrosarcoma

Most extraskeletal myxoid chondrosarcomas show one of four reciprocal translocations: t(9;22)(q22;q12), t(9;17)(q22;q11), t(9;15)(q22;q21), or t(3;9)(q12;q22), with t(9;22) being the most common. These translocations fuse NR4A3 in 9q22-q31.1 with either EWSR1 in 22q12, TAF15 in 17q11, TCF12 in 15q21, or TFG in 3q12.[95-97] Because these fusion genes have not been described in any other tumor type, they represent useful diagnostic markers. The four different fusion partners have unknown prognostic significance.

NR4A3 encodes a ubiquitously expressed orphan nuclear receptor also known as NOR-1, TEC, MINOR, or CHN.[98] The t(9;22) fuses the transactivation domain of EWSR1 to the full length of NR4A3. Analogous to EWSR1-ETS fusions, the EWSR1-NR4A3 fusion protein not only displays strong transcriptional activity, but also regulates RNA splicing.[99]

TAF15, like EWSR1 and FUS, belongs to the TET family, and contains a characteristic 87-amino acid RNA recognition motif implicated in protein-RNA binding.[100] The N-terminal regions of EWSR1, FUS, and TAF15 contain degenerate repeats of the SYGQ motif and mediate powerful transcriptional activation when fused to the heterologous DNA-binding domains of a variety of transcription factors.[101]

By gene profiling, extraskeletal myxoid chondrosarcomas constitute a distinct genomic entity, showing up-regulation of several genes, including *NMB, DKK1, DNER, CLCN3*.[102] *In situ* hybridization confirmed that *NMB* is highly expressed in extraskeletal myxoid chondrosarcoma but not in other sarcoma types, suggesting its potential value as a diagnostic marker. Somewhat surprisingly, the up-regulated genes seen in two different profiling studies had only limited overlap.[96,102]

SIMPLE KARYOTYPE TUMORS ASSOCIATED WITH MUTATIONS

Desmoid Fibromatosis

Desmoid fibromatoses are locally infiltrative, clonal fibroblastic proliferations that arise in the deep soft tissues and never metastasize. Although about 70% result from mutations in *APC* or *CTNNB1*, tumorigenesis may be also be influenced by endocrine and physiologic factors such as pregnancy, trauma, and prior surgery. Desmoids are usually divided into two groups: sporadic desmoids and those in individuals with a heterozygous germline mutation in the adenomatous polyposis coli (*APC*) gene (chromosome 5q). Although germline *APC* mutations also often result in familial adenomatous polyposis,[103] some desmoid patients harboring such a mutation have no polyposis. The desmoids in individuals with a germline *APC* mutation display inactivation of the second copy of *APC*, which usually occurs by point mutation or deletion.[103,104]

Among sporadic desmoids, only a minority display *APC* inactivation. A majority (52%–85%) have an activating point mutation in the β-catenin gene, *CTNNB1*.[105,106] These *CTNNB1* mutations stabilize β-catenin, resulting in its overabundance. β-catenin, a mediator of Wnt signaling, is negatively regulated by APC, so both *APC* inactivation and *CTNNB1* activating mutations result in up-regulation of the Wnt pathway. The specific *CTNNB1* mutation may have prognostic significance; patients with S45F-mutant desmoids were reported to have a 5-year recurrence-free survival of only 23%, compared with 57% for those with T41A-mutant tumors and 65% for those with wild type *CTNNB1*.[106] These results raise the possibility that mutation status might aid in selecting patients for more aggressive therapy.

Based on the findings of *APC* inactivation or activating *CTNNB1* mutations in the majority of patients, the development of small-molecule β-catenin antagonists would be likely to provide significant benefit, particularly for patients with advanced disease in whom surgical resection is not feasible. Although such β-catenin–targeted agents are still in preclinical development, an inhibitor of matrix metalloproteinase, a downstream target of β-catenin, substantially reduced tumor volume and tumor invasion in a transgenic *Apc+/Apc*1638N mouse model of aggressive fibromatosis.[107]

Patients with desmoids were found to have elevated levels of PDGF-AA and PDGF-BB, leading to a trial of the tyrosine kinase inhibitor imatinib in patients with advanced desmoid. Three of 19 patients (16%) had a partial response to treatment and four additional patients had stable disease for more than 1 year; overall, the 1-year tumor control rate was 37%.[108] The response in these tumors was thought to be mediated by inhibition of PDGFRB kinase activity.

COMPLEX SARCOMA TYPES

Well-Differentiated and Dedifferentiated Liposarcoma

Well-differentiated and dedifferentiated liposarcomas represent the most common biological group of liposarcoma. This group is characterized by amplification of 12q, including the oncogenes *MDM2, HMGA2,* and *CDK4*. The amplifications usually occur in double minutes, ring chromosomes, and large marker chromosomes. In addition, the 12q13.2-q23.1 locus often harbors complex rearrangements (Fig. 26.2).[19,109,110] On the basis of the rearrangements and correlated overexpression results, 12q may contain additional driver genes besides *MDM2, HMGA2,* and *CDK4*. The possibilities include *NAV3, WIF1, MDM1, DYRK2, ELK3, DUSP6, YEATS4, TBK1,* and *FRS2,* which were found to be amplified in ~14% to 80% of tumors. Some of these genes are known to be involved in liposarcomagenesis, while others were not previously implicated in this disease or in cancer. Aside from 12q aberrations, dedifferentiated liposarcomas have been found to contain significant amplifications of 1p, 1q, 5p, 6q, and 20q.[19,109,110] Amplification of *JUN* (on 1p32) has been suggested as the explanation for the block in adipocyte differentiation in undifferentiated sarcomas.[111] However, more recent studies suggest that *JUN* is amplified or overexpressed in only a subset of dedifferentiated liposarcomas and that other alterations or activated pathways may be required to induce the dedifferentiated phenotype.[19,112]

Microarray analysis of differentially expressed genes in liposarcoma subtypes compared with normal fat has demonstrated activation of cell-cycle and checkpoint pathways, including the up-regulation of CDK4, MDM2, CDK1, CDC7, cyclin B1, cyclin B2, and cyclin E2 in well-differentiated and dedifferentiated liposarcoma, suggesting that these pathways may be useful as therapeutic targets.[113] In fact, nutlin-3a, a selective MDM2 antagonist, induces apoptosis and inhibits proliferation of dedifferentiated liposarcoma cell lines at concentrations that have no phenotypic effects in normal adipose-derived stem cells.[113] Thus, downstream p53 pathway signaling appears to be much more pronounced in dedifferentiated liposarcoma cell lines with overexpressed MDM2 than in adipose-derived stem cells, and MDM2 antagonists might serve as a effective therapeutics for liposarcomas with *MDM2* amplification while having few effects on normal cells. Furthermore, PD0332991, a selective CDK4/CDK6 inhibitor currently in clinical trials, inhibits proliferation of dedifferentiated liposarcoma cells, inducing G1 cell-cycle arrest.[19] These results provide a rationale for use of MDM2 antagonists and CDK4 inhibitors in patients with well-differentiated and dedifferentiated liposarcoma.

Pleomorphic Liposarcoma

Pleomorphic liposarcoma is the least common liposarcoma subtype, accounting for 5% of all liposarcomas. This subtype is characterized by high chromosome counts and complex structural rearrangements, with numerous unidentifiable marker chromosomes, nonclonal alterations, and polyploidy. This complexity has made the detection of specific recurrent rearrangements difficult.

A high-resolution single nucleotide polymorphism (SNP) array analysis has revealed that pleomorphic liposarcoma harbors multiple regions of significant copy number amplification and deletion.[114] The most common alteration, found in approximately 60% of tumors, was a deletion of 13q14.2-q14.3 that includes the *RB1* tumor suppressor. The next most common event was loss of 17p13.1 including *TP53*. Both *RB1* and *TP53* deletions were a mixture of hemizygous loss and less frequent homozygous deletion. Recently, *TP53* point mutations were found in 17% of pleomorphic liposarcomas.[19] Small molecules that reactivate mutant p53, such as PRIMA-1, are presently undergoing phase 1 trials and may have particular utility for pleomorphic liposarcomas harboring deletion or mutation in *TP53*.

A third genetic alteration identified in SNP analysis was frequent deletions of 17q11.2 including the tumor suppressor *NF1* (neurofibromin 1). Among 24 pleomorphic liposarcomas, nine had genomic loss at this locus, eight of which were hemizygous and one was homozygous. In addition, two tumors (8%) had somatic point mutations in *NF1*, and both these tumors also showed deletion of the wild type allele and correspondingly reduced gene expression. These data indicate a diverse pattern of *NF1* aberrations in approximately 38% of pleo-

morphic liposarcomas[19] and suggest that MEK or mTOR inhibitors may have clinical utility, as loss of NF1 function appears to activate the RAS and mTOR pathways.

Myxofibrosarcoma and Pleomorphic Malignant Fibrous Histiocytoma

Pathologists now regard myxofibrosarcoma as a distinct tumor type with clearly defined criteria for diagnosis.[115–117] Myxofibrosarcoma contains variable degrees of myxoid stroma composed of hyaluronic acid and solid sheets of spindled and pleomorphic (irregularly shaped) tumor cells. Pleomorphic malignant fibrous histiocytoma, however, is less well defined, and it remains controversial whether it represents (1) a pleomorphic sarcoma showing fibroblastic/myofibroblastic differentiation and thus sharing a common set of genomic alterations with myxofibrosarcoma, or (2) an end-stage undifferentiated morphologic pattern with genomic alterations distinct from those of myxofibrosarcoma.

Myxofibrosarcoma

Myxofibrosarcoma, also known as myxoid variant of malignant fibrous histiocytoma, includes a spectrum of malignant fibroblastic lesions with variably myxoid stroma (at least 10%), pleomorphism, and a distinctive curvilinear vascular pattern. At present, little is known about the genetic events specific to myxofibrosarcoma. Cytogenetic data are scarce, with only 49 cases described in the literature.[118] Cytogenetic karyotypes tend to be highly complex, often with multiple numerical and structural rearrangements and with chromosome numbers in the triploid or tetraploid range.[119,120] No specific or consistent chromosomal aberration has emerged, although some chromosomes appear to be more involved than others and ring chromosomes have been reported. In general, karyotype complexity has been greater in high-grade lesions and in recurrences.[120]

In an SNP array analysis of 38 myxofibrosarcomas, approximately 55% of tumors harbored chromosome 5p amplification.[19] This region contains *RICTOR* (the rapamycin-insensitive binding partner of mTOR), *CDH9*, and *LIFR*. Other amplified regions included several discontinuous loci on 1p and 1q spanning *PI4KB*, *ETV3*, and *MCL1*, among others. *MCL1*, an antiapoptotic gene, was concomitantly overexpressed in these tumors. Myxofibrosarcomas also harbored deletions of classic tumor suppressors, including *CDKN2A/CDKN2B*, *RB1*, and *TP53*. These events, in combination with the inactivating mutations detected in *NF1* in 11% and *PTEN* in 3% of myxofibrosarcomas, demonstrate extensive loss of function in several known tumor suppressors.[19]

Pleomorphic Malignant Fibrous Histiocytoma

Over 50% of soft tissue sarcomas occurring in older adults are histologically pleomorphic and high grade. Most have traditionally been classified as malignant fibrous histiocytoma (MFH), which has been regarded as the most common sarcoma in adults.[121,122] MFH was originally defined as a pleomorphic spindle cell malignant neoplasm showing fibroblastic and histiocytic differentiation. More recently, pathologists have accepted that the morphologic pattern known as pleomorphic MFH may be shared by a wide range of malignant neoplasms.[123] Many sarcomas that were previously classified as pleomorphic MFH, on careful immunohistochemical and histopathologic analysis, revealed a specific line of differentiation and could be reclassified as myxofibrosarcoma (30%), myogenic sarcoma (30%), liposarcoma (4%), malignant peripheral nerve sheath tumor (2%), or soft tissue osteosarcoma (3%), and about 30% had no specific line of differentiation or were myofibroblastic.[115] Thus, the term *pleomorphic MFH/sarcoma not otherwise specified* is now reserved for pleomorphic sarcomas that show no definable line of differentiation by current technology.

Because diagnostic criteria have shifted over the years, the genetic aspects of pleomorphic MFH are difficult to evaluate. Among the more than 60 cases in the Mitelman Database of Chromosome Alterations in Cancer published as storiform or pleomorphic MFH or MFH not otherwise specified, the karyotypes are highly complex. The majority of tumors have chromosome numbers in the triploid or tetraploid range, but a few have near-haploid karyotypes.[124–128] No specific aberrations have emerged, but telomeric associations, ring chromosomes, and/or dicentric chromosomes are frequent, although not specific for pleomorphic MFH. Unfortunately many of the cytogenetic and array-based CGH studies to date have included heterogeneous groups of tumors characterized as MFH; these studies typically show loss of 2p24, 2q32, and chromosomes 11, 13, and 16 along with gains of 7p15, 7q32, and 1p31.[129–132] In many of these CGH studies, the copy number profiles of the majority of pleomorphic MFH closely resembled those of leiomyosarcomas[133–135] or pleomorphic or dedifferentiated liposarcomas.[136–138] Mutations and/or deletions of *TP53*, *RB1*, and *INK4a* have been suggested to play a critical role in pleomorphic MFH oncogenesis.[131,133,139–141]

Leiomyosarcoma

Leiomyosarcoma is a malignant tumor composed of cells showing distinct smooth muscle features and typically containing intersecting, sharply marginated groups of spindle cells. Karyotypes tend to be complex, with amplifications, gains, and losses involving multiple chromosomes, and karyotype generally differs between tumors.[142–144] Frequent losses of 1p12-pter, 2p, 13q14-q21 (including the *RB1* tumor suppressor),[145] 10q (including *PTEN*),[146] and 16q and gains of 17p, 8q, and 1q21-31 regions have been observed and have been associated with aggressive clinical behavior. In an analysis of copy number alterations in 27 leiomyosarcomas,[19] deletions, which were more common than amplifications, included well-characterized tumor suppressors like *TP53*, *BRCA2*, *RB1*, and *FANCA*. The most prominent changes were chromosome 10 deletions (approximately 50%-70% of cases) (Fig. 26.2). Indeed, genetic inactivation of *Pten* (human 10q23.21) in smooth muscle in mice recapitulates human leiomyosarcoma,[147] suggesting 10q loss occurs early in leiomyosarcomagenesis. In addition to *PTEN* inactivation, we identified homozygous deletions in *MTOR*. Because PTEN is a repressor of Akt, both these events suggest a critical role for aberrant Akt-mTOR signaling in leiomyosarcoma. Inhibition of mTOR using rapamycin analogues such as everolimus (RAD001) has shown some efficacy in patients with leiomyosarcoma in recent clinical trials.[148] Furthermore, *RB1* deletion is common in leiomyosarcomas, with 70% harboring heterozygous deletions and 8% homozygous deletions. A role for *RB1* deletion in leiomyosarcoma fits with the high frequency of leiomyosarcoma observed in individuals with hereditary retinoblastoma.[149]

Malignant Peripheral Nerve Sheath Tumor

Malignant peripheral nerve sheath tumors (MPNSTs) are highly aggressive soft tissue sarcomas that rarely occur in the general population, but are much more common in patients with the hereditary tumor predisposition syndrome neurofibromatosis type 1 (NF1), which is caused by heterozygous mutations of the *NF1* gene. NF1 patients have a lifetime incidence of MPNST of 8% to 13%.[150] Morphologically, MPNSTs are monomorphic spindle cell tumors often with alternating myxoid and cellular areas. In well-differentiated lesions, tumor cell nuclei are typically buckled, resembling the pattern in neurofibroma. The spindle cells in MPNSTs are typically focally reactive for S100 protein in 50% to 70% of cases.

The *NF1* gene is implicated in sporadic as well as NF1-associated MPNST. In a CGH study, about 70% of sporadic and NF1-associated MPNSTs displayed monoallelic or biallelic loss at the *NF1* locus on 17q.[151] *NF1* encodes neurofibromin, a

Ras GTPase-activating protein; it accelerates Ras–GTP hydrolysis and thus negatively regulates Ras.[152] In individuals with NF1, neurofibromas develop when an unknown cell type in the Schwann cell lineage loses its remaining functional *NF1* gene (by mutation, deletion, or loss of heterozygosity), leading to neurofibromin loss and subsequent activation of Ras signaling.[153–155]

Both sporadic and NF1-associated MPNSTs display complex karyotypes and clonal chromosomal aberrations.[118,156,157] In CGH analyses of MPNSTs, the most frequent minimal regions of gain were 1q24.1-q24.2, 1q24.3-q25.1, 8p23.1-p12, 9q34.11-q34.13, and 17q23.2-q25.3.[158] The 17q gain was associated with poor survival and with the overexpression of genes previously implicated in cancer: *TOP2A*, *ETV4*, *ERBB2*, and *BIRC5*.[158–160]

Recent studies have identified some of the genetic alterations that contribute to malignant transformation of neurofibroma to MPNST and many involve the p19ARF-MDM2-p53,[161] p16INK4A-RB1,[162] and EGFR signaling pathways.[163,164] *TP53* (on 17p13) is frequently inactivated in MPNST through mutations or deletions, correlating with the frequent loss of 17p.[157] Other frequent alterations include rearrangement or loss of 13q14 and 9p21, resulting in inactivation of, respectively, *RB1* and *CDKN2A* (encoding the p16INK4A and p14ARF cell cycle inhibitory proteins). In fact, in a recent genomewide, high-resolution analysis of copy number alterations in NF1-associated MPNST, the most frequently deleted locus (33% of cases) encompassed *CDKN2A*, *CDKN2B*, and *MTAP* genes on 9p21.3.[154]

mTOR has been found to be constitutively activated in both *NF1*-deficient primary cells and *NF1*-deficient Schwann cells derived from human neurofibromas cultured in the absence of growth factors. Furthermore, tumor cell lines derived from NF1 patients, and genetically engineered cells in which NF1 knockdown induces transformation, are highly sensitive to the mTOR inhibitor rapamycin.[165] Finally, in a genetically engineered murine model, rapamycin potently suppresses the growth of aggressive NF1-associated malignancies by suppressing the mTOR target cyclin D1. These results demonstrate that mTOR inhibitors may be an effective targeted therapy for patients with neurofibromatosis and MPNST.

The activation of the Ras/Raf/MAPK pathway in the majority of MPNSTs supported targeting B-Raf with the B-Raf tyrosine kinase inhibitor sorafenib. MPNST cell lines are sensitive to sorafenib at nanomolar concentrations, and this was found to be mediated through inhibition of phospho-MEK and phospho-ERK, suppression of cyclin D1, and hypophosphorylation of RB1 at the CDK4-specific sites, resulting in G1 cell-cycle

arrest.[166] A phase 2 trial of sorafenib in patients with metastatic MPNST was recently completed. Although none of the 12 patients with MPNST had RECIST responses, 3 had stable disease and 2 had regression or cystification of metastatic disease.[167]

Angiosarcoma

Angiosarcomas (ASs) are rare vascular malignancies of endothelial cell differentiation that arise either *de novo* or secondary to radiation therapy or chronic lymphedema. By expression profiling, ASs are characterized by up-regulation of vascular-specific receptor tyrosine kinases, including *TIE1*, *KDR* (*VEGFR2*), *TEK* (*TIE2*), and *FLT1* (*VEGFR1*).[168] Full sequencing of these candidate genes identified mutations in *KDR* in 10% of AS patients, all of whom had tumors in the breast, with or without prior radiation. The observed *KDR* mutations were located in the extracellular immunoglobulinlike C2 domain, transmembrane domain, and kinase domain. *KDR* mutations were typically associated with strong KDR protein expression. No gains in *KDR* copy number were detected, even in tumors that overexpressed KDR protein. KDR mutants expressed in COS-7 cells showed ligand-independent activation of the kinase, which was inhibited with specific KDR inhibitors.[168] In contrast with other sarcoma types, AS showed down-regulation of VEGF ligand expression (VEGFA and VEGFB), in keeping with the constitutive activation of KDR independent of exogenous VEGF.[168] These results provide a basis for the activity of VEGFR-directed therapy in primary and radiation-induced AS.

In a recent array-CGH study, recurrent genetic abnormalities were identified in secondary but not primary AS.[169] The most frequent recurrent changes were high-level amplifications on chromosome 8q24.21 (50%), followed by amplification on 10p12.33 (33%) and 5q35.3 (11%). High-level amplification of *MYC* on 8q24.21 was confirmed by FISH in AS associated with radiation and chronic lymphedema, but not in primary tumors. *MYC* amplification was not found to predispose to higher-grade morphology or increased proliferation. These findings suggest that, despite having similar morphology, primary and secondary AS are genetically distinct.

Solitary Fibrous Tumor and Hemangiopericytoma

Solitary fibrous tumor (SFT) and hemangiopericytoma are closely related histopathologically and have been suggested to represent different aspects of a single biological entity. No consistent aberrations have emerged among the approximately 20 cases of each type that have been investigated by chromosome banding analysis, although one-third of hemangiopericytomas and 10% of SFTs have shown involvement of the 12q13-15 region. The remaining cases reveal gains, losses, or structural rearrangements in several other regions, such as 4q13, 9p22-9p23, and 12q24.[170,171] A homogeneous profile for SFTs has, however, emerged from gene expression profiling.[172] The SFT profile is independent of anatomic location, and is distinct from profiles of other sarcoma types. This finding reinforces clinicopathologic studies that unify pleural and extrapleural SFT as a single biological entity.

The SFT expression profile includes overexpression of several tyrosine kinase receptors, such as *DDR1*, *ERBB2*, and *FGFR1*.[172] Furthermore, overexpression of *IGF2* was uniformly detected in SFT, regardless of anatomic location. *IGF2* is subject to imprinting on the paternal allele in most adult tissues, and *IGF2* overexpresssion in SFTs was related to loss of imprinting. Although IGF2 exerts its function by binding to IGF1R, SFTs do not show up-regulation of IGF1R, and it was suggested that IGF2 signaling occurs through the insulin receptor A pathway.[173] Overexpression of *IGF2* and consequent activation of the insulin receptor may also explain why a subset of SFT patients presents with hypoglycemia. This syndrome, known as *Doege-Potter syndrome*, has been associated with large tumor size and aggressive clinical behavior and is resolved by surgical resection of the lesion.[174]

Although a *PDGFRB* mutation (D850V) was reported in a malignant pleural SFT,[175] none of the 39 SFTs tested subsequently showed mutation in this hot spot, nor did they show up-regulation of PDGFRB mRNA.[172]

FUTURE DIRECTIONS: FUNCTIONAL SCREENS AND NEXT-GENERATION SEQUENCING

New targeted therapies are desperately needed for the ~4,000 patients who die each year in the United States of soft tissue sarcoma.[176] A key challenge will be to identify the alterations that drive sarcomagenesis for each subtype of sarcoma. Once these driver alterations are identified, new small molecules to target them can be sought through a combination of functional screens, high-throughput compound screens, combinatorial chemistry, and structural biology information. Use of next-generation sequencing technologies can vastly expand our knowledge of the mutations, translocations, epigenetic alterations, and aberrant signaling pathways associated with specific sarcoma types and subtypes. The major advantage of next-generation sequencing is its ability to produce enormous amounts of data cheaply—in some cases more than 10^9 short reads per instrument run.[177] Concurrent massively parallel sequencing experiments and integrative analysis now enables genomewide analysis of copy number alterations, structural rearrangements, expressed coding mutations, alternative splice forms, digital expression, chimeric/fusion transcripts, and DNA methylation status. This approach will provide a deeper view of the sarcoma genome than was previously possible. For example, on a single tumor sample it is now possible to resequence all of the protein-coding regions of the human genome, generate detailed transcriptome profiles (RNA–seq),[178] and perform genomewide profiling of epigenetic marks and chromatin structure using other seq-based methods (ChIP–seq, methyl–seq, and DNase–seq).[179] In gene expression studies, microarrays are being replaced by seq-based methods because RNA-seq provides far more precision on transcript levels, alternative splicing, and sequence variation in identified genes. RNA-seq has an additional advantage in that it can identify rare transcripts without prior knowledge of a particular gene.[178–181] These seq-based methods, when integrated with data from high-throughput RNA interference screens in cell lines harboring the genetic alterations found in human sarcoma samples, will substantially enhance our ability to identify and target the critical signaling pathways and proteins driving sarcomagenesis.

"Smart" compounds, reflecting the three-dimensional structure of the targeted protein, may then be designed using high-throughput biochemical screens capable of identifying low-affinity compounds, together with sensitive biophysical techniques such as nuclear magnetic resonance, x-ray diffraction, and protein-ligand cocrystallography.[182–185] The resulting physicochemical data should facilitate virtual screening of library structures for their three-dimensional fit with pharmacophores[186] and speed the discovery of new selective small-molecule inhibitors targeting a signaling pathway essential for sarcoma growth and survival.

Selected References

The full list of references for this chapter appears in the online version.

3. Sandberg AA. Updates on the cytogenetics and molecular genetics of bone and soft tissue tumors: liposarcoma. *Cancer Genet Cytogenet* 2004;155:1–24.

11. Forni C, Minuzzo M, Virdis E, et al. Trabectedin (ET-743) promotes differentiation in myxoid liposarcoma tumors. *Mol Cancer Ther* 2009;8:449–457.

19. Barretina J, Taylor BS, Banerji S, et al. Subtype-specific genomic alterations define new targets for soft tissue sarcoma therapy. *Nature Genetics* 2010;42:715–721.

22. Germano G, Frapolli R, Simone M, et al. Antitumor and anti-inflammatory effects of trabectedin on human myxoid liposarcoma cells. *Cancer Res* 2010;70:2235–2244.

24. Ordonez JL, Osuna D, Herrero D, de Alava E, Madoz-Gurpide J. Advances in Ewing's sarcoma research: where are we now and what lies ahead? *Cancer Res* 2009;69: 7140–7150.

28. Garcia-Aragoncillo E, Carrillo J, Lalli E, et al. DAX1, a direct target of EWS/FLI1 oncoprotein, is a principal regulator of cell-cycle progression in Ewing's tumor cells. *Oncogene* 2008;27:6034–6043.

32. Owen LA, Kowalewski AA, Lessnick SL. EWS/FLI mediates transcriptional repression via NKX2.2 during oncogenic transformation in Ewing's sarcoma. *PLoS One* 2008;3:e1965.

34. Kauer M, Ban J, Kofler R, et al. A molecular function map of Ewing's sarcoma. *PLoS One* 2009;4:e5415.

35. Kovar H. Downstream EWS/FLI1 - upstream Ewing's sarcoma. *Genome Med* 2010;2:8.

39. Toretsky JA, Gorlick R. IGF-1R targeted treatment of sarcoma. *Lancet Oncol* 2010;11:105.

40. Wachtel M, Schafer BW. Targets for cancer therapy in childhood sarcomas. *Cancer Treat Rev* 2010;36:318–321.

41. Erkizan HV, Kong Y, Merchant M, et al. A small molecule blocking oncogenic protein EWS-FLI1 interaction with RNA helicase A inhibits growth of Ewing's sarcoma. *Nat Med* 2009;15:750–756.

43. Gerald WL, Haber DA. The EWS-WT1 gene fusion in desmoplastic small round cell tumor. *Semin Cancer Biol* 2005;15:197–205.

45. Stuart-Buttle CE, Smart CJ, Pritchard S, Martin D, Welch IM. Desmoplastic small round cell tumour: a review of literature and treatment options. *Surg Oncol* 2008;17: 107–112.

49. Haldar M, Randall RL, Capecchi MR. Synovial sarcoma: from genetics to genetic-based animal modeling. *Clin Orthop Relat Res* 2008;466:2156–2167.

53. de Bruijn DR, Nap JP, van Kessel AG. The (epi)genetics of human synovial sarcoma. *Genes Chromosomes Cancer* 2007;46:107–117.

57. Lubieniecka JM, de Bruijn DR, Su L, et al. Histone deacetylase inhibitors reverse SS18-SSX-mediated polycomb silencing of the tumor suppressor early growth response 1 in synovial sarcoma. *Cancer Res* 2008;68:4303–4310.

59. Nielsen TO, West RB. Translating gene expression into clinical care: sarcomas as a paradigm. *J Clin Oncol* 2010;28:1796–1805.

71. Wexler LH, Ladanyi M. Diagnosing alveolar rhabdomyosarcoma: morphology must be coupled with fusion confirmation. *J Clin Oncol* 2010;28:2126–2128.

74. Nishijo K, Chen QR, Zhang L, et al. Credentialing a preclinical mouse model of alveolar rhabdomyosarcoma. *Cancer Res* 2009;69:2902–2911.

75. Fisher C. Soft tissue sarcomas with non-EWS translocations: molecular genetic features and pathologic and clinical correlations. *Virchows Arch* 2010;456:153–166.

82. Stockwin LH, Vistica DT, Kenney S, et al. Gene expression profiling of alveolar soft-part sarcoma (ASPS). *BMC Cancer* 2009;9:22.

84. Stacchiotti S, Tamborini E, Marrari A, et al. Response to sunitinib malate in advanced alveolar soft part sarcoma. *Clin Cancer Res* 2009;15:1096–1104.

85. McArthur GA, Demetri GD, van Oosterom A, et al. Molecular and clinical analysis of locally advanced dermatofibrosarcoma protuberans treated with imatinib: Imatinib Target Exploration Consortium Study B2225. *J Clin Oncol* 2005;23:866–873.

105. Tejpar S, Nollet F, Li C, et al. Predominance of beta-catenin mutations and beta-catenin dysregulation in sporadic aggressive fibromatosis (desmoid tumor). *Oncogene* 1999;18:6615.

106. Lazar AJ, Tuvin D, Hajibashi S, et al. Specific mutations in the beta-catenin gene (CTNNB1) correlate with local recurrence in sporadic desmoid tumors. *Am J Pathol* 2008;173:1518–1527.

108. Heinrich MC, McArthur GA, Demetri GD, et al. Clinical and molecular studies of the effect of imatinib on advanced aggressive fibromatosis (desmoid tumor). *J Clin Oncol* 2006;24:1195–1203.

111. Mariani O, Brennetot C, Coindre JM, et al. JUN oncogene amplification and overexpression block adipocytic differentiation in highly aggressive sarcomas. *Cancer Cell* 2007;11:361–374.

112. Snyder EL, Sandstrom DJ, Law K, et al. c-Jun amplification and overexpression are oncogenic in liposarcoma but not always sufficient to inhibit the adipocytic differentiation programme. *J Pathol* 2009;218:292–300.

113. Singer S, Socci ND, Ambrosini G, et al. Gene expression profiling of liposarcoma identifies distinct biological types/subtypes and potential therapeutic targets in well-differentiated and dedifferentiated liposarcoma. *Cancer Res* 2007;67:6626–6636.

115. Fletcher CD, Gustafson P, Rydholm A, Willen H, Akerman M. Clinicopathologic re-evaluation of 100 malignant fibrous histiocytomas: prognostic relevance of subclassification. *J Clin Oncol* 2001;19:3045–3050.

116. Fletcher CD, Unni KK, Mertens F. Pathology and genetics of tumors of soft tissue and bone. In: Kleihues P, Sobin LH, eds. *World Health Organization Classification of Tumours.* Lyon, France: IARC Press, 2002.

136. Chibon F, Mariani O, Derre J, et al. ASK1 (MAP3K5) as a potential therapeutic target in malignant fibrous histiocytomas with 12q14-q15 and 6q23 amplifications. *Genes Chromosomes Cancer* 2004;40:32–37.

143. Sandberg AA. Updates on the cytogenetics and molecular genetics of bone and soft tissue tumors: leiomyosarcoma. *Cancer Genet Cytogenet* 2005;161:1–19.

144. Yang J, Du X, Chen K, et al. Genetic aberrations in soft tissue leiomyosarcoma. *Cancer Lett* 2009;275:1.

147. Hernando E, Charytonowicz E, Dudas ME, et al. The AKT-mTOR pathway plays a critical role in the development of leiomyosarcomas. *Nat Med* 2007;13:748–753.

149. Kleinerman RA, Tucker MA, Abramson DH, et al. Risk of soft tissue sarcomas by individual subtype in survivors of hereditary retinoblastoma. *J Natl Cancer Inst* 2007;99: 24–31.

152. Cichowski K, Jacks T. NF1 tumor suppressor gene function: narrowing the GAP. *Cell* 2001;104:593–604.

154. Mantripragada KK, de Stahl TD, Patridge C, et al. Genome-wide high-resolution analysis of DNA copy number alterations in NF1-associated malignant peripheral nerve sheath tumors using 32K BAC array. *Genes Chromosomes Cancer* 2009;48:897–907.

155. Upadhyaya M, Kluwe L, Spurlock G, et al. Germline and somatic NF1 gene mutation spectrum in NF1-associated malignant peripheral nerve sheath tumors (MPNSTs). *Hum Mutat* 2008;29:74–82.

163. Keizman D, Issakov J, Meller I, et al. Expression and significance of EGFR in malignant peripheral nerve sheath tumor. *J Neurooncol* 2009;94:383–388.

164. Ling BC, Wu J, Miller SJ, et al. Role for the epidermal growth factor receptor in neurofibromatosis-related peripheral nerve tumorigenesis. *Cancer Cell* 2005;7: 65–75.

165. Johannessen CM, Reczek EE, James MF, et al. The NF1 tumor suppressor critically regulates TSC2 and mTOR. *Proc Natl Acad Sci U S A* 2005;102:8573–8578.

166. Ambrosini G, Cheema HS, Seelman S, et al. Sorafenib inhibits growth and mitogen-activated protein kinase signaling in malignant peripheral nerve sheath cells. *Mol Cancer Ther* 2008;7:890–896.

167. Maki RG, D'Adamo DR, Keohan ML, et al. Phase II study of sorafenib in patients with metastatic or recurrent sarcomas. *J Clin Oncol* 2009;27:3133–3140.

168. Antonescu CR, Yoshida A, Guo T, et al. KDR activating mutations in human angiosarcomas are sensitive to specific kinase inhibitors. *Cancer Res* 2009;69:7175–7179.

169. Manner J, Radlwimmer B, Hohenberger P, et al. MYC high level gene amplification is a distinctive feature of angiosarcomas after irradiation or chronic lymphedema. *Am J Pathol* 2010;176:34–39.

172. Hadju M, Singer S, Maki RG, et al. IGF2 over-expression in solitary fibrous tumours is independent of anatomical location and is related to loss of imprinting. *J Pathol* 2010;221:300–307.

177. Metzker ML. Sequencing technologies—the next generation. *Nat Rev Genet* 2010;11:31–46.

178. Wang Z, Gerstein M, Snyder M. RNA-Seq: a revolutionary tool for transcriptomics. *Nat Rev Genet* 2009;10: 57–63.

180. Mortazavi A, Williams BA, McCue K, Schaeffer L, Wold B. Mapping and quantifying mammalian transcriptomes by RNA-Seq. *Nat Methods* 2008;5:621–628.

182. Strebhardt K, Ullrich A. Paul Ehrlich's magic bullet concept: 100 years of progress. *Nat Rev Cancer* 2008;8: 473–480.

185. Oltersdorf T, Elmore SW, Shoemaker AR, et al. An inhibitor of Bcl-2 family proteins induces regression of solid tumours. *Nature* 2005;435:677–681.

186. Schneider G, Fechner U. Computer-based de novo design of drug-like molecules. *Nat Rev Drug Discov* 2005;4: 649–663.

MOLECULAR BIOLOGY OF INDIVIDUAL CANCERS

CHAPTER 27 CUTANEOUS MELANOMA

LEVI A. GARRAWAY AND LYNDA CHIN

Cutaneous melanoma arises from pigment-producing epidermal melanocytes and is the major cause of mortality among skin malignancies. Its incidence has risen steadily at a rate of 3% per year over the past 25 years,[1] with an estimated 68,130 new cases and 8,700 deaths predicted for the United States alone in 2010. Despite a high cure rate for localized primary melanoma (98.3% 5-year survival rate), its aggressive nature results in rapid metastasis to distant sites and a concomitant drop to a 16% 5-year survival rate. Although exposure to ultraviolet (UV) radiation is a known factor contributing to melanoma development, the exact molecular changes that take place in incipient and progressing tumors are still being elucidated.

Currently, vertical tumor (Breslow) thickness (in millimeters) provides the best single indicator of prognosis. This measurement is augmented by additional parameters, including the presence of ulceration, penetration through cutaneous layers, mitotic rate, evidence of "in transit" metastasis, tumor spread to draining lymph nodes, and the presence of distant metastasis. Although melanoma sometimes arises in pre-existing nevi, recent data have demonstrated that typical nevi represent senescent lesions that may be irreversibly growth arrested.[2] It is therefore plausible that a substantial fraction of melanomas may alternatively emerge from normal melanocytes via deregulation of oncogenes or tumor suppressors implicated in melanocytic transformation (Fig. 27.1). The myriad genes involved with melanoma genesis and progression have been subjected to varying degrees of validation in humans, in model organisms, and in cell culture (Table 27.1). The identification of these genes and their associated genetic pathways influences diagnosis and prognosis and shows considerable promise in aiding targeted therapeutic implementation.

THE CDKN2A LOCUS

As many as 70% of melanomas harbor somatic mutations or deletions affecting the CDKN2A locus on chromosome 9p21.[3,4] This observation, together with the initial identification of germline homozygous deletions of CDKN2A as susceptibility events in familial melanoma kindreds,[5] indicates a central role for this locus in melanoma pathogenesis. This locus contains an unusual gene organization, which allows for two separate transcripts and corresponding tumor suppressor gene products to be produced: p16^{INK4A} and p19^{ARF} (Fig. 27.2). Loss of p16^{INK4A} results in the suppression of retinoblastoma (RB) tumor suppressor activity via increased activation of the CDK4/6-cyclin D1 complex; loss of ARF (p14^{ARF} in human and p19^{ARF} in mouse) down-modulates p53 activity through increased activation of MDM2. Thus, deletion of the entire locus accomplishes the inactivation of two critical tumor suppressor pathways: RB and p53. Homozygous deletion of exons 2 and 3 of the mouse Cdkn2a homolog predisposed to a high incidence of melanomas when combined with an activated H-RAS transgene in melanocytes.[6] Thus, CDKN2A lesions may "prime" melanocytic tissue for neoplasia.

THE RETINOBLASTOMA PATHWAY

The RB pathway is responsible for preventing inappropriate cell cycle entry, and germline heterozygous loss of the RB1 gene triggers retinoblastoma. The tumor-modulating properties of the RB pathway are well established in many solid cancers, and its deregulation in melanoma is evidenced by mutations in INK4A, CDK4, or occasionally RB1 itself, as described below.

INK4A

Human intragenic mutations of INK4A that do not affect the ARF coding region preferentially disrupt the RB pathway and sensitize germline carriers to the development of melanomas.[7] In a mouse model engineered to be deficient only for Ink4a (with intact ARF), melanoma formation was observed in cooperation with an oncogenic

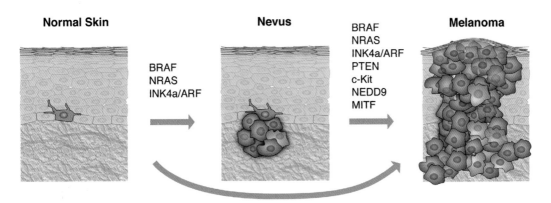

FIGURE 27.1 Validated genes mutated or deregulated in melanoma progression. Progression of normal melanocytes to metastatic melanoma is diagrammed with associated genetic events as a linear process, although in a majority of the cases, melanomas may not arise from a pre-existing nevus. The degree to which the association of each gene has been experimentally validated is shown in Table 27.1.

initiating event (activated H-RAS), albeit with a longer latency than in mice with deletions affecting the entire locus.[8] Notably, the tumors in these mice were also found to harbor either deletion of ARF or mutation of p53. Therefore, while INK4A is a *bona fide* tumor suppressor, additional genetic dysregulation of the p53 pathway seems obligatory for melanoma genesis, at least in the mouse.

MOLECULAR BIOLOGY OF INDIVIDUAL CANCERS

TABLE 27.1

SUMMARY OF VALIDATED GENES INVOLVED IN MELANOMA GENESIS AND PROGRESSION

Methods of Discovery	Melanoma Gene	Proposed Gene Product Behavior	H	E	I	O	K	X	P	M	Ref.
Linkage mapping	INK4A, ARF	Tumor suppressors	•	•	•	•	•	•	•	•	Reviewed in 17
Linkage mapping	NRAS, BRAF	Oncogenes	•	•	•	•	•	•	•	•	Reviewed in 17
Linkage mapping	PTEN	Tumor suppressor	•	•	•	•			•	•	Reviewed in 17
Copy number profiling	NEDD9	Metastasis enhancer	•	•	•		•	•	•		92
Copy number profiling	MITF	Oncogene	•	•	•	•	•		•		75
Expression profiling	WNT5A	Metastasis enhancer		•	•	•	•		•		86
Copy number profiling	GOLPH3	Oncogene	•	•	•	•	•	•	•		100
Copy number profiling	ETV1	Oncogene	•	•	•	•	•	•	•		79
DNA sequencing	ERBB4	Oncogene	•		•	•	•	•			72
RNAi screening	IGFBP7, GAS1	Tumor suppressor / Metastasis suppressor		•	•	•	•	•			101, 102

H, (human gene aberrations) indicates known mutation, amplification, deletion, or focal loss of heterozygosity (LOH) in patients; E, (expression validation) is achieved by reverse transcription-polymerase chain reaction (RT-PCR), Northern, or Western blots; I, (immunohistocompatibility [IHC] or tissue microarrays) refers to histological protein analysis; O, overexpression; K, (knockdown/dominant negative); X, (xenograft) refers to manipulation of gene expression in cell lines; P, (pathway) indicates studies of interactions with putative pathway members; M, (mouse model of melanoma) indicates validation through genetic engineering in mice.

FIGURE 27.2 The unusual genomic structure and products of the *CDKN2A* locus.
A: INK4A and ARF (p14^ARF in human and
p19^ARF in mouse) initiate in different first
exons and share the coding exon 2, but in
an alterative reading frame, thus encoding
two proteins with no amino acid similarity.
The involvement of the neighboring and
related *CDKN2B* locus in the pathology of
melanoma is unclear, although it is often
deleted in conjunction with *CDKN2A*.
(From ref. 3.) **B:** ARF participates in the
p53 pathway by binding to and sequestering the p53 antagonist, MDM2. The loss
of ARF therefore results in the net degradation of p53 by MDM2-mediated ubiquitination. p16^INK4A inhibits the action of
the CDK4/CDK6-cyclin D1 complex in the
retinoblastoma (RB) pathway. The loss of
p16^INK4A results in the phosphorylation
and inactivation of pRB leading to its
uncoupling from the transcription factor
E2F, allowing for transcription of E2F target genes that are required for cell cycle
progression from G_1 to S phase.

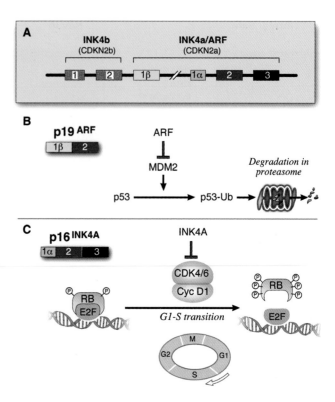

CDK4

CDK4 is a direct target of inhibition by p16^INK4A
(Fig. 27.2) and is a primary regulator of RB activation. Rare germline mutations of *CDK4* that
render the protein insensitive to inhibition by
INK4A (e.g., Arg24Cys) have been identified in a
melanoma-prone kindred.[9] These tumors retain
wild type INK4A function, suggesting that
INK4A is epistatic to CDK4 and that RB pathway deregulation is central to melanoma genesis.
Somatic focal amplifications of *CDK4* are also
observed (albeit rarely) in sporadic melanomas.[10]
Carcinogen treatment induced melanomas in the
animals without somatic Ink4a inactivation, similar to the mutual exclusivity observed in familial
melanoma.[11]

RB1

Germline mutations in *RB1* confer predisposition
to melanoma in patients who have survived bilateral retinoblastoma.[12] These melanomas exhibit
loss of heterozygosity (LOH) of the remaining
wild type RB1 allele. In such patients, estimates of
increased lifetime risk of melanoma range from
4- to 80-fold. Interestingly, the *RB1* gene locus is
frequently deleted in primary cutaneous
melanomas,[13] and RB1 may be subject to genomic
rearrangement in rare instances.[14]

THE p53 PATHWAY

The p53 pathway is critical for maintenance of
the normal genome by regulating a multiplicity of
mechanisms, including cell cycle checkpoints,
DNA damage repair activation, and the appropriate induction of apoptosis. Mutations in the *TP53*
gene occur in over 50% of all tumors. Although
the *TP53* locus is rarely mutated in human
melanomas,[15] this region appears to undergo copy
neutral LOH at enhanced frequency, at least in
advanced tumors.[4] Furthermore, loss of p53 in
mice cooperates with activated H-Ras to induce
melanomas.[16] Thus, while *TP53* is rarely deleted
in human melanomas, inactivation of its pathway
appears critical for melanoma genesis.

ARF

ARF-specific insertions, deletions, and splice
donor mutations have been described in human
melanomas.[17] However, it remains ambiguous
whether the genetic disruption of ARF alone is
sufficient for tumorigenesis. In mouse models,
Arf-specific deletion in conjunction with activated
H-RAS leads to a similar melanoma phenotype as
the *Ink4a*-specific deletion mouse mentioned
above[8]; however, *Arf*-mutant melanomas were
enriched for mutations in the RB pathway.
Notably, upon UV radiation these mice developed

focal amplifications at the *Cdk6* locus,[18] which encodes an orthologue to CDK4. Furthermore, p53 heterozygous mouse melanomas retain Arf, demonstrating their epistatic relationship.[16]

THE MAP KINASE PATHWAY

Extensive genetic and mechanistic studies have unearthed a prevalence of activating mitogen-activated protein kinase (MAPK) pathway mutations across many tumor types. The focal point of MAPK activation is the ERK1/2 kinases, which mediate the transcription of many genes governing cell proliferation and survival (Fig. 27.3). In nontransformed cells, key MAPK effectors have also been shown to regulate differentiation and senescence.

THE RAS FAMILY: H-, N-, AND K-RAS

Increasing evidence shows that the three different members of the classical RAS oncogene family exert functionally separable roles. N-RAS is the most frequently targeted in melanoma (33% of primary and 26% of metastatic samples[19]), followed by H-RAS (mainly in Spitz nevi).[20] Despite their high incidence in other cancer types, K-RAS mutations are rarely observed in melanocytic lesions.[21,22] Interestingly, although N-RAS mutations are found in 54% of congenital nevi, they are rare in dysplastic nevi,[23] implying a distinct evolutionary path from dysplastic nevi to melanoma.

In mouse models, overexpression of activated H-RAS or N-RAS on an Ink4a/Arf-null background results in spontaneous melanoma formation.[6,24] However, while H-RAS-induced

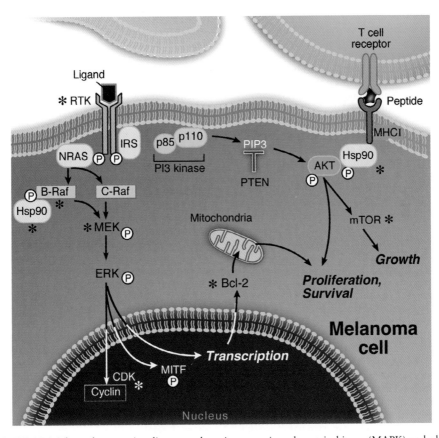

FIGURE 27.3 The melanoma signaling cascades mitogen-activated protein kinase (MAPK) and phosphatidylinositol 3-kinase (PI3K). The MAPK pathway is hyperactivated in melanomas, mainly due to activating mutations in either the NRAS or BRAF genes. The sequential phosphorylations of the downstream MEK and ERK proteins ultimately results in the activation of a number of transcription factors, including MITF, which induce cell proliferation and survival. The PI3K pathway is mainly hyperactivated by loss of the PTEN tumor suppressor, which results in the phosphorylation and activation of the survival gene *AKT* and subsequent stimulation of the mitogenic mammalian target of rapamycin (mTOR) pathway. The relative independence of the MAPK and PI3K pathways is supported by the apparent need for mutations that affect both.

melanomas rarely, if ever, metastasize, N-RAS tumors frequently metastasize to draining lymph nodes and distal organs, in line with the apparent selection for N-RAS over H-RAS mutations in human melanomas. Knockdown of *NRAS* in human melanoma cell lines inhibits their viability, indicating dependency on this oncogene for tumorigenicity.[25] Furthermore, shutting off transgene expression in an inducible H-RAS model caused regression of melanomas that arose following transgene induction, thereby confirming the RAS oncogene dependency in these tumors.[26]

BRAF

Somatic, activating *BRAF* mutations occur at high frequency in melanoma. These mutations are dominated by a single T→A transversion, resulting in a valine to glutamate amino acid substitution (V600E). Although the T→A transversion is not classically associated with UV-induced damage, BRAF mutations appear to be more common in melanomas arising at sites with intermittent exposure to UV.[13,27] On the other hand, melanomas from chronically sun-damaged skin are typically wild type for *BRAF*.[13] BRAF mutations may be an early preneoplastic event, given their high incidence in benign and dysplastic nevi (Fig. 27.1).[28]

BRAF is an immediate downstream target of RAS (Fig. 27.3) in the MAPK pathway. The BRAF(V600E) mutation confers more than 500-fold induction of kinase activity *in vitro*; this dramatic effect may explain why the V600E mutation dominates in BRAF-mutant melanoma. BRAF(V600E) mutations are often observed in conjunction with PTEN loss (see below), implying that dual modulation of MAPK and phosphatidylinositol 3-kinase (PI3K) pathways may promote a fully transformed phenotype.

Extensive data suggest that wild type BRAF operates on a senescence pathway in benign human nevi. Transgenic expression of BRAF(V600E) targeted to melanocytes in zebrafish produced benign nevuslike lesions, whereas invasive melanomas were produced (after extended latency) when crossed into p53 deficient zebrafish.[29] Inducible expression of BRAF(V600E) alone in murine melanocytes resulted in excessive skin pigmentation and the appearance of nevi containing hallmarks of senescence.[30] Human congenital nevi with activating BRAF mutations were shown to express senescence-associated acidic β-galactosidase (SA-β-Gal), the classical senescence-associated marker.[2] This implied that activated BRAF alone is insufficient to induce tumor progression beyond the nevus stage in patients (Fig. 27.1). Interestingly, immunohistochemical staining of nevoid tissues found heterogeneous patterns of INK4A that only partially overlapped with SA-β-Gal, suggesting the presence of INK4A-independent pathway(s) operative in oncogene-induced senescence.

The high prevalence of activating BRAF and NRAS mutations implied that the MAPK cascade might confer a "drugable" melanoma tumor dependency when such mutations were present. This notion was supported by several lines of preclinical evidence, particularly in BRAF(V600E) melanomas. For example, constitutive ERK activation in BRAF[V600E] cells was required for their continued proliferation.[31–33] RNAi knockdown of BRAF in this genetic context inhibited ERK activation, blunted cell growth, and in some cases induced apoptosis *in vitro*.[31,32] BRAF silencing also suppressed anchorage-independent growth and tumor formation in BRAF(V600E) melanomas.[34] As noted above, suppression of NRAS expression in *NRAS*-mutant melanomas resulted in similar growth inhibitory effects.[25] Thus, BRAF or NRAS oncogenic mutations appeared to elaborate a stringent melanoma tumor dependency through aberrant MAPK pathway activation.

In BRAF(V600E) melanomas, the mechanistic basis for oncogene dependency appears to involve both proliferative and apoptotic regulation. Oncogenic *BRAF* inhibits BIM, a pro-apoptotic member of the BCL-2 protein family,[35] and suppression of BRAF activity facilitates translocation of the pro-apoptotic protein BMF to the cytosol in cells harboring the mutation.[36] Moreover, two downstream effectors of RAF signaling—ERK and RSK—were shown to phosphorylate and inhibit the LKB1 tumor suppressor. This results in an inability of LKB1 to activate AMP kinase, which normally down-regulates cell growth under various stress conditions.[37] Thus, activated B-RAF and downstream MAPK effectors appear to augment multiple melanoma cell growth and survival pathways.

The emergence of selective RAF inhibitors has provided an opportunity to evaluate the "drugability" of *BRAF* and *NRAS* oncogene mutations *in vitro* and in the clinical setting. Toward this end, small molecule RAF inhibitors such as PLX4032 potently suppressed the growth of BRAF(V600E) melanoma cells, whereas this inhibitor had little effect on cancer cells lacking this mutation.[38,39] Selective RAF inhibitors also suppressed the formation of BRAF(V600E) tumors in murine xenograft models.[40] These data suggest that stratification of melanomas according to BRAF(V600E) status might be enriched for patients most likely to benefit from small molecule RAF or MEK inhibitors. Recent clinical trial results with selective RAF inhibitors have borne out this prediction. In a phase 1 trial of PLX4032, the overall response rate of BRAF(V600E) melanomas was 90%, with nearly 80% experiencing a partial response by Response Evaluation Criteria in Solid Tumors (RECIST) criteria.[41] NRAS-mutant melanomas did not respond to this agent. Similar results have also been observed with other investigational RAF inhibitors. These initial observations raise the possibility that RAF inhibition may ultimately gain a prominent role in the clinical management of BRAF(V600E) melanomas.

In light of the substantial evidence for "drugable" RAF dependency described above, it was somewhat surprising that selective RAF inhibition showed minimal efficacy against *NRAS*-mutant melanomas both *in vitro* and in early clinical studies. Initial insights into this puzzling discordance emerged from several reports that showed that exposure of RAS-activated cancer cells to selective RAF inhibitors paradoxically increased MAPK signaling, as measured by increased p-MEK and p-ERK levels.[42–44] Biochemical studies revealed that inhibitor-bound BRAF polypeptides retained an ability to form homo- or heterodimers with other (drug-free) RAF molecules, and that this dimerization was associated with MEK phosphorylation in the setting of RAS activation. These provocative results may help explain why some RAF inhibitors fail to inhibit MAPK signaling in cells lacking BRAF(V600E) mutations (e.g., RAS mutant cells). They may also provide a basis for the unexpectedly high incidence (25% to 30%) of keratocanthomas and squamous cell carcinomas that arise in patients treated with selective RAF inhibition.[41]

MEK

Since the MEK1/2 serine-threonine kinases transmit the critical MAPK signal downstream of RAS and RAF, considerable interest has also emerged regarding these kinases in melanoma biology and therapeutics. In contrast to *NRAS* and *BRAF*, MEK1/2 mutations are rare in melanoma (indeed, in cancer in general), although they have occasionally been reported.[45] Nonetheless, pharmacologic MEK inhibition presented another possible therapeutic inroad into *BRAF*- or *NRAS*-mutant melanomas. Robust preclinical evidence favoring this notion derived from a genetic and pharmacologic analysis showing that various MEK inhibitory compounds demonstrated markedly enhanced potency against BRAF(V600E) cancer cells compared to cell lines lacking oncogenic MAPK pathway mutations.[46] In contrast to studies with selective RAF inhibitors, at least some NRAS-mutant melanoma cells were also sensitive to MEK inhibitors, suggesting that the utility of MEK inhibition might extend beyond the BRAF(V600E) context in some cases.[46]

Although initial clinical trial results of MEK inhibition in melanoma were disappointing compared to the RAF inhibitor trials described above, more recent studies have yielded responses in patients with BRAF(V600E) mutations following MEK inhibitor treatment.[47] In addition, molecular analyses have provided an initial glimpse into how mechanisms of resistance might emerge to targeted MAPK pathway inhibition. In one case, a single relapsing focus was resected from a patient who was otherwise responsive to the MEK inhibitor AZD6244[48]; the resistant tumor was found to harbor a somatic *MEK1* mutation capable of conferring resistance to both MEK and BRAF inhibition *in vitro*. These intriguing translational studies have also triggered trials of combined RAF and MEK inhibition as a means to augment the magnitude or duration of clinical responses in BRAF(V600E) melanoma patients. A comprehensive elaboration of resistance to both RAF and MEK inhibition may provide new insights into possible combination therapeutic trials directed against this genetically defined tumor subtype.

THE PHOSPHATIDYLINOSITOL 3-KINASE PATHWAY

The PI3K pathway operates mainly through the downstream activation of the survival kinase AKT (Fig. 27.3), which activates the growth-promoting mammalian target of rapamycin (mTOR) pathway and inhibits proapoptotic effectors such as caspase 9 and BAD. PI3K was capable of replacing N-RAS to induce invasive melanomas in a skin xenograft model.[49] However, unlike the MAPK pathway, genetic alterations specifically targeting components of the PI3K signaling cascade do not occur at high frequency in melanoma.[50]

Several lines of evidence support the cooperative effects of MAPK and PI3K dysregulation in melanoma genesis. For example, transformation of immortalized human melanocytes required the combination of activated BRAF and PI3K, but not BRAF alone, in an artificial skin graft model system.[26] More recently, concomitant expression of oncogenic BRAF together with PTEN silencing in an inducible melanocyte-specific mouse model resulted in robust melanoma development with 100% penetrance.[30,51] These melanomas arose following a short latency and exhibited a high propensity for metastatic dissemination. Together, these data suggest that dysregulated BRAF and PI3K signaling may underpin melanoma genesis in certain subsets of melanomas. Toward this end, a recent study suggested that N-RAS-mutant melanomas may show enhanced reliance on RalGEF signaling,[52] which can be operant downstream of RAS in several contexts.

PTEN

Of the PI3K pathway mutations that do occur, losses of chromosome 10q encompassing PTEN tumor suppressor is the most frequent, the caveat being that additional tumor suppressor(s) may reside in this region (see below). PTEN normally down-regulates phosphorylated AKT via suppression of the second messenger PIP$_3$ (Fig. 27.3). In various genetically engineered mice bearing solid tumors, PTEN loss can be analogous to p53 inactivation, in that one or the other can be gating for oncogenesis. In melanoma, somatic point mutations and homozygous deletions of PTEN are uncommon. Although allelic loss of PTEN is observed only in about 20% of melanoma, loss of expression of PTEN is reported to be in the range of 40% of melanoma tumors,[53] suggesting other mechanisms of its inactivation. Functionally, ectopic expression of PTEN in PTEN-deficient melanoma cells can abolish phospho-AKT activity, induce apoptosis, and suppress growth, tumorigenicity, and metastasis.[50] Correspondingly, heterozygous germline or homozygous somatic inactivation of *Pten* in the mouse strongly promoted tumor formation in multiple cell lineages, a phenotype that was accelerated by the additional deletion of *Ink4a/Arf*.[54] Significantly, these double mutants developed melanoma at low penetrance, consistent with the hypothesis that PTEN inactivation in human melanoma may require additional genetic events such as the commonly associated BRAF(V600E) mutation. As noted above, this hypothesis was recently borne out in a mouse model of simultaneous PTEN loss and oncogenic BRAF induction in melanocytes.[51] The relevance of PTEN inactivation in NRAS-mutant melanomas is less clear; however, studies in genetically engineered mouse models raise the possibility that RAS and PTEN inactivation may also interact to promote melanoma genesis and metastasis.[55]

Many melanomas harbor chromosome arm level hemizygous deletions involving the *PTEN* locus (10q24), although not all are specific to *PTEN*.[4] Thus, other tumor suppressors may exist in this genomic region. The Myc antagonist *MXI* represents one possibility, as *Myc* is amplified or overexpressed in *RAS*-induced *Trp53*-deficient melanomas in the mouse.[16] Other candidate tumor suppressor genes from chromosome 10q include *CUL2* and *KLF6*; both genes are significantly down-regulated in melanomas harboring 10q deletions,[4] although functional evidence that they exert tumor suppressor roles remains scant.

AKT

Elevated phospho-AKT (indicative of activation) has been adversely associated with patient survival[56] and is common in BRAF(V600E) melanomas.[57] Elevated phospho-AKT was particularly manifest in melanoma brain metastases compared to other metastatic sites.[57] Copy number gains of the *AKT3* locus and rare AKT3 point mutations[58] have been detected in melanomas, suggesting that the AKT signaling point itself may be oncogenic.[59] Interestingly, targeted depletion of AKT3 could trigger apoptosis,[59] while AKT1 behaved as a tumor suppressor in melanoma cell lines,[60] raising the possibility of partially nonredundant functions of AKT isoforms.

RECEPTOR TYROSINE KINASES

Receptor tyrosine kinsases (RTKs) are a diverse family of transmembrane kinases that have been implicated in many neoplasms. Several RTKs map to known regions of recurrent melanoma DNA copy number gain or amplification, with corresponding alterations in their expression levels.

c-KIT

The c-Kit gene plays an essential role in melanocyte development, as does its ligand, stem cell factor. Mutation of either results in pigmentation deficiencies, and injection of c-Kit blocking antibody in mice was used to identify the presence of melanocyte stem cells within hair follicles.[61] Numerous immunohistochemical studies have linked progressive loss of c-KIT expression with the transition from benign to primary and metastatic melanomas.[62–64] Thus, at first glance, KIT appeared to be inactivated during melanoma genesis and progression.

However, KIT is somatically activated by point mutations in a specific subset of melanomas that arise within mucosal, acral, or chronic sun-damaged surfaces of the body.[13] High-resolution amplicon melting analyses followed by direct DNA sequencing revealed that three of these mutations harbored a L576P mutation with selective loss of the normal allele.[65] L576P is a known gastrointestinal stromal tumor–associated mutation that maps to the 5′ juxtamembrane domain where most activating KIT mutations cluster.[66] Importantly, these observations suggest the potential utility of c-KIT targeted kinase inhibitors for this subset of previously incurable melanoma patients. Initial case reports have provided preliminary support for this notion.[67] Clinical trials using imatinib are currently under way to determine whether this discovery may represent a major opportunity for targeted therapy in melanoma as previously shown for gastrointestinal stromal tumors.

EPIDERMAL GROWTH FACTOR RECEPTOR FAMILY

The epidermal growth factor receptor (EGFR) activates both the MAPK and PI3K pathways in many cell types. In melanomas, copy number gain of chromosome 7 (where the *EGFR* gene resides) is linked to overexpression of EGFR, despite the lack of focal amplifications.[68] EGFR activation increased the number of visceral metastases in severe combined immunodeficiency (SCID) mouse xenografts without affecting melanoma growth *in vitro*.[69] In the inducible H-RAS mouse model,[26] transcriptomic analysis revealed up-regulation of EGF family ligands including amphiregulin and epiregulin.[70] Furthermore, expression of a dominant negative form of EGFR abolished the tumorigenicity of RAS-driven melanoma cells, indicating that the MAPK pathway is dependent on an uncompromised EGFR signal.[71]

A sequencing-based study of the tyrosine kinome in melanoma found that *ERBB4* mutations may affect as many as 20% of melanomas.[72] Unlike other well-known oncogene mutations, the *ERBB4* mutations identified in this study were mostly nonrecurrent (e.g., the same amino acid or conserved region was rarely affected); however, ERBB4 mutations correlated with increased activation of and dependence on the corresponding protein for viability. If validated by resequencing of large independent sample cohorts, targeted therapeutics against ERBB4 and perhaps other members of the EGFR family may warrant investigation in melanoma.

c-MET

The c-MET gene product and its ligand hepatocyte growth factor/scatter factor (HGF/SF) are known to activate the MAPK pathway, but both have many additional functions. Overexpression of c-MET and HGF is correlated with melanoma progression. Copy gains involving the c-MET locus at 7q33-qter are associated with invasive and metastatic cancers in humans,[73] and elevated MET/HGF expression is correlated with metastatic ability in murine melanoma explants.[47] HGF/SF overexpression in a transgenic mouse model triggered spontaneous melanoma formation after a long latency (up to 2 years); however, time to tumor onset was greatly reduced by exposure to UVB or Ink4a/Arf deficiency.[74] Thus, HGF/MET signaling may play an important role in melanoma genesis and progression. The development of MET inhibitors should allow formal testing of this hypothesis in melanoma patients.

THE MITF PATHWAY

MITF encodes a lineage transcription factor whose function is critical to the survival of normal melanocytes. The identification of *MITF* amplification in melanoma defined this transcription factor as a central modifier of melanoma.[75] In so doing, this discovery identified a novel class of oncogenes termed *lineage survival* oncogenes.[76,77] That is, a tumor may "hijack" extant lineage survival mechanisms in the presence of selective pressures to ensure its own propagation. The elucidation of *MITF* as an oncogene took a cross-tissue approach, wherein the NCI-60 cell line panel representing nine tumor

types was subjected to both gene expression and high-density single-nucleotide polymorphism (SNP) array analysis.[75] A recurrent gain of 3p13–14 significantly segregated melanoma from other tumor classes, with MITF as the only gene in the region showing maximal amplification and overexpression. MITF amplification was subsequently detected in 10% of primary cutaneous and 15% to 20% of metastatic melanomas by fluorescence *in situ* hybridization, correlating with decreased survival in Kaplan-Meier analyses of 5-year patient survival. Exogenous MITF, in combination with activated BRAF, showed transforming capabilities in immortalized primary human melanocytes. Additionally, inhibition of MITF in cell lines showing 3p13–14 amplification reduced growth and survival and conferred sensitivity to certain anticancer drugs. MITF gene disruption leads to coat color defects in mice and pigmentation defects in humans, due to diminished viability of melanocytes. This suggested that MITF was essential for the lineage survival of melanocytes, supporting the contention that it is also critical for the survival of melanomas.

The downstream elements of the MITF pathway include both pigment enzyme genes as well as genes involved in proliferation and survival. MITF intersects with a number of established melanoma pathways, including the transcriptional activation of INK4A, c-Met, and CDK2.[17] Moreover, MITF is activated downstream of both c-Kit and MAPK signaling, via ERK-directed phosphorylation (Fig. 27.3).[78] Additionally, activated BRAF is known to target MITF for proteolytic degradation, which may select for refractory cellular variants harboring amplified MITF. Recently, the ETS transcription factor ETV1 was found to positively regulate MITF expression in melanoma, and *ETV1* may function as an amplified melanoma oncogene in its own right.[79] Furthermore, the mouse Bcl2 proapoptotic gene was shown to be a transcriptional target of MITF.[80] Collectively, these observations place MITF in a central role of melanoma signal integration.

THE WNT PATHWAY

WNT signaling has long been implicated in a variety of cancers. Its activation of downstream transcriptional events has been hypothesized to control lineage commitment and differentiation fates as well as self-renewal properties. The WNT pathway has also been linked to major developmental decisions in neural crest derivatives, with a differentiation bias toward the melanocytic lineage.[81] Additionally, the WNT pathway appears to intersect with MITF functionality at several levels, including direct interactions between MITF and the WNT downstream transcriptional coactivator LEF-1.[82] WNT signaling may augment MITF expression, and MITF may mediate at least a portion of WNT functionality in melanoma.[83]

CTNNB1 and WNT5A

Stabilizing *CTTNB1* mutations that render β-catenin resistant to proteolytic degradation promote tumorigenesis. Such mutations are uncommon in patient samples, despite a high incidence in melanoma cell lines.[84] Nevertheless, a significant fraction of clinical melanoma lesions exhibit immunohistochemical evidence of nuclear β-catenin localization,[85] a hallmark of WNT pathway activation. Additional evidence for the importance of the WNT pathway emerged from gene expression studies that identified a β-catenin-independent Wnt5a signaling pathway correlated with higher grades of clinical melanoma samples.[86] Engineered overexpression of Wnt5a enhanced the *in vitro* invasiveness of melanoma cells, a property suppressed by blockade of the Wnt5a receptor Frizzled-5. Mechanistically, Wnt5a was shown to enhance the action of the PKC pathway, which is believed to control cell adhesion and motility.

THE MC1R PATHWAY

Pigmentation exerts a major influence on skin tumor susceptibility, as it is well documented that fair skin is more sensitive to UV radiation and melanoma genesis. The mechanism underlying this observation is partially explained by the protective effects of melanin, which is produced by melanocytes and distributed to interfollicular keratinocytes. Genetically, the red hair color/pale skin (RHC) phenotype is linked to variant alleles of the melanocyte-specific melanocortin 1 receptor gene (MC1R), which is central to melanin synthesis.[87] The ligand for the G-protein–coupled MC1R is the MSH peptide, which activates downstream signaling consisting of a cAMP-CREB/ATF1 cascade, culminating in the induced expression of MITF. Not all individuals carrying RHC alleles have identical melanin production, yet increased risk for melanoma genesis remains notable regardless,[88] implying that melanin-independent mechanisms might impact the susceptibility of RHC carriers. One possible node is cAMP, the MC1R as second messenger, which may activate pathways incompletely understood at present, such as MAPK and PI3K.[89]

Recent data have implicated the MSH/MC1R pathway in the normal UV pigmentation (tanning) response in skin, a response that is linked to skin cancer (and melanoma) risk in humans. A "redhead" mouse model (frameshift mutation in *MC1R*) was used to demonstrate that the UV-tanning response is dependent on MC1R signaling, because keratinocytes respond to UV by strongly up-regulating expression of MSH. The "fairskin" phenotype was rescued by topical administration of a small molecule cAMP agonist.[90] The resulting dark pigmentation in genetically redhead mice was protective against UV-induced skin carcinogenesis. Subsequent analyses revealed that the p53 tumor suppressor protein may function as a "UV sensor" in keratinocytes, translating UV damage into direct transcriptional stimulation of MSH expression.[91]

THE FAK PATHWAY

NEDD9 was recently demonstrated to enhance the metastatic efficiency of both mouse melanomas and human cell lines by activation of the FAK pathway, which enhances cell motility and adhesion.[92] The discovery of these properties of NEDD9 was enabled by the evolutionary conservation of genetic pathways, which highlighted significant genetic changes when mouse tumors were compared to human melanomas. Array comparative genomic hybridization analysis of metastatic and nonmetastatic tumors derived from the *Ink4a/Arf*$^{-/-}$ inducible H-RAS mouse melanoma model[26] pinpointed an 850 kb minimal common region (MCR) of amplification on chromosome 13. Only one gene in this MCR, *Nedd9*, showed a significant up-regulation in metastatic mouse melanomas but not in normal melanocytes or nonmetastatic melanomas. The syntenic human region, 6p24–25, similarly undergoes copy number gain in 36% of human metastatic but not nonmetastatic melanomas.[92] The cross-species comparison allowed the delimitation of a focal region of interest and designation of NEDD9 as a candidate target of 6p gain in humans.

NEDD9 appears to modulate metastasis activity *in vitro* and *in vivo*. In cell-based assays, invasiveness of human melanoma cells was enhanced or inhibited by overexpression or knockdown of *NEDD9*, respectively. Similarly, knockdown of Nedd9 in metastatic melanoma cells with Nedd9 amplification drastically inhibited distal metastasis to various organs from subcutaneous primary tumor sites. Furthermore, inhibition of FAK itself abolished the invasive potential conferred by NEDD9 in Boyden chamber assays, implicating the entire pathway in metastasis.[92] NEDD9 expression was found to be up-regulated in 50% of primary melanomas when compared to benign nevi, raising the possibility that NEDD9 might confer other biological activities during the early stages of melanoma genesis and that elevated NEDD9 expression might predict a risk of future metastasis.

CANCER STEM CELLS AND MELANOMA

Evidence supporting the biological and therapeutic relevance of a precursor tumor stem cell population has been cited in several tumor types; however, the role of cancer stem cells in melanoma remains controversial. Enthusiasm for a melanoma stem cell model was augmented by a study of ABCB5, an adenosine triphosphate–binding cassette transporter whose homologues have been implicated in stem cell multidrug resistance.[93] Cancer cells expressing high ABCB5 were found to correlate significantly with melanocytic lineage and multidrug resistance in the NCI-60 cell line set.[93,94] Mechanistically, ABCB5 was shown to mediate efflux of the anticancer drug doxorubicin and resistance to melanoma cell killing by this agent via modulation of membrane potential. Notably, the tissue distribution of ABCB5 protein partially colocalized with the putative stem cell marker CD133, suggesting that the drug resistance phenotype might be most closely associated with a long-lived, refractory stem cell population.

Evidence challenging the melanoma stem cell model emerged from xenotransplantation studies in immunocompromised mice. Whereas numerous studies in support of cancer stem cells utilized nonobese diabetic/severe combined immunodeficient (NOD/SCID) mice to show that only approximately 1 of 10,000 tumor cells was capable of tumor initiation, a more recent study employed a more severely immunocompromised strain (NOD/SCID interleukin-2 receptor gamma chain null [Il2rg2/2]).[95] In this setting, more than 1 of 4 melanoma cells were capable of tumor initiation; furthermore, neither ABCB5 nor any other stem cell marker expression could stratify the cells based on tumorigenic efficiency.[95] These results suggest that the "classic" tumor stem cell hypothesis may not fully explain melanoma tumorigenesis; on the other hand, it remains unclear which (if any) xenotransplantation context accurately models the tumor stem cell phenotype. Additional studies are therefore needed to determine the extent to which stem cell features modify melanoma biology or chemotherapeutic response.

CANCER GENOMICS AND TRANSLATION

Advances in sequencing technology have made it possible to obtain the complete genome sequence of entire cancer genomes at ever diminishing costs. Together with developments in computational biology, these advances promise to usher in a new understanding of cancer genome alterations and the tumorigenic mechanisms that result. One of the first cancer genomes to be sequenced was that of a cell line (and its paired normal counterpart) derived from a patient with metastatic melanoma.[96] This effort uncovered more than 33,000 somatic base substitutions, of which 187 were nonsynonymous coding mutations. As expected, most base mutations were C→T transitions indicative of ultraviolet exposure. However, the distribution of mutations across the genome was uneven, with a diminished

prevalence in "gene footprint" areas.[96] This distribution suggested the presence of transcription-coupled DNA repair in these regions. Thus, the complete sequence of this melanoma genome highlighted the mutational and selection dynamics that gave rise to this tumor.

Other studies have investigated the global transcriptional alterations characteristic of melanoma by deploying similar sequencing technologies to characterize cDNA from melanomas (termed RNA-seq). One recent RNA-seq study of ten melanomas (eight "short-term" cultures and two cell lines) identified multiple gene fusions, chimeric transcripts, splice isoforms, and base mutations not previously described.[14] Whereas the gene fusions derived from structural genomic alterations occurred uniquely, several chimeric "read-through" transcripts (transcripts consisting of exons from two adjacent genes) were recurrently detected in different tumors. One such read-through event involved CDK2, a kinase involved in melanoma cell division that is also a transcriptional target of MITF.[14,97]

The high UV-associated base mutation rate in melanoma suggests that nearly 2% of all genes may harbor nonsynonymous coding mutations in a typical cutaneous melanoma, most of which are likely to be "passenger" events with little biological consequence to melanoma genesis or progression. Thus, cataloging all significant genomic alterations that might represent "driver" events (see below) will require not only sequencing hundreds of tumor specimens but also the principled application of increasingly sophisticated analytical methods for data deconvolution. Several large-scale U.S. (Cancer Genome Atlas) and international efforts (International Cancer Genomic Consortium)[98] have taken on the ambitious goal of comprehensively characterizing the genomes of diverse human tumors including melanomas. Thus, it seems certain that the next decade will witness major breakthroughs in melanoma genome characterization that inform the biology and treatment of this malignancy.

Distinguishing "driver" events that may confer transforming activity or dictate prognosis or response to emerging targeted therapeutics will also require intensive functional validation efforts.[99] An example of this was the recent discovery of GOLPH3 as an oncogene in melanoma.[100] Intersection of chromosomal copy number variations (CNVs) in melanoma with those observed in other tumors followed by multilevel functional and clinicopathological validation studies led to the identification of the GOLPH3 gene as a first-in-class Golgi oncogene in a region of recurrent copy number gain.[100] Furthermore, through a broad range of mechanistic and biological studies drawing from model systems as diverse as yeast, mouse, and human, authors showed that GOLPH3 exerts its oncogenic activity in part through regulation of TOR signaling, and that tumor cells with a high level of GOLPH3 exhibited increased sensitivity to mTOR inhibition.[100] In the aggregate, this example highlights the importance of systematic functional validation and detailed biological studies to realize the potential of cancer genomics.

Toward this end, genome-scale functional genetic screens with RNAi have also begun to yield insights in melanoma. For example a systematic RNAi screen found that loss of the secreted protein IGFBP7 could bypass senescence associated with ectopic BRAF(V600E) expression.[101] Moreover, many BRAF(V600E) melanomas showed loss of IGFBP7.[101] In another RNAi study, loss of GAS1 was found to promote melanoma metastases in a murine model, suggesting that GAS1 may function as a metastasis suppressor.[102] While the larger clinical importance of these observations remains to be established, these studies illustrate the power of systematic functional screens to offer new insights into melanoma biology that may ultimately have therapeutic implications.

LOOKING AHEAD

The identification of genetic alterations associated causally or otherwise prominently with melanoma initiation and progression presents the opportunity to exploit the genome for molecular biomarkers of melanoma pathogenesis and progression as well as for targets of therapeutic intervention. The initial success of both targeted therapeutics and immunotherapies that exploit this burgeoning molecular knowledge have paved the way for future rational interventions and in particular therapeutic combinations that may enable more durable clinical responses for many patients with advanced melanoma.

Genome-wide assays for DNA copy number alterations, RNA expression patterns, and increasingly protein activation (phosphorylation) states will continue to inform molecular mechanisms and contribute to melanoma pathogenesis. Within the next several years, many new melanoma cancer genes and effector pathways will likely be discovered through large-scale genome sequencing efforts. Evolving technologies will further uncover additional roles of gene dysregulation, such as epigenetic modification (e.g., methylation) or noncoding RNAs such as microRNAs. The application of sophisticated computational analyses should link these myriad observations so as to allow discovery of cellular networks and modules that exert crucial roles in melanoma genesis, survival, and progression. Finally, application of these types of analyses to relapsing tumor specimens should elaborate the spectrum of mechanisms by which therapeutic resistance emerges, thereby informing additional treatment options. Altogether, the intersection of scientific discovery and therapeutic innovation offers great potential to reduce death and suffering from this malignancy.

Selected References

The full list of references for this chapter appears in the online version.

1. Jemal A, Siegel R, Xu J, Ward E. Cancer statistics, 2010. *CA Cancer J Clin* 2010;60(5):277.
2. Michaloglou C, Vredeveld LC, Soengas MS, et al. BRAFE600-associated senescence-like cell cycle arrest of human naevi. *Nature* 2005;436(7051):720.
4. Lin WM, Baker AC, Beroukhim R, et al. Modeling genomic diversity and tumor dependency in malignant melanoma. *Cancer Res* 2008;68(3):664.
5. Hussussian CJ, Struewing JP, Goldstein AM, et al. Germline p16 mutations in familial melanoma. *Nat Gen* 1994;8(1):15.
6. Chin L, Pomerantz J, Polsky D, et al. Cooperative effects of INK4a and ras in melanoma susceptibility in vivo. *Genes Devel* 1997;11(21):2822.
13. Curtin JA, Fridlyand J, Kageshita T, et al. Distinct sets of genetic alterations in melanoma. *N Engl J Med* 2005;353(20):2135.
14. Berger MF, Levin JZ, Vijayendran K, et al. Integrative analysis of the melanoma transcriptome. *Genome Res* 2010;20(4):413.
15. Chin L. The genetics of malignant melanoma: lessons from mouse and man. *Nat Rev Cancer* 2003;3(8):559.
16. Bardeesy N, Bastian BC, Hezel A, et al. Dual inactivation of RB and p53 pathways in RAS-induced melanomas. *Mol Cell Biol* 2001;21(6):2144.
17. Chin L, Garraway LA, Fisher DE. Malignant melanoma: genetics and therapeutics in the genomic era. *Genes Dev* 2006;20(16):2149.
22. Thomas RK, Baker AC, Debiasi RM, et al. High-throughput oncogene mutation profiling in human cancer. *Nat Genet* 2007;39(3):347.
24. Ackermann J, Frutschi M, Kaloulis K, et al. Metastasizing melanoma formation caused by expression of activated N-RasQ61K on an INK4a-deficient background. *Cancer Res* 2005;65(10):4005.
26. Chin L, Tam A, Pomerantz J, et al. Essential role for oncogenic Ras in tumour maintenance. *Nature* 1999;400(6743):468.
27. Kabbarah O, Chin L. Revealing the genomic heterogeneity of melanoma. *Cancer Cell* 2005;8(6):439.
30. Dhomen N, Reis-Filho JS, da Rocha Dias S, et al. Oncogenic Braf induces melanocyte senescence and melanoma in mice. *Cancer Cell* 2009;15(4):294.
31. Hingorani SR, Jacobetz MA, Robertson GP, Herlyn M, Tuveson DA. Suppression of BRAF(V599E) in human melanoma abrogates transformation. *Cancer Res* 2003;63(17):5198.
32. Wellbrock C, Ogilvie L, Hedley D, et al. V599EB-RAF is an oncogene in melanocytes. *Cancer Res* 2004;64(7):2338.
33. Karasarides M, Chiloeches A, Hayward R, et al. B-RAF is a therapeutic target in melanoma. *Oncogene* 2004;23(37):6292.
34. Hoeflich KP, Gray DC, Eby MT, et al. Oncogenic BRAF is required for tumor growth and maintenance in melanoma models. *Cancer Res* 2006;66(2):999.
37. Zheng B, Jeong JH, Asara JM, et al. Oncogenic B-RAF negatively regulates the tumor suppressor LKB1 to promote melanoma cell proliferation. *Mol Cell* 2009;33(2):237.

40. Tsai J, Lee JT, Wang W, et al. Discovery of a selective inhibitor of oncogenic B-Raf kinase with potent antimelanoma activity. *Proc Natl Acad Sci U S A* 2008;105(8):3041.

41. Flaherty K, Puzanov I, Kim KB, et al. Inhibition of mutated, activated BRAF in metastatic melanoma. *N Engl J Med* 2010;36(9):809–815.

42. Heidorn SJ, Milagre C, Whittaker S, et al. Kinase-dead BRAF and oncogenic RAS cooperate to drive tumor progression through CRAF. *Cell* 2010;140(2):209.

43. Poulikakos PI, Zhang C, Bollag G, Shokat KM, Rosen N. RAF inhibitors transactivate RAF dimers and ERK signalling in cells with wild-type BRAF. *Nature* 2010;464(7287):427.

44. Hatzivassiliou G, Song K, Yen I, et al. RAF inhibitors prime wild-type RAF to activate the MAPK pathway and enhance growth. *Nature* 2010;464(7287):431.

46. Solit DB, Garraway LA, Pratilas CA, et al. BRAF mutation predicts sensitivity to MEK inhibition. *Nature* 2006;439(7074):358.

48. Emery CM, Vijayendran KG, Zipser MC, et al. MEK1 mutations confer resistance to MEK and B-RAF inhibition. *Proc Natl Acad Sci U S A* 2009;106(48):20411.

49. Chudnovsky Y, Adams AE, Robbins PB, Lin Q, Khavari PA. Use of human tissue to assess the oncogenic activity of melanoma-associated mutations. *Nat Genet* 2005;37(7):745.

51. Dankort D, Curley DP, Cartlidge RA, et al. Braf(V600E) cooperates with Pten loss to induce metastatic melanoma. *Nat Genet* 2009;41(5):544.

57. Davies MA, Stemke-Hale K, Lin E, et al. Integrated molecular and clinical analysis of AKT activation in metastatic melanoma. *Clin Cancer Res* 2009;15(24):7538.

61. Nishimura EK, Jordan SA, Oshima H, et al. Dominant role of the niche in melanocyte stem-cell fate determination. *Nature* 2002;416(6883):854.

67. Hodi FS, Friedlander P, Corless CL, et al. Major response to imatinib mesylate in KIT-mutated melanoma. *J Clin Oncol* 2008;26(12):2046.

70. Bardeesy N, Kim M, Xu J, et al. Role of epidermal growth factor receptor signaling in RAS-driven melanoma. *Mol Cell Biol* 2005;25(10):4176.

71. Sibilia M, Fleischmann A, Behrens A, et al. The EGF receptor provides an essential survival signal for SOS-dependent skin tumor development. *Cell* 2000;102(2):211.

72. Prickett TD, Neena SA, Xiaomu Wei, et al. Analysis of the tyrosine kinome in melanoma reveals recurrent mutations in ERBB4. *Nat Genet* 2009;41(10):1127.

73. Bastian BC, LeBoit PE, Hamm H, Brocker E-B, Pinkel D. Chromosomal gains and losses in primary cutaneous melanomas detected by comparative genomic hybridization. *Cancer Res* 1998;58(10):2170.

75. Garraway LA, Widlund HR, Rubin MA, et al. Integrative genomic analyses identify MITF as a lineage survival oncogene amplified in malignant melanoma. *Nature* 2005;436(7047):117.

76. Garraway LA, Sellers WR. From integrated genomics to tumor lineage dependency. *Cancer Res* 2006;66(5):2506.

77. Garraway LA, Sellers WR. Lineage dependency and lineage-survival oncogenes in human cancer. *Nat Rev Cancer* 2006;6(8):593.

79. Jané-Valbuena J, Widlund HR, Perner S, et al. An oncogenic role for ETV1 in melanoma. *Cancer Res* 2010;70(5):2075.

80. McGill GG, Horstmann M, Widlund HR, et al. Bcl2 regulation by the melanocyte master regulator Mitf modulates lineage survival and melanoma cell viability. *Cell* 2002;109(6):707.

81. Dorsky RI, Moon RT, Raible DW. Control of neural crest cell fate by the Wnt signalling pathway. *Nature* 1998;396(6709):370.

86. Weeraratna AT, Jiang Y, Hostetter G, et al. Wnt5a signaling directly affects cell motility and invasion of metastatic melanoma. *Cancer Cell* 2002;1(3):279.

90. D'Orazio JA, Nobuhisa T, Cui R, et al. Topical drug rescue strategy and skin protection based on the role of Mc1r in UV-induced tanning. *Nature* 2006;443(7109):340.

91. Cui R, Widlund HR, Feige E, et al. Central role of p53 in the suntan response and pathologic hyperpigmentation. *Cell* 2007;128(5):853.

93. Schatton T, Murphy GF, Frank NY, et al. Identification of cells initiating human melanomas. *Nature* 2008;451(7176):345.

96. Pleasance ED, Cheetham RK, Stephens PJ, et al. A comprehensive catalogue of somatic mutations from a human cancer genome. *Nature* 2010;463(7278):191.

100. Scott KL, Kabbarah O, Liang MC, et al. GOLPH3 modulates mTOR signalling and rapamycin sensitivity in cancer. *Nature* 2009;459(7250):1085.

101. Wajapeyee N, Serra RW, Zhu X, Mahalingam M, Green MR. Oncogenic BRAF induces senescence and apoptosis through pathways mediated by the secreted protein IGFBP7. *Cell* 2008;132(3):363.

102. Gobeil S, Zhu X, Doillon CJ, Green MR. A genome-wide shRNA screen identifies GAS1 as a novel melanoma metastasis suppressor gene. *Genes Dev* 2008;22(21):2932.

MOLECULAR BIOLOGY OF INDIVIDUAL CANCERS

CHAPTER 28 CENTRAL NERVOUS SYSTEM TUMORS

C. DAVID JAMES, DAVID N. LOUIS, AND WEBSTER K. CAVENEE

Neoplastic transformation in the nervous system is a multistep process in which the normal controls of cell proliferation and cell-cell interaction are suppressed or disabled. This process involves the alteration of several types of genes, including oncogenes, tumor suppressor genes, DNA repair genes, and cell death genes, among others.[1] Our increased knowledge of the molecular genetics that underlie this process has been facilitated by improved methods for detailed and rapid analysis of molecular characteristics of tumors, and information obtained from the application of current technology is beginning to influence the clinical diagnosis and management of CNS cancer. Results from comprehensive analyses of tumor genomes (DNA, DNA modification) and transcriptomes (mRNA, miRNA) are proving especially powerful with regard to applications involving the differential diagnosis of adult malignant gliomas,[2-7] embryonal brain tumors such as medulloblastoma,[8,9] and to the subset of meningiomas that display variable clinical course.[10] In addition to clinical applications, detailed molecular characterizations of CNS tumors continue to help improve our ability to develop increasingly accurate and relevant mouse models of brain tumors,[11] which, in turn, facilitate precise dissection of tumorigenic pathways investigation of therapy-response relationships,[12,13] and improved understanding of the earliest stages of brain tumorigenesis, including the nature of cells that give rise to brain tumors.

NEUROLOGIC TUMOR SYNDROMES

In addition to information obtained through molecular characterizations of sporadically occurring CNS tumors, as well as through cancer stem cell investigations, much of our current understanding of brain tumorigenesis is associated with decades of observation and analysis of inherited cancer predisposition. Neurologic tumor syndromes are accompanied by characteristic panoplies of both neurologic and nonneurologic tumors. A catalog of the major primary brain tumors associated with neurologic tumor syndromes would feature optic nerve gliomas and other astrocytomas in neurofibromatosis type 1 (NF1), ependymomas and meningiomas in neurofibromatosis type 2 (NF2), various malignant gliomas in Li-Fraumeni syndrome, Turcot syndrome and the hereditary glioma pedigrees, and medulloblastomas in Gorlin, Turcot, and Li-Fraumeni syndromes.[14]

Linkage studies that were applied to the initial chromosome regional assignments of the genes associated with these tumor syndromes[15] revealed the *NF1* gene as residing on chromosome 17q, the *NF2* gene on chromosome 22q, and at least one gene for the Turcot syndrome on chromosome 5q (*APC* gene). For the Li-Fraumeni syndrome, mutation analyses identified the *TP53* gene on 17p and the *hCHK2* gene on 22q as being responsible for cancer predisposition. Similarly, germ line mutations of the chromosome 10q-localized *PTEN* gene are responsible for the multicancer Cowden syndrome, and the inactivation of *PTEN* is very common among high malignancy grade astrocytomas in adults.

As has been the case for the examination of tumor DNAs, studies of constitutional DNAs from brain tumor patients for the identification of inherited allelic variants that increase the likelihood of brain tumor occurrence have evolved toward comprehensive investigation, as exemplified by genome-wide association study approaches that have recently revealed possible glioma susceptibility loci. Two recent reports, published simultaneously and independently by multi-institutional consortia, suggested susceptibility loci at 9p21 (CDKN2A-CDKN2B as candidate loci) and 20q13 (RTEL1 as candidate locus reviewed in refs. 16 and 17). Consequently, there appear to be additional CNS tumor predisposing or susceptibility genes, not necessarily associated with definable clinical syndromes, that increase risk for CNS tumor development, and our knowledge of such factors is rapidly expanding from such investigations.

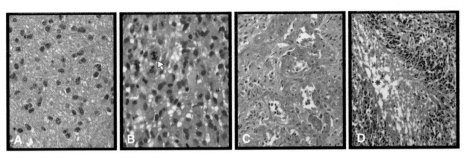

FIGURE 28.1 Examples of grade II (*panel A*), grade III (anaplastic: *panel B*), and grade IV (glioblastoma: *panels C and D*) astrocytoma histopathology. Arrow in panel B shows mitotic figure that is a classification criterion of grade III malignancy. Panels C and D show microvascular proliferation and necrosis with perinecrotic cellular palisading, respectively, which are diagnostic criteria of glioblastoma, grade IV. The asterisk in panel D denotes the necrotic focus.

CNS TUMOR HISTOPATHOLOGY AND MOLECULAR CORRELATES

Diffuse, Fibrillary Astrocytomas

Diffuse, fibrillary astrocytomas are the most common type of primary brain tumor in adults. These tumors are divided histopathologically into three grades of malignancy[14]: World Health Organization (WHO) grade II diffuse astrocytoma, WHO grade III anaplastic astrocytoma, and WHO grade IV glioblastoma (GBM) (Fig. 28.1). WHO grade II diffuse astrocytomas are the most indolent of the spectrum. Nonetheless, these tumors are infiltrative (Fig. 28.1A) and have a marked potential for malignant progression.[18]

Alterations of p53, a tumor suppressor encoded by the *TP53* gene on chromosome 17p, play a key role in the development of at least one-third of all three grades of adult astrocytoma.[19,20] In addition, in higher-grade astrocytomas, p53 function may be deregulated by alterations of other genes, including amplification of *MDM2* or *MDM4* and 9p deletions that result in loss of the p14 product of the *CDKN2A* gene (Fig. 28.2). A recent survey of this pathway demonstrated gene alterations that compromise p53 function in 87% of glioblastoma.[21]

Studies revealing frequent alterations of *TP53* in sporadic astrocytoma are complemented by various model system investigations that support the contribution of p53 inactivation in the early stages of astrocytoma formation. For instance, cortical astrocytes from mice without functional p53 appear immortalized when grown *in vitro* and acquire a transformed phenotype with sustained

TABLE 28.1

COMMON CENTRAL NERVOUS SYSTEM TUMORS AND CORRESPONDING GENE ALTERATIONS[a]

Common Adult Tumors	Frequent Gene and Chromosomal Alterations
Grade II astrocytoma	*IDH1, TP53*
Grade III anaplastic astrocytoma	*IDH1, TP53-**MDM2/4**, CDKN2A-**CDK4/6**-RB*
Grade IV glioblastomas	*TP53-**MDM2/4**, CDKN2A-**CDK4/6**-RB, **EGFR**, PTEN, NF1*
Grade II oligodendroglioma	*IDH1*, chromosome 1p–19q translocations
Grade III oligodendroglioma	*IDH1*, chromosome 1p–19q translocations
Meningioma	*NF2*

Common Pediatric Tumors	Frequent Gene and Chromosomal Alterations
Medulloblastoma	*PTCH, **MYCC**, **MYCN**,* chromosome 17p deletions
Ependymoma	*NF2* (spinal), chromosome 22 deletions (central)
Pilocytic astrocytoma	***KIAA1549-BRAF*** fusion rearrangements

[a]Oncogene alterations are in bold text; tumor suppressor gene alterations are in plain text; functionally related gene alterations have been grouped (e.g., *TP53-**MDM2/4***).

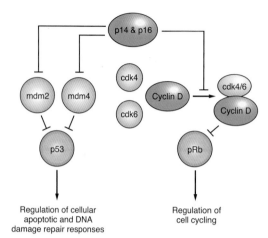

Regulation of cellular
apoptotic and DNA
damage repair responses

Regulation of
cell cycling

FIGURE 28.2 Regulation of p53 and pRb function. p14 and p16 function is inactivated in approximately half of glioblastoma, as well as in a significant fraction of grade III (anaplastic) astrocytoma, due to homozygous deletion of a DNA sequence at chromosomal location 9p21 that encodes each of these tumor suppressors. The genes encoding mdm 2 and 4, as well as for cdk4 and 6, are amplified in some high-grade astrocytomas, and provide alternative genetic mechanisms to the p14 + p16 gene deletions for achieving suppression of p53 and pRb function. The *TP53* and *RB* genes that encode these tumor suppressor proteins are themselves inactivated in many high-grade astrocytomas, and in such instances the gene alterations affecting upstream regulators are not observed. Proteins indicated in green are oncogenic, whereas those indicated in red act as negative regulators of cell growth (tumor suppressors). Percent values indicate gene alteration frequencies, as defined by The Cancer Genome Atlas project.[21]

propagation in defined media.[22] Cortical astrocytes from mice with haploid *TP53* status behave more like wild type astrocytes and only show signs of immortalization and transformation after losing their sole wild type copy of *TP53*.[22] Results associated with p53 inactivation in genetically modified mouse models also support the importance of p53 loss of function in promoting astrocytoma initiation, although such demonstrations have been reported in the context of an accompanying, second gene alteration, such as *NF1* gene inactivation.[23] In total, there is ample evidence provided through numerous avenues of investigation that indicate the importance of compromised p53 function to the formation of astrocytoma.

During the 16 months prior to this writing, it has become well established that mutations of the isocitrate dehydrogenase 1 gene (*IDH1*) occur in a large fraction of grade II and grade III gliomas, irrespective of relative astrocytic versus oligodendroglial histology.[24] The possible consequences of this gene alteration are discussed later, but, notably, antibodies specific to the mutant form of the IDH1 protein can now be used reliably for glioma diagnosis on routine tissue sections.[25] Interestingly, both *TP53* and *IDH1* mutations have been posi-

tively correlated with tumor MGMT methylation, which, in turn, is thought to accelerate G:C to A:T transition mutations. Others have previously noted that gliomas with MGMT methylation have a higher incidence of such mutations in *TP53*,[26] and MGMT methylation has recently been correlated with *IDH1* mutation in glioma,[27] with the most common *IDH1* alteration also being of the G:C to A:T transition type. Thus, it is possible that epigenetic alteration of low-grade glioma genomes, specifically methylation inhibition of MGMT expression, promotes the mutation of genes whose alteration are well established as occurring frequently in low-grade tumors.

Progression to Anaplastic Astrocytoma

The transition from WHO grade II astrocytoma to WHO grade III anaplastic astrocytoma is accompanied by a marked increase in malignant behavior.[14] Although patients with grade II astrocytomas may survive for 5 or more years, patients with anaplastic astrocytomas often die within 2 or 3 years and frequently show progression to GBM. Histologically, the major differences between grade II and grade III tumors are increased cellularity and the presence of mitotic activity (Fig. 28.1B), implying that higher proliferative activity is the hallmark of the progression to anaplastic astrocytoma.

A number of molecular abnormalities have been associated with anaplastic astrocytoma, and several studies indicate that these abnormalities converge on one critical cell-cycle regulatory complex which includes the p16, cyclin-dependent kinase 4 (cdk4), cdk6, cyclin D1, and retinoblastoma (Rb) proteins. The simplest schema suggests that p16 inhibits the cdk6/cyclin D1 and/or cdk4/cyclin D1 complexes, preventing these from phosphorylating Rb, and so ensuring that phospho-Rb (pRb) maintains its brake on the cell cycle (Fig. 28.2).

Chromosome 9p loss occurs in approximately 50% of anaplastic astrocytomas and GBMs, and these 9p alterations target the CDKN2A locus, which encodes the p16 and ARF proteins. The *CDKN2A* gene is inactivated either by homozygous deletion or, less commonly by point mutations or hypermethylation.[28,29] Loss of chromosome 13q occurs in one-third to one-half of high-grade astrocytomas, with the *RB1* gene preferentially inactivated by losses and mutations. *RB1* and *CDKN2A* alterations in primary gliomas are inversely correlated, and rarely occur together in the same tumor. Inactivation of pRb or p16 in mouse astrocytes has been shown to lead to anaplastic astrocytomas.[30] Amplification of the *CDK4* gene, located on chromosome 12q13–14, provides an alternative to subverting cell-cycle control and facilitating progression to GBM in up to 15% of malignant gliomas.[28] Detection of any of the gene alterations known to influence Rb protein function (CDKN2A homozygous deletion, CDK4 amplification, or RB deletion + mutation) is associated with a poor prognosis for anaplastic astrocytoma patients.[31]

Allelic losses on chromosome 19q have been observed in up to 40% of anaplastic astrocytomas and GBMs, indicating a progression-associated glial tumor suppressor gene that maps to 19q13.3, but the gene(s) being targeted for inactivation has is yet to be identified.

Progression to Glioblastoma

GBM is the most malignant grade of astrocytoma, with survival times of substantially less than 2 years for most patients. Histologically, these tumors are characterized by dense cellularity, high proliferation indices, microvascular proliferation (Fig. 28.1C) and focal necrosis (Fig. 28.1D). The highly proliferative nature of these lesions is most likely the result of multiple mitogenic effects. As previously mentioned, at least one such effect is deregulation of the p16-cdk4/6-cyclin D1-pRb pathway of cell-cycle control (Fig. 28.2). The vast majority, if not all, GBM have alterations of this system, whether it involve inactivation of p16 or pRb, or overexpression of cdk4.[9,28,29,32]

Chromosome 10 loss is a frequent finding in GBM, occurring in 60% to 95% of these tumors, and is far less commonly observed in anaplastic astrocytomas. The PTEN tumor suppressor gene at 10q23.3 is clearly one target of the chromosome 10 deletions, with PTEN mutations of the remaining allele identified in up to 30% of GBM, and a lesser percent of GBM having deletion of all or part of their remaining PTEN gene.[21,33] PTEN functions as a 3' phosphoinositol phosphatase that influences cell proliferation through modulation of the PI3-kinase signaling pathway; PTEN also has protein tyrosine phosphatase activity. Results from model system studies, involving approaches such as the introduction of wild type PTEN into glioma cells with inactivated endogenous PTEN, and which results in the suppression of cell growth,[34] or the inactivation of PTEN function in genetically modified mice, which accelerates tumor formation,[30,35] support the loss of PTEN function as a critical step in the development of high-grade astrocytic malignancy.

In contrast to the deletion of tumor suppressor genes such as PTEN, key oncogenes experience increased copy number and/or elevated expression in GBM. A signature example of this is the gene for epidermal growth factor receptor (EGFR), which encodes a transmembrane receptor tyrosine kinase, whose ligands include EGF and transforming growth factor-a. GBMs with EGFR gene amplification display overexpression of EGFR transcript and protein. EGFR amplification is consistently reported in approximately 40% of all GBM,[36] while being amplified at a much lower frequency in anaplastic astrocytomas. GBMs that exhibit EGFR gene amplification have, in nearly all instances, lost genetic material on chromosome 10, and often have CDKN2A deletions.[37] Approximately one-third of those GBM with EGFR gene amplification also have specific EGFR gene rearrangements,[38] which produce truncated molecules that are constitutively activated in the absence of ligand and that enhance tumor cell proliferative properties.[39,40] The most common of the EGFR mutants, EGFRvIII or ΔEGFR, when expressed in mouse astrocytes lacking p16, causes the formation of intracranial tumors that resemble human GBM.[41]

Much of our existing knowledge, reviewed in the previous sections, regarding gene alterations in GBM, was confirmed by results generated from two ambitious projects that combined detailed genome and transcriptome analyses of large series of histopathologically validated GBM. One of these identified mutation of IDH1 in 12% of GBM,[32] an observation that was subsequently extended to grade II and grade III gliomas, among which IDH1 gene alterations are much more common. Our understanding of the roles of mutant IDH proteins in glio-magenesis is at an early stage, but one investigation suggests that these mutations may result in the accumulation of metabolites that activate the hypoxia-induced factor transcription factor,[42] the tumorigenic effects of which are well established.[43] Another suggested that the mutant and wild type IDH1 molecules may combine in a pathway that results in an oncogenic metabolite, 2-hydroxyglutarate.[44]

The second molecular profiling study, from The Cancer Genome Atlas (TCGA) initiative of the National Institutes of Health, confirmed and extended the importance of receptor tyrosine kinases and downstream signaling mediators in GBM by identifying frequent mutation of the NF1 tumor suppressor gene, PI3 kinase regulatory and catalytic subunits, ERBB2, and amplifications of PDGFRA (Fig. 28.3).[21] Previous GBM involvement of this signaling network, as indicated through frequently occurring gene alterations, had primarily been limited to EGFR and PTEN, although each of the individual alterations had been noted in prior publications. This comprehensive study indicated that as many as 88% of GBM have one or more alterations affecting RTK-RAS-PI3K signaling.

The identification of frequent NF1 gene alterations by the TCGA consortium merits special commentary. Activating mutations of RAS, one of the most common gene alterations in human cancer, have long been known to be infrequent in brain tumors, and, therefore, activated RAS has been generally assumed to not play a significant or frequent role in CNS tumor development. Given the new information from TCGA, indicating that NF1 gene inactivation occurs in 15% to 20% of all GBMs, elevated Ras activity is now implicated in a subset of these tumors, with particularly high incidence of inactivation noted in the so-called mesenchymal GBM subtype[45] (see "Subsets of Glioblastoma").

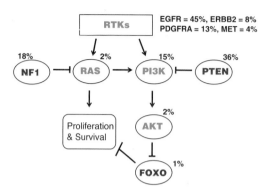

GBM Subclassification Schemes

Primary (de novo, ~90%)	Secondary (~10%)
• Elderly (>62) • EGFR amplification • PTEN inactivation • CDKN2A deletion • Shorter survival	• Younger (<40) • TP53 alteration • IDH1 mutation • Chromosome 19 loss • Longer survival

Mesenchymal	Classical	Proneural	Neural
• 29% • 57.7 yrs • NF1 (+) • IDH1 (-)	• 27% • 55.7 yrs • EGFR (+) • TP53 (-)	• 28% • 51.8 yrs • TP53 (+) • IDH1 (+)	• 16% • 62.8 yrs

FIGURE 28.3 Alterations of RTK/RAS/PI3K signaling in glioblastoma. The third core signaling pathway, at least one element of which is altered in nearly all GBM, as confirmed by The Cancer Genome Atlas (TCGA) project.[9] Receptor tyrosine kinase (RTK) alterations most frequently involve EGFR, with decreasing involvement of PDGFRA, ERBB2, and MET. Downstream signaling mediators RAS and PI3K can be activated by mutation, but are more frequently deregulated by inactivating alterations of the *NF1* and *PTEN* tumor suppressor genes. Percent values indicate gene alteration frequencies, as defined by the TCGA project.

FIGURE 28.4 Current schemes for major subgroup classification of glioblastoma. The primary versus secondary classification is based on the presence or absence of clinical history indicating GBM development from a pre-existing glioma of lesser malignancy, with specific gene alterations found to be associated with such clinical history.[81] Descriptive terms for the lower classification scheme are based on tumor molecular profiles suggesting specific stages of neurogenesis.[58] This classification scheme has recently undergone modification in association with The Cancer Genome Atlas project.[80] +, presence of gene alteration; −, absence of gene alteration.

Subsets of Glioblastoma

Suggesting that all astrocytomas progress through identifiable genetic stages in a linear fashion is an oversimplification. Indeed, it appears as if there are biologic subsets of astrocytomas that reflect the spectrum of clinical heterogeneity observed in these tumors. For instance, approximately one-third of GBM have TP53/chromosome 17p alterations, one-third have *EGFR* gene amplifications, and one-third have neither change.[46]

GBMs with *TP53* mutations that result from the malignant evolution of a lower malignancy grade astrocytic lesion are referred to as secondary (or progressive) GBM. The recently discovered *IDH1* mutations, seen commonly among grade II and III gliomas, similarly show preferential association with GBM that have evolved from lower malignancy grade precursors.[24] In contrast to secondary GBMs, GBMs with *EGFR* amplification may arise *de novo* or rapidly from a pre-existing tumor, without a clinically evident, lower malignancy grade precursor, and are referred to as primary GBM (Fig. 28.4).

Another genomic alteration that defines a significant subset of GBM is the loss of chromosome 10, and in a study using array comparative genomic hybridization (CGH) to identify tumors with chromosome 10 deletion, the analysis of corresponding expression profile data revealed that a novel gene product, the transcript for YKL-40, is significantly up-regulated in tumors with chromosome 10 loss.[47] Whereas the underlying basis of this relationship is yet to be determined, regulation of YKL-40 expression is a matter of interest given the association of

elevated YKL-40 with reduced survival for GBM patients.[48]

In contrast to the use of single biomarkers, such as chromosome 10, or EGFR copy number status, or *TP53* and *IDH1* mutation status for the subclassification of GBM, the comprehensive molecular screening techniques, that generate thousands of data points for each tumor specimen analyzed, and various algorithms (often referred to as *hierarchical clustering*) are proving useful and increasingly popular for identifying patterns associated with clinical or biological properties of interest. An example of this approach, which has served as a paradigm for GBM molecular subclassification, showed that gene expression profiling reproducibly identified three prognostically significant subsets of GBM patients.[49] Descriptive terms for GBM subclassification that were introduced by this study have undergone revision as a result of the TCGA initiative, and currently include classical (proliferative), mesenchymal, proneural, and neural subgroups.[21] These subgroups have strong associations with *EGFR*, *NF1*, and *TP53* + *IDH1* gene alterations, respectively, with the neural subgroup mostly lacking a distinct signature (Fig. 28.4).[45]

Taking into consideration the cumulative results of GBM molecular profiling studies to date, comprehensive molecular characterizations are clearly providing approaches for a clinically relevant classification of GBM that is more robust than achieved using conventional histopathology.[3,4,50] Furthermore, results from transcriptome characterizations have provided insight regarding the molecular biology of this cancer, and have also revealed potential therapeutic targets for the treatment of GBM.

Other Astrocytomas

Pilocytic astrocytoma (PA; WHO grade I) is the most common astrocytic tumor of childhood and differs in its molecular biology, clinical behavior, and histopathology from the diffuse, fibrillary astrocytomas that affect adults. These tumors frequently occur in patients with NF1, and correspondingly, allelic loss of the *NF1* gene on chromosome 17q is observed in approximately half of the PAs from NF1 patients, and nearly all NF1-associated PAs show a lack of NF1 protein expression. Observations derived from the analysis of NF1-associated PAs have shown, however, their distinct gene expression signatures relative to sporadic PAs,[51] suggesting distinct molecular etiologies for sporadic PAs. The recent discovery of a gene alteration that is frequent among sporadic PAs has provided important insight regarding the molecular etiology of these tumors. Specifically, the determination of gene rearrangements and fusions between the *BRAF* and *KIAA1549* genes, have been shown in the majority of PAs examined.[52] Alternative genetic alterations involving *RAF1* and *BRAF* have also been demonstrated in PAs.[53] The demonstration of KIAA1549-BRAF fusion proteins having activated BRAF kinase activity establishes these gene alterations as being oncogenic.[52] However, because PAs do not generally progress to high-grade malignancy, *BRAF* oncogenic activation does not apparently mark these tumors for malignant conversion.

Malignant pediatric astrocytic tumors are histologically similar to their adult counterparts (astrocytomas, anaplastic astrocytomas, and GBMs), and share some of the genetic alterations associated with the adult tumors, especially *TP53* alterations.[54] However, *EGFR* and *PTEN* alterations that are commonly observed among adult grade III and IV astrocytomas do not occur at high incidence among the pediatric cases.[55] Consequently, the molecular basis of high-grade malignancy in many pediatric astrocytomas may well be distinct from that of corresponding adult tumors. Such a possibility is supported by results from a recent study in which a common point mutation of *BRAF* was identified in nearly one-fourth of grade II, III, and IV pediatric astrocytomas.[56] *BRAF* missense mutations are uncommon among adult glioblastomas.[57] Pediatric astrocytomas with *BRAF* alterations were shown as having frequent, accompanying *CDNK2A* homozygous deletion, suggesting a cooperativity between these alterations for contributing to the malignant progression of pediatric astrocytoma.

Oligodendrogliomas and Oligoastrocytomas

Oligodendrogliomas and oligoastrocytomas (mixed gliomas) are diffuse, usually cerebral tumors that are clinically and biologically related to the diffuse, fibrillary astrocytomas.[14] These tumors are less common than diffuse astrocytomas and have generally better prognoses. Patients with WHO grade II oligodendrogliomas, for instance, may have mean survival times of 10 years. In addition, oligodendroglial tumors appear to be differentially chemosensitive, when compared with the diffuse astrocytomas.

Microdissection of the oligodendroglial and astrocytic portions of oligoastrocytomas has shown identical genetic alterations in morphologically distinct portions of individual tumors, suggesting a common underlying molecular biology despite an apparent heterogeneous cellular composition. Allelic losses in oligodendrogliomas and oligoastrocytomas occur preferentially on chromosomes 1p and 19q, affecting 40% to 80% of these tumor types.[58] Because of the frequent loss of these loci in low-grade as well as anaplastic tumors, inactivation of the inferred 1p and 19q tumor suppressor genes has been generally regarded as important to the early stages of oligodendroglial tumorigenesis. The discovery of the majority of these losses being caused by unbalanced translocations between chromosomal arms 1p and 19q implies a scenario in which two tumor suppressor genes could be inactivated through a single event,[59] although target loci have yet to be demonstrated. Alternatively, it has been suggested that the 1p–19q translocations reflect a process of chromatin remodeling that exposes regions of homology that are prone to recombination.[59] In this scenario, the loss of DNA from 1p and 19q would be associated with global chromatin methylation changes, and would suggest an underlying molecular biology of the translocations that is not specifically directed at the deletion of 1p and 19q sequences.

In addition to 1p and 19q deletions, oligoastrocytomas may suffer allelic losses of chromosome 17p, although these losses are not consistently associated with *TP53* mutations. Oncogene amplifications are rare in tumors with oligodendroglial composition, and in total, as well as in contrast to malignant astrocytomas, there is relatively little known regarding the genetic etiology of these tumors, with the exception being the frequent occurrence of *IDH1* mutations, which have been demonstrated as occurring in all grade II and III gliomas, including oligodendrogliomas.[24] Potential associations of such mutations with epigenetic alterations were discussed previously, and it may well be that further insight regarding the molecular etiology of low and intermediate malignancy gliomas will be forthcoming with the maturation of methods for characterizing tumor epigenomes.[60]

Anaplastic oligodendrogliomas have proven to be the first brain tumor for which molecular genetic analysis has had practical clinical ramifications: anaplastic oligodendrogliomas with translocation-associated allelic losses of chromosomes 1p and 19q follow different clinical courses from those tumors that do not have this genetic alteration.[59] Tumors with 1p and 19q loss are usually sensitive to procarbazine, CCNU and vincristine chemotherapy, with nearly 50% of the cases demonstrating complete neuroradiologic responses; correspondingly, patients whose tumors have 1p and 19q loss have median survivals of approximately 10 years.[61] These tumors also appear to have better responses to radiation therapy as well as to temozolomide.[62] On the other hand, anaplastic oligodendrogliomas that lack 1p and 19q loss are only vincristine-sensitive about 25% of the time, and only rarely have complete neuroradiologic responses. As a result, patients whose anaplastic oligodendrogliomas lack 1p and 19q loss have median survivals of approximately 2 years.[61] Recent studies have demonstrated intermediate recurrence-free survival times in those anaplastic oligodendrogliomas that have polysomy for chromosomes 1 and 19 in addition to the typical 1p and 19q losses.[63] At the present time, molecular genetic testing is recommended for: patients diagnosed with anaplastic oligodendrogliomas, small cell malignant tumors in which the differential diagnosis is anaplastic oligodendroglioma versus small cell glioblastoma, and for patients with grade II oligodendrogliomas for whom therapeutic decisions might be influenced by additional knowledge of probable tumor behavior.[58] Thus, molecular genetic analysis of 1p/19q allelic status has become a clinically useful test in neuro-oncology.[64,65]

Ependymomas and choroid plexus tumors

Ependymomas are a clinically diverse group of gliomas that vary from aggressive intraventricular tumors of children to benign spinal cord tumors in adults. Chromosome 22q loss is common in ependymomas, and in spinal ependymomas these losses are associated with mutations of the NF2 gene that resides on chromosome 22.[66] For cerebral ependymomas, the paucity of NF2 mutations[66] suggests that another, as yet unidentified, chromosome 22q gene is critical to the development of the intracranial form of this cancer.

Choroid plexus tumors are also a varied group of tumors that preferentially occur in the ventricular system, ranging from aggressive supratentorial intraventricular tumors of children to benign cerebellopontine angle tumors of adults. Choroid plexus tumors have been reported occasionally in patients with Li-Fraumeni syndrome and rhabdoid predisposition syndrome, raising the possibility of the involvement of the TP53 gene on chromosome

17p or the hSNF5/INI1 gene on chromosome 22q. However, there is no evidence of hSNF5/INI1 point mutations in patients with choroid plexus papilloma, and the mutational status of TP53 have not been extensively studied in these tumors.

CGH studies of ependymoma have confirmed frequent deletions of chromosome 22, and have additionally revealed frequent losses of 6q.[67,68] Recently, array CGH was used in identifying 9q33–34 gains as being associated with ependymoma recurrence and malignant progression.[69] Transcriptome analysis has been applied to multiple series of ependymomas, with the results from one such study indicating potential target genes for the 6q and 22q deletions,[70] the latter of which being especially important to tumors having no apparent involvement of NF2. Another report has shown increased ependymal tumor expression of genes having defined roles in cell proliferation, and suggests that the expression level of these genes may reliably distinguish between ependymomas of grade II and grade III malignancy.[66-71] As has been the case for other types of CNS cancer, gene expression profiling has been used in attempts to identify clinically distinct subsets of ependymoma, with results identifying transcriptional profiles that could distinguish long vs. short-term survivors.[72]

Medulloblastomas

Medulloblastomas are highly malignant, primitive tumors that arise in the posterior fossa, primarily in children. One-third to one-half of all medulloblastomas have an isochromosome 17q on cytogenetic analysis, and corresponding allelic loss of chromosome 17p has been noted on molecular genetic analysis. TP53 mutations, however, are less common than 17p deletions in medulloblastoma, with the majority of 17p losses occurring preferentially at regions telomeric to the TP53 locus, implying the presence of a second, more distal chromosome 17p tumor suppressor gene. For the fraction of medulloblastomas with TP53 mutation, clinical outcomes appear to be unfavorable,[73] thereby supporting determination of medulloblastoma p53 status as an important diagnostic test. In addition to allelic losses on 17p, deletions of chromosome 6q, 8p, 10q, 11, and 16q have also been noted in these tumors. Oncogene amplifications are not common in medulloblastomas, with only MYCC and MYCN shown to be amplified in significant numbers of cases.[74] Copy number gains of the OTX2 gene, which encodes a transcriptional regulator of MYCC,[75] occur in a small proportion of medulloblastomas.[75,76] Gene amplifications and copy number increases may be restricted to the more aggressive large cell and anaplastic subclasses of medulloblastoma.

The discovery of genes underlying two hereditary tumor syndromes has directed attention to signaling pathways involved in medulloblastoma tumorigenesis.[77] Gorlin syndrome (also termed *nevoid basal cell carcinoma syndrome*), a condition characterized by multiple basal cell carcinomas, bone cysts, dysmorphic features, and medulloblastomas arises from defects in *PTCH* (a homolog of the Drosophila *patched* gene) on the long arm of chromosome 9. Medulloblastomas, particularly the nodular desmoplastic variants that are characteristic of Gorlin syndrome, can show allelic loss of chromosome 9q and *PTCH* mutations, and mice that have only one functional copy of the murine *Ptch* gene are predisposed to the development of tumors that are histologically identical to medulloblastoma. The protein encoded by PTCH functions in the pathway regulated by the Sonic hedgehog protein (SHH). Other molecules in this pathway include smoothened (SMO), and rare SMO mutations have been documented in sporadic medulloblastomas. Intriguingly, both germ line and somatic mutations, along with allelic loss, have been identified in SUFU, another member of the SHH pathway that maps to 10q.[78] Alterations in various members of the SHH pathway likely account for the majority of desmoplastic medulloblastomas.

Turcot syndrome, a condition characterized by colonic tumors and brain tumors, is also associated with medulloblastoma; patients with the adenomatous polyposis phenotype may develop medulloblastomas and these patients often have mutations of the *APC* gene on chromosome 5q.[77] The Apc protein operates in the Wnt signaling pathway that includes b-catenin and axin-1, and rare mutations of these genes have been found in sporadic medulloblastomas.

In spite of the contribution of human genetics to our understanding of medulloblastoma development, *PTCH* and *APC* gene alterations, as well as alterations of other genes encoding components of their signaling pathways, are associated with less than 15% of sporadic medulloblastomas, suggesting that the genetic etiology of a significant fraction of these tumors has yet to be determined. The question of whether molecular profiling will provide needed information regarding the genetic etiology of these tumors, as well as provide guidance for the management of medulloblastoma patients, has received substantial attention. A recent study evaluated candidate prognostic markers, selected from medulloblastoma expression data, that were immunohistochemically analyzed for their prognostic value using medulloblastoma tissue arrays. Combined expression of three genes, *MYCC, LDHB,* and *CCNB1,* was able to predict survival in medulloblastoma patients.[79]

Collectively, the results from studies of medulloblastoma genome and transcriptome characterizations suggest that these comprehensive approaches are generating information that will be useful in tumor diagnosis and treatment, and for increasing our understanding of the molecular biology of this cancer.

Meningiomas

Meningiomas are common intracranial tumors that arise in the meninges and compress the underlying brain. Meningiomas are usually benign, but some "atypical" meningiomas may recur locally, and some are frankly malignant.[14] Homozygous inactivation of the chromosome 22 localized *NF2* gene is the rule in the meningiomas of NF2 patients, and *NF2* inactivation is observed in the majority of sporadic fibroblastic and transitional meningioma subtypes.[80] Inactivating *NF2* gene alterations primarily involve immediate truncations, splicing abnormalities or altered reading frames, and result in a lack of, or grossly truncated, proteins.

Approximately 40% of meningiomas have neither *NF2* gene mutations nor allelic loss of chromosome 22q. For these tumors, it is likely that alternative tumor suppressor genes are involved, with potential genomic locations of such genes, including chromosomes 1p, 3p, 5p, 5q, 11, 13, and 17p, as suggested by the results of numerous genetic investigations.

Atypical and malignant meningiomas are not as common as benign meningiomas. Atypical meningiomas often show allelic losses for chromosomal arms 1p, 6q, 9q, 10q, 14q, 17p, and 18q, suggesting the presence of progression-associated genes. Chromosome 10 loss, in particular, has been associated with meningiomas displaying clinically malignant behavior beyond that associated with normal brain invasion alone,[81] which can occur with tumors that are otherwise benign. Chromosome 10 loss as a predictor of meningioma malignancy provides another example of how molecular genetic investigations have clarified grading issues in neuro-oncology. Another study showed a potential correlation between gain of 1q and shorter progression-free survival for patients with atypical meningioma.[10]

Hierarchical clustering of expression profiles has also been used to distinguish high-grade from benign meningiomas.[82,83] Consistent with cytogenetic-based interpretations, the results of such studies have shown that genes on chromosome 1p and 14q are commonly down-regulated in anaplastic meningiomas, and the 14q11.2-localized *NDRG2* gene has been of particular interest because of its decreased expression being associated with meningioma progression.[84] Increased expression of the reverse transcription subunit hTERT (reverse telomerase transcriptase), whose enzymatic activity is critical to chromosome telomere maintenance, may also serve as a potential predictor of meningioma malignancy by its association with tumor recurrence and reduced progression-free survival.

MOLECULAR BIOLOGY OF INDIVIDUAL CANCERS

CURRENT BASIS OF CNS TUMOR TREATMENT AND RESPONSE TO THERAPY

Most therapeutic approaches fail to eradicate entire CNS tumors, and tumor cells that evade primary therapies are responsible for "recurrent" cancer. One concept that is relevant to acquired therapeutic resistance involves tumor initiating cells (also referred to as tumor stem cells), which exist as a subpopulation of cells within individual tumors and that are capable of sustained self-renewal, thereby promoting unlimited tumor growth.[85] Therapeutic targeting of these tumor stem cells may be critically important for the development of curative treatment approaches.[86]

An additional perspective that is proving highly influential for the treatment of cancer involves the individualization of therapy based on specific tumor genome alterations: two examples of this approach that involve the treatment of glioblastoma are described here.

The first example involves a landmark study that demonstrated an association between glioblastoma *MGMT* gene methylation status and tumor response to treatment with the DNA alkylating agent temozolomide.[87] The molecular basis of this relationship may be attributable, in part, to methylguanine methyltransferase (MGMT) gene promoter methylation, observed in approximately 40% of GBM, which markedly down-regulates the synthesis of MGMT transcript and protein. Patients whose glioblastomas had methylated MGMT who received combined radiation and temozolomide therapy survived significantly longer than patients with MGMT-methylated tumors receiving radiation only, or patients whose tumors lacked MGMT methylation and received mono or combination therapy. However, it is also clear that a significant number of glioblastomas treated with temozolomide develop mismatch repair gene defects, most commonly *MSH6* mutations or down-regulation, that lead to a hypermutation phenotype and more rapid progression of disease while being treated with temozolomide.[21,88,89]

Other studies have addressed the relationship between a molecular subset of GBM and therapeutic response involved therapy with EGFR kinase inhibitors, implicating EGFR and PTEN status in predicting response to these inhibitors.[90,91] This interpretation is tenuous, however, as subsequent clinical trials have not demonstrated significant therapeutic effects of these inhibitors, potentially because multiple receptor tyrosine kinases are activated in individual tumors, and the inhibition of one receptor tyrosine kinase, such as EGFR, may contribute to the activation of others.[92,93]

Nonetheless, such studies suggest that current approaches should combine individual tumor biomarker status with corresponding therapies directed against specific biomarkers, or against signaling mediators of the biomarkers. The wealth of GBM biomarker information made available through the TCGA initiative[21] will undoubtedly contribute to the further popularization of this conceptual approach to CNS tumor treatment.

Selected References

The full list of references for this chapter appears in the online version.

1. Louis DN, Pomeroy SL, Cairncross JG. Focus on CNS neoplasia. *Cancer Cell* 2002;1: 125.
4. Nutt CL, Mani DR, Betensky RA, et al. Gene expression-based classification of malignant gliomas correlates better with survival than histological classification. *Cancer Res* 2003;63:1602.
9. Pomeroy SL, Tamayo P, Gaasenbeek M, et al. Prediction of central nervous system embryonal tumour outcome based on gene expression. *Nature* 2002;415:436.
13. Huse JT, Holland EC. Genetically engineered mouse models of brain cancer and the promise of preclinical testing. *Brain Pathol* 2009;19:132.
14. Louis DN, Ohgaki H, Wiestler OD, Cavenee WK, eds. *World Health Organization Histological Classification of Tumours of the Central Nervous System.* Lyon: IARC Press, 2007.
17. Wrensch M, Jenkins RB, Chang JS, et al. Variants in the CDKN2B and TEL1 regions are associated with high-grade glioma susceptibility. *Nat Genet* 2009;41:905.
19. Louis DN, von Deimling A, Chung RY, et al. Comparative study of p53 gene and protein alterations in human astrocytic tumors. *J Neuropathol Exp Neurol* 1993;52:31.

21. Cancer Genome Atlas Research Network. Comprehensive genomic characterization defines human glioblastoma genes and core pathways. *Nature* 2008;455:1061.
22. Bogler O, Huang H-JS, Cavenee WK. Loss of wild-type p53 bestows a growth advantage on primary cortical astrocytes and facilitates their in vitro transformation. *Cancer Res* 1995;55:2746.
23. Reilly KM, Loisel DA, Bronson RT, McLaughlin ME, Jacks T. Nf1;Trp53 mutant mice develop glioblastoma with evidence of strain-specific effects. *Nat Genet* 2000;26:109.
24. Yan H, Parsons DW, et al. IDH1 and IDH2 mutations in gliomas. *N Engl J Med* 2009;360:765.
27. Weller M, Felsberg J, Hartmann C, et al. Molecular predictors of progression-free and overall survival in patients with newly diagnosed glioblastoma: a prospective translational study of the German Glioma Network. *J Clin Oncol* 2009;27: 5743.
28. Ichimura K, Schmidt EE, Goike HM, and Collins VP. Human glioblastomas with no alterations of the CDKN2A (p16INK4A, MTS1) and CDK4 genes have frequent mutations of the retinoblastoma gene. *Oncogene* 1996;13:1065.
29. Ueki K, Ono Y, Henson JW, Efird JT, von Deimling A, Louis DN. CDKN2/p16 or RB alterations occur in the majority of glioblastomas and are inversely correlated. *Cancer Res* 1996;56:150.

30. Xiao A, Wu H, Pandolfi PP, Louis DN, Van Dyke T. Astrocyte inactivation of the pRb pathway predisposes mice to malignant astrocytoma development that is accelerated by PTEN mutation. *Cancer Cell* 2002;1:157.

32. Parsons DW, Jones S, Zhang X, et al. An integrated genomic analysis of human glioblastoma multiforme. *Science* 2008; 321:1807.

34. Furnari FB, Lin H, Huang HS, and Cavenee WK. Growth suppression of glioma cells by PTEN requires a functional phosphatase catalytic domain. *Proc Natl Acad Sci U S A* 1997;94:12479.

35. Kwon CH, Zhao D, Chen J, et al. Pten haploinsufficiency accelerates formation of high-grade astrocytomas. *Cancer Res* 2008;68:3286.

36. Ekstrand AJ, James CD, Cavenee WK, Seliger B, Pettersson RF, Collins VP. Genes for epidermal growth factor receptor, transforming growth factor alpha, and epidermal growth factor and their expression in human gliomas in vivo. *Cancer Res* 1991;51:2164.

37. Hayashi Y, Ueki K, Waha A, Wiestler OD, Louis DN, von Deimling A. Association of EGFR gene amplification and CDKN2 (p16/MTS1) gene deletion in glioblastoma multiforme. *Brain Pathol* 1997;7:871.

38. Ekstrand AJ, Sugawa N, James CD, Collins VP. Amplified and rearranged epidermal growth factor receptor genes in human glioblastomas reveal deletions of sequences encoding portions of the N- and/or C-terminal tails. *Proc Natl Acad Sci U S A* 1992;89:4309.

40. Nishikawa R, Ji XD, Harmon RC, et al. A mutant epidermal growth factor receptor common in human glioma confers enhanced tumorigenicity. *Proc Natl Acad Sci U S A* 1994;91: 7727.

41. Holland EC, Hively WP, DePinho RA, Varmus HE. A constitutively active epidermal growth factor receptor cooperates with disruption of G1 cell-cycle arrest pathways to induce glioma-like lesions in mice. *Genes Dev* 1998;12:3675.

42. Zhao S, Lin Y, Xu W, et al. Glioma-derived mutations in IDH1 dominantly inhibit IDH1 catalytic activity and induce HIF-1alpha. *Science* 2009;324:261.

44. Dang L, White DW, Gross S, et al. Cancer-associated IDH1 mutations produce 2-hydroxyglutarate. *Nature* 2009462: 739.

45. Verhaak RG, Hoadley KA, Purdom E, et al; Cancer Genome Atlas Research Network. Integrated genomic analysis identifies clinically relevant subtypes of glioblastoma characterized by abnormalities in PDGFRA, IDH1, EGFR, and NF1. *Cancer Cell* 201017:98.

46. von Deimling A, von Ammon K, Schoenfeld D, Wiestler OD, Seizinger BR, Louis DN. Subsets of glioblastoma multiforme defined by molecular genetic analysis. *Brain Pathol* 1993;3:19.

49. Phillips HS, Kharbanda S, Chen R, et al. Molecular subclasses of high-grade glioma predict prognosis, delineate a pattern of disease progression, and resemble stages in neurogenesis. *Cancer Cell* 2006;9:157.

50. Maher EA, Brennan C, Wen PY, et al. Marked genomic differences characterize primary and secondary glioblastoma subtypes and identify two distinct molecular and clinical secondary glioblastoma entities. *Cancer Res* 2006;66: 11502.

52. Jones DT, Kocialkowski S, Liu L, et al. Tandem duplication producing a novel oncogenic BRAF fusion gene defines the majority of pilocytic astrocytomas. *Cancer Res* 2008;68: 8673.

54. Pollack IF, Finkelstein SD, Burnham J, et al; Children's Cancer Group. Age and TP53 mutation frerequency in childhood malignant gliomas: results in a multi-institutional cohort. *Cancer Res* 200161:7404.

56. Schiffman JD, Hodgson JG, VandenBerg SR, Flaherty P, Polley MY, Yu M, Fisher PG, Rowitch DH, Ford JM, Berger MS, Ji H, Gutmann DH, James CD. Oncogenic BRAF mutation with CDKN2A inactivation is characteristic of a subset of pediatric malignant astrocytomas. *Cancer Res* 70:512–9, 2010.

58. Reifenberger G, Louis DN. Oligodendroglioma: toward molecular definitions in diagnostic neuro-oncology. *J Neuropathol Exp Neurol* 2003;62:111.

59. Jenkins RB, Blair H, Ballman KV, et al. A t(1;19)(q10;p10) mediates the combined deletions of 1p and 19q and predicts a better prognosis of patients with oligodendroglioma. *Cancer Res* 2006;66:9852.

61. Cairncross JG, Ueki K, Zlatescu MC, et al. Specific chromosomal losses predict chemotherapeutic response and survival in patients with anaplastic oligodendrogliomas. *J Natl Cancer Inst* 1998;90:1473.

64. Ino Y, Betensky RA, Zlatescu MC, et al. Molecular subtypes of anaplastic oligodendroglioma: implications for patient management at diagnosis. *Clin Cancer Res* 2001;7:839.

65. Yip S, Iafrate AJ, Louis DN. Molecular diagnostic testing in malignant gliomas: a practical update on predictive markers. *J Neuropathol Exp Neurol* 2008;67:1.

66. Ebert C, von Haken M, Meyer-Puttlitz B, et al. Molecular genetic analysis of ependymal tumors. NF2 mutations and chromosome 22q loss occur preferentially in intramedullary spinal ependymomas. *Am J Pathol* 1999;155:627.

71. Korshunov A, Neben K, Wrobel G, et al. Gene expression patterns in ependymomas correlate with tumor location, grade, and patient age. *Am J Pathol* 2003;163:1721.

73. Tabori U, Baskin B, Shago M, et al. Universal poor survival in children with medulloblastoma harboring somatic TP53 mutations. *J Clin Oncol* 2010;28:1345.

77. Raffel C. Medulloblastoma: molecular genetics and animal models. *Neoplasia* 2004;6:3102004.

79. de Haas T, Hasselt N, Troost D, et al. Molecular risk stratification of medulloblastoma patients based on immunohistochemical analysis of MYC, LDHB, and CCNB1 expression. *Clin Cancer Res* 2008;14:4154.

80. Wellenreuther R, Kraus JA, Lenartz D, et al. Analysis of the neurofibromatosis 2 gene reveals molecular variants of meningioma. *Am J Pathol* 1995;146:827.

82. Watson MA, Gutmann DH, Peterson K, et al. Molecular characterization of human meningiomas by gene expression profiling using high-density oligonucleotide microarrays. *Am J Pathol* 2002;161:665.

85. Singh SK, Hawkins C, Clarke ID, S et al. Identification of human brain tumour initiating cells. *Nature* 2004;432:396.

86. Bao S, Wu Q, McLendon RE, et al. Glioma stem cells promote radioresistance by preferential activation of the DNA damage response. Nature 2006;444:756.

87. Hegi ME, Diserens AC, Gorlia T, et al. MGMT gene silencing and benefit from temozolomide in glioblastoma. *N Engl J Med* 2005;352:997.

88. Cahill DP, Levine KK, Betensky RA, et al. Loss of the mismatch repair protein MSH6 in human glioblastomas is associated with tumor progression during temozolomide treatment. *Clin Cancer Res* 2007;13:2038.

90. Mellinghoff IK, Wang MY, Vivanco I, et al. Molecular determinants of the response of glioblastomas to EGFR kinase inhibitors. *N Engl J Med* 2005;353:2012.

93. Stommel JM, Kimmelman AC, Ying H, et al. Coactivation of receptor tyrosine kinases affects the response of tumor cells to targeted therapies. *Science* 2007;318:287.

MOLECULAR BIOLOGY OF
INDIVIDUAL CANCERS

CHAPTER 29 CHILDHOOD CANCERS

LEE J. HELMAN AND DAVID MALKIN

The biologic nature of tumors of childhood is clinically, histopathologically, and biologically distinct from that of adult-onset malignancies. Childhood cancers tend to have short latency periods, are often rapidly growing and aggressively invasive, are rarely associated with exposure to carcinogens implicated in adult-onset cancers, and are generally more responsive to standard modalities of treatment, in particular chemotherapy. Most childhood tumors occur sporadically in families with at most a weak history of cancer. In at least 10% to 15% of cases, however, a strong familial association is recognized or the child has a congenital or genetic disorder that imparts a higher likelihood of specific cancer types.[1] Examples of genetic disorders that render a child at increased risk of tumor development include xeroderma pigmentosa, Bloom syndrome, or ataxia-telangiectasia, which predispose to skin cancers, leukemias, or lymphoid malignancies, respectively. In all three cases, constitutional gene alterations that disrupt normal mechanisms of genomic DNA repair are blamed for the propensity to cell transformation. Other hereditary disorders, including Beckwith-Wiedemann syndrome (BWS), von Hippel-Lindau disease, Rothmund-Thomson syndrome, and the multiple endocrine neoplasias types 1 and 2, are thought to be associated with their respective tumor spectra through constitutional activation of molecular pathways of deregulated cellular growth and proliferation. The cancers that occur in these syndromes are generally secondary phenotypic manifestations of disorders that have distinctive recognizable physical stigmata. On the other hand, some cancer predisposition syndromes are recognized only by their malignant manifestations, with nonmalignant characteristics being virtually absent. These include hereditary retinoblastoma, Li-Fraumeni syndrome (LFS), familial Wilms tumor, and familial adenomatous polyposis coli. Each of these presents with distinct cancer phenotypes, and the identified molecular defect is unique for each (Table 29.1). Careful attention to detailed cancer family histories continues to lead to the discovery of new cancer predisposition syndromes and the coincident identification of novel cancer genes.[2]

The study of pediatric cancer and rare hereditary cancer syndromes and associations has led to the identification of numerous cancer genes, including dominant oncogenes, DNA repair genes, and tumor suppressor genes. These genes are important not only in hereditary predisposition but also in the normal growth, differentiation, and proliferation pathways of all cells. Alterations of these genes have been consistently found in numerous sporadic tumors of childhood and led to studies of their functional role in carcinogenesis. The numerous properties of transformed malignant cells in culture or *in vivo* can be explained by the complex abnormal interaction of numerous positive and negative growth-regulatory genes. Pediatric cancers offer unique models in which to study these pathways in that they are less likely to be disrupted by nongenetic factors. The embryonic ontogeny of many childhood cancers suggests that better understanding of the nature of the genetic events leading to these cancers will also augment the understanding of normal embryologic growth and development.

This chapter begins with an outline of tumor suppressor genes—the most frequently implicated class of cancer genes in childhood malignancy. This leads into a discussion of molecular features of retinoblastoma, the paradigm of cancer genetics, followed by analysis of the molecular pathways associated with other common pediatric cancers. Evaluations of the importance of molecular alterations in familial cancers, as well as new approaches in molecular therapeutics, are also addressed.

TUMOR SUPPRESSOR GENES

Faulty regulation of cellular growth and differentiation leads to neoplastic transformation and tumor initiation. Many inappropriately activated growth-potentiating genes, or *oncogenes*, have been identified through the study of RNA tumor viruses and the transforming effects of DNA isolated from malignant cells. However, activated dominant oncogenes themselves do not readily explain a variety of phenomena related to transformation

TABLE 29.1

HEREDITARY SYNDROMES ASSOCIATED WITH CHILDHOOD CANCER PREDISPOSITION

Syndrome	OMIM Entry[a]	Major Tumor Types	Mode of Inheritance	Genes
HEREDITARY GASTROINTESTINAL MALIGNANCIES				
Adenomatous polyposis of the colon	175100	Colon, thyroid, stomach, intestine, hepatoblastoma	Dominant	APC
Juvenile polyposis	174900	Gastrointestinal	Dominant	SMAD4/DPC4
Peutz-Jeghers syndrome	175200	Intestinal, ovarian, pancreatic	Dominant	STK11
GENODERMATOSES WITH CANCER PREDISPOSITION				
Nevoid basal cell carcinoma syndrome	109400	Skin, medulloblastoma	Dominant	PTCH
Neurofibromatosis type 1	162200	Neurofibroma, optic pathway glioma, peripheral nerve sheath tumor	Dominant	NF1
Neurofibromatosis type 2	101000	Vestibular schwannoma	Dominant	NF2
Tuberous sclerosis	191100	Hamartoma, renal angiomyolipoma, renal cell carcinoma	Dominant	TSC1/TSC2
Xeroderma pigmentosum	278730, 278700, 278720, 278760, 278740, 278780, 278750, 133510	Skin, melanoma, leukemia	Recessive	XPA,B,C,D,E,F,G, POLH
Rothmund Thomson syndrome	268400	Skin, bone	Recessive	RECQL4
LEUKEMIA/LYMPHOMA PREDISPOSITION SYNDROMES				
Bloom syndrome	210900	Leukemia, lymphoma, skin	Recessive	BLM
Fanconi anemia	227650	Leukemia, squamous cell carcinoma, gynecological system	Recessive	FANCA,B,C,D$_2$, E,F,G
Shwachman Diamond syndrome	260400	Leukemia/ myelodysplasia	Recessive	SBDS
Nijmegen breakage syndrome	251260	Lymphoma, medullo-blastoma, glioma	Recessive	NBS1
Ataxia telangiectasia	208900	Leukemia, lymphoma	Recessive	ATM
GENITOURINARY CANCER PREDISPOSITION SYNDROMES				
Simpson-Golabi-Behmel syndrome	312870	Embryonal tumors, Wilms tumor	X-linked	GPC3
Von Hippel-Lindau syndrome	193300	Retinal and central nervous hemangio-blastoma, pheochro-mocytoma, renal cell carcinoma	Dominant	VHL
Beckwith-Wiedemann syndrome	130650	Wilms tumor, hepato-blastoma, adrenal carcinoma, rhab-domyosarcoma	Dominant	CDKN1C/NSD1
Wilms tumor syndrome	194070	Wilms tumor	Dominant	WT1
WAGR syndrome	194072	Wilms tumor, gonadoblastoma	Dominant	WT1
Costello syndrome	218040	Neuroblastoma, rhabdomyosarcoma, bladder carcinoma	Dominant	H-Ras

(continued)

MOLECULAR BIOLOGY OF INDIVIDUAL CANCERS

TABLE 29.1

(CONTINUED)

Syndrome	OMIM Entry[a]	Major Tumor Types	Mode of Inheritance	Genes
CENTRAL NERVOUS SYSTEM PREDISPOSITION SYNDROMES				
Retinoblastoma	180200	Retinoblastoma, osteosarcoma	Dominant	*RB1*
Rhabdoid predisposition syndrome	601607	Rhabdoid tumor, medulloblastoma, choroid plexus tumor		*SNF5/INI1*
Medulloblastoma predisposition	607035	Medulloblastoma	Dominant	*SUFU*
SARCOMA/BONE CANCER PREDISPOSITION SYNDROMES				
Li-Fraumeni syndrome	151623	Soft tissue sarcoma, osteosarcoma, breast, adrenocortical carcinoma, leukemia, brain tumor	Dominant	*TP53*
Multiple exostosis	133700, 133701	Chondrosarcoma	Dominant	*EXT1/EXT2*
Werner syndrome	277700	Osteosarcoma, meningioma	Recessive	*WRN*
ENDOCRINE CANCER PREDISPOSITION SYNDROMES				
MEN1	131000	Pancreatic islet cell tumor, pituitary adenoma, parathyroid adenoma	Dominant	*MEN1*
MEN2	171400	Medullary thyroid carcinoma, pheochromocytoma, parathyroid hyperplasia	Dominant	*RET*

WAGR, Wilms tumor, aniridia, genitourinary abnormalities, mental retardation; MEN, multiple endocrine neoplasia.
[a]Online Mendelian Inheritance in Man, http://www.ncbi.nlm.nih.gov/Omim/getmorbid.cgi.
(Adapted from ref. 137.)

and tumor formation. Among these is the suppression of tumorigenicity by fusion of malignant cells with their normal counterparts. If these malignant cells carried an activated dominant oncogene, it would be expected that such a gene would initiate transformation of the normal cells, likely leading to either embryonic or fetal death. The observation is more readily explained by postulating the existence of a factor in the normal cell that acts to suppress growth of the fused malignant cells. Malignant cells commonly exhibit specific chromosomal deletions (Table 29.2). The best example of this occurs in retinoblastoma, a rare pediatric eye tumor in which a small region of the long arm of chromosome 13 is frequently missing. The presumed loss of genes in specific chromosomal regions argues strongly against the concept of a dominantly acting gene being implicated in the development of the tumor. Hereditary forms of cancer are not readily explained by altered growth-potentiating genes. Comparisons between the frequencies of familial

tumors and their sporadic counterparts led Knudson[3] to suggest that the familial forms of some tumors could be explained by constitutional mutations in growth-limiting genes. The resulting inactivation of these genes would facilitate cellular transformation.[4] Such growth-limiting genes were termed *tumor suppressor genes*.

Whereas acquired alterations of dominant oncogenes most commonly occur in somatic cells, mutant tumor suppressor genes may be found either in germ cells or somatic cells. In the former, they may arise *de novo* or be transmitted from generation to generation within a family. The diversity of functions, cellular locations, and tissue-specific expression of the tumor suppressor genes suggest the existence of a complex, yet coordinated, cellular pathway that limits cell growth by linking nuclear processes with the intra- and extracytoplasmic environment. This discussion is limited to those genes for which pediatric tumors are frequently associated.

TABLE 29.2

COMMON CYTOGENETIC REARRANGEMENTS IN SOLID TUMORS OF CHILDHOOD

Solid Tumor	Cytogenetic Rearrangement	Genes[a]
Ewing sarcoma	t(11;22) (q24;q12), +8	EWS(22) FLi-1(11)
Neuroblastoma	del1p32–36, DMs, HSRs, +17q21-qter	N-MYC
Retinoblastoma	del13q14	Rb
Wilms tumor	del11p13, t(3;17)	WT1
Synovial sarcoma	t(X;11) (p11;q11)	SSX(X) SYT(18)
Osteogenic sarcoma	del13q14	?
Rhabdomyosarcoma	t(2;13) (q37;q14), t(2;11),3p-,11p-	PAX3(2) FKHR(13)
Peripheral neuroepithelioma	t(11;22) (q24;q12), +8	EWS(22) FLi-1(11)
Astrocytoma	i(17q)	?
Meningioma	delq22, -22	MN1, NF2, ?
Atypical teratoid/rhabdoid tumor	delq22.11	SNF 5
Germ cell tumor	i(12p)	

[a]Chromosomal location in parentheses.

RETINOBLASTOMA: THE PARADIGM

Retinoblastoma is the prototype cancer caused by mutations of a tumor suppressor gene. It is a malignant tumor of the retina that occurs in infants and young children, with an incidence of approximately 1:20,000.[5] Approximately 40% of retinoblastoma cases are of the heritable form in which the child inherits one mutant allele at the retinoblastoma susceptibility locus (Rb1) through the germ line, and a somatic mutation in a single retinal cell causes loss of function of the remaining normal allele, leading to tumor formation. Tumors are often bilateral and multifocal. The disease is inherited as an autosomal dominant trait, with a penetrance approaching 100%.[6] The remaining 60% of retinoblastoma cases are sporadic (nonheritable), in which both Rb1 alleles in a single retinal cell are inactivated by somatic mutations. As one can imagine, such an event is rare, and these patients usually have only one tumor that presents itself later than in infants with the heritable form. Fifteen percent of unilateral retinoblastoma is heritable[6] but by chance develops in only one eye. Survivors of heritable retinoblastoma have a several 100–fold increased risk of developing mesenchymal tumors such as osteogenic sarcoma, fibrosarcomas, and melanomas later in life.[7] It is thought that several genetic mechanisms may be involved in elimination of the second wild type Rb1 allele in an evolving tumor. These mechanisms include chromosomal duplication or nondisjunction, mitotic recombination, or gene conversion.[8]

The Rb1 gene was eventually mapped to chromosome 13q14.[9] Using Southern blot analysis, it was then possible to demonstrate that the second target gene that led to disease was actually the second copy of the Rb1 locus. Reduction to homozygosity of the mutant allele (or loss of heterozygosity [LOH] of the wild type allele) would lead to the loss of functional Rb1 and account for tumor development.

Using classic cloning techniques, a 4.7-kb complementary DNA fragment was isolated from retinal cells.[10] This gene, Rb1, consisted of 27 exons and encoded a 105-kD nuclear phosphoprotein. As well as being altered in retinoblastoma, this gene and its protein product have been found to be altered in osteosarcomas, small cell lung carcinomas, and bladder, breast, and prostate carcinomas.[10,11] Rb1 plays a central role in the control of cell-cycle regulation, particularly in determining transition from G_1 through S (DNA synthesis) phase in virtually all cell types.

Although it is clear that Rb1 and its protein product play some role in growth regulation, the precise nature of this role remains obscure. In the developing retina, inactivation of the Rb1 gene is necessary and sufficient for tumor formation.[12] It is now clear, however, that these tumors develop as a result of a more complex interplay of aberrant expression of other cell-cycle control genes. In particular, a tumor surveillance pathway mediated by Arf, MDM2, MDMX, and p53 (see later discussion) is activated after loss of Rb1 during development of the retina. Rb1-deficient retinoblasts undergo p53-mediated apoptosis and exit the cell cycle. Subsequently, amplification of the MDMX gene and increased expression of MDMX protein are strongly selected for during tumor progression as a mechanism to suppress the p53 response in Rb1-deficient retinal cells.[13] Not only do these observations provide a provocative biological mechanism for tumor formation in retinoblastoma, but it also offers potential molecular targets for novel therapeutic approaches to this tumor.[14,15] Although the *Rb1* gene is expressed in virtually all mammalian tissues, only in the retina is its inactivation sufficient for tumor initiation. On the other hand, some *Rb1* mutations appear to lead to an attenuated form of the disease, an observation that highlights the variable penetrance in families.[16,17] Outside the retina, *Rb1* inactivation is often a rate-limiting step in tumorigenesis generated by multiple genetic events. The molecular characteristics and potential functional activities of *Rb1* are outlined in detail elsewhere in this volume.

The patterns of inheritance and presentation of retinoblastoma have been well described and the responsible gene identified. The basic mechanisms by which the gene is inactivated are understood, and provocative evidence indicates that the intricate functional interactions of pRB with its binding partners and other cell cycle targets will provide targets for development of novel small molecule therapies.

WILMS TUMOR: THREE DISTINCT LOCI

Wilms tumor, or nephroblastoma, is an embryonal malignancy that arises from remnants of an immature kidney. It affects approximately 1:10,000 children, usually before the age of 6 years (median age at diagnosis, 3.5 years). Five percent to 10% of children present with either synchronous or metachronous bilateral tumors. A peculiar feature of Wilms tumor is its association with nephrogenic rests, foci of primitive but nonmalignant cells whose persistence suggests a defect in kidney development. These precursor lesions are found within the normal kidney tissue of 30% to 40% of children with Wilms tumor. Nephrogenic rests may persist, regress spontaneously, or grow into a large mass that simulates a true Wilms tumor and presents a difficult diagnostic challenge.[18] Another interesting feature of this neoplasm is its association with specific congenital abnormalities, including genitourinary anomalies, sporadic aniridia, mental retardation, and hemihypertrophy. The *WT1* tumor suppressor gene is reduced to homozygosity, at least in part, in a small but highly informative set of sporadic Wilms tumors. In addition, sporadic and hereditary Wilms tumors have been described in which *WT1* is specifically altered.

A genetic predisposition to Wilms tumor is observed in two distinct disease syndromes with urogenital system malformations: the WAGR (Wilms tumor, aniridia, genitourinary abnormalities, mental retardation) syndrome and the Denys-Drash syndrome (DDS)[19] as well as in BWS, a hereditary overgrowth syndrome characterized by visceromegaly, macroglossia, and hyperinsuline-

mic hypoglycemia.[20] These congenital disorders have now been linked to abnormalities at specific genetic loci implicated in Wilms tumorigenesis.

The WAGR syndrome has been correlated with constitutional deletions of chromosome 11q13.[21] Whereas it is now known that the WAGR deletion encompasses a number of contiguous genes, including the aniridia gene *Pax6*,[22] the cytogenetic observation in patients with WAGR was also important in the cloning of the *WT1* gene at chromosome 11p13.[23-25] Characterization of *WT1* demonstrated that this gene spans approximately 50 kb of DNA and contains ten exons. The WT1 protein is a transcription factor. However, the identity of the gene(s) targeted by WT1 during normal kidney development is not known.

The second syndrome closely associated with this locus was initially described by Denys in 1967 and recognized as a syndrome by Drash 3 years later.[26,27] DDS is a rare association of Wilms tumor, intersex disorders, and progressive renal failure.[27] It has been demonstrated that virtually all patients with DDS carry *WT1* point mutations in the germ line.[28]

WT1 is altered in only 10% of Wilms tumors. This observation implies the existence of alternative loci in the etiology of this childhood renal malignancy. One such locus also resides on the short arm of chromosome 11, telomeric of *WT1*, at 11p15. This gene, designated *WT2*, is associated with BWS. Patients with BWS are at increased risk of developing Wilms tumor, as well as other embryonic malignancies, including rhabdomyosarcoma (RMS), neuroblastoma, and hepatoblastoma.[29] The putative *BWS* gene maps to chromosome 11p15 and is tightly linked to the Ha-*ras* oncogene homologue *HRAS-I* and the insulinlike growth factor-2 gene (*IGF-2*). Whether the *BWS* gene and *WT2* are one and the same or two distinct yet closely linked genes remains to be determined. Other genes, including *CDKN1C* (p57KIP2), a maternally expressed gene that encodes a cyclin-dependent kinase inhibitor and negatively regulates cell proliferation,[30] show aberrant methylation in tumors that are associated with cell-cycle deregulation. However, *CDKN1C* is rarely mutated in Wilms tumors.[31] Thus, the search for other genes linked to Wilms tumor continues. Using long-oligonucleotide array comparative genomic hybridization (array CGH), a novel gene termed *WTX* was identified on chromosome Xq11.1. *WTX* is inactivated in one-third of Wilms tumors, and tumors with *WTX* mutations lack *WT1* mutations. Whereas autosomal tumor suppressor genes undergo biallelic inactivation, *WTX* is inactivated by a monoallelic "single-hit" event that targets the single X chromosome in Wilms tumors in males and the active X chromosome in tumors from females.[32] This observation suggests a more important role of the X chromosome in human cancers than had previously been appreciated.[33]

Although linkage studies have indicated that the gene for familial Wilms tumor must be distinct from *WT1* and *WT2*, and from the gene that predisposes to BWS, to date, this gene has been neither cytogenetically localized nor isolated. Whether, of course, the gene for familial Wilms tumor interacts with the gene product of either of the two Wilms tumor suppressor genes has yet to be determined.

Finally, loss of the long arm of chromosome 16 has been observed in approximately 20% of Wilms tumor samples.[34] This observation implicates yet another genetic locus in Wilms tumor. Linkage studies have generally also excluded this locus as the "familial" Wilms tumor gene.[35] However, it is plausible that alterations at 16q can initiate tumorigenesis or be implicated in subsequent steps in the progression of malignancy.

Although both tumors represent classic models of the Knudson "two-hit hypothesis" of tumor development, the spectrum of genetic alterations in Wilms tumor is quite different from that in retinoblastoma. In the latter, there is strong evidence that a single gene is involved whose function is mediated through related cell-cycle control pathway genes, whereas a series of genetic alterations, or at least distinct genetic events, is required for Wilms tumorigenesis. Second, the "single-hit" mechanism of *WTX* inactivation suggests a novel basis for Wilms tumorigenesis; and third, unlike retinoblastoma, which is not associated with other developmental anomalies or congenital abnormalities, patients with Wilms tumor commonly exhibit a spectrum of nonmalignant urogenital, skeletal, and cardiac congenital abnormalities that suggest a dual role of the genes involved in both tumor formation and normal embryonic development.

NEUROFIBROMATOSES

The neurofibromatoses (NFs) comprise two similar entities. NF1 is one of the most common autosomal dominantly inherited disorders, affecting approximately 1 in 3,500 people,[36] and half of them arise from new spontaneous mutations. Carriers of mutant *NF1* are predisposed to a variety of tumors, including optic nerve glioma, neurofibroma and neurofibrosarcoma, malignant schwannoma, or malignant peripheral nerve sheath tumor, astrocytoma, and pheochromocytoma.[37] Occurring with less frequency are leukemias, osteosarcoma, RMS, and Wilms tumor and pediatric gastrointestinal stromal tumors.[38]

Using standard linkage analysis, the *NF1* gene was mapped to chromosomal band 17q11.2 and subsequently cloned.[39] The *NF1* gene is composed of 60 exons spanning 350 kb of the genome and is unusual in that it contains three embedded genes—*OMGP*, *EV12A*, and *EV12B*—of unknown function.[40] The *NF1* gene encodes a 2,818-amino acid protein, termed *neurofibromin*, which is ubiquitously expressed. One region of the gene shows extensive structural homology to the guanosine triphosphatase–activating domain of mammalian guanosine triphosphatase–activating proteins: loss of the protein's activity results in failure of hydrolysis of guanosine triphosphate to guanosine diphosphate by the ras oncoprotein. Loss of neurofibromin function usually results from mutations in one allele of the gene, leading to premature truncation of the protein, followed by absence or mutations of the second allele in tumors. More than one mechanism appears to exist whereby malignant tumors develop in patients with NF.

In addition to structural alterations of both alleles of the *NF1* gene, alternative splicing leading to dysregulation at the level of transcription has also been demonstrated. It appears that the two types of resulting protein may modify the modulation of RAS-regulated signal transduction. This loss of function is thought to lead to elevated levels of the guanosine triphosphate–bound RAS protein that transduces signals for cell division. NF1 is now considered to be one of the RASopathies, a class of developmental disorders caused by activation of the RAS-MAPK pathway.[41] Loss of neurofibromin also is associated with activation of mammalian target of rapamycin (mTOR), suggesting a potential therapeutic target for *NF1*-associated tumors.[42] NF type 2 (*NF2*) is much less frequent than *NF1*, occurring in only one in one million persons. Although it is also inherited as an autosomal dominant disorder with high penetrance, the new mutation rate in *NF2* is low.[43] It is clinically characterized by bilateral acoustic neuromas, spinal nerve root tumors, and meningiomas.

The *NF2* locus was mapped to chromosome 22, band q12,[44] and its 69-kD encoded protein, termed *merlin*, has been shown to be expressed in various tissues, including brain, although not as ubiquitously as *NF1*.[45] The mechanism of tumor formation in *NF2* appears to be in concordance with the Knudson two-hit model, although the mechanism of action of the NF2 protein has not yet been elucidated. Merlin is a member of the ERM (ezrin-radixin-moesin) family of proteins that links cell surface proteins to the cytoskeleton.[46] Although ezrin expression has been linked to metastatic behavior,[47] merlin appears to compete with ezrin activation,[43] and merlin deficiency seems to enhance metastases and promote tumorigenesis through destabilization of adherens junctions.[48] Vestibular schwannomas, a hallmark of NF2, have been shown to signal through epidermal growth factor receptor family receptors, suggesting a potential target for medical therapy in these difficult to manage tumors.[49]

NEUROBLASTOMA

Nonrandom chromosomal abnormalities are observed in more than 75% of neuroblastomas,[50] and many of these are also found in neuroblastoma-derived cell lines. The most common of these is deletion or rearrangement of the short arm of chromosome 1, although loss, gain, and rearrangements of chromosomes 10, 11, 14, 17, and 19 have also been reported. The allelic losses indicate loss of function of as yet unknown tumor suppressor genes in these regions. It is believed that a tumor suppressor gene that lies on band p36 of chromosome 1 is critically important in the pathogenesis and aggressive nature of neuroblastoma. It has been shown that the loss of chromosome 1p is a strong prognostic factor in patients with neuroblastoma, independent of age and stage.[51] Although it is as yet unclear which gene(s) in this region may be directly implicated in neuroblastoma development, aberrant expression of one candidate—p73—which is a member of the p53 tumor suppressor family, has been suggested to play a role in the neuroblastoma cell growth as well as chemotherapy resistance.[52] p73 gives rise to multiple functionally distinct protein isoforms as a result of alternative promoter utilization and alternative mRNA splicing.[53,54] Alternative splicing of the p73 mRNA results in more than seven protein isoforms that differ in the coding sequences of the COOH terminus (TA-p73 $\alpha, \beta, \gamma, \delta, \varepsilon, \zeta, \eta$).

In addition to these COOH-terminal splice forms, three additional forms, Np73α, ΔNp73β, and ΔNp73γ, are transcribed from an alternative promoter located in intron 3. Their protein products lack the NH2-terminal transactivation domain and are thus called ΔNp73. The full-length forms that contain the NH2-terminal transactivation domain are denoted TA. Higher levels of ΔNp73 are associated with an overall worse clinical prognosis, presumably because of the "antiapoptotic" properties of ΔNp73 and its ability to inactivate both TAp73 and p53.[55,56]

Two other unique cytogenetic rearrangements are highly characteristic of neuroblastoma.[57] These structures, homogeneous staining regions and double-minute chromosomes, contain regions of gene amplification. The N-myc gene, an oncogene with considerable homology to the cellular protooncogene c-myc, is amplified within homogeneous staining regions and double-minute chromosomes. Virtually all neuroblastoma tumor cell lines demonstrate amplified and highly expressed N-myc,[58] and N-myc amplification is thought to be associated with rapid tumor progression. Expression of N-myc is increased in undifferentiated tumor cells compared with much lower (or single-copy) levels in more differentiated cells (ganglioneuroblastoma and ganglioneuroma). N-myc expression is diminished in association with the in vitro differentiation of neuroblastoma cell lines.[59] This observation formed the basis for current therapeutic trials demonstrating a survival advantage to patients treated with cis-retinoic acid.[60] Furthermore, a close correlation exists between N-myc amplification and advanced clinical stage.[61]

Although it is clear that altered expression of N-myc contributes to the development of malignancy, it is not yet apparent which cellular functions are altered. The molecular mechanisms underlying regulation of neuroblastoma differentiation may be explained in part through the contribution of other genes and proteins. This is currently under intense investigation through the use of gene expression profiling of N-myc–positive versus –negative tumors.

Neuroblastoma cells that express the high-affinity nerve growth factor receptor trkA[62] can be terminally differentiated by nerve growth factor and may demonstrate morphologic changes typical of ganglionic differentiation. Tumors showing ganglionic differentiation and trk gene activation have a favorable prognosis.[62] In contrast, trkB receptor expression is associated with poor-prognosis tumors and appears to mediate resistance to chemotherapy.[63,64] Resistance to multidrug chemotherapeutic regimens (multidrug resistance) is characteristic of aggressive, poorly responsive N-myc–amplified neuroblastomas. It is interesting to note that expression of the multidrug resistance–associated protein, found to confer multidrug resistance in vitro, is increased in neuroblastomas with N-myc amplification and decreased after differentiation of tumor cells in vitro.[65] It has been demonstrated that high levels of multidrug resistance–associated protein expression are significantly associated with poor outcome, independent of N-myc amplification.[65] Gain of chromosome segment 17q21-qter has been shown to be the most powerful prognostic factor yet.[66] However, no gene has yet been implicated at this site.

A small subset of neuroblastomas is inherited in an autosomal dominant fashion. Until recently, the only gene definitively associated with neuroblastoma risk was PHOX2B, also linked to central apnea.[67] De novo or inherited missense mutations in the tyrosine kinase domain of the ALK (anaplastic lymphoma kinase) gene on chromosome 2p23 have been observed in the majority of hereditary neuroblastoma families, as well as in somatic tumor cells.[68–71] Current phase 1/2 clinical trials with ALK inhibitors substantiate the value of such target identification for novel therapies. The role of other molecular alterations in neuroblastoma continues to be elucidated. In addition to chromosomal loss on chromosome 1p36, unbalanced LOH at 11q23 is independently associated with decreased event-free survival. Alterations at 11q23 occur in almost one-third of neuroblastomas, being most commonly associated with stage 4 disease and age at diagnosis greater than 2.5 years. Both 1p36 LOH and 11q23 LOH were independently associated with decreased progression-free survival in patients with low- and intermediate-risk disease.[72]

Yet another valuable biological marker of clinical significance is telomerase expression and telomere length. In particular, short telomere length is predictive of favorable prognosis, irrespective of disease stage, while long or unchanged telomeres are predictive of poor outcome.[73,74] Telomerase expression, as measured by telomerase reverse transcriptase (hTERT), has been shown to be negative in good-risk neuroblastoma, although it is high in tumors with unfavorable histology.[74] The combined use of these markers—chromosomes 1p and 11q, *N-Myc* amplification, *trkA* and telomerase expression—as prognostic indicators provides a powerful armamentarium with which to develop rational stratified treatment programs for neuroblastoma.

EWING SARCOMA FAMILY OF TUMORS

Ewing sarcoma (ES) is one of the first examples in which the application of molecular diagnostics led to improved tumor classification. ES was first described by James Ewing[75] as a bone tumor characterized by small, blue, round cells and minimal mitotic activity. Turc-Carel et al.[76] identified a recurring reciprocal t(11;22) chromosomal translocation in these tumors in 1983. Investigators subsequently demonstrated a cytogenetically identical t(11;22) in adult neuroblastoma or peripheral primitive neuroectodermal tumor (pPNET), so named because of its histologic similarity to neuroblastoma.[77] Based on the presence of the identical translocation, it was hypothesized that pPNET was related to ES. This translocation breakpoint has been molecularly characterized as an in-frame fusion between a new ES gene, *EWS*, on chromosome 22 and an ETS transcription family member, FLI-1, on chromosome 22.[78–80]

In addition to this fusion transcript being identified in pPNET, other variants, notably the chest-wall Askin tumor and soft tissue ES—previously treated as an RMS because of its location in soft tissue—were also shown to bear the identical fusion transcript. In total, five translocations also have been identified, invariably fusing the *EWS* gene to an ETS family member.[81–84] More than 90% of the ES family of tumors (ESFTs) carry the *EWS-ETS* fusion gene, and a search for *EWS-ETS* by either reverse transcriptase-polymerase chain reaction or fluorescence *in situ* hybridization should be considered standard practice in the diagnostic evaluation of suspected ESFTs. Interestingly, although it was suggested that the specific fusion protein expressed in ESFT has prognostic significance,[85] several prospective studies in the United States and Europe demonstrated no prognostic impact.[86,87] The nature of the novel fusion transcription factor and its downstream targets is currently under intense investigation. One target of the EWS-ETS fusion is repression of the transforming growth factor-β type II receptor,[88] a putative tumor suppressor gene.

Expression profiling analysis has also revealed that p53 is transcriptionally up-regulated by the *EWS-ETS* fusion gene.[89] This is of particular interest because it is now known that expression of *EWS-ETS* can lead to apoptosis, and that additional alterations such as loss of *p53* or *p16* signaling, or both, appear to be necessary components of EWS-ETS–induced transformation.[90] Investigators have now taken advantage of RNA interference technology to inhibit EWS-FLI-1 in Ewing cell lines to identify genes regulated by the fusion in the proper context. Using this approach, *NKX2.2* and *NR0B1* have been found to be a target gene of EWS-FLI-1 that is necessary for oncogenic transformation.[91,92] Recent findings suggest that GGAA microsatellites might mark genes that are up-regulated by EWS-FLI-1 binding.[93]

RHABDOMYOSARCOMA

The two major histologic subtypes of RMS, embryonal and alveolar, have unique histologic appearances as well as distinctive molecular genetic abnormalities, while sharing a common myogenic lineage. Embryonal tumors comprise two-thirds of all RMS and are histologically characterized by a stroma-rich spindle cell appearance. Alveolar tumors comprise approximately one-third of RMS and are histologically characterized by densely packed, small, round cells, often lining a septation reminiscent of a pulmonary alveolus, giving rise to its name. Both histologic subtypes express muscle-specific proteins, including α-actin, myosin, desmin, and MyoD,[94,95] and they virtually always express high levels of IGF-2.[96]

At the molecular level, embryonal tumors are characterized by LOH at the 11p15 locus, which is of particular interest because this region harbors the *IGF-2* gene.[97] The LOH at 11p15 occurs by loss of maternal and duplication of paternal chromosomal material.[98] Although LOH is normally associated with loss of tumor suppressor gene activity, in this instance LOH with paternal duplication may result in activation of *IGF-2*. This occurs because *IGF-2* is now known to be normally imprinted; that is, this gene is normally transcriptionally silent at the maternal allele, with only the paternal allele being transcriptionally active.[99] Thus, LOH with paternal duplication potentially leads to a twofold gene-dosage effect of the IGF-2 locus. Furthermore, in alveolar tumors in which LOH does not occur, the normally imprinted maternal allele has been shown to be re-expressed.[100] Thus, LOH and loss of imprinting in this case may lead to the same functional result—namely, biallelic expression of the normally monoallelically expressed *IGF-2*. However, loss of an as yet unidentified tumor suppressor activity due to LOH also remains a possibility. *HRAS* oncogene is also located at 11p15, and germ line mutations of *HRAS* occur in Costello syndrome, another tumor within the RASopathy family. Patients with Costello syndrome have an increased incidence of embryonal RMS.[101] These data suggest the possibility of cooperativity between *HRAS* mutations and UPD at 11p15 in the development of ERMS.[102]

Alveolar RMS is characterized by a t(2;13) (q35;q14) chromosomal translocation.[103] Molecular cloning of this translocation has identified the generation of a fusion transcription factor, fusing the 5′ DNA-binding region of PAX-3 on chromosome 2 to the 3′ transactivation domain region of *FKHR* gene on chromosome 13.[104] A variant t(1;13) (q36;q14) has been identified in a smaller number of alveolar RMS tumors that fuse the 5′ DNA-binding region of the *PAX-7* gene on chromosome 1 with the identical 3′ transactivation domain of the *FKHR* (Foxo 1A) gene.[105] Fluorescence *in situ* hybridization or reverse transcriptase-polymerase chain reaction can be used to identify these PAX-FKHR fusions. In a review of 171 patients entered into the Intergroup Rhabdomyosarcoma Study Group IV study, the gene fusion was found only in alveolar RMS cases. In the 78 alveolar RMS cases, 55% were PAX3-FKHR+, 22% were PAX7-FKHR+, and 23% were fusion-negative.[106] It has now become clear that these fusion-negative alveolar RMS tumors are clinically and molecularly indistinguishable from embryonal RMS, thus making the presence of the PAX-FKHR fusion a diagnostic criteria for alveolar RMS.[107] The nature of this fusion-derived novel transcription factor and its downstream targets is the subject of active investigation. It also has been suggested that, like ESFT, in which the specific expressed fusion transcript has prognostic significance, the PAX-3–FKHR and the PAX-7–FKHR fusions lead to distinct clinicopathologic entities.[108] The critical role of PAX-3-FKHR in the generation of alveolar RMS has now been recapitulated in a mouse PAX-3-FKHR knock-in model, coupled with either p53 or CDKN2a inactivation.[109]

The PAX-3–FKHR fusion is associated with increased expression of *c-met*.[110] Met is the receptor tyrosine kinase for hepatocyte growth factor/scatter factor and is overexpressed in embryonal and alveolar RMS.[111] A mouse model of embryonal RMS has been generated by expressing a hepatocyte growth factor transgene in Ink4a/Arf-/-mice. The tumors appear to arise from hyperplastic satellite cells (myoblastic precursor cells).[112] The putative role of satellite cells in the pathogenesis of embryonal RMS is supported by a report demonstrating high PAX-7 expression in embryonal RMS compared to alveolar RMS and the association of PAX-7 expression with satellite cells.[113] Other frequently reported genetic alterations that may be common to embryonal and alveolar RMS include activated forms of N- and K-RAS,[114] inactivating *p53* mutations,[115] and amplification and

overexpression of *MDM2, CDK-4, N-MYC*,[116] and *FGFR4* activating mutations.[117]

HEREDITARY SYNDROMES ASSOCIATED WITH TUMORS OF CHILDHOOD

Li-Fraumeni Syndrome

A few hereditary cancer syndromes are associated with the occurrence of childhood as well as adult-onset neoplasms. The paradigm LFS cancer was first described in 1969 from an epidemiologic evaluation of more than 600 medical and family history records of patients with childhood sarcoma.[118] The original description of a kindred with a spectrum of tumors that includes soft tissue sarcomas, osteosarcomas, breast cancer, brain tumors, leukemia, and adrenocortical carcinoma (ACC) has been overwhelmingly substantiated by numerous subsequent studies,[119] although other cancers, usually of particularly early age of onset, are also observed.[120] Germ line alterations of the *p53* tumor suppressor gene are associated with LFS.[121,122] These are primarily missense mutations that yield a stabilized mutant protein. The spectrum of mutations of *p53* in the germ line is similar to somatic mutations found in a wide variety of tumors. Carriers are heterozygous for the mutation, and in tumors derived from these individuals, the second (wild type) allele is frequently deleted or mutated, leading to functional inactivation.[123]

Several comprehensive databases document all reported germ line (and somatic) *p53* mutations and are of particular value in evaluating novel mutations as well as phenotype-genotype correlations.[124] Only 60% to 80% of "classic" LFS families have detectable alterations of the gene. It is not yet determined whether the remainder is associated with the presence of modifier genes, promoter defects yielding abnormalities of *p53* expression, or simply the result of weak genotype-phenotype correlations (i.e., the broad clinical definition encompasses families that are not actual members of LFS). Other candidate predisposition genes, such as *p16, p15, p21, BRCA1, BRCA2*, and *PTEN*, associated with multisite cancer associations have generally been ruled out as potential targets. The role of the hCHK2 checkpoint kinase as an alternative mechanism for functional inactivation of *p53* in LFS has been suggested,[125] although its place as a major contributor to the phenotype has been controversial.[126]

Germ line *p53* alterations have also been reported in some patients with cancer phenotypes that resemble the classic LFS phenotype. Between 3% and 10% of children with apparently sporadic RMS or osteosarcoma have been shown to carry germ line *p53* mutations.[127,128] These patients tend to be younger than those who harbor wild type *p53*. It appears as well that more than 75% of children with apparently sporadic ACC carry germ line *p53* mutations, although in some of these cases, a family history develops that is not substantially distinct from LFS.[129,130] These important findings indicate a broader spectrum of patients at risk of germ line *p53* mutations, and refined criteria for *p53* mutation analysis.[131,132] A striking genotype-phenotype correlation has been observed in a unique subgroup of ACC patients in Brazil in whom the same germ line *p53* mutation at codon 337 has been observed in 35 unrelated kindred.[133] Other cancers typical of LFS are not observed in these families, and the functional integrity of the mutant protein appears to be regulated by alterations in cellular pH,[134] which suggests potential biologic mechanisms in ACC cells by which the *p53* mutation leads to malignant transformation. All these observations suggest that germ line *p53* alterations may be associated with early-onset development of the childhood component tumors of the syndrome.[135] It is not clear what clinical significance these findings have in that no studies of prognostic significance or potential impact on anticancer treatment modalities are reported. Nevertheless, in light of the critical role played by *p53* in the initiation and potentiation of gamma irradiation or chemotherapy-induced DNA damage repair, studies into the effect of such germ line mutations on the potentiation of tumor development related to therapeutic interventions would be important.

The variability in age of onset and type of cancer among LFS families suggests modifier effects on the underlying mutant *p53* genotype. Analysis of mutant genotype-to-phenotype correlations reveals intriguing observations. Nonsense, frameshift, and splice mutations yield a truncated or nonfunctional protein commonly associated with early-onset cancers, particularly brain tumors. Missense mutation in the *p53* DNA binding domain are frequently observed in the setting of breast and brain tumors, while adrenocortical cancers are the only group that are associated with mutations in the non-DNA binding loops. Age of onset modifiers have also now been established. The protein murine double-minute-2 (MDM2) is a key negative regulator of p53 and targets p53 toward proteasomal degradation. The MDM2 single nucleotide polymorphism 309 increases Sp1 transcription factor binding, leading to increased *MDM2* expression levels. Coinheritance of the MDM2 single nucleotide polymorphism 309 T/G isoform is associated with earlier-onset cancer.[136] The earlier age of onset of cancers with subsequent generations in mutant *p53* LFS families suggests genetic anticipation. This observation can be partially explained by several molecular mechanisms including accelerated telomere attrition from generation to generation, absence of the PIN3 polymorphism, or excessive DNA copy number variation in *p53* mutation carriers, all of which may be useful predictive markers of tumor age of onset.[136–138] Thus, although germ line *p53* mutations establish the baseline risk of tumor development in LFS, a complex interplay of modifying genetic cofactors likely defines the specific phenotypes of individual patients.

Beckwith-Wiedemann Syndrome

BWS occurs with a frequency of 1 in 13,700 births. More than 450 cases have been documented since the original reported associations of exomphalos, macroglossia, gigantism, and other congenital anomalies. With increasing age, phenotypic features of BWS become less pronounced. Laboratory findings may include, at birth, hypoglycemia (extremely common), polycythemia, hypocalcemia, hypertriglyceridemia, hypercholesterolemia, and high serum α-fetoprotein levels. Early diagnosis of the condition is crucial to avoid deleterious neurologic effects of neonatal hypoglycemia and to initiate an appropriate screening protocol for tumor development.[139] The increased risk for tumor formation in BWS patients is estimated at 7.5% and is further increased to 10% if hemihyperplasia is present. Tumors occurring with the highest frequency include Wilms tumor, hepatoblastoma, neuroblastoma, and ACC.[20]

The genetic basis of BWS is complex. Various 11p15 chromosomal or molecular alterations have been associated with the BWS phenotype and its tumors.[140] It is unlikely that a single gene is responsible for the BWS phenotype. Because it appears that abnormalities in the region impact an imprinted domain, it is more likely that normal gene regulation in this part of chromosome 11p15 occurs in a regional manner and may depend on various interdependent factors or genes. These include the paternally expressed genes *IGF-2* and *KCNQ10T1* and the maternally expressed genes *H19*, *CDKN1C*, and *KCNQ1*. BWS children who develop rhabdomyosarcoma or hepatoblastoma have epigenetic changes in domain 1, whereas those with Wilms tumor have domain 2 changes or uniparental disomy.[141]

Chromosomal abnormalities associated with BWS are extremely rare, with only 20 cases having been associated with 11p15 translocations or inversions. The chromosomal breakpoint in each of these cases is always found on the maternally derived chromosome 11. This parent-of-origin dependence in BWS suggests that the chromosome translocations disrupt imprinting of a gene in the 11p15 region. On the other hand, BWS-associated 11p15 duplications (approximately 30 reported cases) are always paternally derived, and the duplication breakpoints are heterogeneous.[142] Paternal uniparental disomy, in which two alleles are inherited from one parent (the father), has been reported in approximately 15% of sporadic BWS patients.[143] It is interesting that the insulin/IGF-2 region is always represented in the uniparental disomy, although the extent of chromosomal involvement is highly variable.

Alterations in allele-specific DNA methylation of *IGF-2* and *H19* reflect this paternal imprinting phenomenon.[143] A minority of BWS patients have demonstrable constitutional DNA sequence alterations, the most common of these being *CDKN1C* mutations.[144] Twenty-five percent to 50% of BWS patients exhibit biallelic rather than monoallelic expression of *IGF-2*. Another 50% have epigenetic mutations resulting in loss of imprinting of *KCNQ10T0*. Of interest, epigenetic changes, such as methylation and chromatin modification, occur in many pediatric and adult cancers,[145] indicating the value of the BWS model in understanding the broad scope of molecular changes in cancer. Despite the associated cytogenetic and molecular findings for some patients, no single diagnostic test exists for BWS. This observation is not unlike that described for LFS, or perhaps for other multisite cancer phenotypes, in which the clarity of the phenotype is often weak, making the genetic link cloudy and the likelihood of multiple pathways to tumor formation strong.

Gorlin Syndrome

Nevoid basal cell carcinoma syndrome, or Gorlin syndrome, is a rare autosomal dominant disorder characterized by multiple basal cell carcinomas, developmental defects including bifid ribs and other spine and rib abnormalities, palmar and plantar pits, odontogenic keratocysts, and generalized overgrowth.[146] The Sonic hedgehog (SHH) signaling pathway directs embryonic development of a spectrum of organisms. Gorlin syndrome appears to be caused by germ line mutations of the tumor suppressor gene *PTCH*, a receptor for SHH.[147,148] Medulloblastoma develops in approximately 5% of patients with Gorlin syndrome. Furthermore, approximately 10% of patients diagnosed with medulloblastoma by the age of 2 are found to have other phenotypic features consistent with Gorlin syndrome and also harbor germline *PTCH* mutations.[149] Although Gorlin syndrome develops in individuals with germ line mutations of *PTCH*, a subset of children with medulloblastoma harbor germ line mutations of another gene, *SUFU*, in the SHH pathway, with accompanying LOH in the tumors. Of further note, mice with heterozygous PTC deletions develop RMS.[151] Although RMS is not associated with Gorlin syndrome, the mouse studies suggest a possible link between PTC signaling and RMS.[152]

MALIGNANT RHABDOID TUMORS

Malignant rhabdoid tumors are unusual pediatric tumors that occur as primary renal tumors, but have also been described in lung, liver, soft tissues,

and the central nervous system, where they are often termed *atypical* and *teratoid rhabdoid tumors*.[153] Recurrent chromosomal translocations of chromosome 22 involving a breakpoint at 22q11.2, as well as complete or partial monosomy 22, have been observed, strongly suggesting the presence of a tumor suppressor gene in this area. The *hSNF5/INI1* gene has been isolated and has been shown to be the target for biallelic, recurrent inactivating mutations.[154] The encoded gene product is thought to be involved in chromatin remodeling. Studies have not only demonstrated the presence of inactivating mutations in the majority of malignant rhabdoid tumors (renal or extrarenal) but also in chronic myelogenous leukemia,[155] as well as in a wide variety of other childhood and adult-onset malignancies.[156] An intriguing feature in some individuals with malignant rhabdoid tumors is the observation of germ line mutations, suggesting that this family of tumors may occur as a result of a primary inherited defect in one allele of the *INI1* gene.[157] Further studies of the function of this gene will be important in determining its role in tumorigenesis of this wide spectrum of neoplasms.

PREDICTIVE TESTING FOR GERM LINE MUTATIONS AND CHILDHOOD CANCERS

Several important issues have arisen as a result of the identification of germ line mutations of tumor suppressor genes in cancer-prone individuals and families. These include ethical questions of predictive testing in such families and in unaffected relatives and selection of patients to be tested, as well as the development of practical and accurate laboratory techniques, the development of pilot testing programs, and the role of clinical intervention based on test results. This chapter was not meant to discuss these problems in detail, but one would be remiss to ignore their significance.

For several reasons, testing cannot as yet be offered to the general pediatric population, particularly in light of the demonstrably low carrier rate of the abnormal tumor suppressor genes and the general lack of standardized methods of preclinical screening of carriers. Exceptions to these limitations include screening of gene carriers in families with retinoblastoma, BWS, multiple endocrine neoplasia, familial adenomatous polyposis, and von Hippel-Lindau disease. For some of these diseases, clinical surveillance tools are available, whereas for others, risk-reductive surgery has also been shown to be of value.[158,159] In general, it has been demonstrated that genetic testing does not lead to clinical levels of anxiety, depression, or other markers of psychological distress in the children who are tested, or their parents.[160,161]

However, certain circumstances or personality traits are associated with a greater likelihood of an individual experiencing psychological distress after a positive result.[160] Parents now routinely discuss the options of prenatal diagnosis and preimplantation genetic diagnosis. Multidisciplinary teams must be engaged to provide parents and families the necessary tools with which to approach these ethically challenging decisions.[162,163] The development of screening programs should address aspects of cost, informed consent (particularly where it affects children), socioeconomic impact on the individual tested, consistency in providing results, and counseling. Concerns of risk of employment, health insurance, or life insurance discrimination exist but may be alleviated by congressional legislation to ban such practices.[164]

MOLECULAR THERAPEUTICS

With the identification of alterations in a variety of molecular signaling pathways, including activated growth factor signaling pathways (e.g.,

IGF-2) and altered tumor suppressor pathways (e.g., retinoblastoma), it has become increasingly apparent that these alterations may potentially represent the "Achilles' heel" for these tumors. New agents targeting the tyrosine kinase enzymes that transduce growth factor signals are at various stages of development in early clinical studies. Several IGF-I receptor (IR) antibodies have been tested in ES and rhabdomyosarcoma, and small-molecule IGF-IR kinase inhibitors are entering clinical trials. Several mTOR inhibitors are now approved for treatment of kidney cancer, and these agents are currently being tested in both NF1 as well as in combinations with IGF-IR inhibitors in pediatric sarcomas.

Fusion proteins derived from tumor-specific translocations may themselves represent targets, either as potential neoantigens that could be targeted by cytotoxic T cells or as targets for novel compounds. It is likely that the molecular characterization of pediatric tumors will lead to novel and perhaps more effective treatment approaches in the near future. It is also likely that some of these innovative approaches will at least initially be integrated into standard therapeutic protocols.

MOLECULAR BIOLOGY OF INDIVIDUAL CANCERS

Selected References

The full list of references for this chapter appears in the online version.

3. Knudson AG Jr. Mutation and cancer: statistical study of retinoblastoma. *Proc Natl Acad Sci U S A* 1971;68:820.
8. Cavenee WK, Dryja TP, Phillips RA, et al. Expression of recessive alleles by chromosomal mechanisms in retinoblastoma. *Nature* 1983;305:779.
10. Friend SH, Bernards R, Rogelj S, et al. A human DNA segment with properties of the gene that predisposes to retinoblastoma and osteosarcoma. *Nature* 1986;323:643.
23. Call KM, Glaser T, Ito CY, et al. Isolation and characterization of a zinc finger polypeptide gene at the human chromosome 11 Wilms' tumor locus. *Cell* 1990;60:509
32. Rivera MN, Kim WJ, Driscoll DR, et al. An X chromosome gene, WTX, is commonly inactivated in Wilms tumor. *Science* 2007;315:642.
40. Viskochil D, Buchberg AM, Xu G, et al. Deletions and a translocation interrupt a cloned gene at the neurofibromatosis type 1 locus. *Cell* 1990;62:187.
41. Tidyman WE, Rauen KA. The RASopathies: developmental syndromes of Ras/MAPK pathway dysregulation. *Curr Opin Genet Dev* 2009;19:230.
49. Ammoun S, Cunliffe CH, Allen JC, et al. ErbB/HER receptor activation and preclinical efficacy of lapatinib in vestibular schwannoma. *Neuro Oncol* 2010;12:834.
50. Brodeur GM, Sekhon G, Goldstein MN. Chromosomal aberrations in human neuroblastomas. *Cancer* 1977;40:2256.
51. Caron H, van Sluis P, de Kraker J, et al. Allelic loss of chromosome 1p as a predictor of unfavorable outcome in patients with neuroblastoma. *N Engl J Med* 1996;334:225.
58. Schwab M, Alitalo K, Klempnauer KH, et al. Amplified DNA with limited homology to myc cellular oncogene is shared by human neuroblastoma cell lines and a neuroblastoma tumour. *Nature* 1983;305:245.

59. Thiele CJ, Reynolds CP, Israel MA. Decreased expression of N-myc precedes retinoic acid-induced morphological differentiation of human neuroblastoma. *Nature* 1985;313:404.
61. Schwab M, Ellison J, Busch M, et al. Enhanced expression of the human gene N-myc consequent to amplification of DNA may contribute to malignant progression of neuroblastoma. *Proc Natl Acad Sci U S A* 1984;81:4940.
62. Nakagawara A, Arima-Nakagawara M, Scavarda NJ, et al. Association between high levels of expression of the TRK gene and favorable outcome in human neuroblastoma. *N Engl J Med* 1993;328:847.
68. Mosse YP, Laduenslager M, Longo L, et al. Identification of ALK as a major familial neuroblastoma predisposition gene. *Nature* 2008;455:967.
72. Attiyeh EF, London WB, Mosse YP, et al. Chromosome 1p and 11q deletions and outcome in neuroblastoma. *N Engl J Med* 2005;353(21):2243.
74. Ohali A, Avigad S, Ash S, et al. Telomere length is a prognostic factor in neuroblastoma. *Cancer* 2006;107:1391.
77. Whang-Peng J, Triche T, Knutsen T, et al. Chromosome translocation in peripheral neuroepithelioma. *N Engl J Med* 1984;311:584.
78. Delattre O, Zucman J, Plougastel B, et al. Gene fusion with an ETS DNA binding domain caused by chromosome translocation in human cancers. *Nature* 1992;359:162.
87. van Doorninck JA, Ji L, Schaub B, et al. Current treatment protocols have eliminated the prognostic advantage of type 1 fusions in Ewing sarcoma: a report from the Children's Oncology Group. *J Clin Oncol* 2010;28:1989.
89. Lessnick SL, Dacwag CS, Golub TR. The Ewing's sarcoma oncoprotein EWS/FLI induces a p53-dependent growth arrest in primary human fibroblasts. *Cancer Cell* 2002;1:393.

92. Kinsey M, Smith R, Lessnick SL. NR0B1 is required for the oncogenic phenotype mediated by EWS/FLI in Ewing's sarcoma. *Mol Cancer Res* 2006;4:851.

95. Dias P, Parham DM, Shapiro DN, et al. Myogenic regulatory protein (MyoD1) expression in childhood solid tumors: diagnostic utility in rhabdomyosarcoma. *Am J Pathol* 1990;137:1283.

97. Scrable H, Witte D, Shimada H, et al. Molecular differential pathology of rhabdomyosarcoma. *Genes Chromosomes Cancer* 1989;1:23.

99. Rainier S, Johnson LA, Dobry CJ, et al. Relaxation of imprinted genes in human cancer. *Nature* 1993;362:747.

100. Zhan S, Shapiro DN, Helman LJ. Activation of an imprinted allele of the insulin-like growth factor II gene implicated in rhabdomyosarcoma. *J Clin Invest* 1994; 94:445.

101. Gripp KW. Tumor predisposition in Costello syndrome. *Am J Med Genet C Semin Med Genet* 2005;137C:72.

104. Barr FG, Galili N, Holick J, et al. Rearrangement of the PAX3 paired box gene in the paediatric solid tumour alveolar rhabdomyosarcoma. *Nat Genet* 1993;3:113.

106. Sorensen PH, Lynch JC, Qualman SJ, et al. PAX3-FKHR and PAX7-FKHR gene fusions are prognostic indicators in alveolar rhabdomyosarcoma: a report from the Children's Oncology Group. *J Clin Oncol* 2002;20(11): 2672.

109. Keller C, Arenkiel BR, Coffin CM, El-Bardeesy N, DePinho RA, Capecchi MR. Alveolar rhabdomyosarcomas in conditional Pax3:Fkhr mice: cooperativity of Ink4a/ARF and Trp53 loss of function. *Genes Dev* 2004; 18:2614.

117. Taylor JG 6th, Cheuk AT, Tsang PS, et al. Identification of FGFR4-activating mutations in human rhabdomyosarcomas that promote metastasis in xenotransplanted models. *J Clin Invest* 2009;119:3395

118. Li FP, Fraumeni JF Jr. Rhabdomyosarcoma in children: epidemiologic study and identification of a familial cancer syndrome. *J Natl Cancer Inst* 1969;43:1365.

121. Malkin D, Li FP, Strong LC, et al. Germ line p53 mutations in a familial syndrome of breast cancer, sarcomas, and other neoplasms. *Science* 1990;250:1233.

124. Olivier M, Eeles R, Hollstein M, et al. The IARC TP53 database: new online mutation analysis and recommendations to users. *Hum Mutat* 2002;19:607.

132. Tinat J, Bougeard G, Baert-Desurmont S, et al. 2009 version of the Chompret criteria for Li-Fraumeni syndrome. *J Clin Oncol* 2009;27(26):e108.

133. Ribeiro RC, Sandrini F, Figueiredo B, et al. An inherited p53 mutation that contributes in a tissue-specific manner to pediatric adrenal cortical carcinoma. *Proc Natl Acad Sci U S A* 2001;98:9330.

135. Olivier M, Goldgar DE, Sodha N, et al. Li-Fraumeni and related syndromes: correlation between tumor type, family structure, and TP53 genotype. *Cancer Res* 2003;63: 6643.

138. Shlien A, Tabori U, Marshall CR, et al. Excessive genomic DNA copy number variation in the Li-Fraumeni cancer predisposition syndrome. *Proc Natl Acad Sci U S A* 2008; 105:11264.

142. Henry I, Bonaiti-Pellie C, Chehensse V, et al. Uniparental paternal disomy in a genetic cancer-predisposing syndrome. *Nature* 1991;351:665.

148. Hahn H, Wicking C, Zaphiropoulous PG, et al. Mutations of the human homolog of Drosophila patched in the nevoid basal cell carcinoma syndrome. *Cell* 1996;85:841.

150. Taylor MD, Liu L, Raffel C, et al. Mutations in SUFU predispose to medulloblastoma. *Nat Genet* 2002;31:306.

154. Versteege I, Sevenet N, Lange J, et al. Truncating mutations of hSNF5/INI1 in aggressive paediatric cancer. *Nature* 1998;394:203.

157. Biegel JA, Zhou JY, Rorke LB, et al. Germ-line and acquired mutations of INI1 in atypical teratoid and rhabdoid tumors. *Cancer Res* 1999;59:74.

162. Lammens C, Bleiker Aaronson N, Aaronson N, et al. Attitudes towards pre-implantation genetic diagnosis for hereditary cancer. *Fam Cancer* 2009;8(4):457.

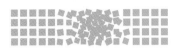

CHAPTER 30 LYMPHOMAS

URBAN NOVAK, LAURA PASQUALUCCI, AND RICCARDO DALLA-FAVERA

The term *lymphoma* identifies a heterogeneous group of biologically and clinically distinct neoplasms that originate from the lymphoid organs and have historically been divided into two distinct categories, namely non–Hodgkin's lymphoma (NHL) and Hodgkin's lymphoma (HL).[1,2] During the past 3 decades, significant progress has been made in elucidating the molecular pathogenesis of lymphoid malignancies as a clonal malignant expansion of B cells (in the majority of cases) or of T cells. The molecular characterization of the most frequent genetic abnormalities associated with lymphoma development has led to the identification of a number of protooncogenes and tumor suppressor genes that are altered in B-cell NHL (B-NHL) and whose abnormal functioning contributes to lymphoma pathogenesis. Relatively less is known about the pathogenesis of T-cell NHL (T-NHL) and HL. This chapter will focus on the molecular pathogenesis of the most common types of lymphoma, including B-NHL, T-NHL, HL, and chronic lymphocytic leukemia/small lymphocytic lymphoma (CLL/SLL), which also derives from mature B cells. Emphasis will be given to the mechanisms of genetic lesion and the nature of the involved genes in relationship to the normal biology of lymphocytes.

THE CELL OF ORIGIN OF LYMPHOMA

Lymphomas originate from mature B cells in approximately 85% of the cases, while the remaining 15% derive from the T-cell lineage. A key concept for the understanding of lymphomagenesis is the relationship between these tumors and the unique DNA modification events that take place in normal lymphocytes in order to enable the production of highly efficient neutralizing antibodies in B cells, and to encode T-cell receptors in T cells.

Normal B-Cell Development and the Dynamics of the Germinal Center Reaction

B lymphocytes are generated from a common pluripotent stem cell in the bone marrow, where precursor B cells first assemble their immunoglobulin heavy chain locus (*IGH*) followed by the light chain loci (*IGL*) through a site-specific process of cleavage and rejoining, known as V(D)J recombination.[3,4] Cells that fail to express a functional (and nonautoreactive) antigen receptor are eliminated within the bone marrow, while B-cell precursors that have successfully rearranged their antibody genes are positively selected to migrate into peripheral lymphoid organs as mature, naive B cells.[5] In most B cells, the subsequent maturation steps are linked to the histologic structure of the germinal center (GC), a highly specialized microenvironment that forms following encounter of naive B cells with a foreign antigen, together with signals from CD4+ T and antigen-presenting cells.[5–7]

The development of the GC can be schematically described as occurring in two stages. First, B cells enter the GC dark zone, which consists of rapidly proliferating centroblasts (CBs) (doubling time <12 hours). In this phase, CBs modify the variable region of their Ig genes (*IgV*) by the process of somatic hypermutation (SHM), which introduces mostly single nucleotide substitutions but also deletions and duplications in order to change their affinity for the antigen.[5,7–10] CBs express elevated levels of BCL6,[11,12] a transcriptional repressor[13] that negatively regulates a broad set of genes, including those involved in (1) B-cell receptor (BCR) and CD40 signaling[14,15]; (2) T-cell mediated B-cell activation[14]; (3) induction of apoptosis[14,16]; (4) response to DNA damage, by modulation of genes involved in the sensing and execution of DNA damage responses[17–20]; (5) multiple cytokine and chemokine signaling pathways, including the ones involved in interferon and transforming growth factor-β responses[14,16]; and (6) plasma cell differentiation, via suppression of the PRDM1/BLIMP1 master regulator.[21–24] This transcriptional program suggests that the BCL6 function is critical to establish the proliferative status of CBs while allowing the execution of DNA modification processes (SHM and class-switch recombination) without eliciting responses to DNA damage, and preventing premature activation and differentiation prior to the selection for the survival of cells producing high affinity antibodies.

In the light zone, CBs are thought to cease proliferation and differentiate into centrocytes (CCs), which are rechallenged by the antigen through the interaction with CD4+ T cells and follicular dendritic cells.[5,6] CCs expressing a BCR with reduced affinity for the antigen are eliminated by apoptosis, while a few cells with high affinity will be stimulated by a variety of signals, including the engagement of their BCR by the antigen itself and the activation of the CD40 receptor by the CD40 ligand present on CD4+ T cells. These signals down-regulate BCL6, allowing the arrest of proliferation and the restoration of DNA damage responses, as well as activation and differentiation capabilities, such that B cells can be selected for survival and differentiation into memory cells and plasma cells.[6,25] In the GC, CCs also undergo class-switch recombination (CSR), a DNA remodeling event that confers distinct effector functions to the antibodies.[26] Both SHM and CSR depend on the activity of the activation-induced cytidine deaminase (AID) enzyme and represent B-cell–specific functions that modify the genome of B cells via mechanisms involving single- or double-strand breaks,[27–29] a notion that will become important in the understanding of the mechanisms generating genetic alterations in B-NHL.

This schematic description is useful to focus on two key concepts for the understanding of B-NHL pathogenesis. First, the activity of SHM, which introduces irreversible DNA changes in the genome, allowed to conclude that most B-NHL types, with the exception of mantle-cell lymphoma (MCL), derive from GC-experienced B cells, as they contain hypermutated IgV sequences, and that clonal expansion occurred within the GC, because the malignant clones contain largely identical mutations, suggesting the derivation from a single founder cell.[30] Second, the most frequent oncogenic events in B-NHL—namely, chromosomal translocations and aberrant somatic hypermutation (ASHM)—result from mistakes in the machinery that normally diversifies the Ig genes during B lymphocyte differentiation, further supporting the GC origin of most B-NHL (Fig. 30.1). Finally, the definition of two distinct phases during GC development reflects stages of B-cell differentiation and function that can to some extent be recognized in different B-NHL subtypes.

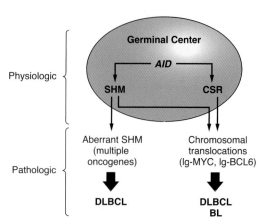

FIGURE 30.1 Model for the generation of genetic lesions during lymphomagenesis. B-NHL–associated genetic lesions appear to be due to mistakes occurring during the physiologic processes of somatic hypermutation and class-switch recombination in the highly proliferative environment of the germinal center (*top*). These include chromosomal translocations, which in most cases juxtapose the *Ig* genes to one of several protooncogenes (e.g., *BCL6* or *MYC*), and aberrant somatic hypermutation of multiple target genes AID, activation-induced cytidine deaminase; SHM, somatic hypermutation; CSR, class-switch recombination.

Normal T-Cell Development

T-cell development proceeds through sequential stages defined according to the expression of the molecules CD4 and CD8. Committed lymphoid progenitors exit the bone marrow and migrate to the thymus as early T-cell progenitors or double-negative 1 (DN1) cells, which lack expression of CD4 and CD8 as well as of the T-cell receptor (TCR).[31] In the thymic cortex, T cells advance through the double-negative stages DN2, DN3, and DN4, while undergoing specific rearrangements at the TCRβ locus in order to acquire

expression of the pre-TCR.[31] Those thymocytes that have successfully recombined the pre-TCR will be selected to further differentiate into double-positive cells (DP; CD4+CD8+), which express a complete surface TCR and can then enter a process of positive and negative selection in the medulla, before exiting the thymus as single positive T cells.[31] The end result of this process is a pool of mature T cells that exhibit coordinated TCR and coreceptor specificities as required for effective immune responses to foreign antigens. Most mature T-NHLs arise from postthymic T cells in the lymphoid organs.

GENERAL MECHANISMS OF GENETIC LESION IN LYMPHOMA

Chromosomal Translocations

Chromosomal translocations are the genetic hallmark of malignancies derived from the hematopoietic system. Lymphoma-associated translocations represent reciprocal and balanced recombination events that occur between two specific chromosomes, are clonally represented in each tumor case, and are often recurrently associated with a given tumor type.

Although the precise molecular mechanisms that are responsible for the generation of translocations remain partially obscure, significant advances have been obtained during the past decade in our understanding of the events that are required for their initiation.[32] It has now been documented that chromosomal translocations occur at least in part as a consequence of mistakes during *Ig* and *TCR* gene rearrangements in B and T cells, respectively. Based on the characteristics of the chromosomal breakpoint, three distinct scenarios can be distinguished: (1) translocations derived from mistakes of the RAG-mediated V(D)J recombination process, as is the case for translocations involving *IGH* and *CCND1* in MCL or *IGH* and *BCL2* in follicular lymphoma (FL)[32–34]; (2) translocations mediated by errors in the AID-dependent CSR process, such as those involving the *Ig* genes and *MYC* in sporadic Burkitt lymphoma (BL)[32]; and (3) translocations occurring as by-products of the AID-mediated SHM mechanism, which also generates DNA breaks, such as those joining the *Ig* and *MYC* loci in endemic BL.[32] Conclusive experimental evidence for the involvement of antibody-associated remodeling events has been recently provided through *in vivo* studies performed in lymphoma-prone mouse models, where the removal of the AID enzyme was sufficient to abrogate the generation of *MYC-IGH* translocations in normal B cells undergoing CSR[35,36] and to prevent the development of GC-derived B-NHL.[37,38]

The common feature of all NHL-associated chromosomal translocations is the presence of a protooncogene in proximity to the chromosomal recombination sites. In most lymphoma types, and in contrast with acute leukemias, the coding domain of the oncogene is not affected by the translocation, but its pattern of expression is altered as a consequence of the juxtaposition of heterologous regulatory sequences derived from the partner chromosome (protooncogene deregulation) (Fig. 30.2). Two distinct types of protooncogene deregulation (i.e., homotopic and heterotopic) can be distinguished. Homotopic deregulation occurs when the protooncogene becomes constitutively expressed in the lymphoma cell, while its expression is tightly regulated in normal lymphoid cells. Conversely, heterotopic deregulation occurs when the protooncogene is not expressed in the normal tumor counterpart and undergoes ectopic expression in the lymphoma. In most types of NHL-associated translocations, the heterologous regulatory sequences responsible for protooncogene deregulation are derived from antigen receptor loci that are expressed at high levels in the target tissue.[32] However, in certain translocations, such as the ones involving BCL6 in diffuse large B-cell lymphoma (DLBCL), different promoter regions from distinct chromosomal sites can be juxtaposed to the protooncogene in individual tumor cases, a concept known as *promiscuous translocations*.[39–46]

Less commonly, B-NHL–associated chromosomal translocations juxtapose the coding regions of the two involved genes to form a chimeric unit that encodes for a novel fusion protein, an outcome typically observed in chromosomal translocation associated with acute leukemia (Fig. 30.2). Examples are the t(11;18) of mucosa-associated lymphoid tissue (MALT) lymphoma and the t(2;5) of anaplastic large cell lymphoma (ALCL). The molecular cloning of the genetic loci involved in most recurrent translocations has led to the identification of a number of protooncogenes involved in lymphomagenesis (Table 30.1).

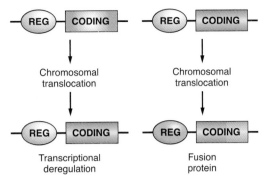

FIGURE 30.2 Molecular consequences of chromosomal translocations. *Top panel*: schematic representation of the two protooncogenes involved in prototypic chromosomal translocations, with their regulatory (REG) and coding sequences. Only one side of the balanced, reciprocal translocations is indicated. *Bottom panel*: two distinct outcomes of chromosomal translocations. In the case of transcriptional deregulation (*left scheme*), the normal regulatory sequences of the protooncogene are substituted with regulatory sequences derived from the partner chromosome, leading to deregulated expression of the protooncogene. In most cases of B-NHL, the heterologous regulatory regions derive from the *Ig* loci. In the case of fusion proteins (*right scheme*), the coding sequences of the two involved genes are joined in frame into a chimeric transcriptional unit that encodes for a fusion protein, characterized by novel biochemical and functional properties.

Aberrant Somatic Hypermutation

The term *aberrant somatic hypermutation* (ASHM) defines a recently identified mechanism of genetic lesion that is uniquely associated with B-NHL, particularly DLBCL, leading to the mutation of multiple non-Ig genes.[47] ASHM has been proposed to derive from a malfunction in the physiologic SHM process, although the mechanism involved in this malfunction has not been identified.

In GC B cells, SHM is tightly regulated both spatially and temporally to introduce mutations only in the rearranged *IgV* genes[8] as well as in the 5′ region of a few other genes, including *BCL6* and the *CD79* components of the B-cell receptor,[48–52] although the functional role of the mutations found in these other genes remains obscure. On the contrary, multiple mutational events were found to affect numerous loci in over

MOLECULAR BIOLOGY OF INDIVIDUAL CANCERS

TABLE 30.1

MOST COMMON GENETIC LESIONS ASSOCIATED WITH NON-HODGKIN'S LYMPHOMA (NHL)

NHL Subtype	Genetic Abnormality	% of Cases Affected	Involved Gene	Functional Consequences	Gene Function
Mantle cell lymphoma	t(11;14)(q13;q32)	95	CCND1	Transcriptional deregulation	Cell-cycle regulation
Burkitt lymphoma	t(8;14)(q24;q32)	80	MYC	Transcriptional deregulation	Control of proliferation and growth
	t(2;8)(p11;q24)	15	MYC	Transcriptional deregulation	
	t(8;22)(q24;q11)	5	MYC	Transcriptional deregulation	
Follicular lymphoma	t(14;18)(q32;q21)	90	BCL2	Transcriptional deregulation	Antiapoptosis
	t(2;18)(p11;q21)	Rare	BCL2	Transcriptional deregulation	
	t(18;22)(q21;q11)	Rare	BCL2	Transcriptional deregulation	
Diffuse large B-cell lymphoma (GCB)	t(8;14)(q24;q32)	10	MYC	Transcriptional deregulation	Proliferation and growth
	t(14;18)(q32;q21)	30	BCL2	Transcriptional deregulation	Antiapoptosis
	t(3;other)(q27;other)	15	BCL6	Transcriptional deregulation	DNA damage responses; differentiation
	EZH2 M	20	EZH2	Unknown	Chromatin remodeling
Diffuse large B-cell lymphoma (ABC)	t(3;other)(q27;other)	25	BCL6	Transcriptional deregulation	DNA damage responses; differentiation
	TNFAIP3 M/D	20	TNFAIP3	Loss of function	Negative NF-κB regulator
	PRDM1 M/D	20	PRDM1	Loss of function	Terminal B-cell differentiation
	CD79B M	18	CD79B	Gain of function	Chronic active BCR signaling
	CARD11 M	9	CARD11	Gain of function	Positive NF-κB regulator
	18q21 amplifications	30	BCL2	Increased gene dosage	Antiapoptosis
Primary mediastinal B cell lymphoma	9p24.1 amplifications	50	JAK2	Increased gene dosage	JAK-STAT pathway regulation
			PDL1, PDL2	Increased gene dosage	Immunomodulatory responses

Disease	Abnormality	Frequency (%)	Gene	Mechanism	Function
MALT lymphoma	t(11;18)(q21;q21)	30	API2-MALT1	Fusion protein	Positive NF-κB regulator
	t(14;18)(q32;q21)	15–20	MALT1	Transcriptional deregulation	Positive NF-κB regulator
	t(3;14)(p13;q32)	10	FOXP1	Transcriptional deregulation	Transcription factor
	t(1;14)(p22;q32)	5	BCL10	Transcriptional deregulation	Positive NF-κB regulator
Lymphoplasmacytic lymphoma	t(9;14)(p13;q32)	50	PAX5	Transcriptional deregulation	B-cell proliferation and differentiation
Anaplastic large cell lymphoma	t(2;5)(p23;q35)	60[a]	NPM/ALK	Fusion protein	Tyrosine kinase
Classic Hodgkin's lymphoma	TNFAIP3 M/D	40[b]	TNFAIP3	Loss of function	Negative NF-κB regulator
	SOCS1 M/D	45	SOCS1	Loss of function	JAK-STAT pathway regulation
	2p13 amplifications	50	REL	Increased gene dosage	Positive NF-κB regulator
	9p24.1 amplifications	50	JAK2	Increased gene dosage	JAK-STAT pathway regulation
			PDL1, PDL2	Increased gene dosage	Immunomodulatory responses

GCB, germinal center B-cell-like; ABC, activated B-cell-like; BCR, B-cell receptor; MALT, extranodal marginal zone lymphoma of mucosa-associated lymphoid tissue; M, mutation; D, deletion.

[a]In the adult population; 85% in childhood.

[b]Sixty percent in Epstein-Barr virus–negative cases.

50% of DLBCL cases, as well as in a few other lymphoma types, including, among others, AIDS-associated B-NHL, primary central nervous system lymphomas, and posttransplant lymphoproliferative disorders.[53–57] The identified target loci comprise more than 10% of the genes transcribed in B cells and include several well-known protooncogenes such as *PIM1* and *MYC,* one of the most frequently altered human oncogenes.[47] These mutations are typically distributed within ~2 Kb from the transcription initiation site (i.e., the hypermutable domain in the Ig locus)[58] and, depending on the genomic configuration of the target gene, may affect nontranslated as well as coding regions, thus altering the response to factors that normally regulate their expression, or changing key structural and functional properties.[47] This is the case of *MYC,* where a significant number of events lead to amino acid changes with proven functional consequences in activating its oncogenic potential. However, a comprehensive characterization of the potentially extensive genetic damage caused by ASHM is still lacking.

Other Mechanisms of Protooncogene Alteration

In addition to chromosomal translocations and ASHM, the structure of protooncogenes and/or their pattern of expression can be altered by gene copy number amplifications and somatic point mutations. Compared with epithelial cancer, only a few genes have been identified so far as specific targets of chromosomal amplification in B-NHL, as exemplified by *REL* and *BCL2* in DLBCL,[59–62] and PD-1 ligands in primary mediastinal B-cell lymphoma (PMBCL).[63] However, the recent introduction of advanced cytogenetic and high-resolution, genome-wide single nucleotide polymorphism array technologies is likely to reveal a more complex scenario, leading to the identification of additional chromosomal sites of amplification. Somatic point mutations may alter the coding sequence of the target protooncogene and thus the biological properties of its protein product, as observed in *MYC* and *BCL2*.[25,64–66] More recently, a number of genes involved in the activation of the NF-κB transcription complex have also been found to harbor oncogenic point mutations in DLBCL,[67,68] leading to constitutive activation of NF-κB.[67,68] Mutations of the *RAS* genes, a very frequent protooncogene alteration in human neoplasia, are virtually absent in lymphomas.[69]

Inactivation of Tumor Suppressor Genes

Until recently, the *TP53* gene, possibly the most common target of genetic alteration in human cancer,[70] remained one of few *bona fide* tumor suppressor genes involved in the pathogenesis of NHL, although at generally low frequencies and restricted to specific disease subtypes, such as BL and DLBCL derived from the transformation of FL or CLL.[71–73] The mechanism of *TP53* inactivation in NHL is similar to that detected in human neoplasia in general, entailing point mutation of one allele and chromosomal deletion or mutation of the second allele.[70] In recent years, additional genes have been identified as targets of biallelic inactivation in B-NHL through specific chromosomal deletions and/or mutations. Two such genes lie on the long arm of chromosome 6 (6q), a region long known to be deleted in a large percentage of aggressive lymphomas, and associated with poor prognosis[74,75]: the *PRDM1/BLIMP1* gene on 6q21, which is biallelically inactivated in ~25% of activated B-cell-like (ABC)-DLBCL cases,[76–78] and the gene encoding for the negative NF-κB regulator *INFAIP3* on chromosome 6q23, which is commonly lost in ABC-DLBCL, PMBCL, and subtypes of marginal-zone lymphoma and HL.[67,79–81]

Deletions of chromosome 13q14.3 represent the most frequent lesions in CLL (>50% of cases)[82,83] and encompass three noncoding elements, namely the *DLEU2/mir-15a/16-1* cluster,[84–87] whose deletion in mice promotes the development of CLL,[88] documenting its pathogenetic role. Tumor suppressor inactivation via epigenetic transcriptional silencing was described for *CDKN2A* (*p16/INK4a*) as an infrequent event in various B-NHL.[89,90] More recently, monoallelic inactivating mutations and deletions were found to affect the acetyltransferase genes *CREBBP* and *EP300* in a significant proportion of DLBCL and FL, suggesting a role as haploinsufficient tumor suppressors.[91] Major efforts are currently ongoing to identify the total complement of genetic lesions that are associated with the development of various lymphoma types by taking advantage of recently developed genome-wide technologies.

Infectious Agents

Viral and bacterial infections have both been implicated in the pathogenesis of lymphoma. At least three viruses are associated with specific NHL subtypes: the Epstein-Barr virus (EBV), the human herpesvirus-8 (HHV-8/KSHV), and the human T-cell leukemia virus type 1 (HTLV-1). Other infectious agents, such as human immunodeficiency virus (HIV), hepatitis C virus (HCV), *Helicobacter pylori,* and *Chlamydophila psittaci,* have an indirect role in NHL pathogenesis by either impairing the immune system and/or providing chronic antigenic stimulation.

EBV was initially identified in cases of endemic African BL[92,93] and subsequently detected also in a fraction of sporadic BL, HIV-related lymphomas and primary effusion lymphomas (PELs).[71,94–100]

On infection of a B lymphocyte, the EBV genome is transported into the nucleus, where it exists predominantly as an extrachromosomal circular molecule (episome).[101] The formation of circular episomes is mediated by the cohesive terminal repeats, which are represented by a variable number of tandem repeats sequence.[101,102] Because of this termini heterogeneity, the number of tandem repeats sequences enclosed in newly formed episomes may differ considerably, thus representing a clonal marker of a single infected cell.[102] Evidence for a pathogenetic role of the virus in NHL infected by EBV is at least twofold. First, it is well recognized that EBV is able to significantly alter the growth of B cells.[101] Second, EBV-infected lymphomas usually display a single form of fused EBV termini, suggesting that the lymphoma cell population represents the clonally expanded progeny of a single infected cell.[71,94] Nonetheless, the role of EBV in lymphomagenesis is still unclear as the virus infects virtually all humans during their lifetime and its transforming genes are commonly not expressed in the tumor cells of BL.

HHV-8 is a gammaherpesvirus initially identified in tissues of HIV-related Kaposi sarcoma[103] and subsequently found to infect PEL cells as well as a substantial fraction of multicentric Castleman disease.[104–107] Phylogenetic analysis has shown that the closest relative of HHV-8 is herpesvirus saimiri, a gamma-2 herpesvirus of primates associated with T-cell lymphoproliferative disorders.[108] Like other gammaherpesviruses, HHV-8 is also lymphotropic and can be found in lymphocytes both *in vitro* and *in vivo*.[103,106,107] Lymphoma cells naturally infected by HHV-8 harbor the viral genome in its episomal configuration and display a marked restriction of viral gene expression, suggesting a pattern of latent infection.[108]

HTLV-1 is a member of the lentivirus group that can immortalize normal T cells *in vitro* and can cause adult T-cell leukemia/lymphoma (ATLL).[109–112] Unlike acutely transforming retroviruses, the HTLV-1 genome does not encode a viral oncogene. Moreover, this retrovirus does not transform T cells by *cis*-activation of an adjacent cellular protooncogene because the provirus appears to integrate randomly within the host genome.[110–112] Rather, the pathogenetic effect of HTLV-1 seems to be due to viral production of a transregulatory protein (HTLV-1 tax) that activates the transcription of several host genes.[113–119]

An association between B-NHL and infection by HCV, a single-stranded RNA virus of the Flaviviridae family, has been proposed because of the increased risk of developing lymphoproliferative disorders among HCV-positive patients.[120] Although the underlying mechanisms remain unclear, current models suggest that chronic B-cell stimulation by antigens associated with HCV infection may induce nonmalignant B-cell expansion, which subsequently evolves into B-NHL by accumulating additional genetic lesions.

A causal link between antigen stimulation by *H. pylori* and MALT lymphoma originating in the stomach is documented by the observation that *H. pylori* can be found in the vast majority of the lymphoma specimens,[121–123] and long-term complete regression of the disease is achieved in 70% of cases on eradication of infection with antibiotics.[124] However, cases with t(11;18)(q21;21) respond poorly to antibiotic eradication.[125]

C. psittaci, an obligate intracellular bacterium, was recently linked to the development of ocular adnexal marginal zone B-cell lymphoma, although variations in prevalence among different geographic areas remain a major investigational issue.[4,126,127] In this indolent lymphoma, *C. psittaci* causes both local and systemic persistent infection, presumably contributing to lymphomagenesis via its mitogenic activity as well as through its ability to promote polyclonal cell proliferation and to induce resistance to apoptosis in the infected cells *in vivo*. Notably, bacterial eradication with antibiotic therapy is often followed by lymphoma regression.[128]

MOLECULAR PATHOGENESIS OF B-CELL NON-HODGKIN'S LYMPHOMA

The following section will focus on well-characterized genetic lesions that are associated with the most common types of B-NHL, classified according to the World Health Organization classification of lymphoid neoplasia.[2] The molecular pathogenesis of HIV-related NHL will also be addressed, while the pathogenesis of other B-cell NHL types remains far less understood.

Mantle Cell Lymphoma

Cell of Origin

MCL is an aggressive disease representing ~5% of all NHL diagnoses and generally regarded as incurable.[2,89] Based on immunophenotype, gene expression profile, and molecular features, such as the presence of unmutated *IgV* genes in most cases, MCL is thought to derive from naïve, pre-GC peripheral B cells located in the inner mantle zone of secondary follicles (Fig. 30.3).

Genetic Lesions

MCL is typically associated with the t(11;14)(q13;q32) translocation that juxtaposes the *IGH* gene on chromosome 14q32 to a region containing the *CCND1* gene (also known as *BCL1*) on chromosome 11q13 (Table 30.1).[129–131] The translocation consistently leads to homotopic deregulation

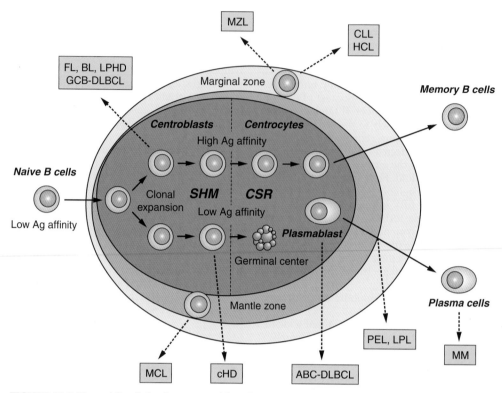

FIGURE 30.3 Normal B-cell development and lymphomagenesis. Schematic representation of a lymphoid follicle, constituted by the germinal center (GC) and the mantle zone, along with the surrounding marginal zone. B cells that have successfully rearranged their *Ig* genes in the bone marrow move to peripheral lymphoid organs as naïve B cells. On encounter with a T-cell–dependent antigen, B cells become proliferating centroblasts in the GC and eventually mature into centrocytes. These events are associated with the activation of somatic hypermutation and class-switch recombination. Only GC B cells with high affinity for the antigen will be positively selected to exit the GC and further differentiate into plasma cells or memory B cells, while low-affinity clones are eliminated by apoptosis. *Dotted arrows* indicate the putative normal counterpart of various lymphoma subtypes, as identified based on the presence of somatically mutated *IgV* genes, as well as on distinctive phenotypic features. MCL, mantle cell lymphoma; FL, follicular lymphoma; BL, Burkitt lymphoma; DLBCL, diffuse large B-cell lymphoma (GCB, germinal center B-cell-like; ABC, activated B-cell-like); CLL, chronic lymphocytic leukemia/ HCL, hairy cell leukemia; MM, multiple myeloma; LPHD, lymphocyte predominance Hodgkin disease; LPL, lympho plasma cytic lymphoma; MZL, marginal zone lymphoma; PEL, primary effusion lymphoma.

and overexpression of cyclin D1, a member of the D-type G_1 cyclins that regulates the early phases of the cell cycle and is normally not expressed in resting B cells.[132–134] By deregulating cyclin D1, t(11;14) is thought to contribute to malignant transformation by perturbing the G_1-S phase transition of the cell cycle.[89] In addition to t(11;14), up to 10% of MCLs overexpress aberrant or shorter cyclin D1 transcripts, as a consequence of secondary rearrangements, microdeletions, or point mutations in the gene 3′ untranslated region.[135–137] These alterations may lead to cyclin D1 overexpression through the removal of destabilizing sequences and the consequent increase in mRNA half-life. Typically, this subset of cases is characterized by high proliferative activity and a more aggressive clinical course.[138] The pathogenetic role of cyclin D1 deregulation in human neoplasia is suggested by

the ability of the overexpressed protein to transform cells *in vitro* and to promote B-cell lymphomagenesis in transgenic mice,[139–141] although a specific animal model that faithfully recapitulates the features of the human MCL is still lacking. Importantly, the frequency and specificity of this genetic lesion, together with the expression of CCND1 in the tumor cells, provide an excellent marker for MCL diagnosis.[2]

Other genetic alterations involved in MCL include frequent biallelic inactivation of the *ATM* gene by genomic deletions and mutations,[142] loss of the *TP53* gene in 20% of patients, where it represents a marker of poor prognosis,[143] and inactivation of the *CDKN2A* gene by genomic deletion, mutation, or hypermethylation in approximately half of the cases belonging to the MCL variant characterized by a blastoid cell morphology.[144] In a small number of cases, *BMI1* is amplified and/

or overexpressed, possibly as an alternative mechanism to the loss of CDKN2A.[138,145]

Burkitt Lymphoma

Cell of Origin

BL is an aggressive lymphoma comprising three clinical variants, namely sporadic Burkitt lymphoma (sBL), endemic Burkitt lymphoma (eBL), and HIV-associated BL, often diagnosed as the initial manifestation of AIDS.[2] The presence of highly mutated IgV sequences that carry the hallmark of SHM,[146–149] together with the expression of a distinct gene expression signature,[150,151] indicates the derivation from a GC B cell.

Genetic Lesions

All BL cases, including the leukemic variants, share a virtually obligatory genetic lesion, that is, chromosomal translocations involving the MYC gene on region 8q24 and one of the Ig loci on the partner chromosome.[152,153] In ~80% of cases, this is represented by the IGH locus, leading to t(8;14)(q24;q32), while in the remaining 20% of cases either IGκ (2p12) or IGλ (22q11) are involved.[152–155] Although fairly homogeneous at the microscopic level, these translocations display a high degree of molecular heterogeneity. The t(8;14) breakpoints are located 5′ and centromeric to MYC, whereas they map 3′ to MYC in t(2;8) and t(8;22).[152–156] Further molecular heterogeneity derives from the exact breakpoint sites on chromosomes 8 and 14 in t(8;14). Translocations of eBL tend to involve sequences on chromosome 8 at an undefined distance 5′ to MYC (>1,000 Kb) and sequences on chromosome 14 within or in proximity to the Ig I$_H$ region.[157,158] In sBL, t(8;14) preferentially involves sequences within or immediately 5′ to MYC (<3 Kb) on chromosome 8, and sequences within the Ig switch regions on chromosome 14.[157,158]

The common consequence of t(8;14), t(2;8), and t(8;22) is the ectopic and constitutive overexpression of the MYC protooncogene,[159–161] which is normally not detected in most proliferating GC B cells.[11] At least two distinct mechanisms are responsible for MYC deregulation, including juxtaposition of the MYC coding sequences to heterologous enhancers derived from Ig loci,[159–161] and structural alterations of the gene 5′ regulatory sequences, which alter the responsiveness to cellular factors controlling its expression.[162] In fact, the MYC exon 1/intron 1 junction, encompassing critical regulatory elements, is either decapitated by the translocation or mutated in the translocated alleles. Oncogenic activation of MYC can also be due to amino acid substitutions within the gene exon 2, encoding for the protein transactivation domain.[64,65] These mutations can abolish the ability of p107, a nuclear protein related to RB1, to suppress MYC activity,[163] or can increase protein stability.[164,165]

MYC is a nuclear phosphoprotein that functions as a sequence specific DNA-binding transcriptional regulator controlling proliferation, differentiation, and apoptosis, all of which are implicated in carcinogenesis.[166,167] In addition, MYC controls DNA replication independent of its transcriptional activity, a property that may promote genomic instability by inducing replication stress.[168] Consistent with its involvement in multiple cellular processes, the MYC target gene network is estimated to include ~15% of all protein-coding genes as well as noncoding RNAs.[167,169] In vivo, MYC is found mainly in heterodimeric complexes with the related protein MAX, and such interaction is required for MYC-induced stimulation of transcription and cell proliferation.[170–176] In B-NHL carrying MYC translocations, constitutive expression of MYC induces transcription of a subset of target genes that have diverse roles in regulating cell growth by affecting DNA replication, energy metabolism, protein synthesis, and telomere elongation.[167,176,177] In addition, deregulated MYC expression is thought to cause genomic instability, thus contributing to tumor progression by facilitating the occurrence of additional genetic lesions.[178] Dysregulation of MYC expression in a number of transgenic mouse models leads to the development of aggressive B-cell lymphomas with high penetrance and short latency.[165,179,180] These mouse models confirm the pathogenetic role of deregulated MYC in B cells, although the resulting tumors tend to be more immature than the human BL, most likely because of the early activation of the promoter sequences used for expression of the MYC transgene.

Cooperating oncogenic events in BL include loss of TP53 by mutation and/or deletion (30% of both sBL and eBL cases),[72] inactivation of CDKN2B by hypermethylation,[181] and deletions of 6q, detected in ~30% of cases, independent of the clinical variant.[74] Additionally, one contributing factor to the development of BL is monoclonal EBV infection, present in virtually all cases of eBL and in ~30% of sBL.[92,94,182,183] The consistent expression of EBER, a class of small RNA molecules, has been proposed to mediate the transforming potential of EBV in BL.[184] However, because EBV infection in BL displays a peculiar latent infection phenotype characterized by negativity of both EBV-transforming antigens LMP1 and EBNA2, the precise pathogenetic role of the virus has remained elusive.[185]

Follicular Lymphoma

FL represents the second most common type of B-NHL, accounting for ~20% of all diagnoses, and the most common low-grade B-NHL.[2] Over time, FL tends to transform into an aggressive lymphoma with a diffuse large cell architecture (Fig. 30.3).[2]

Cell of Origin

FL arises from a GC-derived B cell, as documented by the presence of somatically mutated Ig genes that show evidence of ongoing SHM activity, and by the expression of specific GC B-cell markers such as BCL6 and CD10.[1]

Genetic Lesions

The genetic hallmark of FL is represented by chromosomal translocations affecting the $BCL2$ gene on chromosome band 18q21, which are detected in 80% to 90% of cases independent of cytologic subtype, although less frequent in grade 3 FL[130,186–189] (Table 30.1). In t(14;18), the rearrangement joins the 3' untranslated region of $BCL2$ to an $Ig\ J_H$ segment, resulting in the ectopic expression of BCL2 in GC B cells,[186,187,190–194] where its transcription is normally repressed by BCL6.[16,25] Approximately 70% of the breakpoints on chromosome 18 cluster within the major breakpoint region, while the remaining 5% to 25% map to the more distant minor cluster region, located ~20 kb downstream of the $BCL2$ gene.[186,187,190,191] Rearrangements involving the 5' flanking region of $BCL2$ have been described in a minority of cases.[195] The $BCL2$ gene encodes a 26-kD integral membrane protein that controls the cell apoptotic threshold by preventing programmed cell death[196–199]; BCL2 may thus contribute to lymphomagenesis by inducing resistance of tumor cells to apoptosis independent of antigen selection. Nevertheless, additional genetic aberrations are likely required for malignant transformation, a major role being played by chronic antigen stimulation.[200–202]

More recently, somatic mutations of the polycomb-group oncogene $EZH2$, which encodes a histone methyltransferase responsible for the trimethylation of Lys27 of histone H3 (H3K27), were found in 7% of FL patients.[203] These mutations result in the replacement of a single tyrosine (Tyr641) in the SET domain of the EZH2 protein, and were associated with increased levels of H3K27me3 through a mechanism that involves altered substrate catalytic specificity.[203] However, the precise mechanism by which this amino acid change contributes to tumorigenesis remains to be clarified.

Chromosomal translocations of the $BCL6$ gene are detected in 6% to 14% of all FL cases, and were shown to have a significantly higher prevalence in the group of patients known to eventually transform into aggressive DLBCL.[204–207] Other genetic lesions are also predominantly observed in FL cases that have undergone histologic progression to a high-grade NHL, and

include deletions of chromosome 6 (20% of the cases),[74] $TP53$ mutations (25% to 30%),[73,208–210] inactivation of $CDKN2A$ through deletion, mutation, and hypermethylation (one-third of patients),[144,211] rearrangements of MYC in rare cases,[212] and a variety of copy number aberrations.[213] Overall, the molecular events that lead to the clinical progression of FL remain poorly characterized.

Diffuse Large B-Cell Lymphoma

DLBCL is the most common type of B-NHL, accounting for ~40% of all new diagnoses in adulthood, and includes cases arising *de novo*, as well as cases that derive from the clinical evolution of various, less aggressive B-NHL types (i.e., FL and CLL).[2,214]

Cell of Origin

Over the past decade, the advent of genome-wide gene expression profile technologies has allowed the identification of multiple phenotypic DLBCL subgroups that reflect the derivation from B cells at various differentiation stages. These include at least three well-characterized subtypes: a GC B-cell-like (GCB) DLBCL, which appears to derive from proliferating GC centroblasts; an ABC DLBCL, which shows a transcriptional signature related to plasmablastic B cells presumably blocked during post-GC differentiation; and PMBCL, which is postulated to arise from thymic B cells; the remaining 15% to 30% of cases remain unclassified.[215–218] Stratification according to gene expression profiles has prognostic value, as patients diagnosed with a GCB-DLBCL display a better overall survival compared with ABC-DLBCL,[62] but does not direct differential therapy, and is imperfectly replicated by immunophenotyping or morphology[219,220]; thus, it is not officially incorporated into the World Health Organization classification. A separate classification scheme identified three subsets defined by the expression of genes involved in oxidative phosphorylation, B-cell receptor/proliferation, and tumor microenvironment/host inflammatory response.[221]

Genetic Lesions

The heterogeneity of DLBCL is reflected in the catalogue of genetic lesions that are associated with its pathogenesis. These include balanced reciprocal translocations deregulating the expression of protooncogenes, gene amplifications, chromosomal deletions, single-point mutations, and aberrant somatic hypermutation.[222,223] Notably, most of these abnormalities are preferentially or exclusively associated with individual DLBCL phenotypic subtypes, indicating that

GCB- and ABC-DLBCL use distinct oncogenic pathways.[224]

GCB-DLBCL. Genetic lesions that are specific to GCB-DLBCL include the t(14;18) and t(8;14) translocations, which deregulate the *BCL2* and *MYC* oncogenes in 34% and 10% of cases, respectively[25,62,225–227]; mutations affecting an autoregulatory domain within the BCL6 5'untranslated exon 1[228–230]; mutations of the *EZH2* gene[203]; and deletions of the tumor suppressor *PTEN*.[224] In addition, recent studies have identified frequent monoallelic mutations and deletions inactivating the acetyltransferase genes *CREBBP* and *EP300* predominantly in this subtype of DLBCL, where they affect nearly 40% of cases.[91]

Somatic mutations of the BCL6 5' regulatory sequences are detected in up to 75% of DLBCL cases,[48,231,232] and reflect the activity of the physiologic SHM mechanism that operates in normal GC B cells.[48,49,52] However, functional analysis of numerous mutated *BCL6* alleles revealed that a subset of mutations are specifically associated with DLBCL while being absent in normal GC cells or in other B-cell malignancies.[229] These mutations deregulate *BCL6* transcription by disrupting an autoregulatory circuit through which the BCL6 protein controls its own expression levels via binding to the promoter region of the gene[229,230] or by preventing CD40-induced BCL6 down-regulation in post-GC B cells.[233] Because the full extent of mutations deregulating *BCL6* expression has not been characterized, the fraction of DLBCL cases carrying abnormalities in *BCL6* cannot be determined.

Approximately 50% of all DLBCL are also associated with ASHM.[47] The number and identity of the genes that accumulate mutations in their coding and noncoding regions due to this mechanism varies in different cases and is still largely undefined. However, preferential targeting of individual genes has been observed in the two main COO-defined DLBCL subtypes, with mutations of *MYC* and *BCL2* being found at significantly higher frequencies in GCB-DLBCL, and mutations of *PIM1* almost exclusively observed in ABC-DLBCL. ASHM may therefore contribute to the heterogeneity of DLBCL via the alteration of different cellular pathways in different cases. Mutations and deletions of the *TP53* tumor suppressor gene are mostly detectable in cases originating from the transformation of FL, and are therefore more often associated with chromosomal translocations involving *BCL2* and with a GCB-DLBCL phenotype.[73]

ABC-DLBCL. Several genetic abnormalities are observed almost exclusively in ABC-DLBCL, including amplifications of the *BCL2* locus on 18q24[234,235]; mutations within the NF-κB (*CARD11*, *TNFAIP3/A20*)[67,68] and B-cell receptor signaling (*CD79B*)[236] pathways; inactivating mutations and deletions of *BLIMP1*[76–78]; chromosomal translocations deregulating the *BCL6* oncogene; deletion or lack of expression of the *p16* tumor suppressor gene and, rarely, mutations of the *ATM* gene.[237,238]

Chromosomal translocations affecting band 3q27 cause rearrangements of the *BCL6* gene in up to 35% of all DLBCL cases,[75,205,239] with a twofold higher frequency in the ABC-DLBCL subtype[228] (Table 30.1). These rearrangements juxtapose the intact coding domain of *BCL6* downstream and in the same transcriptional orientation to heterologous sequences derived from the partner chromosome, including *IGH* (14q23), *IGκ* (2p12), *IGλ* (22q11), and at least 20 other chromosomal sites unrelated to the Ig loci.[39–46] The majority of these translocations result in a fusion transcript in which the promoter region and the first noncoding exon of Bcl6 are replaced by sequences derived from the partner gene.[40,240] Because the common denominator of these promoters is a broader spectrum of activity throughout B-cell development, including expression in the post-GC differentiation stage, the translocation prevents the down-regulation of *BCL6* expression that is normally associated with differentiation into post-GC cells. Deregulated expression of a normal *BCL6* gene product may play a critical role by enforcing the proliferative phenotype typical of GC cells while blocking terminal differentiation, as confirmed by a mouse model in which deregulated *BCL6* expression causes DLBCL.[241]

In up to 25% of ABC-DLBCL, the *PRDM1* gene is inactivated by a variety of genetic lesions, including truncating or missense mutations and/or genomic deletions, as well as by transcriptional repression through constitutively active, translocated BCL6 alleles.[76–78] The *PRDM1* gene encodes for a zinc finger transcriptional repressor that is expressed in a subset of GC B cells undergoing plasma cell differentiation and in all plasma cells,[242,243] and is an essential requirement for terminal B-cell differentiation.[244] Thus, *BLIMP1* inactivation may contribute to lymphomagenesis by blocking post-GC B-cell differentiation. Notably, translocations deregulating the *BCL6* gene are virtually never found in *BLIMP1* mutated DLBCLs, suggesting that *BCL6* deregulation and *BLIMP1* inactivation represent alternative oncogenic mechanisms converging on the same pathway (Fig. 30.4).

A predominant feature of ABC-DLBCL is the constitutive activation of the NF-κB signaling pathway, initially evidenced by the selective expression of a signature enriched in NF-κB target genes, and by the requirement of NF-κB for proliferation and survival in ABC-DLBCL cell lines. A number of recent studies have led to the identification of multiple oncogenic alterations affecting positive and negative regulators of

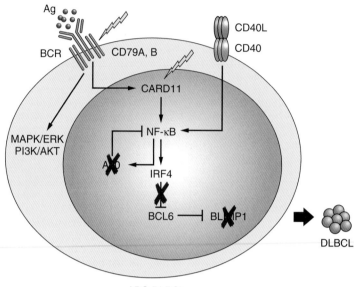

FIGURE 30.4 Pathway lesions in activated B-cell-like diffuse large B-cell lymphoma (ABC-DLBCL). Schematic representation of a germinal center centrocyte, expressing a functional surface B-cell receptor (BCR) and CD40 receptor. In normal B cells, engagement of the BCR by the antigen (spheres) or interaction of the CD40 receptor with the CD40L presented by T cells induce activation of the NF-κB pathway, including its targets IRF4 and A20. IRF4, in turn, down-regulates *BCL6* expression, allowing the release of *BLIMP1* expression, a master plasma cell regulator required for plasma cell differentiation. In ABC-DLBCL, multiple genetic lesions converge on this pathway and disrupt it at multiple levels in different cases (percentages as indicated), presumably contributing to lymphomagenesis by favoring the antiapoptotic and proproliferative function of NF-κB while blocking terminal B-cell differentiation through mutually exclusive deregulation of *BCL6* and inactivation of *BLIMP1*.

NF-κB, specifically in this disease subtype, providing genetic evidence for this phenotypic characteristic. In up to 30% of cases, the *TNFAIP3* gene encoding for the negative regulator A20 is biallelically inactivated by mutations and/or deletions, thus preventing termination of NF-κB responses.[67,79] The tumor suppressor role of A20 was documented by the observation that reconstitution of A20 knockout cell lines with wild type protein induces apoptosis and blocks proliferation, in part due to suppression of NF-κB activity.[67,79] In an additional ~10% of ABC-DLBCL, the *CARD11* gene is targeted by oncogenic mutations clustering in the coiled-coil domain and enhancing its ability to transactivate NF-κB target genes.[67,68] Less commonly, mutations were found in a variety of other genes encoding for NF-κB components, overall accounting for over half of all ABC-DLBCL[67] and suggesting that yet unidentified lesions may be responsible for the NF-κB activity in the remaining fraction of cases. In addition to constitutive NF-κB activity, ABC-DLBCLs display evidence of chronic active BCR signaling, which is associated with somatic mutations affecting the immunoreceptor tyrosine-based activation motif signaling modules of *CD79B* and *CD79A* in 10% of ABC-DLBCL biopsy samples but rarely in other DLBCLs.[236]

PMBCL. PMBCL is a tumor observed most commonly in young female adults, which involves the mediastinum and displays a distinct gene expression profile, largely similar to a particular type of HL.[217,218] A genetic hallmark of both PMBCL and HL is the amplification of chromosomal region 9q24, detected in nearly 50% of patients.[224,245] This relatively large interval encompasses multiple genes of possible pathogenetic significance, including the gene encoding for the *JAK2* tyrosine kinase or the *PDL1* and *PDL2* genes, which encode for inhibitors of T-cell responses.[63,224,245] Besides contributing to lymphomagenesis, elevated expression levels of these genes may partly explain the unique features of these lymphoma types, which are characterized by a significant inflammatory infiltrate. PMBCL also shares with HL the presence of genetic lesions affecting the NF-κB pathway and the deregulated expression of receptor tyrosine kinases.[81,246–248]

Extranodal Marginal Zone Lymphoma of Mucosa-Associated Lymphoid Tissue

Cell of Origin

MALT lymphoma represents the third most common form of B-NHL,[2] and has steadily risen in incidence over the past 2 decades.[249] The presence of rearranged and somatically mutated *IgV* genes,[30,250] together with the architectural relationship with mucosa-associated lymphoid tissue,[2] indicate the post-GC origin of these tumors, possibly from a marginal zone, memory B cell (Fig. 30.3). A critical role for antigen stimulation, particularly in the pathogenesis of gastric MALT lymphoma, is supported by the observation that (1) this disease is associated with chronic infection of the gastric mucosa by *H. pylori* in virtually all cases,[121–123] (2) eradication of *H. pylori* by antibiotic treatment can lead to tumor regression in ~70% of cases,[124,251] and (3) MALT lymphoma cells express autoreactive BCR, in particular to rheumatoid factors.[252,253]

Whether the development of MALT lymphoma arising in body sites other than the stomach is also dependent on antigen stimulation remains an open question. In this respect, it is remarkable that salivary gland and thyroid MALT lymphoma are generally a sequela of autoimmune processes, namely Sjögren syndrome and Hashimoto thyroiditis, respectively.

Genetic Lesions

Of several structural aberrations that are selectively and recurrently associated with MALT lymphoma, most target the NF-κB signaling pathway, suggesting a critical role in the pathogenesis of the disease. The most common one is the t(11;18)(21;21) translocation, which involves the *API2 (BIRC3)* gene on 11q21 and the *MALT1* gene on 18q21,[254,255] and is observed in 25% to 40% of gastric and pulmonary MALT lymphomas.[256–258] API2, a member of the family of Inhibitor of Apoptosis Proteins, plays an evolutionary conserved role in regulating programmed cell death in diverse species. MALT1, together with BCL10 and CARD11, is a component of the CBM ternary complex and plays a central role in BCR and NF-κB signaling activation.[90] Notably, the wild type proteins encoded by these two genes are incapable of activating NF-κB, as opposed to the API/MALT1 fusion protein, suggesting that the translocation may confer a survival advantage to the tumor by leading to inhibition of apoptosis and constitutive NF-κB activation without the need for upstream signaling.[254,255,259] In an additional 15% to 20% of cases, the *MALT1* gene is translocated to the *IGH* locus in t(14;18)(q32;q21).[260,261]

Recurrent abnormalities of chromosomal band 1p22, generally represented by t(1;14)(p22;q32), occur in ~5% of MALT lymphomas and cause deregulated expression of *BCL10*, a cellular homologue of the equine herpesvirus-2 *E10* gene, which encodes an amino-terminal caspase recruitment domain (CARD) homologous to that found in several apoptotic molecules.[262,263] BCL10, however, does not have proapoptotic activity *in vivo*, where it functions as a positive regulator of antigen-induced activation of NF-κB.[90,264,265] Thus, the translocation may provide both antiapoptotic and proliferative signals mediated via NF-κB transcriptional targets. Trisomy 3 represents a recurrent numerical abnormality in MALT lymphomas; however, the genes involved remain presently unknown.[266,267]

A more recently identified translocation associated with, although not restricted to, MALT lymphoma is t(3;14)(p13;q32),[268,269] which leads to deregulated expression of FOXP1, a member of the Forkhead box family of winged-helix transcription factors involved in regulation of Rag1 and Rag2, and essential for B-cell development.[270] Finally, homozygous or hemizygous loss of *TNFAIP3* due to mutations and/or deletions has been reported in 20% of MALT lymphoma patients, where it is mutually exclusive with other genetic lesions, leading to NF-κB activation.[80] Genetic lesions also involved in other lymphoma types include *BCL6* alterations and *TP53* mutations.[271–273]

Chronic Lymphocytic Leukemia/ Small Lymphocytic Lymphoma

Cell of Origin

CLL is a malignancy of mature, resting B lymphocytes, which originates from the oncogenic transformation of a common cellular precursor resembling an antigen-experienced B cell.[274,275] This notion was conclusively demonstrated when gene expression profile studies revealed that, although CLL can express somatically mutated or unmutated *IgV* genes at approximately equal percentages,[276,277] all cases share a homogeneous signature more related to that of CD27+ memory and marginal zone B cells.[278,279] Moreover, analysis of the *Ig* gene repertoire in these patients indicates very similar, at times almost identical, antigen receptors among different individuals.[280–285] This finding, known as *stereotypy*, strongly supports a critical role for the antigen in CLL pathogenesis. The histogenetic heterogeneity of CLL carry prognostic relevance, as cases with mutated *Ig* genes associate with a significantly longer survival.[286,287] Intriguingly, 6% of the normal elderly population develops a monoclonal B-cell lymphocytosis (MBL) that seems to be the precursor to CLL in 1% to 2% of cases.[288]

Genetic Lesions

Different from most mature B-NHLs, and consistent with the derivation from a post-GC or GC-independent B cells, CLL cases are largely devoid of balanced, reciprocal chromosomal translocations.[82,83] On the contrary, CLL is recurrently associated with several numerical abnormalities, including trisomy 12 and monoallelic or biallelic deletion/inactivation of chromosomal regions 17p, 11q, and 13q14 (Table 30.1).[82,83] Of these, deletion of 13q14 represents the most frequent chromosomal aberration, being observed in up to 76% of cases as a monoallelic event, and in 24% of cases as a biallelic event. Interestingly, this same deletion is also found in those with MBL.[288] In all affected cases, the minimal deleted region encompasses a long noncoding RNA (*DLEU2*) and two microRNAs expressed as a cluster, namely miR-15a and miR-16-1.[84,85,87] The causal involvement of 13q14-minimal deleted region–encoded tumor suppressor genes in CLL pathogenesis was recently demonstrated *in vivo* in two animal models that developed clonal lymphoproliferative diseases including MBL, CLL, and DLBCL, at 25% to 40% penetrance.[88] Trisomy 12 is found in approximately 16% of patients evaluated by interphase fluorescent *in situ* hybridization and correlates with a poor survival, but no specific genes have been identified.[289–291] Deletions of chromosomal region 11q22-23 (18% of cases) almost invariably encompass the *ATM* gene and may thus promote genomic instability.[292–294] Because these mutations may occur in the patient germ line, it is thought that they may account, at least in part, for the familial form of the disease. A similar pathogenetic mechanism may be involved in cases with 17p13 genomic deletions (~7%), which include the *TP53* tumor suppressor and are frequently accompanied by mutation of the second allele.[72,295] A higher frequency of *TP53* alterations is observed after transformation of CLL/SLL to Richter syndrome, a highly aggressive lymphoma with a poor clinical outcome.[72]

HIV-Related NHL

The association between an immunodeficiency state and the development of lymphoma has been recognized in several clinical conditions, including congenital (e.g., Wiskott-Aldrich syndrome), iatrogenic (e.g., treatment with immunosuppressor agents), and viral-induced (e.g., AIDS) immunodeficiencies. HIV infection has emerged as a major risk factor for lymphomagenesis, prompting detailed investigations of the molecular pathophysiology of HIV-related NHL, which are primarily classified into three clinicopathologic categories: HIV-related BL, DLBCL, and PEL.[2,296–298] Based on the site of origin, HIV-related NHLs are generally grouped into systemic HIV-related NHL (i.e., DLBCL and BL) and HIV-related PCNSL, which is characterized by a uniform morphology consistent with a diffuse architecture of large cells.[2,296–298]

Cell of Origin

HIV-related NHLs invariably derive from B cells that have experienced the GC reaction, as indicated by the presence of somatically mutated *Ig* and *BCL6* genes, as well as by several phenotypic and genome-wide transcriptional features.[296–298] Based on the presence or absence of immunoblastic features, and on the expression pattern of the BCL6 protein, the EBV-encoded LMP1, and the CD138/syndecan-1 antigen, a proteoglycan associated with the terminal phases of B-cell differentiation, both HIV-related DLBCL and PCNSL can be segregated into two distinct histogenetic categories: cases displaying the BCL6+/CD138−/LMP1− phenotype closely resemble the phenotype of GC B cells; conversely, BCL6−/CD138+/LMP1+ cases are morphologically consistent with immunoblastic lymphoma, plasmacytoid, and reflect a post-GC stage of B-cell differentiation.[296–298] PEL consistently derives from B cells, reflecting a preterminal stage of B-cell differentiation.[105,106,299,300]

Genetic Lesions

The different categories of HIV-related NHL associate with distinctive molecular pathways. Cases of HIV-related BL consistently display activation of MYC by chromosomal translocations that are structurally similar to those found in sporadic BL, while rearrangements of *BCL6* are always absent.[296–298,301] HIV-related BLs also frequently harbor mutations of *TP53* (60%), mutations of the *BCL6* 5′ noncoding regions (60%), and, in 30% of cases, infection of the tumor clone by EBV, although the EBV-encoded antigens LMP1 and EBNA2 are not expressed.[302,303] Stimulation and selection by antigens, frequently represented by autoantigens, appear to be a prominent feature of HIV-related BL.[148,304]

Different from BL, the most frequent genetic alteration detected in HIV-related DLBCL is infection by EBV, which occurs in approximately 60% to 70% of the cases and associates frequently, although not always, with expression of *LMP1*.[71,98,303] Also different from HIV-BL, HIV-related DLBCL displays rearrangements of *BCL6* in 20% of cases.[301] Mutations of *BCL6* 5′ noncoding regions occur in 70% of cases.[305]

All HIV-related PCNSLs harbor EBV infection.[306] However, only the subset of cases with immunoblastic plasmacytoid morphology expresses the LMP1-transforming protein of EBV.[100] HIV-related PCNSLs display evidence of ASHM[54] and harbor oncogenic mutations in the *CARD11* gene (16% of cases),[307] which may explain in part the presence of constitutive NF-κB activity previously recognized in this lymphoma subtype. Although some reports have suggested that HHV-8 may be related to PCNSL pathogenesis in immunocompromised patients, extensive analysis of HIV-related PCNSL has unequivocally ruled out this hypothesis.[308,309]

The last type of HIV-related NHL that has been characterized at the molecular level is represented by PEL, also known as *body cavity–based lymphoma*.[105,106,299] This lymphoma entity is associated with HHV-8 infection in 100% of cases and clinically presents as effusions in the serosal cavities of the body (pleura, pericardium, and peritoneum) in the absence of solid tumor masses.[105,106,299] In addition to HHV-8, cases of PEL frequently carry coinfection of the tumor clone by EBV.[97,99,105,106,299]

MOLECULAR PATHOGENESIS OF T-CELL NHL

Peripheral T-cell lymphomas (PTCLs) encompass a highly heterogeneous and relatively uncommon group of diseases representing 5% to 10% of all cases of NHL worldwide, with significant geographic variation in both incidence and relative prevalence.[2] PTCLs arise from mature postthymic T cells and, according to the clinical presentation of the disease, are listed as leukemic or disseminated, predominantly extranodal, cutaneous, and predominantly nodal.[2] Although the study of T-cell neoplasms is hampered by the rarity of these diseases and the difficulty of collecting homogeneous sample series, significant advances have been made over the past decades in our understanding of their biology, classification, and prognosis.

Adult T-Cell Lymphoma/Leukemia (HTLV-1–Positive)

Cell of Origin

The term ATLL encompasses a spectrum of lymphoproliferative diseases associated with HTLV-1 infection and mainly restricted to southwestern Japan and the Caribbean basin.[2,310] The United States and Europe are considered low-risk areas as less than 1% of the population are HTLV-1 carriers,[311] and only 2% to 4% of seropositive individuals eventually develop ATLL.[2,110,111] Clonal rearrangement of the TCR is evident in all cases, and clonal integration of the virus has been observed.[312,313]

Genetic Lesions

Compared with other mature T-cell tumors, the molecular pathogenesis of ATLL has been eluci-

dated to a wider extent. Particularly, the role of HTLV-1 has been linked to the production of a transregulatory protein (HTLV-1 tax), which markedly increases expression of all viral gene products and transcriptionally activates the expression of certain host genes, including *IL2, CD25* (the α chain of the IL-2 receptor), *c-sis, c-fos,* and *GM-CSF.*[113–117,242] Indeed, a property of ATLL cells is the constitutive high level expression of IL-2 receptors. The central role of these genes in normal T-cell activation and growth, together with the results of *in vitro* studies, support the notion that tax-mediated activation of these host genes represents an important mechanism by which HTLV-1 initiates T-cell transformation.[113] In addition, tax interferes at multiple sites with DNA damage repair functions and with mitotic checkpoints,[118,119,314] consistent with the fact that ATLL cells harbor a high frequency of karyotypic abnormalities.

The long period of clinical latency that precedes the development of ATLL (usually 10–30 years), the small percentage of infected patients who develop this malignancy, and the observation that leukemic cells from ATLL are monoclonal suggest that HTLV-1 is not sufficient to cause the full malignant phenotype.[110–112] A model for ATLL therefore implies an early period of tax-induced polyclonal T-cell proliferation which, in turn, facilitates the occurrence of additional genetic events, leading to the monoclonal outgrowth of a fully transformed cell. In this respect, a recurrent genetic lesion in ATLL is represented by mutations of the *TP53* tumor suppressor gene, which is inactivated in 40% of cases.[315,316]

Peripheral T-Cell Lymphoma, Not Otherwise Specified

This category represents the largest and most heterogeneous group of PTCLs, and includes all cases that lack specific features allowing classification within another entity. The majority of these cases derive from αβ CD4+ T cells and show aberrant defective expression of one or several T-cell–associated antigens.[317] Based on gene expression profile analysis, PTCL not otherwise specified (NOS) as a group appears to be most closely related to activated T cells than to resting T cells, and can be segregated according to similarities with the transcriptional signature of CD4+ and CD8+ T cells. However, no correlation can be observed between gene expression profile and immunophenotype, likely reflecting the variable detection of T-cell antigens in the disease.

Genetic Lesions

Clonal numerical and structural aberrations are found in most PTCL NOS by conventional cytogenetics and in all cases by more sensitive approaches such as array-based methods. For a few loci, correlation between gene copy number and expression has been confirmed, suggesting a pathogenetic role. Candidate genes targeted by copy number gains include *CDK6* on chromosome 7q, *MYC* on chromosome 8, and the NF-κB regulator *CARD11* at 7p22, while losses of 9p21 are associated with reduced expression of *CDKN2A/B*.[318] Chromosomal translocations involving the TCR loci have been reported in rare cases and remain poorly understood because the identity of the translocation partner has not been identified, with few exceptions: the *BCL3* gene, the poliovirus receptor-related 2 (*PVRL2*) gene, found in the t(14;19)(q11;q13) translocation, and the *IRF4* gene, cloned in two cases.[319–321]

Angioimmunoblastic T-Cell Lymphoma

Cell of Origin

Angioimmunoblastic T-cell lymphoma (AITL) is an aggressive disease of the elderly and accounts for about one-third of all PTCL in Western countries.[322] The tumor cells display a mature CD4+CD8–T-cell phenotype, with frequent aberrant loss of one or several T-cell markers, and coexpression of *BCL6* and CD10 in at least a fraction of cells. Recently, gene expression profile studies allowed the conclusive establishment of the cellular derivation of AITL from follicular T-helper cells,[323] as initially suspected based on expression of single markers.[324]

Genetic Lesions

Clonal aberrations have been reported in up to 90% of AITL patients and are mostly represented by chromosomal imbalances, while chromosomal translocations affecting the TCR loci are extremely rare.[318] However, the scarce number of genetic studies performed so far has failed to provide any significant clues regarding the oncogenic pathways involved in AITL.

Cutaneous T-Cell Lymphoma

Genetic lesions are involved in a limited but significant fraction of primary CTCLs showing molecular markers of clonality.[325] Rearrangements of the *NFKB2* gene at 10q24 encode for a protein that lacks the ankyrin regulatory domain required for regulating the physiological NFKB2 nuclear/cytoplasmic distribution, but retains the rel effector domain and can bind kappa B sequences *in vitro*.[326] The translocation may thus contribute to lymphoma development by causing constitutive activation of the NF-κB pathway.

Anaplastic Large Cell Lymphoma

Cell of Origin

ALCL is a distinct subset of T-NHL (~12% of cases) whose normal cellular counterpart has not yet been established.[2,310] The tumor is composed of large pleomorphic cells that exhibit a unique phenotype characterized by positivity for the CD30 antigen and loss of most T-cell markers.[2,327] Based on the expression of a chimeric protein containing the cytoplasmic portion of anaplastic lymphoma kinase (ALK) as a consequence of translocations involving the *ALK* gene, ALCL may be subdivided into two groups, which display distinct transcriptional signatures[328]: the most common and curable ALK-positive ALCL and the more aggressive ALK-negative ALCL.[2,329–331] However, the identification of a common 30-genes predictor that can discriminate ALCL from other T-NHL, independent of ALK status, suggests that these two subgroups are closely related and may derive from a common precursor.[332]

Genetic Lesions

The genetic hallmark of ALK+ ALCL is chromosomal translocations involving band 2p23 and a variety of chromosomal partners, with t(2;5)(p23;q35) accounting for 70% to 80% of the cases.[2,333] Cloning of the translocation breakpoint in t(2;5) demonstrated the involvement of the *ALK* gene on 2p23 and the nucleophosmin (*NPM1*) gene on 5q35.[334] As a consequence, the aminoterminus of NPM is linked in frame to the catalytic domain of ALK, driving transformation through multiple molecular mechanisms[334]: (1) the *ALK* gene, which is not expressed in normal T lymphocytes, becomes inappropriately expressed in lymphoma cells, conceivably because of its juxtaposition to the promoter sequences of *NPM1*, which are physiologically expressed in T cells; and (2) all translocations involving *ALK* produce proteins with constitutive tyrosine activity, due in most cases to spontaneous dimerization induced by the various fusion partners.[333] Constitutive ALK activity, in turn, results in the activation of several downstream signaling cascades, with the JAK-STAT and PI3K-AKT pathways playing central roles.[335–338] The transforming ability of the chimeric NPM/ALK protein has been proven both *in vitro* and *in vivo* in transgenic mouse model.[339–341]

In a minority of cases, fusions other than NPM-ALK cause the abnormal subcellular localization of the corresponding chimeric ALK proteins and the constitutive activation of ALK. Among these alternative rearrangements, the most frequent involve *TPM3* or *TPM4*, *TRK-fused genes*,[342] *ATIC*,[343,344] *CLTCL1*, and *MSN*. No recurrent cytogenetic abnormality has been described in ALK-negative ALCL, and the molecular events responsible for this disease subtype remain largely unknown.

MOLECULAR PATHOGENESIS OF HL

HL is a B-lymphoid malignancy characterized by the presence of scattered large atypical cells—the mononucleated Hodgkin cells and the multinucleated Reed-Sternberg cells (HRS)—residing in a complex admixture of inflammatory cells.[2,345] Based on the morphology and phenotype of the neoplastic cells, as well as on the composition of the infiltrate, HL is segregated into two major subgroups: nodular lymphocyte-predominant HL (NLPHL; ~5% of cases) and classic HL (cHL), comprising the nodular sclerosis, mixed cellularity, and lymphocyte-depletion and lymphocyte-rich variants. Until recently, molecular studies of HL have been hampered by the paucity of the tumor cells in the biopsy (typically <1%, although occasional cases can present >10% HRS cells). However, the introduction of sophisticated laboratory techniques allowing the isolation and enrichment of neoplastic cells has markedly improved our understanding of HL histogenesis.

Cell of Origin

Despite the HRS of cHL cells having lost expression of nearly all B-cell–specific genes,[346–348] both HL types represent clonal expansions of B cells, as revealed by the presence of clonally rearranged and somatically mutated Ig genes.[349,350] In about 25% of cHL cases, nonsense mutations disrupt originally in-frame V_H gene rearrangements (crippling mutations), thereby preventing antigen selection and suggesting that HRS cells of cHL have escaped apoptosis through a mechanism not linked to antigen stimulation.[350]

Genetic Lesions

A number of structural alterations lead to the constitutive activation of NF-κB in cHL. Nearly half of the cases display amplification of *REL,* associated with increased protein expression levels[351,352]; gains or translocations of the positive regulator BCL3 were also reported.[319] More recently, a number of inactivating mutations were found in genes coding for negative regulators of NF-κB, including *NFKBIA* (20% of cases), *NFKBIE* (15%), and *TNFAIP3* (40%).[81,353–355] Notably, *TNFAIP3*-mutated cases are invariably EBV-negative, suggesting that EBV infection may substitute in part for the pathogenetic function of A20 in causing NF-κB constitutive activation.[81,355] Amplification of *JAK2* and inactivating mutations of *SOCS1,* a negative regulator of the JAK-STAT signaling pathway, are often found in NLPHL[245,248]; in an additional large number of cases, constitutive JAK-STAT activity is sustained by autocrine and paracrine signals.[345] BCL6 translocations have been reported in the lymphocytic and histiocytic cells of NLPHD, but only rarely in cHL,[356,357] and translocations of *BCL2* or mutations in positive or negative regulators of apoptosis (e.g., *TP53, FAS, BAD,* and *ATM*) are virtually absent.[345] Finally, an important pathogenetic cofactor in cHL, but not NLPHL, is represented by monoclonal EBV infection, which occurs in approximately 40% of cHL and up to 90% of HIV-related HL, suggesting that infection precedes clonal expansion.[345] Of the viral proteins encoded by the EBV genome, infected HRS cells most commonly express LMP1, LMP2, and EBNA1 but not EBNA2.[345]

Selected References

The full list of references for this chapter appears in the online version.

2. Swerdlow SH, Campo E, Harris NL, et al. *WHO Classification of Tumours of Haematopoietic and Lymphoid Tissues.* Lyon, France: IARC, 2008.
5. Rajewsky K. Clonal selection and learning in the antibody system. *Nature* 1996;381:751–758.
6. Klein U, Dalla-Favera R. Germinal centres: role in B-cell physiology and malignancy. *Nat Rev Immunol* 2008;8: 22–33.
17. Phan RT, Dalla-Favera R. The BCL6 proto-oncogene suppresses p53 expression in germinal-centre B cells. *Nature* 2004;432:635–639.
28. Muramatsu M, Kinoshita K, Fagarasan S, et al. Class switch recombination and hypermutation require activation-induced cytidine deaminase (AID), a potential RNA editing enzyme. *Cell* 2000;102:553–563.
29. Revy P, Muto T, Levy Y, et al. Activation-induced cytidine deaminase (AID) deficiency causes the autosomal recessive form of the Hyper-IgM syndrome (HIGM2). *Cell* 2000; 102:565–575.
35. Ramiro AR, Jankovic M, Eisenreich T, et al. AID is required for c-myc/IgH chromosome translocations in vivo. *Cell* 2004;118:431–438.
37. Pasqualucci L, Bhagat G, Jankovic M, et al. AID is required for germinal center-derived lymphomagenesis. *Nat Genet* 2008;40:108–112.
41. Ye BH, Lista F, Lo Coco F, et al. Alterations of a zinc finger-encoding gene, BCL-6, in diffuse large-cell lymphoma. *Science* 1993;262:747–750.
47. Pasqualucci L, Neumeister P, Goossens T, et al. Hypermutation of multiple proto-oncogenes in B-cell diffuse large-cell lymphomas. *Nature* 2001;412:341–346.
48. Pasqualucci L, Migliazza A, Fracchiolla N, et al. BCL-6 mutations in normal germinal center B cells: evidence of somatic hypermutation acting outside Ig loci. *Proc Natl Acad Sci U S A* 1998;95:11816–11821.
49. Shen HM, Peters A, Baron B, Zhu X, Storb U. Mutation of BCL-6 gene in normal B cells by the process of somatic

hypermutation of Ig genes. *Science* 1998;280:1750–1752.

67. Compagno M, Lim WK, Grunn A, et al. Mutations of multiple genes cause deregulation of NF-kappaB in diffuse large B-cell lymphoma. *Nature* 2009;459:717–721.

68. Lenz G, Davis RE, Ngo VN, et al. Oncogenic CARD11 mutations in human diffuse large B cell lymphoma. *Science* 2008;319:1676–1679.

69. Neri A, Knowles DM, Greco A, McCormick F, Dalla-Favera R. Analysis of RAS oncogene mutations in human lymphoid malignancies. *Proc Natl Acad Sci U S A* 1988;85:9268–9272.

72. Gaidano G, Ballerini P, Gong JZ, et al. p53 mutations in human lymphoid malignancies: association with Burkitt lymphoma and chronic lymphocytic leukemia. *Proc Natl Acad Sci U S A* 1991;88:5413–5417.

76. Mandelbaum J, Bhagat G, Tang H, et al. BLIMP1 is a tumor suppressor gene frequently disrupted in activated B-cell like diffuse large B-cell lymphoma. *Cancer Cell* 2010;18(6):568.

79. Kato M, Sanada M, Kato I, et al. Frequent inactivation of A20 in B-cell lymphomas. *Nature* 2009;459:712–716.

81. Schmitz R, Hansmann ML, Bohle V, et al. TNFAIP3 (A20) is a tumor suppressor gene in Hodgkin lymphoma and primary mediastinal B cell lymphoma. *J Exp Med* 2009;206:981.

82. Dohner H, Stilgenbauer S, Benner A, et al. Genomic aberrations and survival in chronic lymphocytic leukemia. *N Engl J Med* 2000;343:1910–1916.

84. Calin GA, Dumitru CD, Shimizu M, et al. Frequent deletions and down-regulation of micro-RNA genes miR15 and miR16 at 13q14 in chronic lymphocytic leukemia. *Proc Natl Acad Sci U S A* 2002;99:15524–15529.

88. Klein U, Lia M, Crespo M, et al. The DLEU2/miR-15a/16-1 cluster controls B cell proliferation and its deletion leads to chronic lymphocytic leukemia. *Cancer Cell* 2010;17:28–40.

94. Neri A, Barriga F, Inghirami G, et al. Epstein-Barr virus infection precedes clonal expansion in Burkitt's and acquired immunodeficiency syndrome-associated lymphoma. *Blood* 1991;77:1092–1095.

103. Chang Y, Cesarman E, Pessin MS, et al. Identification of herpesvirus-like DNA sequences in AIDS-associated Kaposi's sarcoma. *Science* 1994;266:1865–1869.

130. Tsujimoto Y, Yunis J, Onorato-Showe L, et al. Molecular cloning of the chromosomal breakpoint of B-cell lymphomas and leukemias with the t(11;14) chromosome translocation. *Science* 1984;224:1403–1406.

132. Motokura T, Bloom T, Kim HG, et al. A novel cyclin encoded by a bcl1-linked candidate oncogene. *Nature* 1991;350:512–516.

152. Dalla-Favera R, Bregni M, Erikson J, et al. Human c-myc onc gene is located on the region of chromosome 8 that is translocated in Burkitt lymphoma cells. *Proc Natl Acad Sci U S A* 1982;79:7824–7827.

153. Dalla-Favera R, Martinotti S, Gallo RC, Erikson J, Croce CM. Translocation and rearrangements of the c-myc oncogene locus in human undifferentiated B-cell lymphomas. *Science* 1983;219:963–967.

167. Meyer N, Penn LZ. Reflecting on 25 years with MYC. *Nat Rev Cancer* 2008;8:976–990.

168. Dominguez-Sola D, Ying CY, Grandori C, et al. Non-transcriptional control of DNA replication by c-Myc. *Nature* 2007;448:445–451.

169. Eilers M, Eisenman RN. Myc's broad reach. *Genes Dev* 2008;22:2755–2766.

179. Adams JM, Harris AW, Pinkert CA, et al. The c-myc oncogene driven by immunoglobulin enhancers induces lymphoid malignancy in transgenic mice. *Nature* 1985;318:533–538.

188. Cleary ML, Smith SD, Sklar J. Cloning and structural analysis of cDNAs for bcl-2 and a hybrid bcl-2/immunoglobu-

lin transcript resulting from the t(14;18) translocation. *Cell* 1986;47:19–28.

196. Hockenbery D, Nunez G, Milliman C, Schreiber RD, Korsmeyer SJ. Bcl-2 is an inner mitochondrial membrane protein that blocks programmed cell death. *Nature* 1990;348:334–336.

215. Alizadeh AA, Eisen MB, Davis RE, et al. Distinct types of diffuse large B-cell lymphoma identified by gene expression profiling. *Nature* 2000;403:503–511.

217. Savage KJ, Monti S, Kutok JL, et al. The molecular signature of mediastinal large B-cell lymphoma differs from that of other diffuse large B-cell lymphomas and shares features with classical Hodgkin lymphoma. *Blood* 2003;102:3871–3879.

218. Rosenwald A, Wright G, Leroy K, et al. Molecular diagnosis of primary mediastinal B cell lymphoma identifies a clinically favorable subgroup of diffuse large B cell lymphoma related to Hodgkin lymphoma. *J Exp Med* 2003;198:851–862.

224. Lenz G, Wright GW, Emre NC, et al. Molecular subtypes of diffuse large B-cell lymphoma arise by distinct genetic pathways. *Proc Natl Acad Sci U S A* 2008;105:13520–13525.

229. Pasqualucci L, Migliazza A, Fracchiolla N, et al. Mutations of the BCL6 proto-oncogene disrupt its negative autoregulation in diffuse large B-cell lymphoma. *Blood* 2003;101:2914–2923.

232. Migliazza A, Martinotti S, Chen W, et al. Frequent somatic hypermutation of the 5' noncoding region of the BCL6 gene in B-cell lymphoma. *Proc Natl Acad Sci U S A* 1995;92:12520–12524.

233. Saito M, Gao J, Basso K, et al. A signaling pathway mediating downregulation of BCL6 in germinal center B cells is blocked by BCL6 gene alterations in B cell lymphoma. *Cancer Cell* 2007;12:280–292.

236. Davis RE, Ngo VN, Lenz G, et al. Chronic active B-cell-receptor signalling in diffuse large B-cell lymphoma. *Nature* 2010;463:88–92.

251. Wotherspoon AC. Gastric lymphoma of mucosa-associated lymphoid tissue and *Helicobacter pylori*. *Annu Rev Med* 1998;49:289.

274. Caligaris-Cappio F, Hamblin TJ. B-cell chronic lymphocytic leukemia: a bird of a different feather. *J Clin Oncol* 1999;17:399–408.

278. Klein U, Tu Y, Stolovitzky GA, et al. Gene expression profiling of B cell chronic lymphocytic leukemia reveals a homogeneous phenotype related to memory B cells. *J Exp Med* 2001;194:1625–1638.

279. Rosenwald A, Alizadeh AA, Widhopf G, et al. Relation of gene expression phenotype to immunoglobulin mutation genotype in B cell chronic lymphocytic leukemia. *J Exp Med* 2001;194:1639–1647.

288. Rawstron AC, Bennett FL, O'Connor SJ, et al. Monoclonal B-cell lymphocytosis and chronic lymphocytic leukemia. *N Engl J Med* 2008;359:575.

310. de Leval L, Bisig B, Thielen C, Boniver J, Gaulard P. Molecular classification of T-cell lymphomas. *Crit Rev Oncol Hematol* 2009;72:125–143.

333. Chiarle R, Voena C, Ambrogio C, Piva R, Inghirami G. The anaplastic lymphoma kinase in the pathogenesis of cancer. *Nat Rev Cancer* 2008;8:11–23.

334. Morris SW, Kirstein MN, Valentine MB, et al. Fusion of a kinase gene, ALK, to a nucleolar protein gene, NPM, in non-Hodgkin's lymphoma. *Science* 1994;263:1281–1284.

349. Küppers R, Rajewsky K, Zhao M, et al. Hodgkin disease: Hodgkin and Reed-Sternberg cells picked from histological sections show clonal immunoglobulin gene rearrangements and appear to be derived from B cells at various stages of development. *Proc Natl Acad Sci U S A* 1994;91:10962–10966.

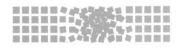

CHAPTER 31 ACUTE LEUKEMIAS

GLEN D. RAFFEL AND JAN CERNY

MOLECULAR BIOLOGY OF INDIVIDUAL CANCERS

Our understanding of the molecular genetics of acute leukemias has improved dramatically over the past decade. Fueled in part by the availability of the complete sequence of the human genome, more than 100 different mutations have been identified that can be causally implicated in the pathogenesis of acute leukemias. At first glance, the plethora of mutations presents a discouraging prospect for the development of molecular targeted therapies. However, far more mutations are identified than there are phenotypes of acute leukemia, and a theme is developed in this chapter that many of these mutations must target similar signal transduction or transcriptional pathways. Thus, it is plausible to consider therapeutic approaches that target these shared pathways of transformation. Although many mutations remain to be identified, those observed thus far have provided critical insights into the pathophysiology of leukemia and the development of novel therapeutic targets.

LEUKEMIC STEM CELL

An important emerging concept in the pathobiology of leukemia is the existence of a "leukemic stem cell." In normal hematopoietic development, there is a rare population of hematopoietic stem cells that have self-renewal capacity and give rise to multipotent hematopoietic progenitors. These multipotent myeloid or lymphoid progenitors do not have self-renewal capacity but mature into normal terminally differentiated cells in the peripheral blood. It is hypothesized that there is a leukemic stem cell that has limitless self-renewal capacity and gives rise to clonogenic leukemic progenitors that do not have self-renewal capacity but are incapable of normal hematopoietic differentiation.

The first convincing evidence in support of the existence of a leukemic stem cell was derived from experiments in which human leukemic cells were injected into immunodeficient NOD-SCID mice (nonobese diabetic mice with severe combined immunodeficiency disease).[1] These data show that the resultant leukemias are derived from as few as 1:1,000 to 1:10,000 cells, indicating that there is a rare population of human leukemic cells that have self-renewal capacity in this assay. These cells have similar immunophenotypes to normal self-renewing hematopoietic progenitors and suggest that the leukemogenic mutation occurs in a hematopoietic stem cell. In support of this hypothesis, clonal cytogenetic abnormalities, such as the t(9;22), have been detected in primitive hematopoietic progenitors such as CD34+/CD38− cells (reviewed in ref. 2).

However, this paradigm has been recently challenged and revised. First, new protocols that enhance engraftment of human leukemia in xenotransplant setting have been described suggesting the importance of homing and the role of microenvironment.[3,4] Data also show that it may be the leukemic oncogenes themselves that confer properties of self-renewal. In a murine system, transduction of the leukemia oncogenes *MLL-ENL* (mixed-lineage leukemia 1-eleven nineteen leukemia), *MOZ-TIF2* (monocytic leukemia zinc finger protein-transcriptional intermediary factor 2), or *MLL-AF9* (mixed-lineage leukemia *ALL1*-fused gene from chromosome 9 protein) can confer properties of self-renewal to purified committed hematopoietic progenitors that have no capacity for self-renewal.[5,6] *MLL-AF9* oncogene-induced leukemia showed that leukemic stem cells account for as high as 25% of the leukemic cells while exhibiting mature myeloid immunophenotype.[7] High frequency of leukemic stem cells have been also described in a murine AML *Sfpi−/−*.[8] *HOX* family and *Notch* genes, frequent mutational targets in acute leukemia, as discussed later in this chapter, are being found to have significant roles in hematopoietic stem cell self-renewal.[9] Secondary mutations may also enable activation of similar self-renewal pathways. For example, analysis of cells from acute myeloid leukemia (AML) blast crisis in chronic myeloid leukemia (CML) shows a shift in the leukemic stem cell to an immunophenotype of a committed myeloid progenitor and concurrent nuclear localization of β-catenin, a process thought to increase stem cell self-renewal.[10] Further investigation will be required to determine to what extent these findings can be extrapolated to other leukemia oncogenes and to human leukemia. One of the major goals is identification of transcriptional programs, genes, and pathways that confer limitless self-renewal and may be targets for therapeutic intervention. In addition, these transcriptional programs may be commandeered to confer properties of self-renewal to adult somatic tissues for therapeutic purposes such as tissue regeneration. For further development of this issue, see Chapter 11.

ELUCIDATION OF GENETIC EVENTS IN ACUTE LEUKEMIA

The search for causative mutations in acute leukemia has accelerated in recent years because of the availability of new means for evaluating genome integrity in leukemic cells. The bulk of known translocations and deletions was found by analyzing conventionally stained chromosomal banding patterns of karyotypes. Classic karyotypic analysis is able to identify lesions with a resolution of 5 to 10 Mb. An improvement on this technique is spectral karyotyping, in which 24 unique dye combinations are used on conjugated probes specific to each chromosome. Mutations can be observed in the resolution of 1 to 2 Mb. This technique is particularly useful in finding otherwise cryptic or complex translocations as chromatin in derivative chromosomes are "painted" to identify their chromosome of origin.

New technologies such as comparative genomic hybridization (CGH) and single nucleotide polymorphism (SNP) arrays allow detailed (<35 kb) mapping of unbalanced insertions or deletions (reviewed in refs. 11 and 12). Array comparative genomic hybridization determines DNA copy gain or loss by comparing the hybridization of sample DNA to a series of clones or oligonucleotides from regions throughout the genome bound to a chip with a normal reference DNA sample. SNP arrays differ in that oligomers of SNP sequences representing known alleles throughout the genome are used in the array to measure changes in expected genotype and copy number. Finally, low-cost, high-throughput sequencing and microarray-based resequencing techniques have allowed identification of new somatic mutations at the single nucleotide level and are making enormous inroads into the pathogenesis, prognosis, and classification of leukemias with "normal" cytogenetics. Sequencing of complete AML genomes has been accomplished and alternative strategies limiting sequencing to the transcriptome or kinase-encoding regions (kinome) to reduce cost and effort are also uncovering new, significant mutations.[13–15] Worldwide initiatives to sequence large numbers of cancer genomes, including leukemia subtypes, are being coordinated and cataloged through the International Cancer Genome Consortium (http://www.icgc.org).[16]

RECURRING CHROMOSOMAL ABNORMALITIES IN ACUTE LEUKEMIA

Nonrandom chromosomal abnormalities can be detected in the majority of cases of acute leukemia using classic high-resolution banding techniques. These include balanced reciprocal chromosomal translocations, such as t(8;21)(q22;q22) or t(15;17)(q22;q21); internal deletions of single chromosomes, such as 5q- or 7q-; gain or loss of whole chromosomes (+8 or −7); or chromosome inversions, such as inv(3), inv(16), or inv(8). Complex chromosomal abnormalities are observed in approximately 15% of *de novo* cases that do not have an antecedent hematologic disorder; this constitutes a clinical group of patients with particularly poor prognoses. Selected recurring cytogenetic abnormalities observed in acute leukemias are annotated in Table 31.1.

Initial insights into the pathobiology of acute leukemias were derived from analysis and molecular cloning of recurring chromosomal translocations.[17] First, it appears that certain genomic loci are associated with specific subtypes of leukemia. For example, more than 40 different recurring translocations target the *MLL* gene locus on chromosome 11q23 and are generally associated with a myelomonocytic or monocytic AML phenotype (FAB M4 or M5). As another example, five different translocations target the retinoic acid receptor alpha locus (RAR-α), including the t(15;17)(q22;q21), which is the most common of these, and are all associated with an acute promyelocytic leukemia (APL) phenotype (FAB M3). Second, it appears that most chromosomal translocations associated with AMLs target transcription factors that are important for normal hematopoietic development. For example, more than a dozen translocations target the core-binding factor (CBF), a heterodimeric transcriptional complex essential for hematopoiesis. The translocations that target *CBF*, such as the t(8;21), result in expression of dominant negative inhibitors of normal CBF function, such as the AML1/ETO fusion. Thus, one consequence of many of these chromosomal translocations in acute leukemias is impaired hematopoietic differentiation. A third general observation has been that fusion genes associated with acute leukemias are necessary but not sufficient to cause acute leukemia.

CHROMOSOMAL TRANSLOCATIONS THAT TARGET CORE-BINDING FACTOR

CBF is targeted by more than a dozen different chromosomal translocations in acute leukemias, including the t(8;21) or inv(16), observed in approximately 20% of AMLs, and the t(12;21), present in approximately 25% of patients with pediatric B-cell acute lymphoblastic leukemia (ALL).[18] Adult patients with CBF leukemias have a favorable prognosis and the TEL/AML1 fusion that is expressed as a consequence of t(12;21) in children confers a favorable prognosis among B-cell ALL.[19]

CBF is a heterodimeric transcription factor composed of the AML1 and CBFβ proteins that is critical for normal hematopoietic development. Loss of function of either subunit results in a complete lack of definitive hematopoiesis.[20,21] The AML1 subunit of CBF contacts DNA but only weakly transactivates target genes as a monomer. When bound to its heterodimeric partner CBFβ, which does not contact DNA itself, transactivation of CBF target genes is dramatically enhanced.[19] CBF transactivates a spectrum of target genes that are important in normal myeloid development, including cytokines (e.g., granulocyte-macrophage colony-stimulating factor) and cytokine receptors (such as M-CSF receptor), as well as in lymphoid development, such as the TCRβ enhancer and the immunoglobulin heavy-chain loci. Because CBF targets genes that are important for normal hematopoietic development, a mutation or gene rearrangement that resulted in loss of function of either *AML1* or *CBFβ* might be expected to impair hematopoietic differentiation.[19]

Compelling evidence has been shown that translocations that target CBF result in loss of function through dominant negative inhibition. The *AML1/ETO* fusion associated with t(8;21) and the CBFβ/SMMHC (smooth muscle myosin heavy chain) fusion associated with inv(16) are dominant negative inhibitors of CBF and impair hematopoietic differentiation. Expression of either the *AML1/ETO* or *CBFβ/SMMHCC* fusion genes from their endogenous promoter in mice completely inhibits the function of the residual AML1 or CBFβ alleles, resulting in a lack of definitive hematopoiesis and resultant embryonic lethality.[20,21] The phenotype observed is the same as that seen in *AML1–/–* or *CBFβ–/–* mice, indicating that the AML1/ETO or CBFβ/SMMHC fusions, respectively, act as complete dominant negative inhibitors of the native proteins. Repression of CBF target genes by the AML1/ETO or CBFβ/SMMHC fusions is mediated by aberrant recruitment of the nuclear corepressor complex, as it is for the PML/RAR-α fusion (reviewed in refs. 22 and 23). Thus, it has been suggested that histone deacetylase, a component of the corepressor complex, may be a therapeutic target for leukemias associated with translocations that target CBF.[24]

Although expression of AML1/ETO leads to alterations of gene expression and hematopoietic cell proliferation leukemia and confers the ability to serially replate in methylcellulose culture (a measure of self-renewal potential), this does not result in development of leukemia in an animal model. However coexpression of an alternatively spliced isoform of the *AML1-ETO* transcript, *AML1-ETO9a*, that includes an extra exon, exon 9a, of the *ETO* gene (*AML1-ETO9a* encodes a C terminally truncated AML1-ETO protein of 575 amino acids) leads to a rapid development of leukemia in a mouse retroviral transduction–transplantation model.[25] The presence of *AML1-ETO9a* closely correlates with presence of activating c-Kit mutations in humans, conferring a poor prognosis.[26] Similarly, expression of CBFβ/SMMHC in adult hematopoietic cells results in leukemia only after a markedly prolonged latency; this latency can be shortened using mutagenesis strategies.[27] Translocations that target *CBF* impair hematopoietic differentiation and confer certain properties of leukemic stem cells, such as the ability to serially replate, but are not sufficient to cause leukemia. In some situations fusion proteins from alternatively spliced isoforms of a chromosomal translocation may work together to induce cancer development.[26]

CHROMOSOMAL TRANSLOCATIONS THAT TARGET THE RETINOIC ACID RECEPTOR ALPHA GENE

The empiric observation that all-*trans*-retinoic acid (ATRA) induces complete responses in patients with APL drove the subsequent cloning of the t(15;17)(q22;q21) fusion gene involving the RAR-α locus. Several groups demonstrated at approximately the same time that the RAR-α (*RARα*) gene on chromosome 17 was fused to a novel partner that was eventually identified as the promyelocytic leukemia (PML) gene.[28–30] Two reciprocal fusion RNA species are produced as a consequence of the translocation, *RARα/PML* and *PML/RARα*. The PML/RAR-α fusion protein contains the zinc finger of PML fused to the DNA- and protein-binding domains of RAR-α. Several other chromosomal translocations associated with an APL phenotype have been cloned and characterized. Each of these targets the *RARα* locus, with fusion to various

TABLE 31.1

SELECTED EXAMPLES OF CYTOGENETIC AND MOLECULAR ABNORMALITIES IN LEUKEMIA

Cytogenetic Abnormality	Genes Involved	Derivation of Abbreviation	Protein Characterization	Disease
FUSIONS INVOLVING THE CORE-BINDING FACTORS (CBFs)				
t(8;21)(q22;q22)	CBFA2T1/ETO (8q22)	Eight twenty-one	Zinc finger protein	AML
	CBFA2/AML1 (21q22)	AML 1	α subunit of CBF complex	
inv(16)(p13q22)	MYH11 (16p13)	Myosin heavy chain 11	Smooth muscle myosin heavy chain	AML
	CBFB/CBFβ (16q22)	CBF-β	β subunit of CBF complex	
t(3;21)(q26;q22)	EVI1 (3q26)	Ecotropic virus integration site 1	Multiple zinc fingers	MDS, AML
	CBFA2/AML1 (21q22)	AML 1	α subunit of CBF complex	CML-BC
t(12;21)(p13;q22)	TEL (12p13)	Translocation ETS leukemia	ETS-related transcription factor	ALL
	CBFA2/AML1 (21q22)	AML 1	α subunit of CBF complex	
FUSIONS INVOLVING MLL				
t(4;11)(q21q23)	AF4 (4q21)	ALL1 fused chromosome 4	Transactivator	ALL, AML
	MLL (11q23)	Mixed-lineage leukemia	Drosophila trithorax homologue	
t(11;19)(q23;p13.3)	MLL (11q23)	Mixed-lineage leukemia	Drosophila trithorax homologue	AML, ALL
	ENL (19p13.3)	ENL	Transcription factor	
t(9;11)(p22;q23)	AF9 (9p22)	ALL1 fused chromosome 9	Nuclear protein, ENL homology	AML, ALL
	MLL (11q23)	Mixed-lineage leukemia	Drosophila trithorax homologue	
t(11;22)(q23;q13)	MLL (11q23)	Mixed-lineage leukemia	Drosophila trithorax homologue	AML
	P300 (22q13)	Protein 300 kD	Adenoviral E1A-associated protein	
t(1;11)(q21;q23)	AF1q (1q21)	ALL1 fused chromosome 1q	No homology to any known protein	AML
	MLL (11q23)	Mixed-lineage leukemia	Drosophila trithorax homologue	
+11 (sole) or normal cytogenetics	MLL (11q23)	Mixed-lineage leukemia	MLL partial tandem duplication	AML
FUSIONS INVOLVING RAR-α				
t(15;17)(q22;q12–21)	PML (15q21)	Promyelocytic leukemia	Zinc finger protein	APL
	RAR-α (17q21)	Retinoic acid receptor-α	Retinoic acid receptor-α	
t(11;17)(q23;q21)	PLZF (11q23)	Promyelocytic leukemia zinc finger	Zinc finger protein	APL
	RAR-α (17q21)	Retinoic acid receptor-α	Retinoic acid receptor-α	
T(5;17)(q32;q21)	NPM1	Nucleophosmin	Chaperone	APL
	RAR-α (17q21)	Retinoic acid receptor-α	Retinoic acid receptor-α	

FUSIONS INVOLVING *E2A*				
t(1;19)(q23;p13.3)	*PBX1* (1q23)	Pre-B transformation 1	Homeodomain	ALL
	E2A (19p13.3)	Early region 2A	bHLH transcription factor	
t(17;19)(q22;p13.3)	*HLF* (17q22)	Hepatic leukemia factor	Leucine zipper	ALL
	E2A (19p13.3)	Early region 2A	bHLH transcription factor	
FUSIONS INVOLVING NUCLEOPORIN GENES AND *HOX* GENES				
t(6;9)(p23;q34)	*DEK* (6p23)	Not relevant to molecule	Transcription factor	AML
	CAN/NUP214 (9q34)	Nuclear pore 214	Nucleoporin	
t(7;11)(p15;p15)	*HOXA9* (7p15)	Homeobox A9	Homeobox protein	AML/MDS
	NUP98 (11p15)	Nuclear pore 98	Nucleoporin	AML
FUSIONS INVOLVING OTT1 AND MAL				
t(1;22)(p13;q13)	*OTT1* (1p13)/*MAL* (22q13)	One twenty-two megakaryocytic acute leukemia	*Spen* homologue unknown / Serum response cofactor	AML (M7)
TRANSLOCATIONS INVOLVING THE IMMUNOGLOBULIN ENHANCER LOCI				
t(8;14)(q24;q32)	*MYC* (8q24)	Myelocytomatosis virus	bHLH/bZIP transcription factor	ALL
	IGH (14q32)	Ig heavy chain	Ig heavy chain promoter	
t(2;8)(p12;q24)	*IGK* (2p12)	Ig κ-chain	Igκ-chain promoter	ALL
	MYC (8q24)	Myelocytomatosis virus	bHLH/bZIP transcription factor	
t(8;22)(q24;q11)	*MYC* (8q24)	Myelocytomatosis virus	bHLH/bZIP transcription factor	ALL
	IGL (22q11)	Ig λ-chain	Igλ-chain promoter	

(continued)

TABLE 31.1

(CONTINUED)

Cytogenetic Abnormality	Genes Involved	Derivation of Abbreviation	Protein Characterization	Disease
TRANSLOCATIONS INVOLVING THE T-CELL RECEPTOR GENES				
t(1;14)(p32;q11)	TAL1/SCL (1p33)	T-cell acute leukemia 1/stem cell leukemia	bHLH transcription factor	ALL
t(1;7)(p32;q34)	TCRα/δ (14q11)	T-cell receptor-α/δ	T-cell receptor promoter	ALL
	TAL1/SCL (1p32)	T-cell acute leukemia 1/stem cell leukemia	bHLH transcription factor	
t(7;9)(q34;q34)	TCRβ (7q34)	T-cell receptor-β	T-cell receptor promoter	ALL
	TCRβ (7q34)	T-cell receptor-β	T-cell receptor promoter	
	TAL2/SCL2 (9q34)	T-cell acute leukemia 2/stem cell leukemia	bHLH transcription factor	
t(7;19)(q34;p13)	TCRβ (7q34)	T-cell receptor-β	T-cell receptor promoter	ALL
	LYL1 (19p13)	Lymphoid leukemia 1	bHLH transcription factor	
t(8;14)(q24;q11)	MYC (8q24)	Myelocytomatosis virus	bHLH/bZIP transcription factor	ALL
	TCRα/δ (14q11)	T-cell receptor-α/δ	T-cell receptor promoter	
t(11;14)(p15;q11)	LMO1 (11p15)	LIM only 1	Zinc finger	ALL
	TCRα/δ (14q11)	T-cell receptor-α/δ	T-cell receptor promoter	
t(11;14)(p13;q11)	LMO2 (11p13)	LIM only 2	Zinc finger	ALL
	TCRα/δ (14q11)	T-cell receptor-α/δ	T-cell receptor promoter	
t(7;10)(q34;q24)	TCRβ (7q34)	T-cell receptor-β	T-cell receptor promoter	ALL
	HOX11 (10q24)	Homeobox 11	Homeobox gene	

AML, acute myeloid leukemia; MDS, myelodysplastic syndrome; CML, chronic myeloid leukemia; ETS, E twenty-six retrovirus; ENL, eleven nineteen leukemia; ALL, acute lympho-blastic leukemia; MLL, mixed-lineage leukemia; APL, acute promyelocytic leukemia; bHLH, basic helix-loop-helix; bZIP, basic region/leucine zipper; Ig, immunoglobulin; LIM, Lin-11, Isl-2, Mec-3 homeodomain.

partners (see Table 31.1). The best studied of these is the PLZF/RAR-α fusion, which also aberrantly recruits the nuclear corepressor complex (Table 31.1). However, in contrast with the PML/RAR-α fusion, ATRA is not able to relieve corepression mediated by the PLZF/RAR-α fusion, and thus is not effective in patients who harbor the t(11;17) associated with this fusion gene.[31]

As with CBF fusions, the PML/RAR-α fusion protein functions as a dominant inhibitory oncogene for RAR-α–interacting proteins, including RXR-α. In addition, the PML/RAR-α fusion interferes with the function of the native PML protein, which is thought to function as a tumor suppressor gene.[32] Collectively, the dominant interfering activities of the PML/RAR-α fusion protein result in a block in differentiation at the promyelocyte stage of development. The clinical response of these patients to ATRA is explained by the ability of this retinoid to bind to the PML/RAR-α fusion protein and reverse repression of target genes required for normal hematopoietic development. The ability of the PML/RAR-α fusion protein to repress transcription is partly due to the aberrant recruitment of the nuclear corepressor complex, including histone deacetylase, suggesting that pharmacologic agents that inhibit histone deacetylases may be useful in therapy of APL.[24,33]

The transforming properties of the *PML/RARα* fusion gene have been tested in murine models. Expression of *PML/RAR-α* in transgenic mice from promoters that direct expression to the promyelocyte compartment result in an APL-like phenotype.[34–36] However, there is approximately a 6-month lag before the development of leukemia, incomplete penetrance of approximately 15% to 30%, and acquired karyotypic abnormalities, all suggesting that second mutations are required for induction of leukemia. In at least some cases, activating mutations in *FLT3*, as discussed later in "Activating Mutations in *FLT3* and *KIT*," may be the additional mutation required. ATRA is efficacious in leukemic animals, expressing both PML/RAR-α and activated FLT3, and this model has allowed for the preclinical testing of novel agents such as arsenic trioxide.[37]

CHROMOSOMAL TRANSLOCATIONS THAT TARGET HOX FAMILY MEMBERS

The large HOX family of transcription factors is important in patterning in vertebrate development and also plays a critical role in normal hematopoietic development (reviewed in ref. 38). *HOX* genes may also be targeted by chromosomal translocations, with examples including the NUP98/HOXA9 and NUP98/HOXD13 fusions,

associated with t(7;11) and t(2;11), respectively (see Table 31.1).[39,40] *HOX* gene expression is tightly regulated during hematopoietic development. HOXA9, for example, is expressed in early hematopoietic progenitor cells but is down-regulated during hematopoietic differentiation and is undetectable in terminally differentiated cells. It has been suggested that unregulated overexpression of the HOXA9 moiety from the constitutively active NUP98 promoter may result in aberrant differentiation. Experimental support for this hypothesis includes the observation that the NUP98/HOXA9 fusion protein can transform 3T3 fibroblasts, an activity that requires the HOXA9 DNA-binding domain.[41]

The contribution of the NUP98 moiety to leukemic transformation is not fully understood. NUP98 is normally a component of the nuclear pore complex and is constitutively and ubiquitously expressed. However, several lines of evidence suggest that NUP98 contributes more than a constitutively activated promoter. For example, NUP98 motifs known as *FG repeats* are essential for transformation and may serve to recruit transcriptional coactivators, such as CBP/p300, to HOXA9 DNA-binding sites.[41] In murine models of leukemia, overexpression of HOXA9 alone is not sufficient to cause AML, but coexpression of HOXA9 with transcriptional cofactors, such as MEIS1, results in efficient induction of AML. Thus, the NUP98 moiety in the context of the NUP98/HOXA9 fusion may serve multiple functions, including provision of an active promoter, and recruitment of transcriptional coactivators such as CBP/p300 that subserve the function of other cofactors such as MEIS1. Epidemiologic evidence that the NUP98 moiety contributes to leukemogenesis includes the observation that there are now a spectrum of fusion proteins involving components of the nuclear pore that are targeted by chromosomal translocations in acute leukemias. These include *NUP98* and *NUP214* fused to a diverse group of partners, including *HOXA9* and *HOXD13*, and the *DDX10*, *PMX1*, *DEK*, and *ABL1* genes, respectively.

It has been hypothesized that dysregulated *HOX* gene expression may be important in leukemias that do not directly target HOX family members. Several proteins that are upstream of HOX expression have been observed as fusion genes associated with AML, the most frequent of these are *MLL* gene rearrangements. More than 40 chromosomal translocations target *MLL* and result in fusions of *MLL* with a broad spectrum of partners. However, a common biologic feature of all of these may be their ability to dysregulate *HOX* gene expression during hematopoietic development. For example, t(12;13) associated with AML results in expression of high levels of CDX2 from the *TEL* locus.[42] CDX2 is a homeotic protein that regulates expression of HOX family members in the colonic epithelium. As in hematopoietic development, *HOX* gene expression is highest in colonic stem cells in the colonic crypts and is down-regulated with maturation. It has been shown that CDX2 and CDX4 can dysregulate HOX expression in hematopoietic progenitors and result in leukemia.[42,43] Evidence to support this includes the ability of CDX2 to induce leukemia in murine retroviral transduction models.[42,43] Although CDX2 is not normally expressed in hematopoietic cells, a family member, CDX4, has been cloned and appears to play a similar role in hematopoietic development as CDX2 does in the gut. Of note, CDX4 in hematopoietic cells appears to either be downstream or epistatic with MLL in regulation of *HOX* gene expression.[44]

Taken together, these data indicate that the NUP98/HOXA9 fusion transforms hematopoietic progenitors in part through dysregulated overexpression and by transactivation mediated through the NUP98 transactivation domain that recruits CBP. However, like other gene rearrangements involving hematopoietic transcription factors, expression of NUP98/HOXA9 alone is not sufficient to cause leukemia. In murine bone marrow transplant models, NUP98/HOXA9 induces AML only after markedly prolonged latencies indicative of a requirement for second mutation.

CHROMOSOMAL TRANSLOCATIONS THAT TARGET THE *MLL* GENE

As noted earlier in "Recurring Chromosomal Abnormalities in Acute Leukemia," the *MLL* locus is involved in more than 40 different chromosomal translocations with a remarkably diverse group of fusion partners,[45,46] and are associated with mostly FAB subtype M4 or M5, and fewer with M2 AML. Patients who have received prior chemotherapy for cancer and develop AML (therapy-related myelodysplastic syndrome [MDS]/AML, t-AML) often have abnormalities in 11q23, especially those patients treated with topoisomerase inhibitors such as etoposide or topotecan. Chromosomal translocations involving band 11q23 result in expression of a fusion gene containing amino-terminal *MLL* sequences fused to a wide variety of partners. There has been no common functional motif or activity ascribed to all partners; however, specific fusions may be associated with specific leukemic phenotypes. The MLL/AF4 fusion associated with t(4;11) is frequently observed in infant leukemias and is associated with an ALL phenotype in more than 90% of cases, whereas the MLL/AF9 fusion associated with the t(9;11) is almost exclusively associated with AML. Certain MLL fusion genes also have prognostic significance. For example, patients with t(9;11)(p22;q23) have a better outcome than those with other translocations involving 11q23.

The *MLL* gene encodes a large, ubiquitously expressed protein. The *Drosophila* protein trithorax, a homologue of *MLL*, regulates patterning and *HOX* gene expression during development. It has been hypothesized, in part based on these observations, that MLL might be required for maintenance of *HOX* gene expression. In support of this hypothesis, mice that lack *Mll* express HoxA7 but are not able to maintain its expression.[47] Mice that have homozygous deficiency for *Mll* have an embryonic lethal phenotype at day 10.5 postconception. Even heterozygous animals have developmental anomalies in the axial skeleton and hematopoietic deficits including anemia.[47] Thus, as for other genes targeted by chromosomal translocations, *MLL* is important for normal hematopoietic development.

The function of *MLL* is not fully understood, but cell culture and murine models have provided some insight into transforming activity of the fusion proteins. The MLL protein of the fusion protein retains the amino terminal AT hooks that facilitate binding to DNA, as well as a methyltransferase domain. With the exception of CBP/p300, the function of the remaining broad spectrum of divergent fusion partners is poorly understood. In fact, the remarkable divergence of partners has suggested that alteration in the *MLL* gene itself is a critical required event for transformation. In support of a central role of *MLL* rearrangement in AML, it has been reported that partial tandem duplications of *MLL* are associated with AML, in particular AML associated with +11.[48] Data demonstrating that MLL is a processed polypeptide provide further support for this hypothesis. MLL is processed by proteolytic cleavage into two component parts by a novel protease called *taspase 1*.[49] Cleavage is required for normal regulation of expression of anterior and posterior *HOX* gene paralogs during development. It has thus been suggested that *MLL* fusion genes, which are not cleavable, may mimic the uncleaved native MLL protein, thereby dysregulating *HOX* gene expression.[50]

MLL fusion genes have transforming properties in serial replating assays in retrovirally transduced hematopoietic progenitors as well as in murine models (reviewed in ref. 45). Although various *MLL* fusions have similar transforming properties *in vitro*, there are distinctive differences in disease penetrance and latency in the murine models, depending on the fusion partner. It is possible that the *MLL* gene rearrangement may be critical for transformation, whereas the fusion partners confer properties related to disease phenotype. The long latency of disease in murine models supports the hypothesis that *MLL* fusions, like the PML/RAR-α and CBF-related fusion proteins, require second mutations to cause leukemia.

As noted in "Leukemic Stem Cell," data indicate that certain *MLL* fusion genes may also confer properties of self-renewal to hematopoietic progenitors. MLL/ENL expression in common myeloid progenitors or granulocyte-monocyte progenitors in a murine system conferred properties of self-renewal, including the ability to serially replate in methylcellulose cultures and to engender a transplantable AML phenotype in recipient animals.[5] Similarly in a mouse model of *MLL-AF9* oncogene-induced leukemia, up to a quarter of the leukemic cells exhibit stem cell behavior.[7] Furthermore the *MLL-AF9*–positive leukemic stem cells are heterogeneous as they give rise to ALL when injected into immunodeficient mice. The same cells cause AML when injected into immunodeficient mice that are transgenic for the human genes *SCF, GM-CSF*, and *IL-3*.[51] These data indicate that leukemogenic mutations may occur in cells that have no intrinsic self-renewal capacity and yet confer these properties by activation of specific transcriptional programs, which may be further modified by clues from microenvironment. These exciting observations provide tools for identification of target genes that confer properties of self-renewal and may have value as therapeutic targets for treatment of leukemia.

CHROMOSOMAL TRANSLOCATIONS THAT INVOLVE TRANSCRIPTIONAL COACTIVATORS AND CHROMATIN REMODELING PROTEINS

Several translocations associated with leukemia involve transcriptional coactivators and chromatin-modifying proteins that have no apparent DNA-binding specificity. These include the MLL/CBP and MOZ/CBP fusions that involve the transcriptional coactivator CBP and the MLL/p300 and MOZ/TIF2 fusions, which involve the coactivators p300 and TIF2, respectively.[52,53] Although TIF2 itself is not known to have histone acetylase transferase (HAT) activity, a hallmark of the coactivators CBP and p300, it has a well-characterized CBP interaction domain that serves to recruit CBP into a complex with MOZ/TIF2.[54] Thus, recruitment of CBP/p300 is a shared theme among this group of fusion genes.

The transcriptional targets and transformation properties of this class of fusion proteins are not fully understood. Transduction of MLL/CBP into primary murine bone marrow cells followed by transplantation results in a long-latency AML, suggesting the need for secondary mutations.[55] MOZ/TIF2 also results in leukemia in a similar model system. MOZ is a HAT protein that contains a nucleosome-binding domain and an acetyl–coenzyme A–binding catalytic domain.

Mutational analysis shows that leukemogenic activity requires MOZ nucleosome-binding activity and CBP recruitment activity, but the MOZ HAT activity is dispensable. These data would be consistent with a CBP gain of function in which CBP is recruited to MOZ nucleosome-binding sites.[54] However, it has also been hypothesized that the leukemogenic potential of this class of fusions may be related to dominant negative interference with CBP/p300 or that the translocation leads to simple loss of function of CBP expressed from one allele. In support of this hypothesis, loss of a single allele of CBP/p300 in the human Rubinstein-Taybi syndrome increases predisposition to malignancies including colon cancer, and mice that are heterozygous for CBP that develop hematopoietic tumors.[56]

t(1;22) TRANSLOCATION ASSOCIATED WITH INFANT ACUTE MEGAKARYOBLASTIC LEUKEMIA

Until recently, little was known about the molecular pathogenesis of acute megakaryoblastic leukemias (AMKLs; FAB M7), partly because of the difficulty in obtaining adequate quantities of material for analysis from densely fibrotic bone marrow. The t(1;22) that is associated with the majority of non–Down syndrome AMKL in infants has been cloned. The translocation results in expression of the *OTT1/MAL* fusion gene.[57,58] *OTT1 (RBM15)* contains three amino-terminal RNA recognition motifs and a Spen paralog and ortholog C terminal motif that is conserved in *Drosophila*. Ott1 deletion in mice reveals multiple roles in hematopoietic development including megakaryocyte growth.[59] The *MAL (MKL1)* gene is a Rho-GTPase-regulated cofactor for serum response factor and controls megakaryocyte development.[60,61] A knock-in mouse model expressing OTT1/MAL is able to recapitulate AMKL and demonstrated that constitutive transcriptional activation from RBPJκ, a downstream Notch effector, is essential for its pathogenesis.[62]

DELETIONS AND NUMERIC ABNORMALITIES IN ACUTE LEUKEMIAS

Deletions of all or part of chromosomes 5 and 7 and trisomy 8 are among the most common chromosomal abnormalities associated with gain or loss of genetic material but are not associated with a specific subtype of AML. They are considerably more frequent in older patients, whereas the frequency of the specific translocations and inversions described previously decreases with age. These same abnormalities (+8, −7, −5/5q-) are more common in patients with an antecedent MDS, therapy-related AML, or exposure to environmental mutagens. Specific translocations or inversions are relatively less common in these patient groups. An exception to this is AML, which develops in patients who have received high doses of etoposide for treatment of a previous malignancy. As noted in "Chromosomal Translocations that Target the *MLL* Gene," translocations involving 11q23 are commonly observed in this setting.

The high frequency of deletions of the long arm of chromosome 5 (5q-) has interest because the genes encoding several hematopoietic growth factors and their receptors are located on this arm, including *GM-CSF* (5q23–31), *IL-3* (5q23–31), and *IL-4* (5q23–31). The *M-CSF* receptor, c-*fms*, and the *PDGFβR* are also on this chromosome, at 5q33. In some 5q- chromosome defects, one or more of these genes may be deleted. An intensive effort has been made to identify putative tumor suppressor genes in several critically deleted regions of chromosome 5q, as well as 7q and 20q (reviewed in ref. 63). In addition, genomic wide loss of heterozygosity screens have identified a spectrum of other smaller recurrent deletions associated with AML.[64]

An RNA-mediated interference (RNAi)-based screen of each gene within the common deleted region led to identification of *RPS14* gene. A partial loss of function of the ribosomal subunit protein RPS14 in normal hematopoietic progenitor cells recapitulated the disease with impaired erythropoiesis and relative preservation of the other lineages. Conversely, a forced expression of *RPS14* rescued the disease phenotype in patient-derived bone marrow cells. In patients with the 5q- syndrome, 1 allele of *RPS14* is deleted, and haploinsufficient expression of *RPS14* has been confirmed in patient samples. These results indicate that the *RPS14* gene is a causal gene in the 5q- syndrome.[65] However, it is conceivable that other genes (on 5q or elsewhere) collaborate with *RPS14* to cause the disease phenotype and eventually to progress to AML. In that regard, the 5q-syndrome region on chromosome 5 should be distinguished from a more centromeric locus on 5q that has been associated with therapy-related and aggressive subtypes of MDS as well as AML, and for which two candidate genes, *CTNNA1* and *EGR1*, have been recently reported.[66,67]

Acquired deletions are a hallmark of cancer and precancerous states. In general, such deletions flag the existence of a tumor suppressor gene conforming to two-hit hypothesis, in which one allele is often deleted and the other allele is inactivated by deletion, mutation, or epigenetic modification. However, the search for the key tumor suppressor gene has been elusive in the 7q or 20q deleted regions in MDS or AML. Several possible explanations can be made for the difficulty in identification of classic tumor suppressors, despite the availability of complete genomic sequence and detailed annotations of expressed sequences in these regions. The residual allele may be affected by epigenetic mutations that interfere with expression, such as promoter or aberrant methylation, or both, but do not affect coding sequence. These types of mutations are more difficult to detect. Alternatively, it is possible that haploinsufficiency for one or more genes in the critically deleted loci is responsible for the MDS/AML phenotype.[68] Haploinsufficiency for the transcription factor AML1 has been reported in a familial leukemia syndrome, and haploid gene dosage is increasingly being identified as a genetic basis for inherited human diseases.[69,70] RNAi-based discovery of the 5q- syndrome gene suggests that haploinsufficient disease genes can be identified with this approach.

CHROMOSOMAL TRANSLOCATIONS THAT RESULT IN OVEREXPRESSION OF OTHERWISE NORMAL GENES

The chromosomal translocations described thus far result in expression of aberrant fusion genes. Chromosomal translocations may also result in overexpression of otherwise normal genes as a result of juxtaposition of a gene not normally expressed in adult hematopoietic tissues adjacent to an active promoter or enhancer. Most of those identified thus far involve the immunoglobulin or T-cell receptor (TCR) enhancer loci, and thus most of these are associated with lymphoid malignancies.

The prototypical example of juxtaposition of an immunoglobulin enhancer locus to an oncogene resulting in B-cell leukemia and lymphoma is the t(8;14)(q24;q32), resulting in overexpression of the *MYC* bHLH/bZIP transcription factor on chromosome 8 because of juxtaposition to the immunoglobulin heavy-chain enhancer on chromosome 14. Similar phenotypes ensue from juxtaposition to other immunoglobulin enhancers in the human genome, such as the Igκ locus on chromosome 2 or the Igλ locus on chromosome 22, and are characterized as B-ALL or lymphoma (Table 31.1). Overexpression of *MYC* from immunoglobulin enhancers in murine models results in B-cell leukemias and lymphomas, confirming a central role for *MYC* overexpression in transformation. However, the mechanism of transformation of *MYC*, and, indeed, a complete understanding of its target genes, is not fully understood. MYC is fully active as a transcription factor when heterodimerized with MAX. MAX is normally a homodimer, or a heterodimer complexed with MAD, which represses transcription. Overexpression of *MYC* is thought to shift the equilibrium in favor of an MYC-MAX homodimer that transactivates genes that confer the leukemic phenotype to B cells.

CHROMOSOMAL TRANSLOCATIONS INVOLVING THE T-CELL RECEPTOR

T-cell leukemias are often associated with overexpression of a number of genes because of juxtaposition to the TCR enhancer loci (*TCRβ* at chromosome 7q34 or *TCRα/δ* at chromosome 14q11). Overexpression is thus associated with T-cell phenotypes, including T-cell ALL and lymphoma. For example, T-cell ALL may be associated with overexpression of bHLH family members that include TAL1/SCL, TAL2/SCL2, LYL1, HOX11, HOX11L2, LMO2, LMO1, and MYC (Table 31.1; reviewed in refs. 71 and 72). In addition to the minority of T-ALL cases with gene rearrangements involving these loci, it has been demonstrated that many patients without evident cytogenetic abnormalities overexpress TAL1, LMO2, HOX11, or HOX11L2.

POINT MUTATIONS IN ACUTE LEUKEMIA

Although intensive effort has focused on chromosomal translocations in leukemia, in part because of their high frequency in various kinds of leukemia, it has become increasingly clear that point mutations play an important role in a spectrum of leukemias (Table 31.2). Ongoing high-throughput sequencing initiatives have identified numerous solitary and recurring somatic point mutations within the various leukemic subtypes. The interpretation of these sequencing data requires the identification of "driver" *versus* "passenger" mutations. Driver mutations cause genetic alterations contributing to leukemic pathophysiology, whereas passenger mutations occur in leukemia cells and are propagated but are not etiologic to the disease.[73] It is therefore essential that newly discovered somatic mutations in leukemia through sequencing studies undergo subsequent biologic validation in an experimental model system.

Oncogenic *RAS* Mutations

Activating mutations in *RAS* may be associated with AML and MDS, typically at codons 12, 13, or 61, or *N*- or *K-RAS*. The reported incidence varies

TABLE 31.2

POINT MUTATIONS IN ACUTE LEUKEMIA

Mutation	Frequency in AML (%)
SIGNAL TRANSDUCTION PATHWAYS—ACTIVATING	
FLT3-ITD	~20–25
FLT3 activation loop	~5–10
RAS (N- and K-)	~15–20
KIT (D816V and D816Y)	~5
PTPN11	<5
MPL (W515L and T487A) (more common in AMKL)	<5
JAK2 and JAK3 (more common in *AMKL*)	<5
TRANSCRIPTION FACTORS—LOSS OF FUNCTION	
C/EBPα (more common in FAB M2)	8–10
RUNX1 (*AML1*; more common in *FAB M2*)	<5
GATA-1 (more common in AMKL in Down syndrome)	<5

AML, acute myeloid leukemia.

widely between studies from 25% to 44% and *RAS* mutations may confer a worse prognosis (reviewed in ref. 74). Considerable effort has been devoted to developing small-molecule inhibitors of RAS activation, with a focus on prenylation inhibitors, including farnesyl transferase and geranyl-geranylation inhibitors that preclude appropriate targeting of activated RAS to the plasma membrane.[75] Specifically targeting activated RAS mutants remains an attractive option, and prenyltransferase inhibitors appear to have activity in AML. However, clinical activity is not correlated with the presence of activating mutations in RAS or even with inhibition of the target farnesyl transferase itself.[75,76] Several possible interpretations can be made of these observations, including the possibility that RAS is activated by mechanisms other than intrinsic point mutations (e.g., constitutively activated tyrosine kinases such as FLT3), or that other proteins that are targets of prenylation are important in leukemia pathogenesis, or that farnesyl transferase inhibitors have off-target effects.

Activating Mutations in Tyrosine Kinases

One of the more exciting recent developments in the pathogenesis of AMLs has been identification and characterization of activating mutations in hematopoietic tyrosine kinases. Substantial evidence has been shown that chromosomal translocations that activate tyrosine kinases can contribute to the pathogenesis of CML syndromes. The most common of these is the *BCR/ABL* gene rearrangement, but other examples include the TEL/ABL, TEL/PDGFβR, TEL/JAK2, H4/PDGFβR, FIP1/PDGFβR, and rabaptin/PDGFβR fusion proteins. However, these fusion genes are only rarely encountered in AMLs. Approximately 1% to 2% of cases of *de novo* AML have the *BCR/ABL* gene rearrangement. In addition, there are very rare cases of disease progression from CML to AML associated with acquisition of second mutations such as the *NUP98/HOXA9*, *AML1/ETO*, or *AML1/EVI1* rearrangement noted in Table 31.1. However, point mutations in the tyrosine kinase activation loop and juxtamembrane (JM) mutations that activate *FLT3* and *c-KIT* have been identified in a significant proportion of AML cases. These findings may have important therapeutic implications with the demonstration of the efficacy of molecular targeting of the ABL kinase in *BCR/ABL*-positive CML and CML blast crisis with imatinib.[77]

Activating mutations in *FLT3* have been reported in approximately 30% to 35% of cases of AML.[78] In 20% to 25% of cases, internal tandem duplications (ITDs) of the JM domain result in constitutive activation of FLT3. These can range in size from a few to more than 50 amino acids and are always in frame. Because of the extensive variability in size and exact position of the repeats within the JM domain, it has been hypothesized that these are loss-of-function domains that impair an autoinhibitory domain, resulting in constitutive kinase activation in the absence of ligand. In support of this, the crystallographic structure of FLT3 demonstrates a 7 amino acid extension of the JM domain that intercalates into the catalytic domain, thereby precluding kinase activation.[79] It is likely that ITD mutations in this region would disrupt structure of the autoinhibitory domain, resulting in kinase activation. In an additional 5% to 10% of cases, so-called activating loop mutations occur near position D835 in the tyrosine kinase.[80] Several large studies have confirmed the frequency of these mutations in adult and pediatric AML populations and the fact that mutations in *FLT3* appear to confer a poor prognosis.[81-83] High-throughput sequencing of AML patient samples lacking known FLT3 mutations revealed nine novel acquired mutations resulting in amino acid changes within the extracellular, JM, and activation domains; however, only four of the nine changes were driver mutations capable of kinase activation and conferring growth factor independence, thus emphasizing the need for biologic validation of sequencing data.[84]

FLT3 mutations may occur in conjunction with known gene rearrangements, such as *AML1/ETO*, *PML/RARα*, CBFβMYH11, or MLL. Analogous activating loop mutations at position D816 have also been reported in *C-KIT* in approximately 5% of cases of AML. Activating mutations in the thrombopoietin receptor, MPLW515L, originally identified in myelofibrosis with myeloid metaplasia, and MPLT487A have been observed in both primary cases of AMKL and those secondary to myeloid metaplasia.[85-87]

The Janus kinase family (JAK1-3) of nonreceptor tyrosine kinases, in addition to involvement in translocation-derived fusions such as TEL/JAK2, have been found to contain activating point mutations. JAK kinases are important signaling intermediaries of multiple hematopoietic cytokine receptors and downstream effectors such as STAT proteins.[88] *JAKV617F*, originally identified as a causative mutation in *polycythemia vera*, is also seen to a minor extent in AML.[89] Additional mutations in *JAK2* and *JAK3* have been isolated in AMKL.[87,90,91] Mutations in *JAK1*, 2, or 3 are found in approximately 11% of *BCR/ABL*-negative childhood acute lymphoid leukemia and were often concurrent with deletion of the IKAROS lymphoid-specific transcription factor and the CDKN2A/B tumor suppressor.[92] As sequencing efforts continue, it is probable the list of activating kinase mutations will dramatically increase. As kinases are proving to be relatively amenable to targeted therapy, the opportunities for treatment tailored to these activated kinases should likewise expand.

MUTATION IN TUMOR SUPPRESSOR GENES

Wilms' tumor gene was originally described as a tumor suppressor gene in patients with WAGR (Wilms' tumor predisposition-aniridia-genitourinary-mental retardation).[93] *WT1* is found in adult tumors from different origin, and these tumors arise in tissues that normally do not express *WT1*. It has therefore been suggested that expression of *WT1* might play an oncogenic role in these tumors (reviewed in ref. 94). *WT1* is located at the chromosome 11p and encodes for a transcription factor with N-terminal transcriptional regulatory domain and C-terminal zinc finger domain (exon 7 to 10). The expression of *WT1* inversely correlates with the degree of differentiation in the hematopoietic system as it is present in CD34+ cells and absent in mature leukocytes.[94,95] *WT1* functions as a potent transcription regulator of genes important for cell survival and cell differentiation. The disruption of *WT1* function promotes stem cell proliferation and hampers differentiation.[94] Although the precise role of *WT1* in normal and malignant hematopoiesis remains to be further elucidated, it seems to have a dual role in leukemia.[96]

The wild type form of *WT1* is highly (75% to 100%) expressed in a variety of acute leukemias.[97] Consistent with the function of an oncogene is the pattern of *WT1* expression in CML, where low levels are found in the chronic phase but are frequently increased in the accelerated and blast crisis phase.[98] High levels of *WT1* in patients after chemotherapy is associated with poor prognosis.

WT1 can act as a tumor suppressor in mice.[99] Mutation of the *WT1* gene can be detected in approximately 10% of normal karyotype AMLs.[100,101] Mutations that cluster to exon 7 (mostly frameshift mutations resulting from insertions and deletions) and exon 9 (mostly substitutions) are associated with poor clinical outcome.[101–103] These data are examples of *WT1* as a tumor suppressor. On the other hand, a recent study has analyzed mutations within the entire *WT1* coding sequence in a very large cohort of young adults with normal karyotype AML. Contrary to the previous observations,[101–103] *WT1* mutations had no prognostic impact.[104] The different results from these large studies could be explained by the variable biological role of *WT1* in AML, possible differences in therapy, and other patient characteristics. It is therefore desirable that testing for *WT1* mutations becomes part of the risk assessment in future clinical trials to resolve these discrepancies.

TP53 is a tumor suppressor that induces cell-cycle arrest in a response to apoptotic cell death or DNA repair due to genotoxic substances, oncogenes, hypoxia, DNA damage, or ribonucleotide depletion.[105] Inactivation of *TP53* plays an important role during neoplastic transformation in solid tumors and also during progression of hematologic malignancies.[106–108] Animal experiments suggest that the loss of one *TP53* allele could be sufficient for tumorigenesis.[109] This could be relevant for the development of leukemia in patients with single *TP53* deletion. The loss of 17p in AML is often accompanied by a *TP53* mutation resulting in a loss of heterozygosity.[110,111] Another possibility is the inactivation of downstream mediators of *TP53*, which affect not only cell-cycle arrest but also DNA repair and apoptosis. Alternatively, overexpression of genes inhibiting or promoting degradation of TP53 can be considered; for example, *MDM2* gene amplifications have been detected in B-CLL.[112] *TP53* deletion can be present as a loss of 17p as a part of a complex aberrant karyotype or as a single chromosomal aberration, both resulting in a poor clinical outcome.[110,113–115]

The incidence of *TP53* aberrations is high in AML with a complex aberrant karyotype (up to 70%),[110] but relatively rare in other AML groups (2% to 9%),[83,110,116] and *TP53* mutations without cytogenetic alteration are to rare events.[111,117] Low-risk AML t(8;21) or inv(16) is not associated with *TP53* deletion. There is significant positive association between *TP53* deletion and other high-risk chromosomal aberrations such as del(5q), and monosomy 5 and 7.[115,118] Molecular risk factors *FLT3-ITD* and *NPM1* mutation do not seem to cluster with the *TP53* deletion in complex karyotype patients.[115] *TP53*-deleted cells have greater resistance to various conventional antileukemic drugs.[119] Although published data of multidrug-resistance gene expression showed negative influence on therapy response in complex aberrant patients,[120] the association of *TP53* deletion and *MDR1* expression has been confirmed for CML, but not for AML.[121] Hence, an independent mechanism of resistance needs to be considered.[115] Taken together, *TP53* deletion is a high-risk factor conveying a poor outcome, and further studies are necessary to provide and evaluate alternative therapies.

ACTIVATING MUTATIONS OF NOTCH

NOTCH1 is a component of an evolutionarily conserved pathway shown to direct T-cell lineage determination in early and late stages of lymphocyte development as well as play a role in hematopoietic stem cell self-renewal (reviewed in ref. 122). NOTCH1 is a heterodimeric transmembrane receptor. Ligand binding to NOTCH1 allows proteolytic cleavage of the heterodimerization domain (HD) by γ-secretase of the C-terminal intracellular domain (ICN), which then localizes to the nucleus to function as a transactivator. Involvement of NOTCH1 in T-ALL had been observed with the rare t(7;9)(q34;q34.3) in which translocation of TCRβ locus into the *NOTCH1* gene results in the expression of the truncated, transcriptionally active ICN.

Recently, a series of point mutations in NOTCH1 were identified in over half of all T-ALL cases[123] (reviewed in ref. 124). These mutations clustered in two primary locations, the HD and the proline, glutamate, serine, and threonine-rich (PEST) domain. The missense mutations within the HD domain make NOTCH1 more amenable to γ-secretase–mediated cleavage, thus enhancing activation. The PEST domain controls the rate of degradation of the activated ICN. PEST domain mutants are primarily small insertions/deletions into the reading frame causing deletion of all or part of the domain and extending the half-life of the activated ICN. Fortuitously, γ-secretase inhibitors (GSIs) had already undergone significant clinical development from the involvement of γ-secretase in processing the pathogenic β-amyloid peptide associated with Alzheimer dementia. Initial clinical trials of GSIs in T-ALL have shown minimal effects on disease and significant gastrointestinal toxicity.[125] Use of GSIs in combination with agents affecting alternative pathways may provide synergism and improve efficacy. Treatment of a mouse model of T-ALL with GSIs and corticosteroids has demonstrated that GSIs are capable of abrogating corticosteroid resistance in established cell lines as well as limiting GSI-mediated gut toxicity.[126]

MUTATIONS ALTERING LOCALIZATION OF NPM1

NPM1 (*nucleophosmin1*) encodes a protein that acts as a molecular chaperone between the nucleus and cytoplasm. It is involved in multiple cellular processes including regulation of TP53/ARF pathways, ribosome biogenesis, and duplication of centrosomes. *NPM1* had been previously identified in acute leukemias as a translocation fusion partner with *RAR* and *MLF* as well as with *ALK* in anaplastic large cell lymphoma. Aberrant cytoplasmic localization of *NPM1* has been observed in 25% to 30% of adult AML and is associated with point mutations within exon 12, which are hypothesized to enhance a nuclear export motif within the expressed protein.[127] The mechanism by which mutated *NPM1* causes leukemia is not clear; however, the cytoplasmic localization of *NPM1* is thought to be intrinsic to its altered function.[128] *NPM1* mutations are found more frequently in AML with normal karyotypes (50% to 60%) and more apt to have *FLT3-ITD* mutations as well. Among normal cytogenetic AMLs, the presence of cytoplasmic *NPM1* in the absence of the *FLT3-ITD* is associated with a more favorable prognosis.[128]

LOSS-OF-FUNCTION POINT MUTATIONS IN *AML1*, *C/EBPα*, AND *GATA-1*

AML1 (also known as *RUNX1*, *CBFA2*) is a frequent target of translocations in human leukemias. In addition to frequent involvement of *AML1* as a consequence of chromosomal translocations, it has been determined that loss-of-function mutations in *AML1* are responsible for the inherited leukemia syndrome FPD/AML (familial platelet disorder with propensity to develop acute myelogenous leukemia).[69,129] In addition, approximately 3% to 5% of sporadic cases of AML harbor loss-of-function mutations in *AML1*,[69,130] with a higher frequency in M0 AML (25%) and in AML or MDS with trisomy 21. It is not known whether loss-of-function mutations in *AML1* confer the favorable prognosis associated with translocations involving the *AML1* gene.

C/EBPα is a 42-kDa hematopoietic transcription factor that is required for normal myeloid lineage development. Because many translocations associated with AML phenotypes result in loss of function of hematopoietic transcription factors, it has been hypothesized that *C/EBPα* may also be a target for loss-of-function mutations in human leukemia. Two major types of *C/EBPα* point mutations have been described in AML: short frame-shifting mutations in the region encoding the amino-terminus causing expression of a shortened 30-kDa protein with dominant negative activity and in-frame insertions or deletions in the region of the carboxy-terminus that alter the DNA-binding or dimerization domains causing loss of function.[131] Thus, these mutations would be predicted to impair hematopoietic differentiation. Although the bulk of *C/EBPα* occur in patients with normal cytogenetics, overall and progression-free survival is closer to the favorable rather than intermediate prognostic group.[132] Therefore, *C/EBPα* mutational status may provide a more accurate risk assessment for normal cytogenetic AML.

GATA-1 mutations are associated with a subset of AMKLs (FAB M7), in particular leukemias arising in patients with Down syndrome (constitutional trisomy 21). These mutations result in early termination of the full-length GATA-1 protein; however, translation of a short form, GATA-1s, from an alternate initiation codon occurs. GATA-1s is theorized to function as either a hypomorphic or dominant negative allele and dysregulation of GATA-1 pathways is thought to contribute to leukemogenesis.[133,134] *GATA-1* mutations are often seen in a tansient myeloproliferative disorder that precedes Down syndrome–associated AMKL, suggesting that *GATA-1* mutation is an early event.[133] *GATA-1* mutations thus far have only been associated with Down syndrome and have not been observed in other infant AMKLs, including those with the t(1;22) described earlier in "t(1;22) Translocation Associated with Infant Acute Megakaryoblastic Leukemia."

MUTATION OF LYMPHOID DEVELOPMENT GENES IN ALL

Analysis of pediatric acute leukemia samples through a combination of high-resolution SNP arrays and genomic sequencing revealed numerous cryptic translocations, small deletions, and point mutations affecting genes required for B-cell commitment and differentiation.[135] These genes include *PAX5*, *E2A*, *EBF1*, *LEF1*, *IKAROS*, and *AIOLOS*, and their mutations predominantly produce haploinsufficiency resulting in hypomorphic expression. Forty percent of acute precursor B-cell leukemias possessed mutation of at least one gene required for B-cell development, and 31.7% specifically had mutations within the *PAX5* gene.

Because of the requirement of these factors for normal early to late precursor B development, the immunophenotypic stage most closely related to the leukemias, it is hypothesized that loss of normal expression levels leads to a block in differentiation, a critical step in leukemogenesis.[135]

MUTATIONAL COMPLEMENTATION GROUPS IN ACUTE LEUKEMIAS

Several lines of evidence indicate that more than one mutation is necessary for the pathogenesis of acute leukemia. First, there is evidence for acquisition of additional cytogenetic abnormalities with disease progression from CML to AML (i.e., CML blast crisis). Published examples of progression in *BCR/ABL*-positive CML include acquisition of t(3;21) *AML1/EVI1*, t(8;21) *AML1/ETO*, or t(7;11) *NUP98/HOXA9* gene rearrangements. Progression of chronic myelomonocytic leukemia to AML in a patient with the *TEL/PDGFβR* gene rearrangement was associated with acquisition of a t(8;21) *AML1/ETO* gene rearrangement.[136] Second, expression of the AML1/ETO or CBFβ/MYH11

fusion proteins in murine models is not sufficient to cause AML.[27,137] Chemical mutagens must be used in these contexts to generate second mutations that cause the AML phenotype. Third, evidence indicates that in some cases the *TEL/AML1* gene rearrangement associated with pediatric ALL may be acquired *in utero*, but ALL does not develop until years later, indicating a requirement for a second mutation.[138] Fourth, AML develops in transgenic mice that express the PML/RAR-α fusion protein only after a long latency of 3 to 6 months, with incomplete penetrance, indicating a need for a second mutation.[34–36]

The genetic epidemiology of AML provides important clues to the nature of the collaborating mutations. One broad complementation group in AML (Fig. 31.1) is composed of mutations that activate signal transduction pathways. These include activating mutations in *FLT3*, *RAS*, and *KIT* and, more rarely, the *BCR/ABL* and *TEL/PDGFβR* fusion associated with disease progression in CML. These can be viewed as a complementation group because even though they are collectively present in approximately 50% of cases of AML, they rarely, if ever, occur together in the same patient.

A second complementation group, typified by translocations involving hematopoietic transcription

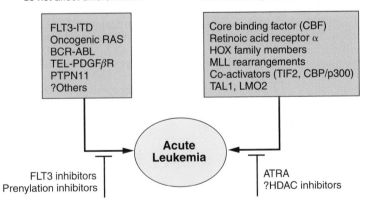

FIGURE 31.1 Cooperating mutations in acute leukemia. Leukemia is composed of two broad complementation groups, defined by lack of concurrence of any two mutations in the same complementation group in the same patient. One group is characterized by activating mutations in signal transduction pathways, such as FLT3-ITD or oncogenic N-RAS. When expressed alone, these mutations confer a proliferative or survival advantage, or both, but do not affect differentiation. The second group exemplified by AML1/ETO or PML/RAR-α are associated with impaired differentiation and the ability to confer properties of self-renewal to hematopoietic progenitors. Together, the complementation groups collaborate to engender the acute leukemia phenotype. This model has important therapeutic implications in that each of the complementation groups can be potentially targeted for therapeutic intervention, such as small-molecule inhibitors of FLT3 or RAS, or agents that override the block in differentiation, such as all-*trans*-retinoic acid (ATRA) or possibly histone deacetylase (HDAC) inhibitors.

factors, includes *AML1/ETO, CBFβ/SMMHC, PML/RARα, NUP98/HOXA9,* and *MLL* gene rearrangements, and *MOZ/TIF2,* and they are never observed together in the same leukemia. In general, this second class of mutations impairs hematopoietic differentiation and may confer properties of self-renewal to the leukemic stem cell but is not sufficient to cause leukemia when expressed alone (see "Recurring Chromosomal Abnormalities in Acute Leukemia"). However, one mutation from each of these two complementation groups often coexists in the same leukemia. For example, activating mutations in *FLT3* or *RAS* have been observed in association with virtually all of the fusion genes in the second class described earlier.[139]

Support has also been given for the hypothesis of collaborating classes of leukemia oncogenes derived from analysis of genotypes of CML patients who progress to AML. Some cases of *BCR/ABL*-positive CML progress to AML associated with acquisition of the t(7;11) translocation associated with expression of the *NUP98/HOXA9* fusion gene discussed earlier. As another example, TEL/PDGFβR-positive chronic myelomonocytic leukemia may progress to AML associated with acquisition of the t(8;21) translocation related to expression of the AML1/ETO fusion. These cases of disease progressions from CML to AML imply that constitutively activated tyrosine kinases cooperate with mutations in hematopoietic transcription factors to cause the AML phenotype.

These findings suggest a hypothesis for the pathogenesis of AML in which there are two broad classes of cooperating mutations (Fig. 31.1).[139] One class, exemplified by activating mutations in *FLT3* or *RAS,* confer either a proliferative or survival advantage, or both, to hematopoietic progenitors but do not affect differentiation. These mutations do not confer self-renewal capacity as assessed in part by the ability to serially replate in culture or to serially transplant disease in murine models.[140,141] A second class of mutations, exemplified by *AML1/ETO, CBFβ/SMMHC, PML/RARα, NUP98/HOXA9,* and *MLL* gene rearrangements, and *MOZ/TIF2* serve primarily to impair hematopoietic differentiation and confer properties of self-renewal. Together, these cooperating mutations induce the AML phenotype characterized by enhanced proliferative and survival advantage, impaired differentiation, and limitless self-renewal capacity. Experimental evidence supports this model of cooperativity in murine models between BCR/ABL and NUP98/HOXA9,[142] TEL/PDGFβR and AML1/ETO,[143] and FLT3/ITD and PML/RAR-α.[144] These findings have important therapeutic implications in that it may be possible to target both classes of mutations. For example, in APL with activating mutations in *FLT3,* it may be possible to target FLT3 with small-molecule inhibitors and PML/RAR-α with ATRA (see Fig. 31.1).

CONCLUSION

The quest to elucidate the essential pathophysiologic changes involved in leukemogenesis has been accelerated with the use of newer technologies such as high-resolution mapping and high-throughput sequencing. It is now possible to identify specific molecular pathways complementing known recurrent translocations as well as gain insight into the mechanisms underlying normal karyotype leukemias. Not only can these novel mutations be used for more accurate prognostication, but they also provide an opportunity for drug development, targeting the essential pathways dysregulated in leukemia. As the availability of pathway-targeted therapeutics increases, interrogation of a patient's leukemia for alterations at the genomic level may allow individualized therapy addressing the pathways responsible for leukemic cell survival, proliferation, and differentiation, which ideally would improve treatment efficacy and reduce therapy-related morbidity and mortality.

Selected References

The full list of references for this chapter appears in the online version.

1. Bonnet D, Dick JE. Human acute myeloid leukemia is organized as a hierarchy that originates from a primitive hematopoietic cell. *Nat Med* 1997;3:730.
3. Saito Y, Kitamura H, Hijikata A, et al. Identification of therapeutic targets for quiescent, chemotherapy-resistant human leukemia stem cells. *Sci Transl Med* 2007;2(17):17.
6. Huntly BJ, Shigematsu H, Deguchi K, et al. MOZ-TIF2, but not BCR-ABL, confers properties of leukemic stem cells to committed murine hematopoietic progenitors. *Cancer Cell* 2004;6:587–596.

7. Somervaille TCP, Cleary ML. Identification and characterization of leukemia stem cells in murine MLL-AF9 acute myeloid leukemia. *Cancer Cell* 2006;10:257–268.
9. Huntly BJ, Gilliland DG. Leukaemia stem cells and the evolution of cancer-stem-cell research. *Nat Rev Cancer* 2005;5:311–321.
10. Jamieson CH, Ailles LE, Dylla SJ, et al. Granulocyte-macrophage progenitors as candidate leukemic stem cells in blast-crisis CML. *N Engl J Med* 2004;351:657–667.
13. Ley TJ, Mardis ER, Ding L, et al. DNA sequencing of a cytogenetically normal acute myeloid leukaemia genome. *Nature* 2008;456:66.

14. Loriaux MM, Levine RL, Tyner JW, et al. High-throughput sequence analysis of the tyrosine kinome in acute myeloid leukemia. *Blood* 2008;111:4788.

16. International Cancer Genome Consortium. International network of cancer genome projects. *Nature* 2010;464:993–998.

17. Rowley JD. The role of chromosome translocations in leukemogenesis. *Semin Hematol* 1999;36:59–72.

18. Koschmieder S, Halmos B, Levantini E, Tenen DG. Dysregulation of the C/EBP{alpha} differentiation pathway in human cancer. *J Clin Oncol* 2009;27:619–628.

26. Jiao B, Wu CF, Liang Y, et al. AML1-ETO9a is correlated with C-KIT overexpression/mutations and indicates poor disease outcome in t(8;21) acute myeloid leukemia-M2. *Leukemia* 2009;23:1598.

32. Salomoni P, Pandolfi PP. The role of PML in tumor suppression. *Cell* 2002;108:165–170.

33. Scaglioni PP, Pandolfi PP. The theory of APL revisited. *Curr Top Microbiol Immunol* 2007;313:85–100.

37. Tallman MS, Nabhan C, Feusner JH, Rowe JM. Acute promyelocytic leukemia: evolving therapeutic strategies. *Blood* 2002;99:759–767.

38. Abramovich C, Humphries RK. Hox regulation of normal and leukemic hematopoietic stem cells. *Curr Opin Hematol* 2005;12:210–216.

45. Eguchi M, Eguchi-Ishimae M, Greaves M. Molecular pathogenesis of MLL-associated leukemias. *Int J Hematol* 2005;82:9–20.

46. Slany RK. The molecular biology of mixed lineage leukemia. *Haematologica* 2009;94:984–993.

51. Wei J, Wunderlich M, Fox C, et al. Microenvironment determines lineage fate in a human model of MLL-AF9 leukemia. *Cancer Cell* 2008;13:483.

56. Kung AL, Rebel VI, Bronson RT, et al. Gene dose-dependent control of hematopoiesis and hematologic tumor suppression by CBP. *Genes Dev* 2000;14:272–277.

62. Mercher T, Raffel GD, Moore SA, et al. The OTT-MAL fusion oncogene activates RBPJ-mediated transcription and induces acute megakaryoblastic leukemia in a knockin mouse model. *J Clin Invest* 2009;119:852–864.

64. Sweetser DA, Chen CS, Blomberg AA, et al. Loss of heterozygosity in childhood de novo acute myelogenous leukemia. *Blood* 2001;98:1188.

65. Ebert BL, Pretz J, Bosco J, et al. Identification of RPS14 as a 5q(-) syndrome gene by RNA interference screen. *Nature* 2008;451:335.

69. Song WJ, Sullivan MG, Legare RD, et al. Haploinsufficiency of CBFA2 causes familial thrombocytopenia with propensity to develop acute myelogenous leukaemia. *Nat Genet* 1999;23:166–175.

71. Armstrong SA, Look AT. Molecular genetics of acute lymphoblastic leukemia. *J Clin Oncol* 2005;23:6306–6315.

72. O'Neil J, Look AT. Mechanisms of transcription factor deregulation in lymphoid cell transformation. *Oncogene* 2007;26:6838–6849.

73. Stratton MR, Campbell PJ, Futreal PA. The cancer genome. *Nature* 2009;458:719–724.

75. Lancet JE, Karp JE. Farnesyltransferase inhibitors in hematologic malignancies: new horizons in therapy. *Blood* 2003;102:3880–3889.

76. Braun BS, Shannon K. Targeting Ras in myeloid leukemias. *Clin Cancer Res* 2008;14:2249–2252.

84. Frohling S, Scholl C, Levine RL, et al. Identification of driver and passenger mutations of FLT3 by high-throughput DNA sequence analysis and functional assessment of candidate alleles. *Cancer Cell* 2007;12:501–513.

85. Pardanani AD, Levine RL, Lasho T, et al. MPL515 mutations in myeloproliferative and other myeloid disorders: a study of 1182 patients. *Blood* 2006;108:3472–3476.

86. Hussein K, Bock O, Theophile K, et al. MPLW515L mutation in acute megakaryoblastic leukaemia. *Leukemia* 2009;23:852–855.

88. Baker SJ, Rane SG, Reddy EP. Hematopoietic cytokine receptor signaling. *Oncogene* 2007;26:6724–6737.

91. Walters DK, Mercher T, Gu TL, et al. Activating alleles of JAK3 in acute megakaryoblastic leukemia. *Cancer Cell* 2006;10:65–75.

92. Mullighan CG, Downing JR. Genome-wide profiling of genetic alterations in acute lymphoblastic leukemia: recent insights and future directions. *Leukemia* 2009;23:1209.

94. Hohenstein P, Hastie ND. The many facets of the Wilms' tumour gene, WT1. *Hum Mol Genet* 2006;15:R196.

96. Yang L, Han Y, Saurez Saiz F, Minden MD. A tumor suppressor and oncogene: the WT1 story. *Leukemia* 2007;21:868–876.

97. Miyagi T, Ahuja H, Kubota T, et al. Expression of the candidate Wilm's tumor gene, WT1, in human leukemia cells. *Leukemia* 1993;7:970–977.

101. Summers K, Stevens J, Kakkas I, et al. Wilms' tumour 1 mutations are associated with FLT3-ITD and failure of standard induction chemotherapy in patients with normal karyotype AML. *Leukemia* 2007;21:550–551.

102. Virappane P, Gale R, Hills R, et al. Mutation of the Wilms' tumor 1 gene is a poor prognostic factor associated with chemotherapy resistance in normal karyotype acute myeloid leukemia: the United Kingdom Medical Research Council Adult Leukaemia Working Party. *J Clin Oncol* 2008;26:5429–5435.

103. Paschka P, Marcucci G, Ruppert AS, et al. Wilms' tumor 1 gene mutations independently predict poor outcome in adults with cytogenetically normal acute myeloid leukemia: a Cancer and Leukemia Group B Study. *J Clin Oncol* 2008;26:4595–4602.

105. Vousden KH, Lu X. Live or let die: the cell's response to p53. *Nat Rev Cancer* 2002;2:594.

109. Venkatachalam S, Shi Y-P, Jones SN, et al. Retention of wild-type p53 in tumors from p53 heterozygous mice: reduction of p53 dosage can promote cancer formation. *EMBO J* 1998;17:4657–4667.

110. Haferlach C, Dicker F, Herholz H, et al. Mutations of the TP53 gene in acute myeloid leukemia are strongly associated with a complex aberrant karyotype. *Leukemia* 2008;22:1539–1541.

115. Seifert H, Mohr B, Thiede C, et al. The prognostic impact of 17p (p53) deletion in 2272 adults with acute myeloid leukemia. *Leukemia* 2009;23:656.

122. Radtke F, Wilson A, MacDonald HR. Notch signaling in hematopoiesis and lymphopoiesis: lessons from *Drosophila*. *Bioessays* 2005;27:1117–1128.

123. Weng AP, Ferrando AA, Lee W, et al. Activating mutations of NOTCH1 in human T cell acute lymphoblastic leukemia. *Science* 2004;306:269–271.

124. Grabher C, von Boehmer H, Look AT. Notch 1 activation in the molecular pathogenesis of T-cell acute lymphoblastic leukaemia. *Nat Rev Cancer* 2006;6:347–359.

125. DeAngelo DJ, Stone JR, Silverman LB, et al. A phase I clinical trial of the Notch inhibitor MK-0752 in patients with T-cell acute lymphoblastic leukemia/lymphoma (T-ALL) and other leukemias. *ASCO Meeting Abstracts* 2006:6585.

126. Real PJ, Tosello V, Palomero T, et al. Gamma-secretase inhibitors reverse glucocorticoid resistance in T cell acute lymphoblastic leukemia. *Nat Med* 2009;15:50–58.

127. Falini B, Mecucci C, Tiacci E, et al. Cytoplasmic nucleophosmin in acute myelogenous leukemia with a normal karyotype. *N Engl J Med* 2005; 352:254.

131. Mueller BU, Pabst T. C/EBPalpha and the pathophysiology of acute myeloid leukemia. *Curr Opin Hematol* 2006;13:7–14.

133. Wechsler J, Greene M, McDevitt MA, et al. Acquired mutations in GATA1 in the megakaryoblastic leukemia of Down syndrome. *Nat Genet* 2002;32:148–152.

134. Malinge S, Izraeli S, Crispino JD. Insights into the manifestations, outcomes, and mechanisms of leukemogenesis in Down syndrome. *Blood* 2009;113:2619–2628.

135. Mullighan CG, Goorha S, Radtke I, et al. Genome-wide analysis of genetic alterations in acute lymphoblastic leukaemia. *Nature* 2007;446:758–764.

144. Kelly LM, Kutok JL, Williams IR, et al. PML/RARalpha and FLT3-ITD induce an APL-like disease in a mouse model. *Proc Natl Acad Sci U S A* 2002;99:8283.

CHAPTER 32 CHRONIC LEUKEMIAS

ANUPRIYA AGARWAL, JOHN C. BYRD, AND MICHAEL W. DEININGER

Chronic myeloid leukemia (CML) and chronic lymphocytic leukemia (CLL) are very different diseases and yet share important clinical features. Both are usually diagnosed in an indolent stage characterized by expansion of differentiating cells that can last for several, sometimes many years. In both, the acquisition of additional mutations promotes progression to advanced therapy-refractory disease and both are incurable with currently available drug therapy. In this chapter, we will discuss the key pathogenetic mechanisms of CML and CLL, with emphasis on recent data and potential therapeutic implications.

CHRONIC MYELOID LEUKEMIA

CML is caused by BCR-ABL, a constitutively active tyrosine kinase generated as the result of a reciprocal translocation between chromosomes 9 and 22. The annual incidence of CML is 1.3 to $1.5/10^5$, with a slight male preponderance, but no significant differences across ethnicities. The only established CML risk factor is exposure to ionizing radiation, evident from studies in survivors of the nuclear explosions in Japan and patients exposed to thorotrast or radiotherapy. During the initial chronic phase (CP) cellular differentiation and function are largely maintained, therapy is effective and mortality is low. Without effective treatment the disease invariably progresses to blastic phase (BP), a rapidly fatal acute myeloid or lymphoid leukemia.

Pathogenesis

The first cases of what was probably CML were described by Bennett and Virchow in the mid 1840s.[1] In 1960, Philadelphia cytogeneticists Nowell and Hungerford[2] described a "minute" chromosome 22 in CML cells that became known as the *Philadelphia chromosome* (Ph). In 1973, Janet Rowley[3] discovered that Ph is in fact the result of a reciprocal translocation between chromosomes 9 and 22 [t(9;22) (q34;q11)]. The genes juxtaposed by the translocation were sub-

sequently identified as *ABL* (Abelson) on 9q34[4] and breakpoint cluster region (*BCR*) on chromosome 22q11 (Fig. 32.1). The next critical discoveries were that the constitutive tyrosine kinase activity of BCR-ABL is required for cellular transformation and that the clinical disease was reproducible in a murine model.[5,6] According to the World Health Organization the presence of BCR-ABL in the context of a myeloproliferative neoplasm is diagnostic of CML, although the translocation is also found in a subset of patients with acute lymphoblastic leukemia (ALL) and rare cases of acute myeloid leukemia (AML).

Molecular Anatomy of the BCR-ABL Junction

The breakpoints within *ABL* occur upstream of exon 1b, downstream of exon 1a, or, more frequently, between the two. Regardless of the exact breakpoint location, splicing of the primary transcript yields an mRNA in which *BCR* sequences are fused to *ABL* exon a2. Breakpoints within *BCR* localize to one of three breakpoint cluster regions (*bcr*). More than 90% of CML patients and one-third of Ph+ ALL patients express the 210kDa isoform of BCR-ABL, in which the break occurs in the 5.8-kb major breakpoint cluster region (M-*bcr*), which spans exons e12-e16 (formerly exons b1-b5). Alternative splicing gives rise to either b2a2 (e13a2) or b3a2 (e14a2) transcripts.[5] In remaining Ph+ ALL patients and in rare CML cases, the breakpoints are further upstream in the 54.4-kb minor breakpoint cluster region (m-*bcr*), generating an e1a2 transcript that is translated into p190^BCR-ABL.[7] A third breakpoint downstream of exon 19 in the micro breakpoint cluster region (μ-*bcr*) gives rise to an e19a2 BCR-ABL mRNA and p230^BCR-ABL and is associated with neutrophilia.

Other BCR-ABL variants, including b2a3, b3a3, e1a3, e6a2 or e2a2, have been observed in isolated cases.[8] Deletions flanking the breakpoints are detected in a subset of patients, which confer a poor prognosis to patients on interferon therapy, but probably not on imatinib.[9–11] The reciprocal ABL-BCR transcript, although

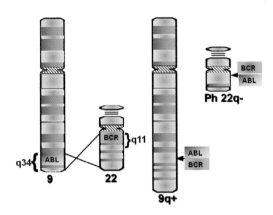

FIGURE 32.1   Schematic representation of the t(9;22) (q34;q11) translocation that creates the Philadelphia (Ph) chromosome. The *ABL* and *BCR* genes reside on the long arms of chromosome 9 and 22, respectively. As a result of the (9;22) translocation, the *BCR-ABL* gene is formed on the derivative of chromosome 22 (22q–, Ph chromosome), while the reciprocal *ABL-BCR* resides on the derivative of 9q+.

detectable in approximately two-thirds of patients, does not seem to play any significant role in pathogenesis.[12]

Functional Domains of BCR-ABL and Kinase Activation

p210[BCR-ABL] contains several distinct domains (Fig. 32.2).[13] The N-terminal coiled-coil domain of BCR allows BCR-ABL dimerization, which is critical for kinase activation. The p210[BCR-ABL] protein also retains the serine/threonine kinase and Rho guanine nucleotide exchange factor homology (Rho-GEF) domains of BCR, which are deleted in p190[BCR-ABL], which may explain the differences in disease phenotype associated with the two variants. In contrast to BCR, the ABL sequence is almost completely retained, including SRC homology domains 2 and 3, the tyrosine kinase domain, a proline-rich sequence, and a

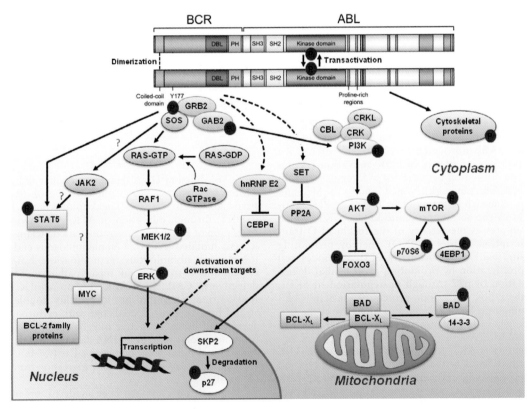

FIGURE 32.2   *BCR-ABL* domain structure and simplified representation of molecular signaling pathways activated in CML cells. Following dimerization of *BCR-ABL*, autophosphorylation generates docking sites on *BCR-ABL* that facilitate interaction with intermediary proteins such as GRB2. CrkL and CBL are also direct substrates of *BCR-ABL* that are part of a multimeric complex (*purple*). These *BCR-ABL*–dependent signaling complexes in turn lead to activation of multiple pathways whose net result is enhanced survival, inhibition of apoptosis, and perturbation of cell adhesion and migration. A subset of these pathways and their constituent transcription factors (*blue*), serine/threonine-specific kinases (*green*), cell-cycle regulatory protein (*yellow*), and apoptosis-related proteins (*red*) are shown. Several pathways were identified that are responsible for CML stem cell maintenance and/or *BCR-ABL*–mediated disease transformation (*orange*).

large C terminus with nuclear localization signal, DNA-binding, and actin-binding domains. The N-terminal "cap" region of ABL negatively regulates kinase activity by binding to a hydrophobic pocket at the basis of the kinase domain, which in the Ib isoform is mediated by N-terminal myristoylation. It is believed that the replacement of the cap with BCR sequences contributes to constitutive kinase activation.

Signal Transduction

Numerous substrates and binding partners of BCR-ABL have been identified (Fig. 32.2). Current efforts are directed at linking these pathways to the specific phenotypic defects that characterize CML, such as increased proliferation, decreased apoptosis, defective adhesion to bone marrow stroma, and genetic instability.[14] As comprehensive review of the multiple implicated pathways is beyond the scope of this chapter, we will focus on those for which strong evidence supports a rate-limiting role in disease pathogenesis.

Phosphatidylinositol-3 Kinase (PI3K)

PI3K is activated by autophosphorylation of tyrosine 177, which generates a high-affinity docking site for the SH2 domain of the GRB2 adapter, which in turn recruits GAB2 into a complex that activates PI3K.[15,16] Consistent with a critical role of the Y177/GRB2/GAB2 axis, mutation of tryosine 177 to phenylalanine or lack of GAB2 abrogates myeloid leukemia.[16] An alternative pathway of PI3K activation is complex formation between its p85 regulatory subunit, CBL, and CrkL, which bind to the SH2 and proline-rich domains of BCR-ABL.[17] PI3K activates the serine-threonine kinase AKT, which suppresses the activity of the forkhead O transcription factors (FOXO), thereby promoting survival.[18,19] Additionally PI3K enhances cell proliferation by promoting proteasomal degradation of p27 through up-regulation of SKP2, the F-Box recognition protein of the SCF^{SKP2} E3 ubiquitin ligase; absence of SKP2 from the leukemia cells prolongs survival in a murine CML model.[20] Another important outlet of PI3K signaling is AKT-dependent activation of mTOR, which leads to the constitutive phosphorylation of ribosomal protein p70S6 kinase and 4E-BP1, which enhance protein translation and cell proliferation.[21,22]

RAS/Mitogen-activated Protein Kinase (MAPK) Pathways

GRB2-mediated recruitment and activation of SOS promotes exchange of GTP for GDP on RAS.[15,23] GTP-RAS activates MAP kinase, promoting proliferation. Signaling from RAS to MAPK involves the serine-threonine kinase RAF-1[24,25] and RAC, another GTP–GDP exchange factor.[26] A crucial role for the latter is supported by the fact that lack of RAC1/2 delays BCR-ABL leukemia in a murine model.[27]

Janus Kinase (JAK) Signal Transducer and Activator of Transcription (STAT) Pathway

BCR-ABL activates STAT5 through direct phosphorylation or indirectly through phosphorylation by HCK, a SRC family kinase, or JAK2.[28,29] Active STAT5 induces the transcription of anti-apoptotic proteins like MCL-1 and BCL-X$_L$.[30] Initial experiments in mice failed to demonstrate a critical role for STAT5.[31] However, it was subsequently established that the mice used in this study were not null for STAT5, but expressed an N terminally deleted protein with partially retained function. In contrast, complete lack of STAT5 abrogates both myeloid and lymphoid leukemogenesis.[32]

Cytoskeletal Proteins

BCR-ABL phosphorylates several proteins involved in adhesion and migration, including FAK, paxillin, p130CAS and HEF1. This and activation of RAS[15,33] are thought to impair integrin-mediated adhesion of CML progenitors to stroma and extracellular matrix, causing premature circulation as well as abnormal proliferation of Ph+ progenitors.[34]

DNA Repair

BCR-ABL impairs DNA damage surveillance by various mechanisms. For example, BCR-ABL has been shown to suppress checkpoint kinase 1 (CHK1) through inhibition of ATR[35] or down-regulation of BRCA1, a substrate of ataxia telangiectasia mutated (ATM).[36] Nonhomologous end-joining and homologous recombination, both critical double-strand break repair pathways, are defective in CML. BCR-ABL also up-regulates RAD51, inducing rapid but low-fidelity double-strand break repair on challenge with cytotoxic agents and induces reactive oxygen species that promote chronic oxidative DNA damage, double-strand breaks and point mutations. Lastly, telomere length decreases with disease progression from CP to BP.[37]

Although progress has been made to understand the extraordinary complexity of BCR-ABL signaling, a complete picture is still elusive. To overcome the limitations of investigating single pathway, quantitative proteomics is being used to establish a comprehensive picture of BCR-ABL signaling.[38] These results suggest that cellular processes in CML, rather than relying on a single pathway, use integrated networks to fully realize their leukemogenic potential.

Murine Models of CML

The most commonly used murine model of CML is retroviral expression of BCR-ABL in bone marrow followed by transplantation into lethally irradiated syngeneic recipients, which develop a CML-like myeloproliferative neoplasm.[39] Recently, an inducible transgenic mouse model has been developed, in which conditional BCR-ABL expression is under the control of the 3′ enhancer of the murine stem cell leukemia (SCL) gene. This model serves as a promising new tool for studying leukemogenic mechanisms in hematopoietic stem cells during disease initiation and progression.[40] Lastly, xenograft models use various strains of immunodeficient mice for engraftment of primary CML cells.[41] The problem with xenograft models is that the engraftment of CP cells is low, probably because of their compromised interactions with the microenvironment as a result of species differences in cytokines and adhesion molecules. More promising results have been obtained by injecting CML cells directly into the livers of newborn mice.[42]

CML Stem Cell

The origin of CML in a pluripotent hematopoietic stem cell (HSC) was elegantly demonstrated in the late 1970s in studies showing clonality of granulocytes, erythrocytes, and platelets of female patients heterozygous for glucose-6-phosphate dehydrogenase, a polymorphic X-chromosomal gene.[43] BCR-ABL does not confer self-renewal, implying that Ph must be acquired by an HSC already endowed with this capacity.[44] For unknown reasons the main cellular expansion occurs in the progenitor cell compartment, while at least initially the majority of HSC are Ph-negative.[45] Serial xenograft studies have shown that CML leukemia stem cells (LSCs) reside within the quiescent CD34+38− fraction of bone marrow cells. Significant progress has recently been made by the identification of the IL-1 receptor-associated protein (IL-1RAP) as a surface marker specifically expressed on CD34+38− CML HSC.[45a] If confirmed, this will enable studies into the biology of these cells. Several genes were shown to have a critical role for leukemia-initiating cells maintenance in CML, including promyelocytic leukemia,[46] the hematopoietic-specific Rac2 GTPase,[47] smoothened, which is an essential component of the hedgehog pathway,[48] and β-catenin. The fact that these genes are also critical for maintenance and self-renewal of normal HSCs may be an obstacle to exploiting them as therapeutic targets.

Progression to Blastic Phase

Disease progression is believed to be due to the accumulation of molecular abnormalities that lead to a loss of terminal differentiation capacity of the leukemic clone, which however continues to depend on BCR-ABL activity. BCR-ABL mRNA and protein levels are higher in BP than in CP cells, including CD34+ granulocyte macrophage progenitors (GMPs), which are expanded in BP.[49] Another mechanism that enhances BCR-ABL activity in BP is inactivation of PP2A through up-regulation of SET, which in turn inhibits the PP2A phosphatase and its substrate protein tyrosine phosphatase I (SHP1). As SHP1 normally promotes BCR-ABL degradation through dephosphorylation, its reduced activity stabilizes BCR-ABL.[50]

The most striking feature of BP, the loss of differentiation capacity, suggests that the function of key myeloid transcription factors must be compromised. Occasionally, the differentiation block can be ascribed to mutations that result in the formation of dominant-negative transcription factors such as AML1-EVI or NUP98-HOXA9, which block differentiation or favor preferential growth of immature precursors.[51–53] Isolated cases of myeloid transformation have been associated with the acquisition of core binding factor mutations typical of AML. A more universal mechanism appears to be the BCR-ABL–induced down-regulation of CCAAT/enhancer binding protein-α (CEBPα) through the stabilization of the translational regulator heterogeneous nuclear ribonucleoprotein E2 (hnRNP E2), which is low or undetectable in CP but readily detectable in BP CML.[54] Interestingly, dominant-negative mutations of CEBPα are fairly common in AML,[55] but rare in CML-BP.[56]

Aberrant activation of Wnt/β-catenin signaling is believed to contribute to CML progression by conferring self-renewal capacity to GMPs. Activated β-catenin regulates self-renewal by undergoing translocation to the nucleus where it interacts with lymphoid enhancer factor/T-cell factor and regulates the transcription of genes such as Myc and Cyclin D1.[57] The acquisition of self-renewal by GMPs is expected to greatly increase the pool of LSCs in BP. Interestingly, expression microarray studies have implicated β-catenin activation not only in disease progression but also in resistance to tyrosine kinase inhibitors, supporting the view that drug resistance and disease progression share a common genetic basis.[58,59] This has implications for prognostication as well as for the development of strategies to prevent progression and overcome resistance.

Conclusions

BCR-ABL orchestrates an integrated network of signaling pathways that upend the physiological control of proliferation, cell death, DNA repair and microenvironment interaction, and lead to the clinical phenotype of CML.

Cooperation with additional genetic events that accumulate over time inevitably leads to BP and drug resistance. Although significant progress has been made toward understanding transformation and disease progression, much remains to be learned. The availability of genome-wide scanning tools will undoubtedly accelerate this process and hopefully lead to the discovery of new therapeutic targets to eliminate CML LSC, overcome drug resistance unless effective therapy is initiated early on, and improve the prognosis of patients whose disease has progressed to BP.

CHRONIC LYMPHOCYTIC LEUKEMIA

CLL is one of the most common types of leukemia in adults and has a relatively consistent immunophenotype including dim-surface immunoglobulin expression, CD19, CD20, CD23 along with the pan T-cell marker CD5.[60] The impact on overall survival in young and elderly patients with CLL is quite substantial. Patients with a diagnosis under the age of 50 have a median expected lifespan of 12.3 years, which compares to 31.2 years in an age-matched control group.[61] Although younger patients have poor outcome and shortened survival with CLL, several recent studies have also identified elderly patients as a high-risk group for poor survival following treatment.[62–65] A small subset of CLL patients have indolent disease for many years and do not require therapy or intervention. Improving our understanding of the origin, biology, and progression of CLL will best help define both risk stratification of patients and also identify potential new treatments for this disease.

Origin of CLL

Attempts to identify the origin of CLL with respect to a normal B-cell counterpart has also occurred and remains a controversial area.[66–68] Unlike most other B-cell lymphomas and leukemia with the exception of mantle cell lymphoma, CLL expresses typical mature B-cell markers with coexpression of CD5. This prompted many to hypothesize that CLL may be derived from CD5+ B cells whose immunoglobulin (Ig)V_H is unmutated. However, the overall phenotype of CLL with expression of CD5, CD23, and CD19, and low levels of sIgM or IgD is not observed in any other type of normal B-cell counterpart. Additionally, investigators identified that approximately 40% of CLL cases are IgV$_H$ unmutated, whereas the remainder are IgV$_H$ mutated.[69,70] These two groups also were shown to have distinct clinical features, prompting the hypothesis that CLL may represent two distinct diseases.[69,70]

Two sentinel articles examining mRNA gene expression profiling in CLL and normal B cells provided similar findings, suggesting CLL is in fact one disease with a common CLL gene signature.[71,72] The first, by Klein et al.,[71] examined cDNA gene expression profiles derived from IgV$_H$ unmutated, IgV$_H$ mutated, and normal B cells derived from different stages of differentiation. A nonsupervised analysis of gene expression profile demonstrated that IgV$_H$ mutated and unmutated CLL cases were not distinguished in any manner among a common profile typical of CLL. This CLL profile in the majority of samples had best resemblance to postgerminal center memory B cells and lacked any similarity to naive B cells, CD5+ B cells, and germinal center centroblasts. A supervised analysis of IgV$_H$ unmutated and mutated CLL did demonstrate distinct genes that could separate these two clinical subsets of CLL.

A second article, published concurrently by Rosenwald et al.,[72] demonstrated similar findings of a common CLL phenotype described by Klein et al. as compared with other normal B cells and B-cell malignancies. In particular, the CLL gene phenotype was not shared by CD5+ normal B cells, thereby providing collaborating evidence that this is likely not the CLL cell of origin. Using a nonsupervised analysis of CLL samples, IgV$_H$ unmutated and mutated samples were intermingled. However, supervised analysis of IgV$_H$ unmutated and mutated CLL identified a number of genes differentially expressed in the former group related to B-cell receptor signaling and proliferation. In particular, ZAP-70 (zeta-chain associated protein kinase) overexpression was overexpressed in IgV$_H$ unmutated CLL as compared with IgV$_H$ mutated CLL.[73–76]

Subsequent studies have suggested that ZAP-70 expression may partly explain why IgV$_H$ unmutated CLL patients have more active evidence of B-cell receptor signaling on ligation of the B-cell receptor.[77–79] Multiple studies confirming both the clinical prognostic significance of IgV$_H$ mutational status and/or ZAP70 expression have subsequently been reported. IgV$_H$ and/or ZAP70 represent very strong independent variables in predicting early disease progression, treatment remission duration, and survival of CLL patients. Unfortunately, the extreme variability in measurement of ZAP-70 expression among different investigators has limited full application of this biomarker clinically.

Chromosomal Abnormalities in the Pathogenesis of CLL

In CLL, conventional metaphase cytogenetics can identify chromosomal aberrations in only 20% to 50% of cases because of the low in vitro mitotic activity of CLL tumor cells.[80] Early nonstimulated metaphase karyotype studies of CLL demonstrated abnormalities in descending frequency of occurrence, including trisomy 12, deletions at 13q14, structural aberrations of 14q32, and deletions of 11q, 17p, and 6q.[81] In addition, complex karyotype (three or more abnormalities) occur in approximately 15% of patients and were noted in these early studies to predict for rapid disease progression, Richter's transformation, and inferior survival.[82–84] The use of CD40L or combination of interleukin (IL)-2 and cytosine-phosphate-guanosine (CpG) stimulation prior to metaphase analysis has also been reported with identification of translocations in 33 of 96 patients (34%) that were both balanced and unbalanced, which is associated with significantly shorter median time from diagnosis to requiring therapy and overall survival.[85] Subsequent comparative genomic hybridization (CGH) and global single nucleotide polymorphism (SNP) array studies in CLL have confirmed these deletions and also other chromosomal deletions in CLL.[86–88] Increasing aberrations in these same studies of CGH or SNP arrays have been associated with more aggressive disease.

Given the limitation of standard or stimulated karyotype analysis and inability to feasibly analyze patients by CGH or SNP arrays, interphase cytogenetics of known abnormalities are used to identify common, clinically significant aberrations in CLL. The largest study of interphase cytogenetics resulted in improved sensitivity to detect partial trisomies (12q12, 3q27, 8q24), deletions (13q14, 11q22-23, 6q21, 6q27, 17p13), and translocations (band 14q32) in more than 80% of all cases. In a large study of 325 patients by Dohner et al.,[89] a hierarchical model consisting of five genetic subgroups was constructed on the basis of regression analysis of CLL patients with chromosomal aberrations. The patients with a 17p deletion had the median survival time of 32 months and shortest treatment-free interval (TFI) of 9 months, whereas patients with 11q deletion followed closely with 79 months and 13 months, respectively.[89] The favorable 13q14 deletion group had a long TFI of 92 months and a median survival of 133 months, while the group without detectable chromosomal anomalies and those with trisomy 12 fell into the intermediate group with median survival of 111 and 114 months. Their TFI was 33 and 49 months, respectively. Based on this pivotal study, CLL patients are prioritized in a hierarchical order (deletion 17p13 > deletion 11q22-q23 > trisomy 12 > no aberration > deletion 13q14).[89] Of interest, patients with high-risk interphase cytogenetic abnormalities or other complex abnormalities are almost always found to have IgVH unmutated or ZAP-70–positive CLL.[90] The impact of high-risk interphase cytogenetics relative to disease progression, outside its association with IgVH unmutated CLL, remains uncertain.

Gene Mutation or Deletion Versus Epigenetic Silencing in the Pathogenesis of CLL

In many types of cancer including leukemia and lymphoma, the presence of activating mutations of specific oncogenes and also inactivating mutations and/or deletions of tumor suppressor genes directly contribute to the pathogenesis of the disease. In CLL only a few known tumor suppressor genes have been noted to be mutated or deleted in tumor cells. Of these, the p53 tumor suppressor gene has been the most rigorously studied based on it being one of the most commonly silenced genes in cancer. Deletions of the p53 gene are generally noted to occur in 3% to 10% of patients at diagnosis and generally occur as part of loss of large regions in del(17p13).[89,91] Mutations of p53 are also relatively uncommon and occur in a similar low proportion of CLL patients. The presence of deletion and mutation of p53 is more common but not uniform, with a proportion of patients having only one of the aberrations. Outcome in all studies is negatively influenced by the presence of a del(17p13.1), whereas only a subset of studies have shown that loss of p53 predicts aggressive disease course with rapid progression to time requiring therapy and inferior survival.[92–97] Both del(17p) and p53 mutations become more frequent as the disease progresses.[96] Overall, this suggests that loss of p53 function by mutation or deletion may be an important contributor to disease progression, but it likely does not contribute to the early pathogenesis of the disease. Indirect inactivation of p53 by mutation of ATM also occurs in CLL and correlates with more rapid disease progression.[93,98–100] Similar to p53, loss of ATM becomes more frequent with disease progression and also is likely a late event in the pathogenesis of this disease.

Whereas enhanced B-cell receptor signaling and ZAP-70 expression has been shown to contribute to the pathogenesis of CLL, efforts to identify mutations in this pathway have been limited. A screen of the tyrosine kinase kinome in selected exons that encode the kinase domain was reported from 95 CLL patients in whom 65 different kinases were examined based on relevance to B-cell biology.[101] No somatic tumor-associated mutations were found. The estimated frequency of mutations in the CLL genome based on this study was less than one mutation per 6.21 Mb DNA. The low proportion of mutations fall well under that observed in most solid tumors and also supports that gene mutations may not be a major contributor to the pathogenesis of this disease.

Finally, efforts to identify mutations in commonly deleted gene regions in CLL have been undertaken. Greatest attention has been placed on the most common del(13q14), where no protein coding gene mutation has been observed. However, the Croce group in 2002 identified that the microRNAs miR15 and miR16 resided in the minimally deleted region that was lost in approximately 70% of CLL patients.[102] MicroRNAs are small noncoding RNAs that effectively inhibit translation or induce degradation of numerous genes based on partial complementarity to site at the 3′ untranslated region of mRNA. Further support for the role of miR16.1 in the pathogenesis of CLL came from identification of both germ line mutations in a small number of CLL patients with a history of familial CLL.[103] Additionally, it was noted that New Zealand Black mice that develop both autoimmune disease and an indolent murine CLL and also have an acquired point mutation in the 3′ flanking sequence of microRNA mir-16-1.[104] The linkage of the mir-15a/16-1 complex to the development of murine CLL in a spontaneous mouse model suggests that mir-15a/16-1 is at least one of the molecular aberrations responsible for CLL. Klein et al.,[105] in a recent article, have demonstrated that a mouse with deletion of the miR15/miR16 region also develops a disease similar to human CLL, confirming the ultimate importance of this miR cluster in the development of CLL. These findings related to miRs and absent mutations suggest that miRs and other forms of epigenetic silencing, as opposed to mutational silencing of genes, are likely much more important in the pathogenesis and progression of CLL.

The role of microRNA and other noncoding genes in transcriptional and translational silencing of genes in CLL is now widely expanding. A subsequent study has demonstrated miR15 and miR16 target genes involved in disrupting apoptosis (bcl-2).[106] Multiple additional studies have demonstrated several other known important genes in the pathogenesis of CLL. Similarly, other forms of epigenetic silencing are also being shown to be relevant. Examples of alternative forms of epigenetic silencing can occur via promoter CpG methylation, recruitment of specific corepressor complexes, or recruitment of specific chromatin remodeling ATPase screening of CLL patients demonstrate distinct patterns of methylation by several groups.[107–110] Multiple oncogenes (bcl-2, TCL1, ZAP70)[111–113] have been shown to be aberrantly hypomethylated (hence expressed), whereas tumor suppressor genes (DAPK1, SFRP1, ID4, and PTPRO)[114–117] are hypermethylated (hence silenced), suggesting promoter methylation is one important key to gene regulation as part of malignant transformation. The current model for gene silencing likely involves loss of gene transcriptional activity followed by methylation.[118,119]

CLL and Proliferation

For many decades, CLL was viewed as a nonproliferating leukemia whose pathogenesis was driven solely by disrupted apoptosis and extended tumor cell survival. This paradigm was in part perpetuated based on the nonproliferating blood compartment. However, as with normal B cells, it has come to be recognized that CLL cell proliferation likely occurs in sites where microenvironment stimulation can occur, such as the lymph node and bone marrow. In such sites, proliferation centers are observed with a high proportion of dividing CLL cells that are often surrounded by either T cells or accessory stromal cells capable of providing cytokine costimulation.[120,121] Advances in technology including oral intake of heavy water have come forward to accurately measure all body compartments of CLL and assess the birth rate of CLL tumor cells *in vivo* in patients.[122] These studies have demonstrated a broad range of proliferation of CLL cells that varies based on disease state and also IgV$_H$ mutational status.[123,124] As one might expect, this same proliferation rate identified through heavy water studies in CLL was also shown to be predictive of disease progression. Collectively, these studies have at least partially discredited the theory that CLL is purely an accumulative disease, and rather focused study on specific compartments of the body that have very different biologic features of proliferation.

CLL and Disrupted Apoptosis

As the normal cell from which the disease CLL is derived is uncertain, it is quite difficult to equivalently compare to know if a difference in spontaneous apoptosis exists. However, several studies derived from CLL do provide evidence that apoptosis at least *in vivo* is disrupted. Despite the rarity of *Bcl-2* gene rearrangement in B-CLL, overexpression of *Bcl-2* mRNA and bcl-2 protein expression is common and has been shown to contribute to both disrupted spontaneous apoptosis and also *ex vivo* drug resistance.[112,125–128] Similarly, other antiapoptotic bcl-2 family member proteins including MCL-1, A1, and BCL-XL have also been shown to be elevated either in resting CLL or in CLL cells exposed to soluble and contact factors present in the microenvironment and they also contribute to drug resistance.[129–131]

Finally, a host of transcription factors involving the NFκB,[132] WNT,[133] hedgehog,[134] and JAK/STAT[135] signaling pathway have been shown to be constitutively active and also to contribute to disrupted apoptosis and drug resistance in CLL. In particular, differential activation of NF-kappa B activation in CLL[119,136–139] as compared with normal resting B cells and its relevant prognostic significance[140–142] with respect to predicting outcome and also its positive role in regulating many of the antiapoptotic genes up-regulated in CLL has generated particular interest.

B-cell Receptor Signaling in CLL

Identification of the divergent natural history of CLL based on IgVH mutational status, ZAP-70 expression, and associated enhanced B-cell receptor signaling has raised interest in the role of this in the pathogenesis of CLL.[77–79,143] Activation of the proximal lyn kinase and also downstream syk has been demonstrated in CLL.[144–146] Additionally, increased activity of the PI3-kinase pathway as measured by both lipid kinase activity and also baseline phosphorylation of p-AKT has been preliminarily reported.[147,148] Complementing this finding, a recent study demonstrated that mature memory B-cell development was in great part dependent on the PI3-kinase pathway.[149] A recent study using the isoform-specific inhibitor of PI3-kinase-δ demonstrated that much of the survival protection generated by the microenvironment from stromal cells, cytokines (CD40L, IL-6, TNF-α), and fibronectin contact is mediated via PI3-Kinase δ isoform signaling.[150] Of great interest has been the transition of these B-cell receptor kinase pathway inhibitors to clinical trials. Here, with syk, PI3-kinase δ isoform inhibitors, and BTK inhibitors they have demonstrated dramatic and often rapid clinical responses with relatively favorable toxicity profile in CLL patients. The success of such therapeutics further emphasizes the importance of BCR signaling in the pathogenesis of CLL.

Progression of CLL: Role of Genomic Instability and Clonal Evolution

Two small studies of previously untreated patients have been examined for features associated with clonal evolution and have noted this to be more frequent in patients with IgVH unmutated status[151] or those expressing the surrogate marker for IgVH mutational status, ZAP70.[91] The smaller of these studies noted clonal evolution to occur more commonly among those patients with progression.[151] One recently published study in which patients with long telomere length were more likely to have IgVH mutated disease and del(13q14), whereas those with del(11q22.3), del(17p13.1), complex karyotype (more than abnormalities) and IgVH unmutated disease were likely to have extended telomeres.[152] Furthermore, one small study suggested long telomere length among patients with IgVH unmutated disease could identify patients with an expected extended progression-free survival.[153] The contribution of clonal evolution, telomere length, and global hypomethylation in CLL progression will require further study.

Conclusion

A significant amount of data has been produced concerning the pathogenesis of CLL. Emerging from such work is the importance of epigenetics in the progression of CLL from normal B cells and also enhanced B-cell receptor signaling. Murine mouse models have demonstrated the importance of NF-κB, Bcl-2, TCL1, and loss of miR 15, MiR 16, and Leu2 in the pathogenesis of CLL. It is likely that current lines of investigation, along with emerging technologies related to whole-genome signaling, global proteomic assessment, and miR profiling, will lead to further advances in risk stratification and improvement in CLL therapy.

MOLECULAR BIOLOGY OF INDIVIDUAL CANCERS

Selected References

The full list of references for this chapter appears in the online version.

1. Deininger MW. Chronic myeloid leukemia: an historical perspective. *American Society of Hematology Education Program Book,* 50th Anniversary Review. 2008:418.
2. Nowell PC, Hungerford DA. Chromosome studies on normal and leukemic human leukocytes. *J Natl Cancer Inst* 1960;25:85.
3. Rowley JD. A new consistent chromosomal abnormality in chronic myelogenous leukaemia identified by quinacrine fluorescence and Giemsa staining. *Nature* 1973;243:290.
5. Groffen J, Stephenson JR, Heisterkamp N, et al. Philadelphia chromosomal breakpoints are clustered within a limited region, bcr, on chromosome 22. *Cell* 1984;36:93–99.
6. Daley GQ, Van Etten RA, Baltimore D. Induction of chronic myelogenous leukemia in mice by the P210bcr/abl gene of the Philadelphia chromosome. *Science* 1990;247:824–830.
7. Melo JV. The diversity of BCR-ABL fusion proteins and their relationship to leukemia phenotype. *Blood* 1996;88:2375–2384.

9. Huntly BJ, Guilhot F, Reid AG, et al. Imatinib improves but may not fully reverse the poor prognosis of patients with CML with derivative chromosome 9 deletions. *Blood* 2003;102:2205.
12. Melo JV, Gordon DE, Cross NC, et al. The ABL-BCR fusion gene is expressed in chronic myeloid leukemia. *Blood* 1993;81:158–165.
16. Sattler M, Mohi MG, Pride YB, et al. Critical role for Gab2 in transformation by BCR/ABL. *Cancer Cell* 2002;1:479–492.
18. Naka K, Hoshii T, Muraguchi T, et al. TGF-beta-FOXO signalling maintains leukaemia-initiating cells in chronic myeloid leukaemia. *Nature* 2010;463:676.
20. Agarwal A, Bumm TG, Corbin AS, et al. Absence of SKP2 expression attenuates BCR-ABL-induced myeloproliferative disease. *Blood* 2008;112:1960.
23. Kardinal C, Konkol B, Lin H, et al. Chronic myelogenous leukemia blast cell proliferation is inhibited by peptides that disrupt Grb2-SoS complexes. *Blood* 2001;98:1773–1781.
29. Ilaria RL, Jr., Van Etten RA. P210 and P190(BCR/ABL) induce the tyrosine phosphorylation and DNA binding activity of multiple specific STAT family members. *J Biol Chem* 1996;271:31704.

32. Hoelbl A, Schuster C, Kovacic B, et al. Stat5 is indispensable for the maintenance of bcr/abl-positive leukaemia. *EMBO Mol Med* 2010;2:98–110.

33. Verfaillie CM, Hurley R, Zhao RC, et al. Pathophysiology of CML: do defects in integrin function contribute to the premature circulation and massive expansion of the BCR/ABL positive clone? *J Lab Clin Med* 1997;129:584–591.

34. Ramaraj P, Singh H, Niu N, et al. Effect of mutational inactivation of tyrosine kinase activity on BCR/ABL-induced abnormalities in cell growth and adhesion in human hematopoietic progenitors. *Cancer Res* 2004;64:5322–5331.

35. Melo JV, Barnes DJ. Chronic myeloid leukaemia as a model of disease evolution in human cancer. *Nat Rev Cancer* 2007;7:441–453.

38. Brehme M, Hantschel O, Colinge J, et al. Charting the molecular network of the drug target Bcr-Abl. *Proc Natl Acad Sci U S A* 2009;106:7414.

39. Pear WS, Miller JP, Xu L, et al. Efficient and rapid induction of a chronic myelogenous leukemia-like myeloproliferative disease in mice receiving P210 bcr/abl-transduced bone marrow. *Blood* 1998;92:3780–3792.

40. Koschmieder S, Gottgens B, Zhang P, et al. Inducible chronic phase of myeloid leukemia with expansion of hematopoietic stem cells in a transgenic model of BCR-ABL leukemogenesis. *Blood* 2005;105:324–334.

41. Agliano A, Martin-Padura I, Mancuso P, et al. Human acute leukemia cells injected in NOD/LtSz-scid/IL-2Rgamma null mice generate a faster and more efficient disease compared to other NOD/scid-related strains. *Int J Cancer* 2008;123:2222–2227.

43. Fialkow PJ, Jacobson RJ, Papayannopoulou T. Chronic myelocytic leukemia: clonal origin in a stem cell common to the granulocyte, erythrocyte, platelet and monocyte/macrophage. *Am J Med* 1977;63:125–130.

44. Huntly BJ, Shigematsu H, Deguchi K, et al. MOZ-TIF2, but not BCR-ABL, confers properties of leukemic stem cells to committed murine hematopoietic progenitors. *Cancer Cell* 2004;6:587–596.

46. Ito K, Bernardi R, Morotti A, et al. PML targeting eradicates quiescent leukaemia-initiating cells. *Nature* 2008;453:1072.

48. Zhao C, Chen A, Jamieson CH, et al. Hedgehog signalling is essential for maintenance of cancer stem cells in myeloid leukaemia. *Nature* 2009;458:776–779.

50. Perrotti D, Neviani P. ReSETting PP2A tumour suppressor activity in blast crisis and imatinib-resistant chronic myelogenous leukaemia. *Br J Cancer* 2006;95:775–781.

57. Jamieson CH, Ailles LE, Dylla SJ, et al. Granulocyte-macrophage progenitors as candidate leukemic stem cells in blast-crisis CML. *N Engl J Med* 2004;351:657–667.

58. McWeeney SK, Pemberton LC, LoWWriaux MM, et al. A gene expression signature of CD34+ cells to predict major cytogenetic response in chronic-phase chronic myeloid leukemia patients treated with imatinib. *Blood* 2010;115:315–325.

59. Radich JP, Dai H, Mao M, et al. Gene expression changes associated with progression and response in chronic myeloid leukemia. *Proc Natl Acad Sci U S A* 2006;103:2794–2799.

60. Matutes E, Wotherspoon A, Catovsky D. Differential diagnosis in chronic lymphocytic leukaemia. *Best Pract Res Clin Haematol* 2007;20:367–384.

69. Hamblin TJ, Davis Z, Gardiner A, et al. Unmutated Ig V(H) genes are associated with a more aggressive form of chronic lymphocytic leukaemia. *Blood* 1999;94:1848–1854.

70. Damle RN, Wasil T, Fais F, et al. Ig V gene mutation status and CD38 expression as novel prognostic indicators in chronic lymphocytic leukemia. *Blood* 1999;94:1840–1847.

71. Klein U, Tu Y, Stolovitzky GA, et al. Gene expression profiling of B cell chronic lymphocytic leukemia reveals a homogeneous phenotype related to memory B cells. *J Exp Med* 2001;194:1625–1638.

72. Rosenwald A, Alizadeh AA, Widhopf G, et al. Relation of gene expression phenotype to immunoglobulin mutation genotype in B cell chronic lymphocytic leukemia. *J Exp Med* 2001;194:1639.

75. Rassenti LZ, Huynh L, Toy TL, et al. ZAP-70 compared with immunoglobulin heavy-chain gene mutation status as a predictor of disease progression in chronic lymphocytic leukemia. *N Engl J Med* 2004;351:893–901.

77. Chen L, Apgar J, Huynh L, et al. ZAP-70 directly enhances IgM signaling in chronic lymphocytic leukemia. *Blood* 2005;105:2036–2041.

85. Mayr C, Speicher MR, Kofler DM, et al. Chromosomal translocations are associated with poor prognosis in chronic lymphocytic leukemia. *Blood* 2006;107:742–751.

89. Dohner H, Stilgenbauer S, Benner A, et al. Genomic aberrations and survival in chronic lymphocytic leukemia. *N Engl J Med* 2000;343:1910–1916.

91. Shanafelt TD, Witzig TE, Fink SR, et al. Prospective evaluation of clonal evolution during long-term follow-up of patients with untreated early-stage chronic lymphocytic leukemia. *J Clin Oncol* 2006;24:4634.

101. Brown JR, Levine RL, Thompson C, et al. Systematic genomic screen for tyrosine kinase mutations in CLL. *Leukemia* 2008;22:1966–1969.

102. Calin GA, Dumitru CD, Shimizu M, et al. Frequent deletions and down-regulation of micro- RNA genes miR15 and miR16 at 13q14 in chronic lymphocytic leukemia. *Proc Natl Acad Sci U S A* 2002;99:15524–15529.

103. Calin GA, Ferracin M, Cimmino A, et al. A MicroRNA signature associated with prognosis and progression in chronic lymphocytic leukemia. *N Engl J Med* 2005;353:1793–1801.

104. Raveche ES, Salerno E, Scaglione BJ, et al. Abnormal microRNA-16 locus with synteny to human 13q14 linked to CLL in NZB mice. *Blood* 2007;109:5079–5086.

105. Klein U, Lia M, Crespo M, et al. The DLEU2/miR-15a/16-1 cluster controls B cell proliferation and its deletion leads to chronic lymphocytic leukemia. *Cancer Cell* 2010;17:28–40.

116. Raval A, Tanner SM, Byrd JC, et al. Downregulation of death-associated protein kinase 1 (DAPK1) in chronic lymphocytic leukemia. *Cell* 2007;129:879.

119. Chen SS, Raval A, Johnson AJ, et al. Epigenetic changes during disease progression in a murine model of human chronic lymphocytic leukemia. *Proc Natl Acad Sci U S A* 2009;106:13433–13438.

124. Messmer BT, Messmer D, Allen SL, et al. In vivo measurements document the dynamic cellular kinetics of chronic lymphocytic leukemia B cells. *J Clin Invest* 2005;115:755–764.

132. Furman RR, Asgary Z, Mascarenhas JO, et al. Modulation of NF-kappa B activity and apoptosis in chronic lymphocytic leukemia B cells. *J Immunol* 2000;164:2200–2206.

150. Herman SE, Gordon AL, Wagner AJ, et al. The phosphatidylinositol 3-kinase-{delta} inhibitor CAL-101 demonstrates promising pre-clinical activity in chronic lymphocytic leukemia by antagonizing intrinsic and extrinsic cellular survival signals. *Blood* 2010;116:2078–2088.

151. Stilgenbauer S, Sander S, Bullinger L, et al. Clonal evolution in chronic lymphocytic leukemia: acquisition of high-risk genomic aberrations associated with unmutated VH, resistance to therapy, and short survival. *Haematologica* 2007;92:1242.

Note: Page locators followed by *f* and *t* indicate figure and table, respectively.